a **LANGE** clinical manual

Neonatology:

Management, Procedures, On-Call Problems, Diseases and Drugs

3rd Edition

Editor

Tricia Lacy Gomella, M.D.
Attending in Neonatology
Francis Scott Key Medical Center
Instructor in Pediatrics
The Johns Hopkins University School of Medicine
Baltimore, Maryland

Associate Editors

M. Douglas Cunningham, M.D.
Professor of Clinical Pediatrics and Neonatology
Department of Pediatrics
University of California, Irvine, College of Medicine
Director, Infant Special Care Unit
Saddleback Memorial Medical Center
Laguna Hills, California

Fabien G. Eyal, M.D.
Associate Professor of Pediatrics
The Johns Hopkins University School of Medicine
Chairman, Department of Neonatology
Francis Scott Key Medical Center
Baltimore, Maryland

Consulting Editor

Karin E. Zenk, PharmD, FASHP
Associate Adjunct Professor of Pediatrics, University of California, Irvine,
College of Medicine; Pharmacist-Specialist in Pediatrics, University of
California, Irvine, Medical Center (Orange); Associate Clinical Professor of
Pharmacy, University of California, San Francisco, School of Pharmacy

APPLETON & LANGE
Stamford, Connecticut

Copyright © 1994 by Appleton & Lange
Paramount Publishing Business and Professional Group
Previous Editions copyright © 1988, 1992 by Appleton & Lange

98 / 10 9 8 7 6 5 4

Prentice Hall International (UK) Limited, *London*
Prentice Hall of Australia Pty. Limited, *Sydney*
Prentice Hall Canada, Inc., *Toronto*
Prentice Hall Hispanoamericana, S. A., *Mexico*
Prentice Hall of India Private Limited, *New Delhi*
Prentice Hall of Japan, Inc., *Tokyo*
Simon & Schuster Asia Pte. Ltd., *Singapore*
Editora Prentice Hall do Brasil Ltda., *Rio de Janeiro*
Prentice Hall, *Englewood Cliffs, New Jersey*

ISBN 0-8385-1331-X
ISSN 0697-6295
Acquisitions Editor: Martin Wonsiewicz
Production Editor: Christine Langan
Designer: Elizabeth Schmitz

PRINTED IN THE UNITED STATES OF AMERICA

ISBN 0-8385-1331-X

9 780838 513316 90000

To my twin sons, Leonard and Patrick and singletons Andrew and Michael

Contents

Section V. Diseases And Disorders

Contributors

Marilee C. Allen, MD
[Follow-up of High-Risk Infants]
Associate Professor of Pediatrics, Division of Neonatology, The Johns Hopkins University School of Medicine, Baltimore, Maryland

Gad Alpan, MD
[Infant of Drug-Abusing Mother]
Associate Professor of Pediatrics, The Johns Hopkins University School of Medicine, and Assistant Director of Neonatology, Johns Hopkins Bayview Medical Center, Baltimore, Maryland

Michael R. Barsotti, MD
[Fluids and Electrolytes]
Assistant Clinical Professor, Division of Neonatal/Perinatal Medicine, Department of Pediatrics, University of California, Irvine, College of Medicine

Linda Becker, RN, MPH
[Perinatal Isolation Guidelines]
Kaiser Fontana Hospital, A Kaiser Foundation Hospital, Fontana, California

Dilip Bhatt, MD
[Perinatal Isolation Guidelines]
Director, Division of Neonatology, Kaiser Fontana Hospital, A Kaiser Foundation Hospital, Fontana, California

Veeraiah Chundu, MD
[Hyperbilirubinemia, Exchange Transfusion]
Assistant Clinical Professor, Division of Neonatal/Perinatal Medicine, Department of Pediatrics, University of California, Irvine, College of Medicine

Carol M. Cottrill, MD
[Cardiac Abnormalities, Arrhythmia]
Professor of Pediatrics, Division of Cardiology, Department of Pediatrics, University of Kentucky College of Medicine, Lexington, Kentucky

M. Douglas Cunningham, MD
[Management of the Extremely Low Birth Weight Infant During the First Week of Life, Department of Pediatrics, Respiratory Management]
Professor of Clinical Pediatrics and Neonatology, University of California, Irvine, College of Medicine; Director, Infant Special Care Unit, Saddleback Memorial Medical Center, Laguna Hills, California.

William C. Cvetnic, MD
[Patent Ductus Arteriosus, Persistent Pulmonary Hypertension (Persistent Fetal Circulation)]
Associate Professor of Pediatrics, Obstetrics/Gynecology and Reproductive Services, Medical Director, NICU, Magee Women's Hospital, University of Pittsburgh, School of Medicine

Nirmala S. Desai, MD
[Intrauterine Growth Retardation (Small-for-Gestational-Age Infant)]
Professor of Pediatrics, Division of Neonatology, University of Kentucky, College of
Medicine, Lexington, Kentucky

Victoria Welge Elbin, RNC
[Management of the Extremely Low Birth Weight Infant During the First Week of Life]
Administrative Coordinator, Infant Special Care Unit, Saddleback Memorial Medical
Center, Laguna Hills, California

Armida Esparza, MD
[Thyroid Diseases]
Assistant Clinical Professor, Division of Neonatal/Perinatal Medicine, Department of
Pediatrics, University of California, Irvine, College of Medicine; Director, Special
Care Nursery, Fountain Valley Regional Hospital, Fountain Valley, CA

Fabien G. Eyal, MD
[Nutrition]
Associate Professor of Pediatrics, The Johns Hopkins University School of
Medicine, and Chairman, Department of Neonatology, Johns Hopkins Bayview
Medical Center, Baltimore, Maryland

Bruce Filmer, MBBS
[Renal Diseases]
Chief, Pediatric Urology, Al DuPont Institute, Wilmington, Delaware, and Associate
Professor, Department of Urology, Jefferson Medical College of Thomas Jefferson
University, Philadelphia, Pennsylvania

Dana Gascay, RN, BSN
[Perinatal Isolation Guidelines] Kaiser Fontana Hospital, A Kaiser Foundation
Hospital, Fontana, California

Christine A. Gleason, MD
[Resuscitation of the Newborn, Extracorporeal Membrane Oxygenation (ECMO)]
Associate Professor, Department of Pediatrics, The Johns Hopkins University
School of Medicine, and Director, Neonatal Intensive Care Unit, The Johns Hopkins
Hospital, Baltimore, Maryland

Tricia Lacy Gomella, MD
[Prenatal Testing, Assessment of Gestational Age, Newborn Physical Examination,
Temperature Regulation, Neonatal Radiology, Procedures, On-Call Problems
(Patient Management Problems), Transient Tachypnea of the Newborn]
Attending in Neonatology, Johns Hopkins Bayview Medical Center, Instructor in
Pediatrics, The Johns Hopkins University School of Medicine, Baltimore, Maryland

Janet E. Graeber, MD
[Retinopathy of Prematurity]
Associate Professor of Pediatrics, Department of Pediatrics, West Virginia University
School of Medicine, Morgantown, West Virginia

George W. Gross
[Neonatal Radiology]
Associate Professor of Radiology and Pediatrics, Director of Pediatric Radiology,
Jefferson Medical College of Thomas Jefferson University, Philadelphia,
Pennsylvania

Bryan D. Hall, MD
[Common Multiple Congenital Anomaly Syndromes]
Professor of Pediatrics and Chief, Division of Genetics and Dysmorphology,
University of Kentucky College of Medicine, Lexington, Kentucky

Charles R. Hamm, Jr., MD
[High-Frequency Ventilation]
Assistant Professor of Pediatrics, Division of Neonatology, Department of Pediatrics
University of South Alabama, Mobile, Alabama

Mark Damian Harris, MD
[Rickets and Disorders of Calcium and Magnesium Metabolism]
Instructor in Pediatrics, The Johns Hopkins University School of Medicine, and
Attending in Neonatology, Johns Hopkins Bayview Medical Center, Baltimore,
Maryland

C. Kirby Heritage, MD
[Infant of Diabetic Mother]
Assistant Clinical Professor of Pediatrics, Wright State School of Medicine, and
Attending in Neonatology, Miami Valley Hospital, Dayton, Ohio

Marcus C. Hermansen, MD
[Thrombocytopenia and Platelet Dysfunction, Hydrocephalus, Intraventricular
Hemorrhage]
Associate Professor of Pediatrics, Medical College of Pennsylvania, Philadelphia;
Director of Neonatology, Allegheny General Hospital, Pittsburgh, Pennsylvania

Bonnie Boyer Hudak, M.D.
[Bronchopulmonary Dysplasia]
Assistant Professor of Pediatrics, Division of Pediatric Pulmonary and Neonatology,
Childrens Hospital of Buffalo, Buffalo, New York

William G. Keyes, MD, PhD
[Multiple Gestation]
Attending in Neonatology, Northside Hospital, and Pediatric Intensivist,
Department of Intensive Care Medicine, Scottish Rite Childrens Medical Center,
Atlanta, Georgia

Debra Kulp-Hugues, MD
Chief Resident, Department of Urology, Jefferson Medical College of Thomas
Jefferson University, Philadelphia, Pennsylvania

Michael Langbaum, MD
[Inborn Errors of Metabolism With Acute Neonatal Onset]
Assistant Professor of Pediatrics, Department of Pediatrics, The Johns Hopkins
University School of Medicine, and Attending, Department of Neonatology, Johns
Hopkins Bayview Medical Center, Baltimore, Maryland

Barbara Leighton MD
[Obstetric Anesthesia and the Neonate]
Associate Professor, Department of Anesthesiology and Co-Director of Obstetric
Anesthesia, Jefferson Medical College of Thomas Jefferson University, Philadelphia,
Pennsylvania

Drew Litzenberger, MD
[Infant Transport]

Co-Director of Neonatology, Memorial Mission Medical Center, Asheville, North Carolina

Robert Meyer, Jr, MD
[Perinatal Isolation Guidelines]
Division of Neonatology, Kaiser Fontana Hospital, A Kaiser Foundation Hospital, Fontana, California

Ronald A. Naglie, MD
[Infectious Diseases]
Assistant Clinical Professor, Division of Neonatal/Perinatal Medicine, Department of Pediatrics, University of California, Irvine, College of Medicine

Sally Padilla, RN, BS, CIC
[Perinatal Isolation Guidelines]
Infection Control Practitioner, Kaiser Fontana Hospital, A Kaiser Foundation Hospital, Fontana, California

Ambadas Pathak, MD
[Neonatal Seizures]
Assistant Professor of Pediatrics, The Johns Hopkins University School of Medicine, and Head, Division of Newborn Medicine, Greater Baltimore Medical Center, Baltimore, Maryland

Thomas H. Pauly, MD
[Air Leak Syndromes, Apnea and Periodic Breathing]
Associate Professor, Department of Pediatrics, Chief, Division of Neonatology, University of Kentucky College of Medicine, Lexington, Kentucky

Andrew R. Pulito, MD
[Surgical Diseases of the Newborn]
Professor of Surgery, University of Kentucky College of Medicine, and Chief, Division of Pediatric Surgery, University of Kentucky, Lexington, Kentucky

J. Laurence Ransom, MD
[ABO Incompatibility, Anemia, Polycythemia and Hyperviscosity, Rh Incompatibility]
Director of Neonatal Medicine and Consultant in Pediatric Hematology, The Moses H. Cone Memorial Hospital, Greensboro, North Carolina; Clinical Associate Professor of Pediatrics, University of North Carolina, Chapel Hill, North Carolina

G. Mark Shoptaugh, MD
[Exchange Transfusion, Hyperbilirubinemia]
Attending Neonatologist, Department of Pediatrics, Maricopa County Medical Center, Phoenix, Arizona

Melinda Slack, MD
[Meconium Aspiration]
Director of Neonatology, St. John's Regional Health Center, Springfield, Missouri

Michael W. Stelling, MD
[Ambiguous Genitalia]
Assistant Professor of Pediatrics, Department of Pediatrics, University of Kentucky College of Medicine, Lexington, Kentucky

Feizal Waffarn, MD
[Necrotizing Enterocolitis]
Assistant Professor of Pediatrics in Residence, Division of Neonatal/Perinatal Medicine, Department of Pediatrics, University of California, Irvine, College of Medicine

Betty Lou Eilers Walfman, MD
[Hyaline Membrane Disease (Respiratory Distress Syndrome)]
Director, Intensive Care Nursery, Humana Women's Hospital, Indianapolis, Indiana

Jacki Williamson, RNC, MSN
[Perinatal Isolation Guidelines]
Kaiser Fontana Hospital, A Kaiser Foundation Hospital, Fontana, California

Linda L. Yang, MD
[Perinatal Asphyxia, Neural Tube Defects]
Assistant Clinical Professor, Division of Neonatal/Perinatal Medicine, Department of
Pediatrics, University of California, Irvine, College of Medicine

Karin E. Zenk, PharmD, FASHP
[Commonly Used Medications, Effects of Drugs and Substances on Lactation and
Breast-Feeding, Effects of Drugs and Substances Taken During Pregnancy,
Emergency Medications and Therapy for Neonates]
Associate Adjunct Professor of Pediatrics, University of California, Irvine, College of
Medicine; Pharmacist-Specialist in Pediatrics, University of California, Irvine, Medical
Center (Orange); Associate Clinical Professor of Pharmacy, University of California,
San Francisco, School of Pharmacy

Preface

The second edition of Neonatology proved to be very successful as a practical manual, both in the United States and overseas, providing the opportunity to update this third edition.

Many chapters in the third edition of this manual have been extensively updated and revised. The format of the manual has remained essentially the same, except Section II, Advanced Management, has now been incorporated into Section I. Section I, Basic Management of the Neonate, includes topics that involve daily care of the premature and term infants. The new Ballard exam has been added, high frequency oscillatory ventilation is discussed and new topics like the use of nitric oxide in respiratory support is included. The old Section II, Advanced Management, has been incorporated into Section I, since the majority of those topics now involve routine management of the neonate. Surfactant and high frequency ventilation are commonplace in the NICU, and the challenges of the management of extremely low birthweight infants are encountered with increasing frequency.

Section II, Procedures, discusses the procedures used in neonatal intensive care units. The section has been updated and an expanded section on the use of intraosseous infusions has been added.

Section III, On Call Problems (Patient Management Problems), has been extensively updated to keep pace with current therapy. It continues to be one of the popular sections because of its practicality.

Section IV, Diseases and Disorders, has been extensively revised to reflect new information published over the last several years.

Section V, Neonatal Pharmacology, has combined the commonly used medications and antibiotics in alphabetical order to facilitate finding a specific drug. The new chapters from the second edition, Effects of Drugs or Substances on Lactation and Breastfeeding and Effects of Drugs or Substances Taken During Pregnancy have been updated to keep current.

The management principles and protocols in the update of this manual are not based on practices at only one institution. Contributors are from all over the United States, and the associate editor and consulting editor are from the West Coast and East Coast, respectively. I feel this has enabled us to produce a manual that is not institution-specific but reflects a cross section of contemporary approaches to neonatal management.

Neonatology is a relatively young and rapidly evolving pediatric sub specialty. If treatment protocols vary from center to center, we have identified them as *controversial*. This clearly indicates to the reader that specific institutions may not treat the same problem in the same way and that different approaches may have been used successfully at other institutions.

The authors and editors have made every effort to assure timely and accurate guidelines in this manual. However, it is impossible to list every clinical situation or institution-specific approach to diagnosis and treatment.

My sincerest thanks to the contributors, the editorial staff at Appleton & Lange, and my family for their continued support of this project.

I welcome suggestions and comments about this manual. Letters should be addressed to:

Tricia Lacy Gomella, MD
c/o Appleton & Lange
25 Van Zant Street
East Norwalk, CT 06855

1 Prenatal Testing

AMNIOCENTESIS

Amniotic fluid can be analyzed for prenatal diagnosis of congenital defects and determination of fetal lung maturity. Testing for congenital abnormalities is usually done at 14–16 weeks' gestation. A sample of amniotic fluid is removed under ultrasound guidance. Fetal cells contained in the fluid can be grown in tissue culture for genetic study. This is indicated (1) in women over 35 years of age because of the increased incidence of trisomy 21; (2) in those who have already had a child with a chromosomal abnormality; (3) in those in whom X-linked disorders are suspected; and (4) to rule out inborn errors of metabolism.

CHORIONIC VILLUS SAMPLING

Chorionic villus sampling (CVS) is a technique for first trimester genetic studies. Chorionic villi are withdrawn either through a needle that is inserted through the abdomen and the into the edge of the placenta or through a catheter that is inserted through the vagina and cervix into the placenta. The cells obtained are identical to those of the fetus and are grown and analyzed. CVS can be performed in the first trimester (usually between 9–12 weeks' gestation) and results can be obtained more quickly, thus enabling the patient to have a diagnosis before the end of the first trimester. Indications are the same as for amniocentesis. The risk of pregnancy loss may be higher with CVS than with amniocentesis, but studies have not shown a statistically significant difference. Reported complications after CVS can include pregnancy loss, limb abnormalities, and chromosomal mosaicism.

BIOPHYSICAL PROFILE

The biophysical profile (Table 1–1) is used to assess fetal well-being. A 30-minute ultrasound examination is performed to measure 5 parameters: fetal breathing movements, gross fetal body movements, fetal tone, reactive fetal heart rate, and amniotic fluid volume. A score of 8–10 is considered normal, a score of 4–6 indicates possible poor fetal well-being, and a score of 0–2 is a strong indication of poor fetal well-being.

TABLE 1–1. BIOPHYSICAL PROFILE*

Variable	Normal (2)	Abnormal (0)
Fetal breathing	One episode > 30 seconds in 30 minutes	None or episode < 30 seconds in 30 minutes
Body movement	Three or more movements in 30 minutes	Two or less movements in 30 minutes
Fetal tone	One episode of active limb or trunk extension with flexion	No movement
Nonstress test	Reactive	Nonreactive
Amniotic fluid	One pocket of amniotic fluid 1 cm or more	No fluid pockets or pocket < 1 cm

*Scoring system used to assess fetal well-being, as described in text.

Based on guidelines from Manning F et al: Fetal biophysical profile scoring: A prospective study in 1,184 high-risk patients. *Am J Obstet Gynecol* 1981;40:289.

FETAL HEART RATE MONITORING

Fetal heart rate monitoring may be internal (direct)—electrode attached to fetal scalp—or external (indirect)—electrode attached to maternal abdomen. The baseline heart rate, beat-to-beat variability, and periodic heart rate are measured.

I. **Baseline fetal heart rate.** The baseline fetal heart rate is the rate that is maintained apart from periodic variations caused by uterine contractions. The **normal fetal heart rate** is 120–160 beats/min. **Fetal tachycardia** is present at 160 beats/min or more. Causes of fetal tachycardia include maternal or fetal infection, fetal hypoxia, thyrotoxicosis, and maternal use of drugs such as parasympathetic blockers or betamimetic agents. **Moderate fetal bradycardia** is defined as a heart rate of 100–120 beats/min with normal variability. **Severe fetal bradycardia** is a heart rate of less than 100 beats/min. The most common cause of bradycardia is hypoxia; other causes include hypothermia, complete heart block, and maternal use of drugs such as beta blockers.

II. **Beat-to-beat variability.** In the normal mature fetus, there are slight rapid fluctuations in the interval between beats (beat-to-beat variability). An **amplitude range** (baseline variability) **> 6 beats/min indicates normal beat-to-beat variability** and suggests the absence of fetal asphyxia. Absence of variability may be caused by severe asphyxia, anencephaly, complete heart block, and maternal use of drugs such as magnesium sulfate or morphine.

III. **Periodic fetal heart rate.** The periodic fetal heart rate is the rate that occurs during uterine contractions. There are 3 types of decelerations (Fig 1–1).

A. **Early decelerations.** Early decelerations (decelerations of head compression) occur secondary to vagal reflex tone, which follows minor, transient fetal hypoxic episodes. These are benign and not associated with fetal compromise.

B. **Late decelerations.** Two types of late decelerations are described.

1. **Reflex late decelerations.** These are seen in the setting of normal fetal heart rate variability. They are associated with a sudden insult (eg, maternal hypotension) that affects a normally oxygenated fetus and signifies uteroplacental insufficiency. The normal variability of the fetal heart rate signifies that the fetus is physiologically compensated.

2. **Late decelerations with loss of beat-to-beat variability ("myocardial hypoxia late decelerations").** These are associated with decreased or absent fetal heart rate variability. They result from prolonged asphyxia and signify "fetal decompensation," which may be seen with preeclampsia and intrauterine growth retardation (IUGR).

C. **Variable decelerations.** These are vagal in origin and are most frequently associated with umbilical cord compression. They are classified as severe when the fetal heart rate is below 60 beats/min, the deceleration is longer than 60 seconds in duration, or the fetal heart rate is 60 beats/min below baseline. If beat-to-beat variability is maintained, the fetus is compensated physiologically and oxygenated normally. If severe variable decelerations are present for more than 30 minutes, the fetus may be decompensated, and maneuvers such as maternal oxygen supplementation and maternal positioning in the left lateral decubitus position may improve placental circulation and should be attempted.

FETAL SCALP BLOOD SAMPLING

Fetal scalp blood sampling is used to determine the fetal acid-base status. This procedure can be performed only after rupture of the membranes. It is contraindicated in cases of known blood dyscrasias, infection due to herpesvirus, or obvious chorioamnionitis. A blood sample is obtained from the fetal presenting part (usually the scalp but sometimes the buttocks), and the fetal blood pH is determined. A pH of 7.25 or greater has been shown to correlate (with 92% accuracy) with a 2-minute Apgar score of 7 or greater. A pH of less than 7.15 correlates with a 2-minute Apgar score of less than 6 (80% accuracy). The following results are usually used as a standard protocol.

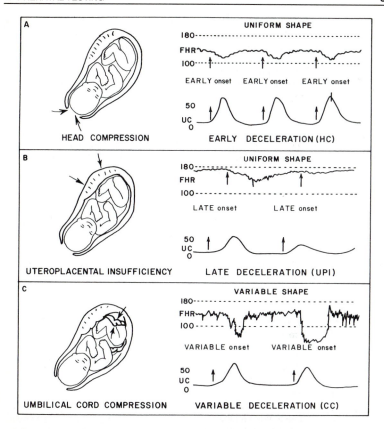

FIGURE 1–1. Examples of fetal heart rate monitoring. UC = uterine contraction (mm Hg); FHR = fetal heart rate in beats per minute (bpm). *(Modified and reproduced, with permission, from McCrann JR, Schifrin BS: Fetal monitoring in high-risk pregnancy.* Clin Perinatol *1974;**1**:149.)*

pH > 7.25: Normal result; fetus is probably normal.

pH < 7.20: Abnormal result; fetus is acidotic. If this result occurs in the absence of maternal acidosis, and a repeat test done 10 minutes after the first one reveals the same or more acidotic pH, delivery is indicated.

pH between 7.20 and 7.25: The test should be repeated. Decisions regarding delivery depend on the clinical situation.

Complications of this test are scalp infections (< 1% of infants) and soft tissue damage to the scalp.

TESTS OF FETAL LUNG MATURITY

I. **Lecithin:sphingomyelin (L:S) ratio.** Lecithin, a saturated phosphatidylcholine (the condensation product of a phosphatidic acid and choline), can be measured specifically in amniotic fluid and is a principal active component of surfactant. It is manufactured by type II alveolar cells. Sphingomyelin is a phospholipid found predominantly in body tissues other than the lungs. The L:S ratio compares levels of lecithin (which increase in late gestation) to levels of sphingomyelin (which remain constant). The L:S ratio is usually 1:1 by 31–32 weeks' gestation and 2:1 by 35 weeks' gestation. The following are guidelines to L:S ratios.

- **L:S 2:1 or greater:** Lungs are mature (98% accuracy). Only 2% of these infants will develop respiratory distress syndrome.
- **L:S 1.5–1.9:1:** 50% will develop respiratory distress syndrome.
- **L:S less than 1.5:1:** 73% will develop respiratory distress syndrome.

Some disorders are associated with delayed lung maturation, and higher than normal L:S ratios must be present before lung maturity has been reached. The 2 most common are diabetes mellitus (L:S ratio of 3:1 is usually accepted as indicating maturity) and Rh isoimmunization associated with hydrops fetalis.

Acceleration of mature L:S ratios is seen in sickle cell disease, maternal narcotic addiction, prolonged rupture of the membranes, chronic maternal hypertension, IUGR, and placental infarction. Differences may also occur in various racial groups.

II. **Phosphatidylglycerol measurement.** Phosphatidylglycerol appears in amniotic fluid at about 35 weeks, and levels increase at 37–40 weeks. This substance is a useful marker for lung maturation. It is reported as either present or absent.

III. **TDx Fetal Lung Maturity (TDx FLM).** This test (available from Abbott Laboratories, North Chicago, IL) measures the relative concentrations of surfactant and albumin (milligrams of surfactant per gram of albumin) in amniotic fluid and gives a result that helps assess fetal lung maturity. TDx FLM has advantages over L:S ratio because less technical expertise is required. This test can be performed more easily and results are obtained more quickly. Results are interpreted in the following ways:

> **< 30 mg/g:** The lungs are definitely immature.
>
> **30–50 mg/g:** The infant is at risk for immature lungs (other conditions may weigh more heavily on whether to deliver).
>
> **50–70 mg/g:** The situation should be treated with caution pending further studies.
>
> **> 70 mg/g:** The likelihood of respiratory distress syndrome (RDS) is small.

NONSTRESS TEST

The nonstress test (NST) is used to detect fetal hypoxia. Fetal well-being is confirmed if there is an increase in the fetal heart rate in response to fetal activity. The baseline fetal heart rate is measured by external monitoring devices. Fetal movements and heart rate are then recorded for 20 minutes.

Decreased fetal movements can occur with fetal sleep, central nervous system depressants, chronic smoking, and medications such as propranolol.

The following guidelines can be used.

I. **Reactive test.** A normal fetal baseline heart rate is present, and there are at least 4 fetal movements in 20 minutes. The heart rate accelerates by at least 15 beats/min during fetal movement. This result indicates that the fetus is usually normal.

II. **Nonreactive test.** No fetal movements occur during a 20-minute period, or there is no acceleration of the fetal heart rate with fetal movements. This result is associated with a poor outcome and should be followed up with the oxytocin challenge test (see below).

III. **Uncertain reactivity.** Fewer than 4 fetal movements occur within a 20-minute period, or the fetal heart rate accelerates less than 15 beats/min during fetal movement. The nonstress test should be repeated, or the oxytocin challenge test should be performed.

CONTRACTION STRESS TEST

The **contraction stress test (CST)** is used to assess a fetus at risk for uteroplacental insufficiency. A monitor is placed on the mother's abdomen to continuously record the fetal heart rate and uterine contractions. An adequate test consists of more than 3 contractions, each lasting at least 40–60 seconds, within a period of 10 minutes. If sufficient contractions do not occur, oxytocin is administered by intravenous pump at a rate of 0.5 mU/min until adequate contractions occur. If oxytocin is needed to produce contractions for the contraction stress test, it is called **oxytocin challenge test (OCT).** Normally, the fetal heart rate increases in response to a contraction and no decelerations occur during the contraction. If late decelerations occur during contractions, uteroplacental insufficiency is probably present.

The CST is contraindicated in patients with placenta previa, those who have had a previous cesarean section with a vertical incision, and those who are at high risk for preterm delivery (premature rupture of the membranes, multiple gestation, incompetent cervix).

Test results are interpreted as follows.

 I. **Negative (normal) test.** No late decelerations occur during adequate uterine contractions. The baseline fetal heart rate is normal. This result is associated with a good fetal outcome. A repeat test is usually performed in 1 week.
 II. **Positive (abnormal) test.** Persistent late decelerations occur during adequate uterine contractions. This result can signify poor fetal outcome, perinatal death, meconium-stained amniotic fluid, or respiratory distress (low 5-minute Apgar score). If the test is positive, delivery is usually recommended.
 III. **Equivocal (suspicious) test.** Intermittent late decelerations occur with adequate uterine contractions. The test should be repeated within 24 hours; most repeat tests will be negative.

ULTRASOUND TESTING

Ultrasound examination is used in the following circumstances.

 I. **To estimate gestational age and weight.** The following parameters are used:
   A. **To determine crown-rump length.** Measurements are most accurate in the first 12 weeks of gestation, with a margin of 3–5 days. Measurements are more difficult to make later in pregnancy as the fetus assumes a more curled-up position.
   B. **To determine biparietal diameter.** Measurement of the biparietal diameter is most accurate at 12–18 weeks' gestation. The measurement is made from the outer edge of one side of the skull to the inner edge of the opposite side.
   C. **To determine femur length.** The femur is measured from the greater trochanter to the distal metaphyses and plotted against a graph for age assessment.
   D. **To determine abdominal circumference.** This measurement is an indication of gestational age and is an accurate indication of IUGR.
 II. **To follow fetal intrauterine growth and detect IUGR.**
 III. **To assess fetal movements and breathing activity.**
 IV. **As an adjunct to amniocentesis and intrauterine transfusion.**
 V. **To help guide the choice of method of delivery.** Detection of gross anomalies with ultrasonography can be used to decide on the type of delivery and support personnel needed (eg, anencephaly, gastroschisis, multiple gestation).
 VI. **To determine amniotic fluid volume**
   A. **Oligohydramnios** (lack of amniotic fluid) is associated with a major anomaly 15% of the time. Renal agenesis and prune-belly syndrome are the most common, along with amniotic fluid leak, severe cardiac disease, and chylothorax. The kidneys can be seen with ultrasonography at 15 weeks and the bladder at 16 weeks.
   B. **Polyhydramnios (hydramnios)** (excess of amniotic fluid) is associated with major anomalies 15% of the time. It is associated with anencephaly, neural tube defects, bowel obstruction such as duodenal atresia, multiple gestation, nonimmune hydrops fetalis, and exstrophy of the bladder.
 VII. **To determine fetal death.** Ultrasound findings of absence of cardiac motion, scalp edema, and overlapping of cranial bones indicate fetal death.
 VIII. **To determine fetal sex.**
 IX. **To detect fetal heart motion.** Fetal heart activity can be detected at 7–8 weeks.

  X. To assess the placenta for location.
 XI. To guide fetal surgeons, for example, in surgical intervention for fetal hydronephrosis.
XII. To evaluate uterine size and shape.
XIII. To rule out placenta previa and abruptio placentae in cases of vaginal bleeding.

REFERENCES

Manning FA et al: Fetal biophysical profile scoring: A prospective study in 1184 high-risk patients. *Am J Obstet Gynecol* 1981;140:289.

Russell JC et al: Multicenter evaluation of TDx test for assessing fetal lung maturity. *Clin Chem* 1989;35:1005.

Stone JL, Lockwood CJ: Amniocentesis and chorionic villus sampling. *Curr Opin Obstet Gynecol* 1993;5:211.

2   Delivery Room Management

OBSTETRIC ANESTHESIA AND THE NEONATE

During birth, the status of the fetus is influenced by many factors. One major factor is obstetric analgesia and anesthesia. Care in choosing analgesic and anesthetic agents can often prevent depression in the newborn, especially in high-risk deliveries.

I. **Placental transfer of drugs.** Drugs administered to the mother may affect the fetus via placental transfer or (less commonly) may cause a maternal disorder that affects the fetus (eg, maternal drug-induced hypotension may cause fetal hypoxia). All anesthetic and analgesic drugs cross the placenta to some degree. Passive diffusion is the usual mechanism, and since most agents are highly permeable, they are also flow-dependent.

Most anesthetic and analgesic drugs have a high degree of lipid solubility, a low molecular weight (< 500), and variable protein-binding and ionization capabilities. These characteristics cause them to be transferred rapidly across the placenta. Local anesthetics and narcotics (which are lipid-soluble and have low ionization) cross the placenta easily, whereas neuromuscular blocking agents (highly ionized) are transferred much more slowly.

II. **Analgesia in labor**
   A. **Inhalation analgesia.** Inhalation analgesia is rarely used in the USA. Entonox (50% O_2 and 50% N_2O) is widely used in other countries. Amounts used are generally much lower than those used in general anesthesia.
   B. **Pudendal block and paracervical block.** Paracervical block may be associated with severe fetal bradycardia caused by uterine vasoconstriction and is now rarely used. If a paracervical block is performed, fetal heart rate monitoring must be used. Pudendal blocks have little direct effect on the fetus. However, seizures have been reported with several local anesthetic agents used for both pudendal and paracervical blocks. Paracervical blocks are used in the first stage of labor and pudendal in the second stage of labor.
   C. **Opioids.** All opioids are rapidly transferred to the fetus and cause dose-related respiratory depression and alterations in the Apgar score and neurobehavioral scores.
      1. **Meperidine (Demerol)** causes severe neonatal depression (as measured by Apgar scoring) if the drug is administered more than 1 hour before delivery. If meperidine is given within 1 hour of birth, there is no significant difference in the neonate when compared to controls (Shnider, 1964). Depression is manifested as respiratory acidosis, decreased oxygen saturation, decreased minute ventilation, and increased time to sustained respiration. Fetal normeperidine (a meperidine metabolite that may cause significant central nervous system depression) increases with longer intervals between drug administration and delivery. Levels are highest at 4 hours after intravenous administration of the drug to the mother. The half-life of meperidine is 13 hours in neonates, whereas the half-life of normeperidine is 62 hours (Moore, 1973).
      2. **Morphine** has a delayed onset of action and perhaps causes more neonatal depression than meperidine (Jouppila, 1982).
      3. **Butorphanol (Stadol)** and **nalbuphine (Nubain)** are agonist-antagonist narcotic agents. They are thought to cause less respiratory depression than morphine, particularly when used in high doses.
      4. **Pentazocine (Fortral)** is said to have a lower rate of placental transfer than meperidine, but most studies have not shown significant differences in the severity of neonatal depression caused by the 2 drugs.

D. Opioid antagonist (naloxone [Narcan]). The effect of naloxone given intramuscularly may last for 48 hours in the fetus. When the drug is injected into the umbilical vein, effects may last for only 30 minutes. With maternal reversal of narcotic, some researchers have shown temporary improvement in neonatal depression due to opioid effect.

E. Sedatives and tranquilizers
1. **Barbiturates.** Barbiturates cross the placenta rapidly and can have pronounced neonatal effects lasting for days. These include somnolence, flaccidity, hypoventilation, and failure to feed. Effects are intensified if opioids are used simultaneously.
2. **Benzodiazepines (diazepam [Valium], lorazepam [Ativan], midazolam [Versed]).** These agents cross the placenta rapidly and equilibrate within minutes after intravenous administration. Fetal levels are often higher than maternal levels. Diazepam given in low doses (< 10 mg) may cause decreased beat-to-beat variability and tone but has little effect on Apgar scores or blood gas levels. Larger doses of diazepam may persist for days and can cause hypotonia, lethargy, decreased feeding, and impaired thermoregulation, with resulting hypothermia. All benzodiazepines share these features; however, diazepam is the most thoroughly studied of the benzodiazepine series. In addition to the above adverse effects, benzodiazepines are less frequently used because they induce childbirth amnesia in the mother, which can be distressing. Midazolam may be used to induce general anesthesia. Anesthetic induction with midazolam is safe for the mother, although low 1-minute Apgar scores and transient neonatal hypotonia may be seen.
3. **Phenothiazines.** Phenothiazines are rarely used today, because they may induce hypotension via central alpha blockade. Phenothiazines are sometimes combined with a narcotic ("neuroleptanalgesia"). Innovar, a combination drug containing the narcotic fentanyl and droperidol, may be safe because of the relatively short half-life of the agents.
4. **Ketamine (Ketaject, many others).** Ketamine may be used for dissociative analgesia or anesthesia. Doses greater than 1 mg/kg may be dangerous, causing neonatal depression and uterine hypotonia. Much smaller doses are normally used in labor (0.1–0.2 mg/kg) and are relatively safe, producing minimal effects in the mother and neonate.

F. Lumbar epidural analgesia. Lumbar epidural analgesia is the most frequently used invasive anesthetic technique for childbirth. Lumbar epidural analgesia is safely administered regional anesthesia that may be beneficial to the fetus. Maternal catecholamine levels may be reduced (catecholamines cause prolonged incoordinate labor and decreased uterine blood flow), leading to diminished maternal hyperventilation and improved fetal oxygen delivery. Vasospasm of uterine arteries in pregnancy-induced hypertension may be relieved (Jouppila, 1982; Shnider, 1979).

Continuous administration of a local anesthetic (eg, bupivicaine, lidocaine) through a catheter placed in the epidural space at the L2 or L3 interspace is usually used. Alternatively, repeated injections through the catheter (so-called topping-off technique) may be used. Epinephrine is sometimes added to prolong the effect and decrease systemic absorption of the agents. Small doses of an opioid may also be added; these have no effect on the neonate. Maternal hypotension caused by sympathetic blockade is easily treated with fluid administration or small doses of ephedrine given intravenously.

G. Caudal epidural analgesia. Caudal epidural analgesia blocks the sacral nerve roots and is excellent for relief of pain in the second stage of labor. There is a high incidence of pelvic floor relaxation with less rotation of the neonate's head. Systemic absorption of anesthetic agents is greater than with lumbar epidural anesthesia. Caudal epidural analgesia is not efficient during the first stage of labor because large doses are needed to block the T11–12 nerve roots. Because of reports of fetal intracranial injections of anesthetic, this technique is becoming less popular.

H. Saddle block. Use of saddle block, a form of low spinal block, is decreasing. It is generally safe for the neonate, provided the block stays low to avoid maternal hypotension. In this technique, a spinal anesthetic is given, and the mother sits up so that the hyperbaric agent settles low in the spinal cord around the conus medullaris. Saddle block is best for the second stage of labor.

I. Local anesthetics. All of the regional anesthetic/analgesic techniques (eg, epidural, spinal) and local blocks (eg, pudendal) depend on the use of local anesthetic agents. Bupivicaine is the most commonly used agent due to its longer half-life.

1. **Lidocaine (Xylocaine).** Placental transfer of lidocaine is significant, but Apgar scores are usually not affected (Abboud, 1982).

2. **Bupivacaine (Marcaine).** Bupivacaine is theoretically less harmful than lidocaine for the fetus because it has a higher degree of ionization and protein-binding than lidocaine. Reports of maternal toxicity leading to convulsions and cardiac arrest after inadvertent intravascular injection have been reported.

3. **Chloroprocaine (Nesacaine).** After systemic absorption, chloroprocaine is rapidly broken down by pseudocholinesterase, so very little reaches the placenta or fetus. Neurobehavioral studies indicate no difference between controls and neonates whose mothers have been given chloroprocaine. Recent reformulation of this agent may increase its use (the earlier formulation was linked to some cases of neurotoxicity).

4. **Mepivacaine (Carbocaine).** Mepivacaine has been largely abandoned in neonatology because of its adverse effects, in particular, lower neurobehavioral scores and higher fetal serum levels of the agent.

J. Psychoprophylaxis. The **Lamaze technique** of prepared childbirth involves instruction in a series of classes for prospective parents. The process of childbirth is explained, and exercises, breathing techniques, and relaxation techniques are taught to relieve labor pain. However, the popular assumption that the neonate benefits if the mother receives no drugs during childbirth is not necessarily justified. Pain and discomfort may cause psychological stress and hyperventilation in the mother and have a profoundly negative impact on the neonate; supplemental anesthesia may be needed. Fifty to 70% of women who have learned the Lamaze method request drugs or an anesthetic block at the time of delivery. **Other psychoprophylaxis techniques** include transcutaneous electric nerve stimulation (TENS), hypnosis, and acupuncture, but these are not currently in widespread use.

III. Anesthesia for cesarean delivery. Regional anesthesia is becoming the technique of choice for cesarean deliveries, but in certain circumstances, general anesthesia is used. If *immediate* delivery is needed, general anesthesia is often used because it has the shortest induction time. However, immediate delivery is usually not mandatory, so regional anesthesia is commonly used.

A. Lumbar epidural anesthesia. Placental transfer of local anesthetics may occur (see above). Maternal hypotension may occur, but preloading the mother with crystalloids usually helps avoid this problem. Use of epidural anesthesia is clearly advantageous to the fetus. There are minimal drug effects, which can be detected only by detailed neurobehavioral testing.

B. Spinal anesthesia. Spinal anesthesia (injection of agent directly into cerebrospinal fluid) uses a lower dose than does epidural anesthesia (infiltration of the epidural space). Maternal and fetal drug levels have been detected but are about one-third those of epidural anesthesia. Hypotension may occur rapidly but can be prevented by administering 1.5–2.0 L balanced salt solution intravenously or by infusing prophylactic intravenous ephedrine. Spinal anesthesia has a shorter induction time than the other regional techniques, so it is preferred for emergency situations. In most studies, the Early Neonatal Neurobehavioral Score (ENNS) (see p 11) is more normal following spinal anesthesia than general anesthesia for cesarean section.

C. General anesthesia. There is a trend away from use of general anesthesia, but it is still used in certain circumstances. These include strong patient preference, emergency delivery (eg, in cases of hemorrhage, cord prolapse, or fetal distress), and contraindications to regional anesthesia (eg, maternal coagulo-pathy, maternal neurologic problems, sepsis, or infection).

After induction of anesthesia, the mother is usually maintained on a combination of nitrous oxide and oxygen with low doses of other agents such as halothane. Opioids or benzodiazepines are rarely given until the cord is clamped.

1. **Agents used in general obstetric anesthesia**
   a. **Surgical premedication.** Premedications traditionally used in surgery are rarely given. Atropinics (used to decrease oral secretions) are seldom used. Glycopyrrolate (Robinul) crosses the placenta much less readily than atropine or scopolamine. Fetal tachycardia and loss of beat-to-beat variability may occur. Cimetidine (Tagamet) and ranitidine (Zantac) (H₂ receptor antagonists) are used by some to decrease gastric volume and increase the pH of gastric secretions as prophylaxis against aspiration pneumonitis. The neonate is not affected by these agents.
   b. **Thiopental (Pentothal).** Thiopental, up to 4 mg/kg, is used for induction of general anesthesia. This dosage exposes the fetus to low concentrations, which are usually achieved within 2–3 minutes. Metabolites may affect fetal brain waves (as seen on EEG) for several days and depress the sucking response. Fetal outcome, as measured by Apgar scoring, is not affected by doses of less than 4 mg/kg.
   c. **Ketamine.** Ketamine is used in doses of less than 1 mg/kg for induction of anesthesia. Neonatal neurobehavioral test scores are slightly better than those of infants of mothers who received thiopental.
   d. **Muscle relaxants.** Muscle relaxants, which are highly ionized, cross the placenta in small amounts and have little effect on the neonate.
      (1) **Succinylcholine (Anectine, many others)** crosses the placenta in minimal amounts. In twice-normal doses, it is detectable in the fetus, but no respiratory effects are seen until the dose is 5 times normal or both mother and fetus have abnormal pseudocholinesterase.
      (2) **Pancuronium (Pavulon) and tubocurarine (Tubarine)** do not affect the neonate. These agents are currently rarely used.
      (3) **Atracurium (Tracrium) and vecuronium (Norcuron)** are fairly new agents that are shorter acting. Atracurium may be safer due to its spontaneous degradation, not relying on renal or hepatic clearance.
   e. **Nitrous oxide** has rapid placental transfer. With inhaled concentrations of greater than 50% nitrous oxide, fetal outcome is proportionate to the interval between induction and delivery (the longer the interval, the worse the fetal status). Prolonged administration of high concentrations of nitrous oxide results in low Apgar scores because of central nervous system depression and perfusion hypoxia. Concentrations of up to 50% are safe, but neonates need supplemental oxygen after delivery, especially if the interval between induction and delivery is long.
   f. **Halogenated anesthetic agents (isoflurane [Forane], enflurane [Ethrane], halothane [Fluothane])** are used to maintain general anesthesia. Beneficial effects include decreased catecholamines and increased uterine blood flow when compared to nitrous oxide alone. Low concentrations of these agents usually do not cause neonatal depression. If depression is seen, it is usually transient, since these volatile agents are readily excreted. These agents cause much more neonatal respiratory depression in compromised fetuses. Higher doses may halt labor by causing decreased uterine contractility (Crawford, 1984). When used, the lowest effective level is chosen and the agent is promptly discontinued at the point of delivery to help decrease uterine atony and further blood loss.
2. **Neonatal effects of general anesthesia.** Failure of endotracheal intubation or aspiration with associated maternal hypoxia can cause deleterious fetal effects. Maternal hyperventilation (Paco₂ < 20 mm Hg) leads to fetal hypoxia and acidosis because of decreased placental blood flow and a shift in the

oxyhemoglobin curve. Aortocaval compression may occur during general anesthesia, resulting in decreased placental perfusion (the mother should be positioned with the left side slightly tilted down to help prevent this). Intubation will increase oxygen saturation of maternal blood up to 300 mm Hg; this will increase oxygen tension and saturation of fetal blood.

3. **Interval between incision of the uterus and delivery.** Incision and manipulation of the uterus cause reflex uterine vasoconstriction, resulting in fetal asphyxia. Long intervals between incision and delivery (> 90 seconds) are associated with significant lowering of Apgar scores. If the interval is longer than 180 seconds, lower Apgar scores and fetal acidosis occur in both regional and general anesthesia (Datta, 1981). Epidural blockade may decrease reflex vasoconstriction, so the length of the interval is of less importance. The interval may be prolonged with breech delivery, multiple delivery, or preterm delivery; if there is scarring of the uterus due to a previous delivery or operation; or if the fetus is large.

4. **Regional versus general anesthesia**
   a. **Apgar scores.** Early studies showed that neonates were less depressed on 1- and 5-minute Apgar scores with regional than with general anesthesia (Benson, 1965). Refinements in general anesthetic techniques lower Apgar scores at 1 minute only. This generally represents transient sedation (ie, temporary neonatal general anesthesia) rather than asphyxia. If the interval between induction and delivery is short, there is less difference between the effects of regional and general anesthesia. If a prolonged delivery time is anticipated, regional anesthesia is preferred because the neonate is less sedated. It is important to note that low Apgar scores secondary to sedation do not have the negative prognostic value of low Apgar scores secondary to asphyxia provided that the neonate is adequately resuscitated.
   b. **Acid-base status.** The differences in acid-base status are minimal and probably not significant. Infants of diabetic mothers may be less acidotic with general than with regional anesthesia, particularly spinal anesthesia, because of the higher incidence of hypotension with regional anesthesia and exacerbation of uteroplacental insufficiency seen in diabetics.
   c. **Neurobehavioral examinations** are used to detect subtle changes in the neonate in the first few hours after birth that may be missed by Apgar scoring or acid-base assessment. After delivery, there is a 1-hour period of alertness, followed by a 3- to 4-hour period of deep sleep and decreased responsiveness. The **Early Neonatal Neurobehavioral Score (ENNS)** was initially developed to detect neurobehavioral changes 2–8 hours after birth (the half-life of most local anesthetics). These changes are usually manifested as decreased tone or decrement in an otherwise alert infant. The **Neonatal Neurologic and Adaptive Capacity Score (NNACS)** uses portions of the ENNS, Brazelton Neonatal Behavioral Assessment Scale, and Amiel-Tison Neurologic Examination. This score is more weighted toward assessment of neonatal tone and is helpful in differentiating abnormalities caused by birth trauma rather than depression. Early neurobehavioral examinations show clear-cut advantages of regional over general anesthesia. Although infants of mothers receiving spinal and epidural anesthesia had similar results at 15 minutes, by 2 hours the epidural group had lower scores. This probably reflects higher local anesthetic uptake. However, there are no significant differences in long-term studies comparing regional and general anesthesia.

RESUSCITATION OF THE NEWBORN

Approximately 4 million infants are born in the USA each year in about 5000 hospitals, only 15% of which have neonatal intensive care facilities (Standards and Guidelines for Cardiopulmonary Resuscitation and Emergency Cardiac Care, 1986). Approximately 6% of newborns require some form of resuscitation. This cannot always be anticipated in time to transfer the mother before delivery to a facility with specialized neonatal support. Therefore, every hospital with a delivery suite should have an organized, skilled resuscitation team and appropriate equipment available (Table 2–1) (Ballard, 1991; Bloom, 1990). An overview of resuscitation is presented in Figure 2–1.

I. Normal physiologic events at birth. Normal transitional events at birth begin with initial lung expansion, generally requiring large, negative intrathoracic pressures, followed by a cry (expiration against a partially closed glottis). Umbilical cord clamping is accompanied by a rise in blood pressure and massive stimulation of the sympathetic nervous system. With onset of respiration and lung expansion, pulmonary vascular resistance falls, followed by a gradual (over minutes to hours) transition from fetal to adult circulation, with closure of the foramen ovale and ductus arteriosus.

II. Abnormal physiologic events at birth. The asphyxiated newborn infant undergoes an abnormal transition. A rhesus monkey model has been used to study changes in physiologic parameters during asphyxiation and resuscitation (Dawes, 1968). Shortly after acute asphyxiation (the cord is clamped while the head is held in a bag filled with saline), the monkey fetus has **primary apnea,** during which spontaneous respirations can be induced by appropriate sensory stimuli. This lasts for about 1 minute, and the fetus then begins deep gasping for 4–5 minutes, ending with the "last gasp." This is followed by a period of **secondary apnea,** during which spontaneous respirations cannot be induced by sensory stimuli. Death occurs if secondary apnea is not reversed by vigorous ventilatory support within several minutes. Because one can never be certain whether an apneic newborn has primary or secondary apnea, resuscitative efforts should proceed as though secondary apnea were present. This experimental model of acute total

---

TABLE 2–1. EQUIPMENT FOR NEONATAL RESUSCITATION

STANDARD EQUIPMENT SETUP
Radiant warmer
Stethoscope
Oxygen source with warmer and humidifier
Suction source, suction catheter, meconium "aspirators"
Nasogastric tubes
Apparatus for bag-and-mask ventilation
Ventilation masks
Laryngoscope (handles, blades, and batteries)
Endotracheal tubes (2.5, 3, 3.5, and 4.0 mm)
Intravenous fluids (10% dextrose, normal saline, Ringer's lactate)
Drugs:
   Epinephrine (1:10,000 solution)
   Naloxone hydrochloride (0.4 mg/mL or 1.0 mg/mL)
   Sodium bicarbonate (0.5 meq/mL)
   Volume expanders (5% albumin, 0-negative whole blood [cross-matched against the mother's blood])
Clock
Syringes, hypodermic needles, and tubes for collection of blood samples
Equipment for umbilical vessel catheterization
Micro blood gas analysis availability
Warm blankets
ADDITIONAL EQUIPMENT SETUP
All of the above plus the following:
   Pressure manometer for use during ventilation
   Oxygen blender
   Heart rate and blood gas monitoring equipment
   Umbilical vessel catheter setup (ready to insert)
   Transcutaneous oxygen tension or saturation monitor
   Blood gas laboratory immediately available
   Apgar timer
   Camera
   Plastic bags for "micro-premies"
   Humidified gas

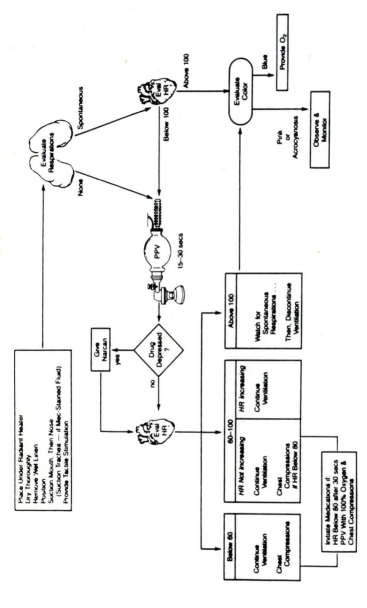

FIGURE 2-1. Overview of resuscitation in the delivery room. *Reproduced with permission. Textbook of Neonatal Resuscitation, 1987, 1990. Copyright American Heart Association.*

13

asphyxia is comparable to an umbilical cord prolapse. A more common clinical occurrence is prolonged partial asphyxia (eg, with maternal hemorrhage or severe placental insufficiency). Resuscitative measures are the same for both clinical scenarios, but the outcome is often worse following prolonged partial asphyxia in utero.

III. **Preparation for high-risk delivery.** Preparation for a high-risk delivery is often the key to a successful outcome. Cooperation between the obstetric staff and the pediatric staff is important. Knowledge of potential high-risk situations and appropriate interventions is essential (Table 2–2). It is useful to have an estimation of weight and gestational age, so that drug dosages can be calculated and the appropriate endotracheal tube and umbilical catheter size chosen (Table 2–3). While waiting for the infant to arrive, it is useful to think through potential problems, steps that may be undertaken to correct them, and which member of the team will handle each step.

IV. **Assessment of need for resuscitation.** The Apgar score (Appendix B) is assigned at 1, 5, and, occasionally, 10–20 minutes after delivery. It gives a fairly objective retrospective idea of how much resuscitation a term infant required at birth and the infant's response to resuscitative efforts. It is not particularly useful during resuscitation. During those long, tense moments, assessment of heart rate, skin color, and respiratory activity provides the quickest and most accurate evaluation of the need for continuing resuscitation. For preterm infants, Apgar scores may be particularly misleading (even in assessment of response to resuscitation) because of developmental differences in tone and response to stimulation.

   A. **Heart rate.** The heart rate is ideally monitored by a cardiotachometer via electrodes taped to the chest. Most often, however, evaluation is done by listening to the apical beat or feeling the pulse by lightly grasping the base of the umbilical cord. The evaluator should tap out each beat so that all team members can hear it. If no heart rate can be heard or felt, ventilatory efforts should be halted for a few seconds so that this finding can be verified by another team member.

   B. **Skin color.** Assessment of skin color may be difficult when there is severe bruising, especially in preterm infants. Marked acrocyanosis may also complicate the picture. Looking at the mucous membranes of the mouth may be helpful under these circumstances. Bluish coloring indicates central cyanosis; oxygen supplementation or assisted ventilation is needed. Pinkish membranes indicate normal oxygen levels, and resuscitation may not be needed.

   C. **Respiratory activity.** Assessment of respiratory activity is made by observing chest movement or listening for breath sounds. If there is no respiratory effort or the effort is poor, the infant needs respiratory assistance, either by manual stimulation or bag-and-mask ventilation.

V. **Technique of resuscitation**

   A. **Ventilatory resuscitation**

      1. **General measures**

         a. **Suctioning.** First, nasal and oropharyngeal secretions should be partially removed with a brief period of suctioning, either with a bulb syringe or a suction catheter. More prolonged suctioning delays resuscitation and may cause a profound vagal response in the infant (Cordero, 1971).

TABLE 2–2. SOME HIGH-RISK SITUATIONS FOR WHICH RESUSCITATION MAY BE ANTICIPATED

High-Risk Situation	Primary Intervention
Preterm delivery	Intubation, lung expansion
Thick meconium	Endotracheal suction
Acute fetal or placental hemorrhage	Volume expansion
Use of narcotics in labor	Administration of naloxone
Hydrops fetalis	Intubation, paracentesis, and/or thoracentesis
Polyhydramnios: gastrointestinal obstruction	Nasogastric suction
Oligohydramnios: pulmonary hypoplasia	Intubation, lung expansion
Maternal infection	Administration of antibiotics
Maternal diabetes	Early glucose administration

TABLE 2-3. EXPECTED BIRTH WEIGHT (50TH PERCENTILE) AT 24–38 WEEKS' GESTATION

Gestational Age (weeks)	Birth Weight (g)
24	700
26	900
28	1100
30	1350
32	1650
34	2100
36	2600
38	3000

Modified and reproduced, with permission, from Battaglia FC, Lubchenco LO: A practical classification of newborn infants by weight and gestational age. *J Pediatr* 1967;**71**:159.

    b. Mechanical ventilation. Most infants can be adequately ventilated with a bag and mask, provided that the mask is the correct size with a close seal around the mouth and nose and provided there is appropriate flow of oxygen to the bag (Fig 2–2). The stomach should be emptied during and after prolonged bag-and-mask ventilation.

    c. Endotracheal intubation. Endotracheal intubation should be performed when indicated. However, multiple unsuccessful attempts at intubation by inexperienced persons may make a bad situation worse, and in such situations, it may be best to continue mask ventilation until experienced help arrives. Absolute indications for aggressive ventilatory support with endotracheal intubation are difficult to list here, since institutional guidelines and clinical situations vary widely. The procedure for endotracheal intubation and some general guidelines are discussed in Chapter 18.

  2. Specific measures

    a. Term infant with meconium staining. Infants born through thick meconium may aspirate this inflammatory material in utero (gasping), during delivery, or immediately after birth. The sickest of these infants have usually aspirated in utero and generally also have reactive pulmonary vasoconstriction. Gregory and associates (1974) were among the first to show

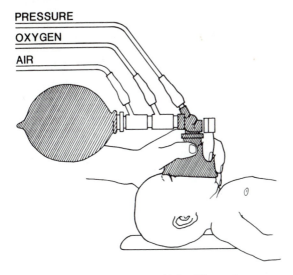

FIGURE 2–2. Bag-and-mask ventilation of the neonate.

that endotracheal suctioning at birth was beneficial. More recently, the American Academy of Pediatrics (AAP) and the American Heart Association (AHA) have suggested using **clinical judgment** in deciding whether or not aggressive endotracheal suctioning is necessary for "thin" meconium or for vigorous, crying infants. Meconium aspiration is discussed in detail in Chapter 67.

(1) **Hypopharyngeal suctioning should be started as soon as the head is delivered, before the infant has started to cry.** Deep suctioning should be avoided because it may result in acute laryngospasm.

(2) **Endotracheal suctioning.** Subsequently, **endotracheal intubation is performed and suction applied directly to the endotracheal tube.** Suctioning can be done directly from the wall unit via a connector to the endotracheal tube, or a suction catheter can be attached to the wall suction unit and inserted down the endotracheal tube. Suction is applied as the endotracheal tube is slowly withdrawn.

(3) **If meconium has been suctioned "below the cords," suctioning should be repeated after reintubation.**

(4) **The procedures described above may continue for up to 2 minutes after delivery, but then other resuscitative measures (particularly, ventilation and oxygenation) must begin.**

(5) **Supplemental oxygen.** Infants born through thick meconium may have experienced prolonged partial asphyxia in utero and may have developed pulmonary vascular constriction, leading to pulmonary hypertension after delivery. It is wise, therefore, to provide generous amounts of supplemental oxygen to these infants.

(6) **If meconium-stained fluid** is reported at less than 34 weeks' gestation, one of the following situations should be suspected:
  (a) The fetus is a growth-retarded term infant.
  (b) The fluid may actually be purulent (consider *Listeria* or *Pseudomonas*).
  (c) The fluid may actually be bile-stained (consider proximal intestinal obstruction).

b. **Term infant with perinatal asphyxia**
  (1) **A term infant with a heart rate of less than 100 beats/min and no spontaneous respiratory activity needs immediate lung expansion and supplemental oxygen provided by bag-and-mask ventilation.** Initially, the lungs should be slowly expanded (5–10 breaths) with peak inflating pressures of 25–30 cm water. If this is not successful in stimulating spontaneous respiratory effort or an improved heart rate, the ventilation rate should be increased to 40–60 breaths/min and peak inflating pressures maintained as high as necessary to expand the lungs. If bag-and-mask ventilation is ineffective or if prolonged positive-pressure ventilation is necessary, endotracheal intubation is indicated. If effective spontaneous respiratory effort results, the infant may be extubated and closely observed while breathing supplemental oxygen.

  (2) **A term infant with a heart rate of more than 100 beats/min but with poor skin color and weak respiratory activity requires stimulation (rubbing the back is often effective), supplemental oxygen blown across the face, and, occasionally, bag-and-mask ventilation to expand the lungs.** Most of these infants will respond with improved skin color and good spontaneous respiratory effort by 5 minutes of age.

c. **Preterm infant.** Preterm infants weighing less than 1200 g most often require immediate lung expansion in the delivery room. Ventilatory support measures should proceed as described for the asphyxiated term infant, with several important differences:

(1) If intubation is required, a smaller endotracheal tube is selected (2.5 or 3 mm internal diameter).

(2) Although high peak inflating pressures may initially be needed to expand the lungs, as soon as the lungs "open up," the pressure should be quickly decreased to as low as 10–15 cm of water by the end of the resuscitation if the clinical course permits.

(3) If available, one of several forms of liquid surfactant may be administered intratracheally as prophylaxis for hyaline membrane disease (see Chap 6).

B. Cardiac resuscitation. During delivery room resuscitation, efforts should be directed first to assisting ventilation and providing supplemental oxygen. A sluggish heart rate will usually respond to these efforts.

1. If the heart rate continues to be less than 80 beats/min by 30 seconds of age, in spite of ventilatory assistance, chest compression should be initiated. The thumbs are placed on the mid sternum just below a line connecting the nipples, while the palms of the hands encircle the torso and support the back (Fig 2–3). The sternum is compressed ½– ¾ inch (1.3–1.9 cm) at a regular rate of 120 compressions/min. The heart rate should be checked periodically and chest compression discontinued when the heart rate is > 80 beats/min.

2. An infant with no heart rate (a true Apgar = 0) who does not respond to ventilation and oxygenation may be considered stillborn. Prolonged resuscitative efforts are a matter for ethical consideration. (Jain, 1991).

C. Drugs used in resuscitation. (See also Emergency Drugs, Inside Front and Back Covers.) The AAP's *Textbook of Neonatal Resuscitation* recommends giving medications if the heart rate remains less than 80 beats/min despite adequate ventilation and chest compressions for a minimum of 30 seconds.

1. Route of administration

a. The endotracheal tube is the fastest route for administration of epinephrine in the delivery room (Lindemann, 1982). Absorption may be impaired if the tube is obstructed or malpositioned.

b. The umbilical vein is the preferred route for drug administration in the delivery room. A 3.5F or 5F umbilical catheter should be inserted just until blood is easily withdrawn (usually less than 5 cm); this should avoid inadvertent placement in the hepatic or portal vein.

c. Alternate routes of administration include peripheral venous and interosseous.

2. Drugs

a. Epinephrine may be necessary during resuscitation when adequate ventilation, oxygenation, and chest compression have failed and the heart rate is still less than 80 beats/min. This drug causes peripheral vasoconstriction, enhances cardiac contractility, and increases the heart rate. The dose is 0.1–0.3 mL/kg of 1:10,000 solution given intravenously or by endotracheal tube. This may be repeated every 5 minutes. If an endotracheal tube is used, the solution should be diluted 1:1 with normal saline.

b. Volume expanders. Hypovolemia should be suspected in any infant requiring resuscitation, particularly when there is evidence of acute blood loss with extreme pallor despite adequate oxygenation, poor peripheral pulse volume despite a normal heart rate, long capillary refill times, or poor response to resuscitative efforts. Appropriate volume expanders include O-negative whole blood (cross-matched against the mother's blood), 10 mL/kg; 5% albumin, 10 mL/kg; and Ringer's lactate and normal saline, 10 mL/kg. All are given intravenously over a 5- to 10-minute period.

c. Naloxone hydrochloride. Naloxone (Narcan) is a narcotic antagonist and should be administered to an infant with respiratory depression unresponsive to ventilatory assistance whose mother has received narcotics within 4 hours before delivery. One major exception to this recommendation is the newborn infant of a drug-addicted mother. These infants

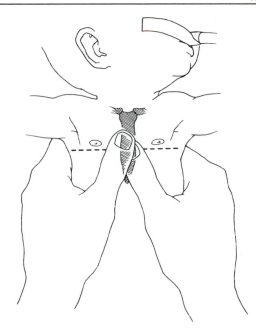

FIGURE 2–3. Technique of external cardiac massage (chest compression) in the neonate. Note the position of the thumbs on the mid sternum, just below the midline.

should never receive Narcan because acute withdrawal symptoms may develop. The AAP has recently issued a change in the dosage of Narcan (*Pediatrics* 1989;**83**:803). The new intravenous or intratracheal dosage for Narcan is 0.1 mg/kg. Two concentrations of naloxone are available: 0.4 mg/mL and 1.0 mg/mL. Neonatal Narcan (0.02 mg/mL) is no longer available. The dose may be repeated every 5 minutes as necessary. It should be emphasized that the half-life of Narcan is shorter that the half-life of narcotics.

d. **Dextrose.** The blood glucose concentration should be checked within 30 minutes after delivery in asphyxiated term infants, infants of diabetic mothers, and preterm infants, especially those whose mothers received tocolysis with ritodrine. Large boluses of dextrose should be avoided, even when the blood sugar is less than 25 mg/dL. To avoid wide swings in blood glucose, give a small bolus of 10% dextrose in water (1–2 mL/kg intravenously), and then begin an intravenous infusion of 10% dextrose at a rate of 4–6 mg/kg/min (80–100 mL/kg/day).

e. **Sodium bicarbonate** is usually not useful during the acute phase of neonatal resuscitation. Without adequate ventilation and oxygenation, it will not improve the blood pH. After prolonged resuscitation, however, sodium bicarbonate may be useful in correcting documented metabolic acidosis. Give 1–2 meq/kg intravenously (usually over a period of 30 minutes).

f. **Atropine and calcium.** Although previously used during resuscitation of the asphyxiated newborn, atropine and calcium are no longer recommended by the AAP or AHA. Current evidence does not support their effectiveness during delivery room resuscitation.

D. **Other supportive measures**
  1. **Temperature regulation.** Although some degree of cooling in a newborn infant is desirable because it provides a normal stimulus to respiratory effort, excessive cooling increases oxygen consumption and exacerbates acido-

sis. This is a problem especially for preterm infants, who have thin skin, decreased stores of body fat, and increased body surface area. Heat loss may be prevented by the following measures.

a. Dry the infant thoroughly immediately after delivery.

b. Maintain a warm delivery room.

c. Place the infant under a prewarmed radiant warmer. See also Chapter 5. Cover preterm infants with plastic wrap or a plastic bag up to the neck.

2. Preparation of the parents for resuscitation. Initial resuscitation usually occurs in the delivery room with one or both parents present. It is helpful to prepare the parents in advance, if possible. Describe what will be done, who will be present, who will explain what is happening, where the resuscitation will take place, where the father should stand, why crying may not be heard, and where the baby will be taken after stabilization.

REFERENCES

Abboud TK et al: Maternal, fetal, and neonatal responses after epidural anesthesia with bupivacaine, 2-chloroprocaine, or lidocaine. *Anesth Analg* 1982;**61**:638.

American Academy of Pediatrics Committee on Drugs: Emergency drug doses for infants and children and naloxone use in newborns: Clarification. *Pediatrics* 83:**803;** 1989.

Ballard RA: Resuscitation in the delivery room. Chapter 22 in: *Schaffer and Avery's Diseases of the Newborn,* 6th ed. Taeusch HW, Ballard RA, and Avery ME (editors). Saunders, 1991.

Benson RC et al: Fetal compromise during elective cesarean section. *Am J Obstet Gynecol* 1965;**91**:645.

Bland, BAR et al: Comparison of midazolam and thiopental for rapid sequence induction for elective cesarean section. *Anesth Analg* 1987;**66**:1165.

Bloom RS, Cropley C: *Textbook of Neonatal Resuscitation.* American Heart Association, American Academy of Pediatrics, 1990.

Caritis SN et al: Fetal acid-base state following spinal or epidural anesthesia for cesarean section. *Obstet Gynecol* 1980;**56**:610.

Cordero L Jr, Hon EH: Neonatal bradycardia following nasopharyngeal stimulation. *J Pediatr* 1971;**78**:441.

Crawford JS: Caesarean section. Chapter 5 in: *Principles and Practice of Obstetric Anesthesia,* 5th ed. Blackwell, 1984.

Datta S et al: Neonatal effect of prolonged anesthetic induction for cesarean section. *Obstet Gynecol* 1981;**58**:331.

Dawes GS: *Foetal & Neonatal Physiology.* Year Book, 1968.

Dubowitz LM .et al: Clinical assessment of gestational age in the newborn infant. *J Pediatr* 1970;**77**:1.

Gregory GA et al: Meconium aspiration in infants: A prospective study. *J Pediatr* 1974;**85**:848.

Jain L et al: Cardiopulmonary resuscitation of apparently stillborn infants: Survival and long-term outcome. *J Pediatr* 1991; **118**:778.

Jouppila P et al: Lumbar epidural analgesia to improve intervillous blood flow during labor in severe preeclampsia. *Obstet Gynecol* 1982;**59**:158.

Kang YG, Abouleish E, Caritis S: Prophylactic intravenous ephedrine infusion during spinal anesthesia for cesarean section. *Anesth Analg* 1982;**61**:839.

Kuhnert BR et al: Effects of low doses of meperidine on neonatal behavior. *Anesth Analg* 1985;**64**:335.

Lindemann R: Endotracheal administration of epinephrine during cardiopulmonary resuscitation. (Letter.) *Am J Dis Child* 1982;**136**:753.

Moore J, McNabb TG, Glynn JP: The placental transfer of pentazocine and pethidine. *Br J Anaesth* 1973;**45(Suppl):**798.

Ravlo O et al: A randomized comparison between midazolam and thiopental for elective cesarean section anesthesia: II. Neonates. *Anesth Analg* 1989;**68**:234.

Sepkoski CM: Neonatal neurobehavior: Development and its relation to obstetric anesthesia. *Clin Anaesthesiol* 1986;**4**:209

Shnider SM; Moya F: Effects of meperidine on the newborn infant. *Am J Obstet Gynecol* 1964;**89**:1009.

Shnider SM et al: Uterine blood flow and plasma norepinephrine changes during maternal stress in the pregnant ewe. *Anesthesiology* 1979;**50**:524.

Standards and guidelines for cardiopulmonary resuscitation and emergency cardiac care. 6. Neonatal advanced life support. *JAMA* 1986;**255**:2969.

Usher R et al: Judgment of fétal age. 2. Clinical significance of gestational age and objective measurement. *Pediatr Clin North Am* 1966;**13**:835.

3 Assessment of Gestational Age

Gestational age can be determined prenatally by the following techniques: date of last menstrual period, date of first reported fetal activity (quickening usually occurs at 16–18 weeks), first reported heart sounds (10–12 weeks by ultrasonic doppler), and ultrasound examination (very accurate if obtained before 20 weeks' gestation). Techniques for determining gestational age in the immediate postnatal period are discussed in this chapter.

I. **Classification.** Infants are classified as **preterm** (< 37 weeks), **term** (37–41⁶⁄₇ weeks), or **posterm** (≥ 42 weeks). Refinements developed in neonatal assessment have provided additional classifications based on a combination of features.

    A. **Small for gestational age (SGA)** is defined as 2 standard deviations below the mean weight for gestational age or below the 10th percentile (see Appendix F). See Chapter 62, Intrauterine Growth Retardation, for a full discussion. SGA is commonly seen in infants of mothers who have hypertension or preeclampsia or those who smoke. This condition has also been associated with TORCH (**to**xoplasmosis, **r**ubella, **c**ytomegalovirus, **h**erpes simplex) infections (see p 7), chromosomal abnormalities, and other congenital malformations.

    B. **Appropriate for gestational age (AGA).** See Appendix F.

    C. **Large for gestational age (LGA)** is defined as two standard deviations above the mean weight for gestational age or above the 90th percentile (see Appendix F). LGA can be seen in infants of diabetic mothers (see Chapter 60), in infants with Beckwith's syndrome, in constitutionally large infants with large parents, or in infants with hydrops fetalis (see p 275).

II. **Methods of determining postnatal gestational age**

    A. **Rapid delivery room assessment.** The most useful clinical signs in differentiating among premature, borderline mature, and full-term infants are (in order of usefulness): creases in the sole of the foot, size of the breast nodule, nature of scalp hair, cartilaginous development of the earlobe, and scrotal rugae and testicular descent in males. These signs and findings are listed in Table 3–1, which enables one to make a rapid assessment at delivery.

    B. **New Ballard Score (NBS).** The Ballard maturational score has been expanded and updated to include extremely premature infants. It has been renamed the New Ballard Score. The score now spans from –10 (correlating with 20 weeks' gestation) to a score of 50 (correlating with 44 weeks' gestation). It is best performed at less than 12 hours of age if the infant is less than 26 weeks' gestation. If the infant is greater than 26 weeks' gestation, there is no optimal age of examination up to 96 hours.

        1. **Accuracy.** The examination is accurate whether the infant is sick or well to within 2 weeks of gestational age. It overestimates gestational age by 2–4 days in infants between 32 and 37 weeks' gestation.

        2. **Criteria.** The examination consists of 6 neuromuscular criteria and 6 physical criteria. The neuromuscular criteria are based on the understanding that passive tone is more useful than active tone in indicating gestational age.

        3. **Procedure.** The examination is administered twice by 2 separate examiners to ensure objectivity, and the data are entered on the chart (Fig 3–1). This form is available in most nurseries. The examination consists of 2 parts, [neuromuscular maturity and physical maturity.] The 12 scores are totaled and maturity rating is expressed in weeks of gestation, estimated by using the chart provided on the form. Part 2 of the form (Fig 3–2) is then used to

TABLE 3-1. CRITERIA FOR RAPID GESTATIONAL ASSESSMENT AT DELIVERY

	36 Weeks and Earlier	37–38 Weeks	39 Weeks and Beyond
Creases in soles of feet	One of 2 transverse creases; posterior three-fourths of sole smooth	Multiple creases; anterior two-thirds of heel smooth	Entire sole covered with creases, including heel
Breast nodule*	2 mm	4 mm	7 mm
Scalp hair	Fine and woolly; fuzzy	Fine and woolly; fuzzy	Coarse and silky; each hair single-stranded
Earlobe	No cartilage	Moderate amount of cartilage	Stiff earlobe with thick cartilage
Testes and scrotum	Testes partially descended; scrotum small, with few rugae	?	Testes fully descended; scrotum normal size, with prominent rugae

*The breast nodule is not palpable before 33 weeks. Underweight full-term infants may have retarded breast development.
Modified and reproduced, with permission, from Usher R, McClean F, Scott KB: Judgment of fetal age. *Pediatr Clin North Am* 1966; 3:835.

MATURATIONAL ASSESSMENT OF GESTATIONAL AGE (New Ballard Score)

NAME _____ DATE/TIME OF BIRTH _____ SEX _____

HOSPITAL NO. _____ DATE/TIME OF EXAM _____ BIRTH WEIGHT _____

RACE _____ AGE WHEN EXAMINED _____ LENGTH _____

APGAR SCORE: 1 MINUTE _____ 5 MINUTES _____ 10 MINUTES _____ HEAD CIRC. _____

EXAMINER _____

NEUROMUSCULAR MATURITY

NEUROMUSCULAR MATURITY SIGN	SCORE							RECORD SCORE HERE
	-1	0	1	2	3	4	5	
POSTURE								
SQUARE WINDOW (Wrist)	>90°	90°	60°	45°	30°	0°		
ARM RECOIL		180°	140°-180°	110°-140°	90°-110°	<90°		
POPLITEAL ANGLE	180°	160°	140°	120°	100°	90°	<90°	
SCARF SIGN								
HEEL TO EAR								

TOTAL NEUROMUSCULAR MATURITY SCORE

SCORE
Neuromuscular _____
Physical _____
Total _____

MATURITY RATING

score	weeks
-10	20
-5	22
0	24
5	26
10	28
15	30
20	32
25	34
30	36
35	38
40	40
45	42
50	44

PHYSICAL MATURITY

PHYSICAL MATURITY SIGN	SCORE							RECORD SCORE HERE
	-1	0	1	2	3	4	5	
SKIN	sticky friable transparent	gelatinous red translucent	smooth pink visible veins	superficial peeling &/or rash, few veins	cracking pale areas rare veins	parchment deep cracking no vessels	leathery cracked wrinkled	
LANUGO	none	sparse	abundant	thinning	bald areas	mostly bald		
PLANTAR SURFACE	heel-toe 40-50 mm:-1 <40 mm:-2	>50 mm no crease	faint red marks	anterior transverse crease only	creases ant. 2/3	creases over entire sole		
BREAST	imperceptible	barely perceptible	flat areola no bud	stippled areola 1-2 mm bud	raised areola 3-4 mm bud	full areola 5-10 mm bud		
EYE/EAR	lids fused loosely: -1 tightly: -2	lids open pinna flat stays folded	sl. curved pinna; soft; slow recoil	well-curved pinna; soft but ready recoil	formed & firm instant recoil	thick cartilage ear stiff		
GENITALS (Male)	scrotum flat, smooth	scrotum empty faint rugae	testes in upper canal rare rugae	testes descending few rugae	testes down good rugae	testes pendulous deep rugae		
GENITALS (Female)	clitoris prominent & labia flat	prominent clitoris & small labia minora	prominent clitoris & enlarging minora	majora & minora equally prominent	majora large minora small	majora cover clitoris & minora		
						TOTAL PHYSICAL MATURITY SCORE		

Reference
Ballard JL, Khoury JC, Wedig K, et al. New Ballard Score, expanded to include extremely premature infants. J Pediatr 1991; 119:417-423. Reprinted by permission of Dr. Ballard and Mosby Year Book, Inc.

GESTATIONAL AGE (weeks)

By dates _____
By ultrasound _____
By exam _____

FIGURE 3-1. Maturational assessment of gestational age (New Ballard Score). (Reproduced, with permission, from Ballard JL et al: New Ballard Score, expanded to include extremely premature infants. J Pediatr 1991;119:417–423).

CLASSIFICATION OF NEWBORNS (BOTH SEXES)
BY INTRAUTERINE GROWTH AND GESTATIONAL AGE [1,2]

NAME _____

HOSPITAL NO. _____

RACE _____

DATE OF BIRTH _____

DATE OF EXAM _____

SEX _____

BIRTH WEIGHT _____

LENGTH _____

HEAD CIRC. _____

GESTATIONAL AGE _____

WEIGHT PERCENTILES

LENGTH PERCENTILES

24

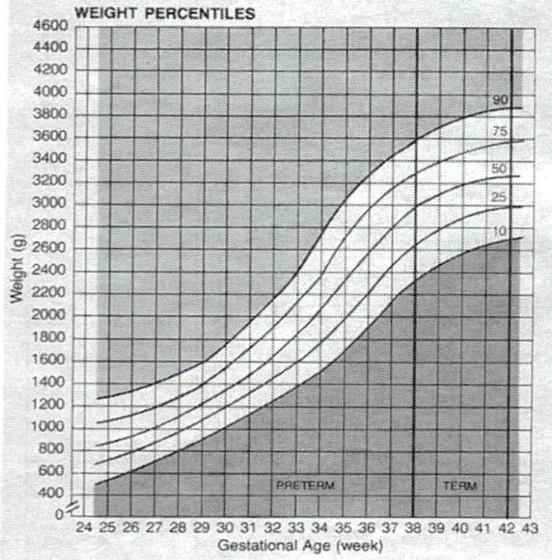

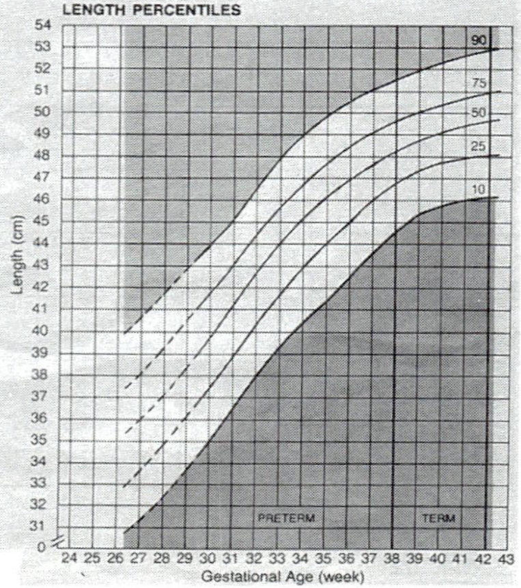

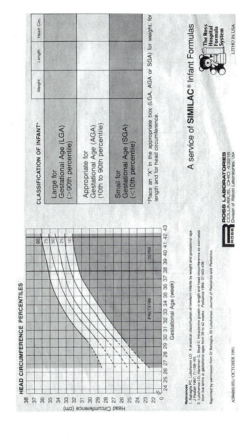

FIGURE 3–2. Classification of newborns (both sexes) by intrauterine growth and gestational age. *(Reproduced, with permission, from Battaglia FC, Lubchenco LO: A practical classification of newborn infants by weight and gestational age. J Pediatr 1967;**71**:159–163; and Lubchenco LO, Hansman C, Boyd E: Intrauterine growth in length and head circumference as estimated from live births at gestational ages from 26 to 42 weeks. Pediatrics 1966;**37**:403–408.)*

plot gestational assessment against length, height, and head circumference to determine if the baby is SGA, AGA, or LGA. These are the so-called **Lubchenco charts.** These charts are in the process of being updated to include the extremely premature infants but are not available at the time of publication. The current Lubchenco charts should be used until revised ones become available.

   (1) Posture. Score 0 if the arms and legs are extended, and 1 beginning flexion of the knees and hips, arms extended; determine other scores based on the diagram.

   (2) Square window. Flex the hand on the forearm between the thumb and index finger of the examiner. Apply sufficient pressure to get as much flexion as possible. Visually measure the angle between the hypothenar eminence and the ventral aspect of the forearm. Determine the score based on the diagram.

   (3) Arm recoil. Flex the forearms for 5 seconds; then grasp the hand and fully extend the arm and release. If the arm returns to full flexion, give a score of 4. For lesser degrees of flexion, score as noted on the diagram.

   (4) Popliteal angle. Hold the thigh in the knee-chest position with the left index finger and the thumb supporting the knee. Then extend the leg by gentle pressure from the right index finger behind the ankle. Measure the angle at the popliteal space and score accordingly.

   (5) Scarf sign. Take the infant's hand and try to put it around the neck posteriorly as far as possible over the opposite shoulder and score according to the diagram.

   (6) Heel to ear. Keeping the pelvis flat on the table, take the infant's foot and try to put it as close to the head as possible without forcing it. Grade according to the diagram.

 b. Physical maturity. These characteristics are scored as shown in Fig 3–1.

   (1) Skin. Carefully look at the skin and grade according to the diagram. Extremely premature infants have sticky, transparent skin and score a −1.

   (2) Lanugo hair is examined on the infant's back, between, and over the scapulae.

   (3) Plantar surface. Measure foot length from the tip of the great toe to the back of the heel. If the results are less than 40 mm, then give a score of −2. If it is betwen 40–50 mm, assign a score of −1. If the measurement is greater than 50 mm and no creases are seen on the plantar surface, then give a score of 0. If there are creases, then score accordingly.

   (4) Breast. Palpate any breast tissue and score.

   (5) Eye/Ear. This section has been expanded to include criteria that apply to the extremely premature infant. Loosely fused eyelids are defined as closed, but gentle traction opens them. Score this as −1. Tightly fused eyelids are defined as inseparable by gentle traction. Base the rest of the score on open lids and the examination of the ear.

   (6) Genitalia. Score according to the diagram.

C. Direct ophthalmoscopy. Another method for determination of gestational age uses direct ophthalmoscopy of the lens. Before 27 weeks, the cornea is too opaque to allow visualization; after 34 weeks, atrophy of the vessels of the lens occurs. Therefore, this technique allows for accurate determination of gestational age at 27–34 weeks only. The pupil must be dilated under the supervision of an ophthalmologist, and the assessment must be performed within 24–48 hours of birth before the vessels atrophy. The following grading system is used as shown in Fig 3–3.

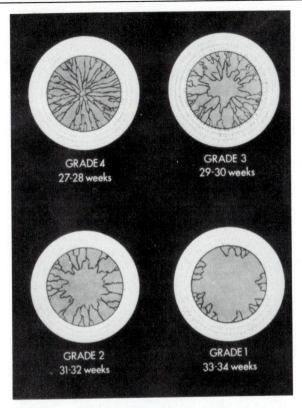

FIGURE 3–3. Grading system for assessment of gestational age by examination of the anterior vascular capsule of the lens. *(Reproduced, with permission, from Hittner HM, Hirsch NJ, Rudolph AJ: Assessment of gestational age by examination of the anterior vascular capsule of the lens.* J Pediatr *1977;**91**:455.)*

1. **Grade 4:** 27–28 weeks. Vessels cover the entire anterior surface of the lens or the vessels meet in the center of the lens.
2. **Grade 3:** 29–30 weeks. Vessels do not meet in the center but are close. Central portion of the lens is not covered by vessels.
3. **Grade 2:** 31–32 weeks. Vessels reach only to the middle-outer part of the lens. The central clear portion of the lens is larger.
4. **Grade 1:** 33–34 weeks. Vessels are seen only at the periphery of the lens.

REFERENCES

Amiel-Tison C: Neurological evaluation of the maturity of newborn infants. *Arch Dis Child* 1968;**43**:89.

Ballard JL, Novak KK, Driver M: A simplified score for assessment of fetal maturation of newly born infants. *J Pediatr* 1979;**95**:769.

Ballard JL et al: New Ballard Score, expanded to include extremely premature infants. *J Pediatr* 1991;**119**:417.

Dubowitz LM et al: Clinical assessment of gestational age in the newborn infant. *J Pediatr* 1970;**77**:1.

Farr V et al: The definition of some external characteristics used in the assessment of gestational age in the newborn infant. *Dev Med Child Neurol* 1966;**8:**657.

Hittner HM, Hirsch NJ, Rudolph AJ: Assessment of gestational age by examination of the anterior vascular capsule of the lens. *J Pediatr* 1977;**91:**455.

Usher R et al: Judgement of fetal age. 2. Clinical significance of gestational age and objective measurement. *Pediatr Clin North Am* 1966;**13:**835.

4 Newborn Physical Examination

The newborn infant should undergo a complete physical examination within 24 hours of birth. It is easier to listen to the heart and lungs first when the infant is quiet. Warming the stethoscope before using decreases the chance of making the infant cry.

I. **Vital signs**

    A. **Temperature.** Indicate if the temperature is rectal (which is usually 1 degree higher than oral), oral, or axillary (which is usually 1 degree lower than oral).

    B. **Respirations.** The normal respiratory rate in a newborn is 40–60 breaths/min.

    C. **Blood pressure.** Blood pressure correlates directly with gestational age, postnatal age of infant, and birth weight. See Appendix C for normal blood pressure curves.

    D. **Pulse rate.** The normal rate is 100–180 beats/min (bpm) in the newborn (usually 120–160 bpm awake; 70–80 bpm asleep). The heart rate increases in the normal infant with stimulation.

II. **Head circumference, length, weight, and gestational age**

    A. **Head circumference and percentile** (see Appendix F, Growth Charts). Place the measuring tape around the front of the head (above the brow [the frontal area]) and the occipital area. The tape should be above the ears. This is known as the occipitofrontal circumference, which is normally 32–37 cm at term.

    B. **Length and percentile** (see Growth Charts, Appendix F).

    C. **Weight and percentile** (see Growth Charts, Appendix F).

    D. **Assessment of gestational age** (see Chapter 3)

III. **General appearance.** Observe the infant and record the general appearance (eg, activity, skin color, obvious congenital abnormalities).

IV. **Skin**

    A. **Color**

        1. **Plethora (deep, rosy red color).** Plethora is more common in infants with polycythemia but can be seen in an over-oxygenated or overheated infant. It is best to obtain a central hematocrit on any plethoric infant.

        2. **Jaundice (yellowish color).** With jaundice, bilirubin levels are usually higher than 5 mg/dL. This condition is abnormal in infants less than 24 hours old and may signify Rh incompatibility, sepsis, and TORCH (**to**xoplasmosis, **r**ubella, **c**ytomegalovirus, **h**erpes simplex) infections (see p 345). After 24 hours, it may result either from these diseases or such common causes as ABO incompatibility or physiologic causes.

        3. **Pallor (washed-out, whitish appearance).** Pallor may be secondary to anemia, birth asphyxia, shock, or patent ductus arteriosus. **Ductal pallor** is the term sometimes used to denote pallor associated with patent ductus arteriosus.

        4. **Cyanosis**

            a. **Central cyanosis** (bluish skin, including the tongue and lips). Central cyanosis is caused by low oxygen saturation in the blood. It may be associated with congenital heart or lung disease.

            b. **Peripheral cyanosis** (bluish skin with pink lips and tongue). Peripheral cyanosis may be associated with methemoglobinemia. **Methemoglobinemia** occurs when hemoglobin oxidizes from the ferrous to the ferric form; the blood actually can have a chocolate hue. Methemoglobin is incapable of transporting oxygen or carbon dioxide. This disorder can be caused by exposure to certain drugs or chemicals (nitrates or nitrites) or may be hereditary (eg, NADH-methemoglobin reductase deficiency, hemoglobin M disease). Treatment for infants is with methylene blue.

    c. **Acrocyanosis** (bluish hands and feet only). Acrocyanosis may be normal for an infant who has just been born (or within the first few hours after birth) or one who is experiencing cold stress. If the condition is seen in an older infant with a normal temperature, decreased peripheral perfusion secondary to hypovolemia should be considered.

  5. Extensive bruising may be associated with a prolonged and difficult delivery and may result in early jaundice.

  6. "Blue on pink" or "pink on blue." Whereas some infants are pink and well-perfused, and others are clearly cyanotic, some do not fit either of these categories. They may appear bluish with pink undertones or pink with bluish undertones. This coloration may be secondary to poor perfusion, inadequate oxygenation, inadequate ventilation, or polycythemia.

  7. Harlequin coloration (clear line of demarcation between an area of redness and an area of normal coloration). The cause is usually unknown. The coloration can be benign and transient (usually less than 20 minutes' duration) or it can be indicative of shunting of blood (persistent pulmonary hypertension, coarctation of the aorta). There can be varying degrees of redness and perfusion. The demarcating line may run from the head to the belly, dividing the body into right and left halves, or it may develop in the dependent half of the body when the newborn is lying on one side.

  8. Mottling (lacy red pattern) may be seen in a normal infant or one with cold stress, hypovolemia, or sepsis. Persistent mottling, referred to as **cutis marmorata**, is found in infants with Down's syndrome, trisomy 13, or trisomy 18.

B. Rashes

  1. Milia. Milia is a rash in which tiny, sebaceous, retention cysts are seen. The whitish, pinhead-sized concretions are usually on the chin, nose, forehead, and cheeks. These benign cysts disappear within a few weeks.

  2. Erythema toxicum. In erythema toxicum, numerous small areas of red skin are seen, with a yellow-white papule in the center. Lesions are most noticeable at 48 hours after birth but may appear as late as 7–10 days. Wright's staining of the papule reveals eosinophils. This benign rash resolves spontaneously.

  3. Candida albicans rash. *Candida albicans* diaper rash appears as erythematous plaques with sharply demarcated edges. Satellite bodies (pustules on contiguous areas of skin) are also seen. Usually the skin folds are involved. Gram's stain of a smear or 10% potassium hydroxide preparation of the lesion reveals budding yeast spores, which are easily treated with Nystatin ointment or cream applied to the rash 4 times daily for 7–10 days.

  4. Transient neonatal pustular melanosis is characterized by 3 different stages of lesions that may appear over the entire body: pustules, ruptured vesicopustules with scaling, and hyperpigmented macules. This benign, self-limiting condition requires no specific therapy.

  5. Acne neonatorum. The lesions are typically seen over the cheeks, chin, and forehead and consist of comedones and papules. The condition is usually benign and requires no therapy; however, severe cases may require treatment with mild keratolytic agents, such as 3% sulfur salicylic acid.

C. Nevi. Hemangiomas near the eyes, nose or mouth that interfere with vital functions or sight may need surgical intervention.

  1. Macular hemangioma ("stork bites"). A macular hemangioma is a true vascular nevus normally seen on the occipital area, eyelids, and glabella. The lesions disappear spontaneously within the first year of life.

  2. Port-wine stain (nevus flammeus) is usually seen at birth, does not blanch with pressure, and does not disappear with time. If the lesion appears over the forehead and upper lip, then **Sturge-Weber syndrome** (port-wine stain over the forehead and upper lip, glaucoma, and contralateral Jacksonian seizures) must be ruled out.

3. **Mongolian spot.** Mongolian spots are dark blue or purple bruiselike macular spots usually located over the sacrum. Usually present in 90% of blacks and Asians, they occur in less than 5% of white children. They disappear by 4 years of age.

4. **Cavernous hemangioma.** A cavernous hemangioma usually appears as a large, red, cystic-appearing, firm, and ill-defined mass that may be found anywhere on the body. The majority of these lesions regress with age, but some require corticosteroid therapy. In more severe cases, surgical resection may be necessary. If associated with thrombocytopenia, **Kasabach-Merritt syndrome** (thrombocythemia associated with a rapidly expanding hemangioma) should be considered. Transfusions of platelets and clotting factors are usually required in patients with this syndrome.

5. **Strawberry hemangioma (macular hemangioma).** Strawberry hemangiomas are flat, bright red, sharply demarcated lesions, that are most commonly found on the face. Spontaneous regression usually occurs (70% disappearance by 7 years of age).

V. **Head.** Note the general shape of the head. Inspect for any cuts or bruises secondary to forceps or fetal monitor leads. Transillumination can be done for severe hydrocephaly and hydranencephaly.

A. **Anterior and posterior fontanelles.** The anterior fontanelle usually closes at 9–12 months and the posterior fontanelle at 2–4 months. A large anterior fontanelle is seen with hypothyroidism and may also be found in infants with skeletal disorders such as osteogenesis imperfecta, hypophosphatasia, and chromosomal abnormalities or who are small for gestational age. A bulging fontanelle may be associated with increased intracranial pressure, meningitis, or hydrocephalus. Depressed (sunken) fontanelles are seen in newborns with dehydration. A small anterior fontanelle may be associated with hyperthyroidism, microcephaly, or craniosynostosis.

B. **Molding.** Molding is a temporary asymmetry of the skull resulting from the birth process. Most often seen with prolonged labor and vaginal deliveries, it can be seen in cesarean deliveries if the mother had a prolonged course of labor before delivery. A normal head shape is usually regained within 1 week.

C. **Caput succedaneum.** Caput succedaneum is a diffuse edematous swelling of the soft tissues of the scalp that may extend across the suture lines. It is secondary to the pressure of the uterus or vaginal wall on areas of the fetal head bordering the caput. Usually it resolves within several days.

D. **Cephalhematoma** is a subperiosteal hemorrhage that *never* extends across the suture line. It can be secondary to a traumatic delivery or forceps delivery. X-ray films or CT scans of the head should be obtained if an underlying skull fracture is suspected (approximately 5% of all cephalhematomas). Hematocrit and bilirubin levels should be followed in these patients. Most cephalhematomas resolve in 6 weeks. Aspiration of the hematoma is rarely necessary.

E. **Increased intracranial pressure.** The following signs are evident in an infant with increased intracranial pressure: bulging anterior fontanelle, separated sutures, paralysis of upward gaze (setting-sun sign), and prominent veins of the scalp. The increased pressure may be secondary to hydrocephalus, hypoxic-ischemic brain injury, intracranial hemorrhage, or subdural hematoma.

F. **Craniosynostosis.** Craniosynostosis is the premature closure of one or more sutures of the skull. It should be considered in any infant with an asymmetric skull. On palpation of the skull, a bony ridge over the suture line may be felt, and inability to freely move the cranial bones may occur. X-ray studies of the head should be performed, and surgical consultation may be necessary.

G. **Craniotabes,** a benign condition, is a softening of the skull that usually occurs around the suture lines and disappears within days. If the area is over most of the skull, then it may be secondary to a calcium deficiency, and osteogenesis imperfecta and syphilis should be ruled out.

VI. Neck. Eliciting the rooting reflex (see p 36) causes the infant to turn its head and allows easier examination of the neck. Palpate the sternocleidomastoid for a hematoma and the thyroid for enlargement, and check for thyroglossal duct cysts. A short neck is seen in Turner's, Noonan's, and Klippel-Feil syndromes.

VII. Face. Look for obvious abnormalities. Note the general shape of the nose, mouth, and chin. The presence of hypertelorism (eyes widely separated) or low-set ears should be noted.

   A. Facial nerve injury. Unilateral branches of the facial (VII) nerve are most commonly involved. There is facial asymmetry with crying. The corner of the mouth droops and the nasolabial fold is absent in the paralyzed side. If the palsy is secondary to trauma, most symptoms disappear within the first week of life, but sometimes resolution may take several months. If the palsy persists, then absence of the nerve needs to be ruled out.

VIII. Ears. Look for unusual shape or abnormal position. The normal position is determined by drawing an imaginary horizontal line from the inner and outer canthus of the eye across the face, perpendicular to the vertical axis of the head. If the helix of the ear lies below this horizontal line, the ears are designated as low-set. Low-set ears are seen with many congenital anomalies (most commonly Treacher Collins, triploidy, and trisomy 9 and 18 syndromes, and fetal aminopterin effects). Preauricular skin tags (papillomas), which are benign, are often seen. Hairy ears are seen in infants of diabetic mothers. Gross hearing can be assessed when an infant blinks to loud noises.

IX. Eyes. Check the red reflex with an ophthalmoscope. If a cataract is present, opacification of the lens and loss of the reflex is apparent. Congenital cataracts require early evaluation by an ophthalmologist. The sclera, which is normally white, can have a bluish tint if the infant is premature because the sclera is thinner in these infants than in terms infants. If the sclera is deep blue, **osteogenesis imperfecta** should be ruled out.

   A. Brushfield's spots (salt-and-pepper speckling of the iris) are often seen with Down's syndrome.

   B. Subconjunctival hemorrhage. Rupture of small conjunctival capillaries can occur normally but is more common after a traumatic delivery. This condition is seen in 5% of newborn infants.

   C. Conjunctivitis. (See Chapter 31.)

X. Nose. If unilateral or bilateral choanal atresia is suspected, verify the patency of the nostrils with gentle passage of a nasogastric tube. Infants are obligate nose breathers, therefore, if they have bilateral choanal atresia, they will present with severe respiratory distress. Nasal flaring is indicative of respiratory distress. Sniffling and discharge are typical of congenital syphilis.

XI. Mouth. Examine the hard and soft palate for evidence of a cleft palate. A short lingual frenulum (tongue-tie) may require surgical treatment.

   A. Ranula. A ranula is a cystic swelling in the floor of the mouth. Most disappear spontaneously.

   B. Epstein's pearls. These keratin-containing cysts, which are normal, are located on the hard and soft palate and resolve spontaneously.

   C. Mucocele. This small lesion on the oral mucosa occurs secondary to trauma to the salivary gland ducts. It is usually benign and subsides spontaneously.

   D. Natal teeth are usually lower incisors. X-rays are needed to differentiate the two types because management is different.

      1. Predeciduous teeth. Supernumerary teeth are found in 1 in 4000 births. They are usually loose and the roots are absent or are poorly formed. Removal is necessary to avoid aspiration.

      2. True deciduous teeth. These teeth are true teeth that erupt early. They occur in about 1 in 2000 births. They should not be extracted.

   E. Macroglossia. Enlargement of the tongue can be congenital or acquired. Localized macroglossia is usually secondary to congenital hemangiomas.

Macrosomia can be seen in **Beckwith's syndrome** (macroglossia, giantism, omphalocele, severe hypoglycemia), or **Pompe's disease** (type II glycogen storage disease).

F. Frothy or copious saliva is commonly seen in infants with an esophageal atresia with tracheoesophageal fistula.

G. Thrush. Oral thrush, which is common in newborns, is a sign of infection due to *C albicans*. Whitish patches appear on the tongue, gingiva, or buccal mucosa. Thrush is easily treated with nystatin suspension, 0.1–1.0 mL applied to each side of the mouth, often with a cotton-tipped swab, 3–4 times per day for 7 days.

XII. Chest

A. Observation. First note if the chest is symmetrical. An asymmetric chest may signify a tension pneumothorax. Tachypnea, sternal and intercostal retractions, and grunting on expiration indicate respiratory distress.

B. Breath sounds. Listen for presence and equality of breath sounds. A good place to listen is in the right and left axillae. Absent or unequal sounds may indicate pneumothorax or atelectasis. Absent breath sounds with the presence of bowel sounds indicates a diaphragmatic hernia; a stat x-ray and emergency surgical consultation is recommended.

C. Pectus excavatum. Pectus excavatum is a sternum that is altered in shape. Usually this condition is of no clinical concern.

D. Breasts in a newborn are usually 1 cm in diameter in term male and female infants. They may be abnormally enlarged (3–4 cm) secondary to the effects of maternal estrogens. This effect, which lasts less than one week, is of no clinical concern. A usually white discharge may be present that is commonly referred to as "witch's milk."

XIII. Heart. Observe for heart rate, rhythm, quality of heart sounds, active precordium, and presence of a murmur. The position of the heart may be determined by auscultation. Abnormal sinus syndromes are described on p 172.

A. Murmurs may be associated with the following conditions.

1. Ventricular septal defect (VSD), the most common heart defect, accounts for approximately 25% of congenital heart disease. Typically a loud, harsh, blowing pansystolic murmur is heard (best heard over the lower left sternal border). Symptoms such as congestive heart failure usually do not begin until after 2 weeks of age, and typically are present from 6 weeks to 4 months. The majority of these defects close spontaneously by the end of the first year of life.

2. Patent ductus arteriosus (PDA) is a harsh, continuous, machinery-type, or "rolling thunder," murmur which usually presents on the second or third day of life, localized to the second left intercostal space. It may radiate to the left clavicle or down the left sternal border. A hyperactive precordium is also seen. Clinical signs include wide pulse pressure and bounding pulses.

3. Coarctation of the aorta, a systolic ejection murmur, radiates down the sternum to the apex and to the interscapular area. It is often loudest in the back.

4. Peripheral pulmonic stenosis. A systolic murmur is heard bilaterally in the anterior chest, in both axillas, and across the back. It is secondary to the turbulence caused by disturbed blood flow because the main pulmonary artery is larger than the peripheral pulmonary arteries. This usually benign murmur may persist up to 3 months of age. It may also be associated with rubella syndrome.

5. Hypoplastic left heart syndrome. A short, midsystolic murmur usually presents anywhere from day 1–21. A gallop is usually heard.

6. Tetralogy of Fallot typically is a loud and harsh systolic or pansystolic murmur heard best at the left sternal border. The second heart sound is single.

7. Pulmonary atresia

a. With VSD. An absent or soft systolic murmur with the first heart sound is followed by an ejection click. The second heart sound is loud and single.

    b. With intact intraventricular septum. Most frequently, there is no murmur and a single second heart sound is heard.

  8. Tricuspid atresia. A pansystolic murmur along the left sternal border with a single second heart sound is typically heard.

  9. Transposition of the great vessels is more common in males than in females.

    a. Isolated (simple). Cardiac examination is often normal, but cyanosis and tachypnea are present along with a normal chest x-ray film and ECG.

    b. With VSD. The murmur is loud, pansystolic, and heard best at the lower left sternal border. The infant typically presents with congestive heart failure at 3–6 weeks' of life.

  10. Ebstein's disease. A long systolic murmur is heard over the anterior portion of the left chest. A diastolic murmur and gallop may be present.

  11. Truncus arteriosus. A systolic ejection murmur, often with a thrill, is heard at the left sternal border. The second heart sound is loud and single.

  12. Single ventricle. A loud systolic ejection murmur with a loud, single second heart sound is heard.

  13. Atrial septal defects (ASDs)

    a. Ostium secundum defect rarely presents with congestive heart failure in infancy. A soft systolic ejection murmur is best heard at the upper left sternal border.

    b. Ostium primum defect rarely occurs in infancy. A pulmonary ejection murmur and early systolic murmur are heard at the lower left sternal border. A split second heart sound is heard.

    c. Common atrioventricular canal presents with congestive heart failure in infancy. A harsh systolic murmur is heard all over the chest. The second heart sound is split if pulmonary flow is increased.

  14. Anomalous pulmonary venous return

    a. Partial. Findings are similar to those for ostium secundum defect (see **XIII.a.13.a**).

    b. Total. With a severe obstruction, no murmur may be detected on examination. With a moderate degree of obstruction, a systolic murmur is heard along the left sternal border, and a gallop murmur is heard occasionally. A continuous murmur along the left upper sternal border over the pulmonary area may also be audible.

  15. Congenital aortic stenosis. A coarse systolic murmur with a thrill is heard at the upper right sternal border and can radiate to the neck and down the left sternal border. If left ventricular failure is severe, the murmur is of low intensity. Symptoms that occur in infants only when the stenosis is severe are pulmonary edema and congestive heart failure.

  16. Pulmonary stenosis (with intact ventricular septum). If the stenosis is severe, a loud systolic ejection murmur is audible over the pulmonary area and radiates over the entire precordium. Right ventricular failure and cyanosis may be present. If the stenosis is mild, a short pulmonary systolic ejection murmur is heard over the pulmonic area along with a split second heart sound.

B. Palpate the pulses (femoral, pedal, radial, and brachial). Bounding pulses can be seen with patent ductus arteriosus. Absent or delayed femoral pulses are associated with coarctation of the aorta.

C. Check for signs of congestive heart failure. Signs may include hepatomegaly, gallop, tachypnea, wheezes and rales, tachycardia, and abnormal pulses.

XIV. Abdomen

  A. Observation. Obvious defects may include an **omphalocele,** where the intestines are covered by peritoneum and the umbilicus is centrally located, or a **gastroschisis,** where the intestines are not covered by peritoneum (the defect is usually to the right of the umbilicus). A **scaphoid abdomen** may be associated with a diaphragmatic hernia.

B. **Auscultation.** Listen for bowel sounds.

C. **Palpation.** Check the abdomen for distention, tenderness, or masses. It is most easily palpated when the infant is quiet or during feeding. In normal circumstances the liver can be palpated 1–2 cm below the costal margin and the spleen tip at the costal margin. Hepatomegaly can be seen with congestive heart failure, hepatitis, or sepsis. Splenomegaly is found with cytomegalovirus (CMV) or rubella infections or sepsis. The kidneys (especially on the right) can often be palpated. Kidney size may be increased with polycystic disease, renal vein thrombosis, or hydronephrosis. Abdominal masses are more commonly related to the urinary tract.

XV. **Umbilicus.** Normally, the umbilicus has two arteries and one vein. The presence of only two vessels (one artery, one vein) could indicate renal or genetic problems (most commonly trisomy 18). If the umbilicus is abnormal, ultrasonography of the abdomen is recommended. In addition, inspect for any discharge, redness, or edema around the base of the cord that may signify a patent urachus or omphalitis. The cord should be translucent; a greenish-yellow color suggests meconium staining, usually secondary to fetal distress.

XVI. **Genitalia.** Any infant with ambiguous genitalia should not undergo gender assignment until a formal endocrinology evaluation has been performed (see Chapter 53). A male with any question of a penile abnormality should not be circumcised until evaluated by a urologist or pediatric surgeon.

A. **Male.** Check for dorsal hood, hypospadias, epispadias, or chordee. Normal penile length at birth is greater than 2 cm. Newborn males always have a marked phimosis. Determine the site of the meatus. Hydroceles are common and usually disappear by 1 year of age. Palpate the testicles and examine for groin hernias. Observe the color of the scrotum. A bluish color may suggest testicular torsion and requires immediate surgical consultation.

B. **Female.** Examine the labia and clitoris. A mucosal tag is commonly attached to the wall of the vagina. Discharge from the vagina is common and is often blood-tinged secondary to maternal estrogen withdrawal. If the labia are fused and the clitoris is enlarged, adrenal hyperplasia should be suspected. A large clitoris can be associated with maternal drug ingestion. Labia majora at term are enlarged.

XVII. **Lymph nodes.** Palpable lymph nodes, usually in the inguinal and cervical areas, are found in approximately 33% of normal neonates.

XVIII. **Anus and rectum.** Check for patency of the anus to rule out imperforate anus. Check the position of the anus. Meconium should pass within 48 hours of birth.

XIX. **Extremities.** Examine the arms and legs, paying close attention to the digits and palmar creases.

A. **Syndactyly,** abnormal fusion of the digits, most commonly involves the third and fourth fingers and second and third toes. A strong family history exists. Surgery is performed when the neonates are older.

B. **Polydactyly** is supernumerary digits on the hands or the feet. This condition is associated with a strong family history. An x-ray film of the extremity is usually obtained to verify if any bony structures are present in the digit. If there are no bony structures, a suture can be tied around the digit until it falls off. If bony structures are present, surgical removal is necessary. Axial extra digits are associated with heart anomalies.

C. **Simian crease.** A single transverse palmar crease is most commonly seen in Down's syndrome but is occasionally a normal variant.

D. **Talipes equinovarus** (clubfoot) is more common in males. The foot is turned downward and inward, and the sole is directed medially. If this problem can be corrected with gentle force, it will resolve spontaneously. If not, orthopedic treatment and follow-up is necessary.

    E. Metatarsus varus is adduction of the forefoot. This condition usually corrects spontaneously.

XX. Trunk and spine. Check for any gross defects of the spine. Any abnormal pigmentation or hairy patches over the lower back should increase the suspicion that an underlying vertebral abnormality exists. A sacral or pilonidal dimple may indicate a small meningocele or other anomaly.

XXI. Hips. Congenital hip dislocation occurs in approximately 1 in 800 live births. More common in white females, this condition is more likely to be unilateral and involve the left hip. Two clinical signs of dislocation are asymmetry of the skin folds on the dorsal surface and shortening of the affected leg.

    Evaluate for congenital hip dislocation by using the **Ortolani and Barlow maneuvers.** Place the infant in the frog leg position. Abduct the hips by using the middle finger to apply gentle inward and upward pressure over the greater trochanter (Ortolani's sign). Adduct the hips by using the thumb to apply outward and backward pressure over the inner thigh (Barlow's sign). (Some clinicians suggest omitting the Barlow maneuver because this action may contribute to hip instability by stretching the capsule unnecessarily.) A click of reduction and a click of dislocation is elicited in infants with hip dislocation. If this disorder is suspected, radiographic studies and orthopedic consultation should be obtained.

XXII. Nervous system. First, observe the infant for any abnormal movement (eg, seizure activity) or excessive irritability. Then, evaluate the following parameters.

  A. Muscle tone
    1. Hypotonia. Floppiness and head lag are seen.
    2. Hypertonia. Increased resistance is apparent when the arms and legs are extended. Hyperextension of the back and tightly clenched fists are often seen.

  B. Reflexes. The following reflexes are normal for a newborn infant:
    1. Rooting reflex. Stroke the lip and corner of cheek with a finger and the infant will turn in that direction and open the mouth.
    2. Glabellar reflex (blink reflex). Tap gently over the forehead and the eyes will blink.
    3. Grasp reflex. Place the finger in the palm of the infant's hand and the infant will grasp the finger.
    4. Neck righting reflex. Turn the infant's head to the right or left and movement of the contralateral shoulder should be obtained in the same direction.
    5. Moro reflex. Support the infant behind the upper back with one hand, then drop the infant back 1 cm or more to the mattress but not on the mattress. This should cause abduction of both arms and extension of the fingers. Asymmetry may signify a fractured clavicle, a hemiparesis, or brachial plexus injury.

  C. Cranial nerves. Note the presence of gross nystagmus, the reaction of the pupils, and the ability of the infant to follow moving objects with its eyes.

  D. Movement. Check for spontaneous movement of limbs, trunk, face, and neck. A fine tremor is usually normal. Clonic movements are not normal and may be seen with seizures.

  E. Peripheral nerves
    1. Erb-Duchenne paralysis involves injury to the fifth and sixth cervical nerves. The shoulder is rotated with the forearm supinated and elbow extended ("waiter's tip" position). The grasping function of the hand is preserved. This condition can be associated with diaphragm paralysis.
    2. Klumpke's paralysis involves the seventh and eighth cervical nerves and the first thoracic nerve. The hand is flaccid with little or no control. If the sympathetic fibers of the first thoracic root are injured, ipsilateral ptosis and miosis can occur.

  F. General signs of neurologic disorders

1. **Symptoms of increased intracranial pressure** (bulging anterior fontanelle, dilated scalp veins, setting-sun sign) (see p 31)
2. **Hypotonia or hypertonia.**
3. **Irritability or hyperexcitability.**
4. **Poor sucking and swallowing reflexes.**
5. **Shallow, irregular respirations.**
6. **Apnea.**
7. **Apathy.**
8. **Staring.**
9. **Seizure activity** (sucking or chewing of the tongue, blinking of eyelids, eye rolling, hiccups).
10. **Absent, depressed, or exaggerated reflexes.**
11. **Asymmetrical reflexes.**

5 Temperature Regulation

The newborn infant must be kept warm and dry to prevent heat loss and its consequences. For this reason, a **neutral thermal environment** should be maintained. At this temperature the least amount of oxygen consumption and metabolic expenditure is needed for the infant to maintain a normal body temperature (see Figs 5–1 and 5–2 and Table 5–1). The **normal skin temperature** in the neonate is 36.0–36.5 °C (96.8–97.7 °F). The **normal core temperature** is 36.5–37.5 °C (97.7–99.5 °F).

I. **Hypothermia.** Preterm infants are predisposed to heat loss because they have less subcutaneous fat, an increased ratio of surface area to body weight, and reduced glycogen and brown fat stores. In addition, they have hypotonia and are therefore unable to curl up to keep warm as a normal infant would.

A. **Mechanisms of heat loss** in the newborn include:

1. **Radiation.** Radiation is heat loss from the infant (warm object) to a colder object in the room.

2. **Conduction.** Conduction is direct heat loss from the infant to the surface with which it is in contact.

3. **Convection.** Convection is heat loss from the infant to the air.

4. **Evaporation.** Heat may be lost by water evaporation from the skin of the infant (especially likely immediately after delivery).

B. **Consequences of hypothermia**

1. **Hypoglycemia** secondary to depletion of glycogen stores.

2. **Metabolic acidosis** caused by peripheral vasoconstriction with anaerobic metabolism and acidosis.

3. **Hypoxia** with increased oxygen demands.

4. **Decreased growth with increased metabolic rate.**

5. **Clotting disorders.** Pulmonary hemorrhage can accompany severe hypothermia.

6. **Shock** with resulting decrease in systemic arterial pressure, decrease in plasma volume, and decreased cardiac output.

7. **Apnea.**

8. **Intraventricular hemorrhage.**

C. **Prevention and treatment of hypothermia.** Because earlier studies revealed that rapid rewarming caused convulsions, apnea, and worsening of the metabolic acidosis, the trend has been to rewarm slowly. One later investigation on rapid versus slow rewarming of hypothermic low birthweight infants showed that the infants who were rapidly rewarmed (2.7–19 hours [rapid group] and 1–3 days [slow group]) had a lower death rate. In another study, no difference between the two groups in the incidence of death, apnea, or seizures was apparent. The difference in the death rate did not reach statistical significance.

Although the subject is still controversial, more clinicians are leaning toward more rapid rewarming. One recommendation is to rewarm at a rate of one degree Celsius per hour unless the infant weighs less than 1200 grams, the gestational age is less than 28 weeks, or the temperature is less than 32.0 °C (89.6 °F) and the infant can be rewarmed more slowly (rate not to exceed 0.6 degrees C per hour).

1. **Equipment**

a. **Closed incubator.** Incubators are usually used for infants who weigh less than 1800 grams. One disadvantage of incubators is that they make observing a sick infant closley or performing any type of procedure difficult. In addition, temperature changes due to sepsis may be masked by

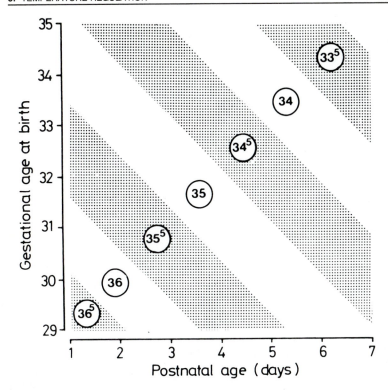

FIGURE 5–1. Neutral thermal environment during the first week of life, based on gestational age. *(Reproduced with permission from Sauer PJJ, Dane HJ and Visser HKA. New standards for neutral thermal environment of healthy very low birthweight infants in week one of life. Arch Disease in Childhood, 1984, 59:18–22.)*

the automatic temperature control system of closed incubators. Infants can be weaned from incubators when their body temperatures can be maintained at an environmental temperature of less than 30.0 °C (usually when the body weight reaches about 1800 grams). Enclosed incubators maintain a constant body temperature using one of the following devices.

(1) **Servocontrolled skin probe** attached to the abdomen of the infant. If the temperature falls, additional heat is delivered as the target skin temperature is reached, and the heating unit turns off automatically. A potential disadvantage is that overheating may occur if the skin sensor is loose.

(2) **Air temperature control device.** With this device, the temperature of the air in the incubator is increased or decreased depending on the measured temperature of the infant. Use of this mode requires constant attention from a nurse and is usually used in older infants.

(3) **Air temperature probe.** A probe that hangs in the incubator near the infant and maintains a constant air temperature. There is less temperature fluctuation with this probe.

b. **Radiant warmer.** The radiant warmer is typically used for very unstable infants or during the performance of medical procedures. The temperature can be maintained in the "servo mode" (ie, by means of a skin probe) or the "nonservo mode" (also called "manual mode") which maintains a

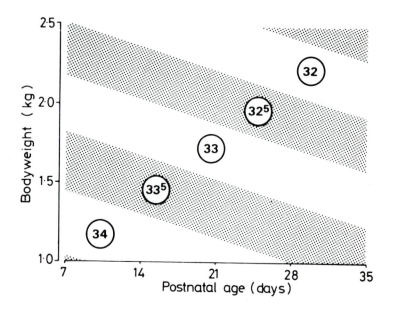

FIGURE 5–2. Neutral thermal environment from day 7–35 (in °C), based on body weight. *(Reproduced with permission from Sauer PJJ, Dane HJ and Visser HKA. New standards for neutral thermal environment of healthy very low birthweight infants in week one of life. Arch Disease in Childhood, 1984, **59**:18–22.)*

constant radiant energy output regardless of the infant's temperature. If the radiant warmer is used in the manual mode, the infant needs to be observed very carefully to avoid overheating.

2. **Temperature regulation in the normal term infant** (weight: > 2500 g)
   a. Place the infant under a **preheated radiant warmer** immediately after delivery.
   b. **Dry** the infant completely to prevent evaporative heat loss.

TABLE 5–1. APPROXIMATE NEUTRAL THERMAL ENVIRONMENT IN INFANTS WHO WEIGH MORE THAN 2500 GRAMS OR GREATER THAN 36 WEEKS' GESTATION. FOR INFANTS UNDER 2500 GRAMS OR LESS THAN 36 WEEKS, SEE FIGURES 5–1 AND 5–2.

Age	Temperature in °C
0–24 hours	31.0–33.8
24–48 hours	30.5–33.5
48–72 hours	30.1–33.2
72–96 hours	29.8–32.8
4–14 days	29.0–32.6
> 2 weeks	(Data not established, but in general, the smaller the infant, the higher the temperature)

(Based on data from Scopes J, Ahmed I: Range of initial temperatures in sick and premature newborn babies. *Arch Dis Child* 1966:**41**:417.)

    c. Cover the head with a cap.

    d. Place the infant, **wrapped in blankets,** in a crib.

    Note: Studies have shown that normal term infants can be wrapped in warm blankets and go directly into their mother's arms without any significant heat loss.

3. Temperature regulation in the sick term infant. Follow the same procedure as for the term infant except place the infant under a radiant warmer with temperature servoregulation.

4. Temperature regulation in the premature infant (weight 1000–2500 g)

    a. For an infant who weighs 1800–2500 g with no medical problems, use of a crib, cap, and blankets is usually sufficient.

    b. For an infant who weighs 1000–1800 g:

        (1) A **well infant** should be placed in a closed incubator with servocontrol.

        (2) A **sick infant** should be placed under a radiant warmer with servocontrol.

5. Temperature regulation in the very low birthweight infant (weight: < 1000 g). Either the radiant warmer or the incubator can be used, depending on the individual situation.

    a. Radiant warmer

        (1) Use servocontrol with the temperature for abdominal skin set at 37.0 °C.

        (2) Cover the infant's head with a cap.

        (3) Use an inner heat shield. The humidity level under the heat shield should be 40–50%.

        (4) Place plastic wrap (eg, Saran Wrap) loosely over the infant.

        (5) Use a black mattress cover to absorb heat.

        (6) Maintain an inspired air temperature of the hood or ventilator of at least 34.0–35.0 °C.

        (7) Place a heating pad (K-pad) under the infant that has an adjustable temperature within 35.0–38.0 °C. To maintain thermal protection, it can be set between 35.0–36.0 °C. If the infant is hypothermic, it can be increased to 37.0–38.0 °C (controversial).

        (8) If the temperature cannot be stabilized, move the infant to a closed incubator.

    b. Closed incubator

        (1) Use servocontrol with the temperature for abdominal skin set at 36.5 °C.

        (2) Use a double-walled incubator if possible.

        (3) Cover the infant's head with a cap.

        (4) Keep the humidity level at 40–50% or higher.

            Note: Excessive humidity and dampness of the clothing and incubator can lead to excessive heat loss or accumulation of fluid and possible infections.

        (5) Keep the temperature of the ventilator at 34.0–35.0 °C or higher.

        (6) Line the ends of the incubator with aluminum foil if needed.

        (7) Place a heated mattress (K-pad) under the infant that has an adjustable temperature within 35.0–38.0 °C. For thermal protection, it can be set between 35.0–36.0 °C. For warming a hypothermic infant, it can be set as high as 37.0–38.0 °C.

        (8) Place plastic wrap loosely over the infant.

        (9) If the temperature is difficult to maintain, try increasing the humidity level.

II. Hyperthermia. Hyperthermia is defined as a temperature that is greater than the normal core temperature of 37.5 °C.

    A. Differential diagnosis

        1. Environmental causes. Excessive temperature, overheating, overbundling, incubator in sunlight, loose probe, servocontrol set too high on radiant warmer, etc.

2. **Infection.** Bacterial or viral infections (eg, herpes).
3. **Dehydration.**
4. **Maternal fever in labor.**
5. **Drug withdrawal.**
6. **Unusual causes**
   a. Hyperthyroid crisis or storm.
   b. Drug effect (eg, prostaglandin E1).
   c. Riley-Day syndrome (periodic high fevers secondary to defective temperature regulation).

B. **Consequences of hyperthermia.** Hyperthermia can cause several problems in the neonate, including tachycardia, tachypnea, irritability, apnea, periodic breathing, dehydration, acidosis, brain damage, and death.

C. **Treatment**
1. **Turn down any heat source.**
2. **Remove excess clothing.**
3. **Treat underlying cause** such as sepsis, dehydration, etc.
4. **Additional measures for older infants** with significant temperature elevation
   a. Tepid water sponge bath.
   b. Acetaminophen, 5–10 mg/kg/dose orally or rectally every 4 hours.

REFERENCES

Sarman I, Can G, Tunnell R: Rewarming preterm infants on a heated, water-filled mattress. *Arch Dis Child* 1989;**64:**687.

Sauer PJJ, Dane HJ, Visser HKA: New standards for neutral thermal environment of healthy very low birthweight infants in week one of life. *Arch Disease Child* 1984;**59:**18.

Scopes J, Ahmed I: Range of initial temperatures in sick and premature newborn babies. *Arch Dis Child* 1966;**41:**417.

Tafari N, Gentz J: Aspects on rewarming newborn infants with severe accidental hypothermia. *Acta Paediatr Scand* 1974;**63:**595.

6 Respiratory Management

Management of infants with respiratory distress requires a broad base of general physiologic support, biophysical monitoring of vital functions and effective ventilatory support. Mechanical ventilation of neonates is constantly changing as new devices have become available and new ventilation strategies have been developed for neonatal care. Likewise, new monitoring techniques and pharmacologic adjuncts are available for ventilatory support. This section seeks to incorporate recent advances into a comprehensive approach for newborn respiratory management.

I. **General physiologic support**
   A. **Fluid therapy.** Maintenance of normal fluid and electrolyte balance is essential to respiratory care. Electrolyte and colloid supplementation are required for maintenance of normal pulmonary perfusion and ventilation. Hypovolemia and poor cadiac output or hypervolemia and pulmonary edema are equally deleterious to pulmonary function.
   B. **Humidity.** The environmental humidity should be maintained at 40%. A thermal neutral environment for minimal oxygen consumption requires 50 percent ambient humidity. Optimal humidity minimizes insensible fluid and body heat losses.
   C. **Body temperature.** Normal body temperature of 36.5–37.5°C (97.7–99.5°F) is essential to respiratory management. Loss of normal body temperature profoundly affects acid-base balance, resulting in metabolic acidosis and increased oxygen consumption. Both consequences increase the need for ventilatory support. Extremes of body temperature cause arterial oxygen determinations to be erroneously high or low.
   D. **Skin care.** The integrity of the skin is important for maintenance of both fluid balance and body temperature. Loss of intact skin also leads to increased risk for systemic infection. Minimal use of adhesives (tapes, leads, patches) and careful protection of skin over bony prominences is essential.
   E. **Body position.** Positioning of respiratory care patients is important for optimal management. Unplanned changes of body position may alter endotracheal tube placement. Prolonged supine positioning ultimately leads to posterior lung segment atelectasis. Lateral positioning during mechanical ventilation can assist in improving atelectatic lobes or regions of interstitial emphysema. Lastly, prone positioning of infants has been shown to greatly enhance ventilation by allowing greater total lung expansion and facilitating drainage of secretions.
   F. **Airway management.** Adequate measures for maintaining patency of the airways includes: positioning, suctioning of secretions, postural drainage, chest vibration and gentle percussion. Additionally, securing the endotracheal tube and comfortable placement of nasal prongs are important.
   G. **Gastrointestinal.** Decompression of the stomach improves diaphragmatic excursion. An indwelling nasogastric tube for gastric decompression and decreased bowel gas may be needed. Adequate hydration maintains softness of stool for passage and further decompression of the abdomen.
   H. **Calories.** Parenteral alimentation by peripheral intravenous fluids or central line can begin as soon as acid-base balance is achieved and normal renal function established. Although adequate calorie intake is not possible early in the course of respiratory distress, early feedings by gavage of small volumes (1–2 mL q3–4 hours) is possible near the end of the first week of life for most infants receiving mechanical ventilation. Early enteral feeds stimulate alimenta-

tion and set the stage for steady advancement of feedings. Feeds by gavage should not begin until bowel sounds and stool passage are well documented.

II. **Monitoring.** Multiple means of monitoring cardiovascular and pulmonary status are available, and are required for adequate management of infants in respiratory distress.

    A. **Blood gases.** Management of ventilation, oxygenation and changes of acid-base status are most accurately determined by **arterial blood gas studies.**

        1. Arterial blood gas studies are the most standardized and accepted measure of respiratory status, especially for the oxygenation of low birth weight infants. They are considered invasive monitoring and require arterial puncture or an indwelling arterial line. Access is now considered routine by umbilical artery or peripherally in the radial, ulnar or posterior tibial artery.

        2. Arterial blood gases may vary according to gestational age, age of infant at time of sampling and ongoing ventilatory care. Examples of typical normal values for infants are given in Table 6–1.

        3. Calculated arterial blood gas indices for determining progression of respiratory distress:

            a. **Alveolar-to-arterial gradient (A-a DO$_2$).** of greater than 600 mmHg for successive blood gases over 6 hours is associated with greater than 80% mortality in most infants if treatment and ventilation do not become effective (Fig 6–1). Formula for A-a DO$_2$:

$$A = PaO_2 \text{ mmHG } P_IO_2 - \frac{Paco_2}{R(0.8)} - PaO_2$$
$$PiO_2 = FiO_2 \ (\ PB - PH_2O)$$
$$760 \text{ mmHg} \quad 47 \text{ mmHg}$$

            b. **Arterial-to-alveolar ratio (a/A ratio)** is also an index for effective respiration. The a/A ratio is the most often used index for evaluation of response to surfactant therapy and is used as an indicator for inhaled nitric oxide therapy for pulmonary hypertension (Fig 6–2).
            Formula for a/A ratio:

$$\frac{a}{A} = \frac{PaO_2 \text{ mm Hg}}{PaO_2 = PiO_2 - Paco_2}$$
$$PiO_2 = FiO_2 \ (PB \quad - \quad PH_2O)$$
$$760 \text{ mmHg} \quad 47 \text{ mmHg}$$

    B. **Venous blood gases.** Determination of values is the same as for arterial blood gases, but interpretation is different. The pH values are slightly lower and Paco$_2$ values are slightly higher, while PaO$_2$ values are of little clinical value if taken from peripheral venous sites.

    C. **Capillary blood gases.** Sampling of "arterialized" capillary blood may provide helpful clinical information, but they are the least accurate. Arterializing of capillary blood is simply warming of the infant's heel just prior to sampling. The pH and Pco$_2$ values are usually slightly lower than venous and may vary consider-

---

TABLE 6–1. NORMAL RANGE OF ARTERIAL BLOOD GAS VALUES FOR TERM AND PRETERM INFANTS AT NORMAL BODY TEMPERATURE AND ASSUMING NORMAL BLOOD HEMOGLOBIN CONTENT

	Pao$_2$	Paco$_2$	pH	HCO$_3$	BE/BD
Term	80–95 mmHg	35–45	7.32–7.38	24–26	± 3.0
Preterm (30–36 weeks gestation)	60–80	35–45	7.30–7.35	22–25	± 3.0
Preterm (less than 30 weeks gestation)	45–60	38–50	7.27–7.32	19–22	± 4

Values for PaO$_2$, PaCO$_2$, and pH are measured directly by electrodes. Bicarbonate (HCO$_3$) and base excess/deficit values are calculated from nomograms of measured values at normal (14.8–15.5 mg/dL) hemoglobin content and body temperature (37°C) and assuming hemoglobin saturation of 88 percent or greater.

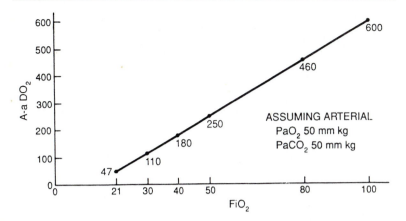

FIGURE 6–1. Progression of A-a DO_2 values for a hypothetical infant with arterial blood gases of PaO_2 50 mmH_g and $Paco_2$ 50 mmH_g at sea level with 50 percent humdity. Mechanical ventilatory support would become necessary at an A-a DO_2 of 250 mmH_g.

ably from one site to another. Capillary blood gases are not valid for evaluating the state of oxygenation of an infant.

D. Mixed venous blood oxygen saturation (SVO_2). Monitoring of SVO_2 is receiving more attention in neonatal respiratory care. Sampling requires slightly more blood than arterial samples and the availability of a co-oximeter. Sample site in infants is ideally through an unbilical vein catheter placed at the level of the right atrium. SVO_2 of 85 percent or greater is associated with poor tissue extraction of oxygen, systemic shunting and poor tissue perfusion. Fiber optic venous catheters via umbilical veins may provide continuous SVO_2 monitoring in the future.

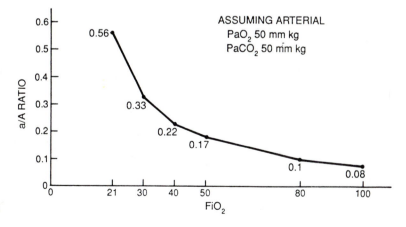

FIGURE 6–2. Progressive decline of a/A ratios for a hypothetical infant as in Figure 6–1. Note the rapid change of values early in respiratory distress (between FiO_2 of 24 and 40 percent). a/A ratios are preferred because of the rapid change in trend heralding respiratory failure.

E. Transcutaneous blood gas monitoring. All transcutaneous techniques require correlation periodically with arterial blood gas determinations.

1. **Transcutaneous oxygen (tcPO$_2$)** monitoring measures the partial pressure of oxygen from the skin surface by an electrochemical sensor known as the Clark polarographic electrode. The electrode heats the skin to 43–44°C and contact is maintained through a conducting electrolyte solution and an oxygen permeable membrane.

   a. **Limitations** include: recalibration daily, relocation to different skin sites every 4–6 hours, irritation or injury to a premature infant's skin secondary to adhesive rings and thermal burns. Additional limitations are related to poor skin perfusion caused by shock, acidosis, hypoxia, hypothermia, edema or anemia.

   b. **Other disadvantages** are related to high cost of technician time and materials for relocation of electrode and recalibration. Also, tcPO$_2$ has limited or no use for extremely low birth weight infants because of skin injury.

   c. **Advantages** are that tcO$_2$ is non-invasive and has a high degree of accuracy over a range of 30–150 mmHg PaO$_2$.

2. **Trancutaneous carbon dioxide monitoring (tcPCO$_2$)** is usually accomplished simultaneously by a single lead enclosed with a tcPO$_2$ electrode. The tcPCO$_2$ electrode (Stowe-Severinghaus) operates by tissue–CO$_2$-equilibration across the skin and generation of an electrical charge proportional to the change in pH of the contact electrolyte solution.

   a. **Limitations** of the tcPCO$_2$ include all of those associated with tcPO$_2$ monitoring. Moreover, it is less reliably correlated to arterial Paco$_2$. Calibration and response times are longer for tcPO$_2$.

   b. **Advantages.** tcPCO$_2$ is non-invasive and can trend changes in Paco$_2$ in chronic respiratory conditions over protracted periods of time.

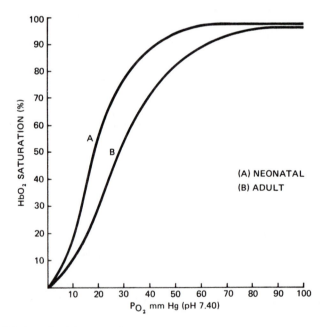

FIGURE 6–3. Comparison between normal mean oxyhemoglobin dissociation curves of **(A)** term infants at birth and **(B)** adults. The pH is 7.40. (Modified and reproduced, with permission, from Sherwood WC, Cohen A (editors): *Transfusion Therapy: The Fetus, Infant, and Child.* Masson, 1980.)

       c. Disadvantages are poor correlation to actual $Paco_2$, slow response, and need for frequent technical support.

  3. Pulse oximetry (SaO_2). The pulse oximeter utilizes a photo sensor on the skin to measure the percentage of oxygen saturation of hemoglobin available for oxygen transport. It is affected by the oxyhemoglobin dissociation curve. A higher saturation for a given oxygen tension (curve shifted to the left) occurs with alkalosis, hypothermia, fetal hemoglobin, high altitude, and hypometabolism. A lower saturation for a given oxygen tension (curve shifted to the right) occurs with acidosis, hyperthermia, hypermetabolism, and hypercarbia. Fig 6–3 compares hemoglobin saturation in adults and infants at birth, while Fig 6–4 illustrates a series of infant pulse oximetry studies correlating SaO_2 and PaO_2. Table 6–2 shows oxygen saturation of arterial blood (SaO_2) as a function of PaO_2 and pH, and is useful in the interpretation of pulse oximeter readings.

       a. Limitations include poor correlation of SaO_2 to PaO_2 at upper and lower PaO_2 values. SaO_2 of 88–93% corresponds to PaO_2 of 50–80 mmHg. For infants with high or low saturations arterial blood gas correlation is needed.

       b. Advantages include minimal damage to skin, and required manual calibration. SaO_2 by pulse oximetry is less affected by skin temperature and perfusion than $tcPO_2$.

       c. Disadvantages include the tendency of patient movement and excessive external lighting to skew readings and that there is no correction of SaO_2 for abnormal hemoglobin (such as methemoglobin).

F. End-tidal CO_2 monitoring ($PetCO_2$). Expired breath analysis by infrared spectroscopy for CO_2 content gives close correlation to $Paco_2$. Similar techniques for neonates are increasing in availability and give rapid information for changes in CO_2 unlike the slow response of $tcPCO_2$.

  1. Limitations include the rather large adapter to endotracheal tube and poor

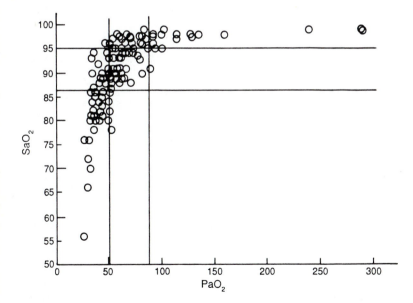

FIGURE 6–4. Range of SaO_2 versus PaO_2 by pulse oximetry on a group of monitored neonates (Adapted from Cunningham MD, et al., *J Perinatal* 8:333, 1988, with premission).

TABLE 6–2. SaO$_2$ AS A FUNCTION OF PO$_2$ and pH^{a,b}

PO$_2$	pH				
	7.30	7.35	7.40	7.45	7.50
			SaO$_2$		
120	98	98	98	98	99
100	97	97	97	98	98
90	96	96	97	97	97
80	95	95	96	96	97
70	92	93	94	95	95
65	91	92	93	94	94
60	88	90	91	92	93
55	85	87	89	90	91
50	81	83	85	87	88
45	76	78	80	83	85
40	69	71	74	77	79
35	61	63	66	69	72
30	51	54	57	60	62
20	29	32	34	36	39
10	7	8	9	10	11

[a] Assuming a temperature of 37° C, normal levels of 2,3-DPG, a PaCO$_2$ of 40 mm Hg, and adult hemoglobin.
[b] This graph is merely a reference tool and is not to be used for deriving precise values of PO$_2$ or pH from the Ohmeda Biox saturation readings.
Reproduced, with permission, from the Ohmeda Company, Boulder, Colorado.

response if respiratory rate is above 60 BPM and poor response if humidity of inspired air is excessive.

2. **Advantages** are that it is a non-invasive technique with high correlation to arterial PaCO$_2$. It is most helpful as a monitoring technique in the stage of weaning infants from mechanical ventilation.

3. **Disadvantages** are related to various disease states. High ventilation perfusion mismatch such as intrapulmonary shunts, uneven ventilation or increased dead space are conditions that would give unreliable PetCO$_2$ values. Generally, a/A ratios of less than 0.3 negate PetCO$_2$ monitoring.

G. **Lung surfactant.** Studies of respiratory status involve determination of lung surfactant constituents. Surfactant phospholipids and phospholipid profiles are obtained either intrapartum by amniocentesis (see Chap 1) for lecithin, sphingomyelin and phosphatidylglycerol. Additionally, newborn gastric or tracheal aspirates can be used for the same determination. The significance of these studies points to lung maturity, expectations regarding need for respiratory support, and the need for surfactant replacement therapy.

1. **Amniotic fluid** lung/surfactant (L/S) ratios of 2:1 or greater by 2-dimensional thin layer chromatography confirm fetal lung maturity in nearly all non-diabetic pregnancies. L/S ratios of 2.5:1 or greater are preferred for declaring fetal lung maturity in diabetic pregnancies.

2. **Gastric contents** aspirated in the first hour of life closely reflect amniotic fluid studies for L/S ratios. Tracheal aspirates in the first hours of life tend to have higher L/S ratios due to lesser amounts of sphingomyelin in the aspirate.

3. **Phosphatidylglycerol (PG)** presence in increasing amounts also signifies lung maturity beyond 35 weeks' gestation in all pregnancies.

H. **Monitoring of vital signs and other physiologic parameters.** The infant with respiratory distress may have derangements of other organ functions. Comprehensive monitoring requires that physical measurements as well as biochemical and electrophysical monitoring be incorporated into the overall information of the patient.

1. **Physical examination** for color and respiratory effort, as well as auscultation of lungs for equality of breaths is important. Additionally, the cardiac, neurologic and abdominal examinations are required. Abdominal distention cannot be overlooked in an infant with respiratory distress.

2. **Blood pressure (BP)** requires frequent monitoring. Either mean value or systolic/diastolic pressures should be obtained. Volume replacement or vasopressor therapy are often required for neonates with severe respiratory distress. Standard nomograms for blood pressure (see Appendix C) are available for comparative data.

3. **Central venous pressure (CVP).** Increasingly the umbilical vein catheter at the level of the right atrium is available for CVP monitoring. Levels of 4–6 cm H_2O are generally taken as normal; however, the range is 2–8 cm H_2O.

4. **Urine output** is a critical value in overall assessment of a neonate in respiratory failure. A urine output of 1.5–2.5 mL/kg/hr signifies good cardiac output, adequate intravascular volume with normal CVP and normal mean BP values. Also of importance is urine specific gravity; fluctuating values of 1.006 to 1.012 are indicators of normal urine formation.

5. **Body weight.** Consistent with urine output is the need for daily (or twice daily) body weights to determine changes that may signify fluid retention or excessive insensible losses. In-bed electronic scales should be standard equipment for sick neonates requiring mechanical ventilation.

6. **Monitoring blood studies** for hemoglobin, hematocrit, calcium, sodium, potassium, chloride, blood urea nitrogen and creatinine are all related to managing respiratory failure and maintaining satisfactory cardiovascular and renal function.

I. **Monitoring mechanical ventilation.** Although there are many different types of infant ventilators, only a few devices and means for monitoring events during mechanical breath cycles are available. Monitoring is limited to conventional mechanical ventilation (CMV) using time-cycled/pressure-limited or volume-controlled infant ventilators.

1. **Inspired oxygen.** Fraction of inspired oxygen (FiO_2) is a percentage of oxygen available for inspiration. It is expressed either as a percentage (21–100) or as a decimal (0.21–1.00). Battery operated oxygen analyzers are a standard for monitoring oxygen therapy for infants. They consist of electrochemical cells calibrated by ambient or inspired oxygen concentrations up to 100%. During mechanical ventilation, an in-line oxygen analyzer with a ventilator circuit for continuous read-out of the oxygen concentration flowing to the infant is preferable. Further management of oxygen therapy requires:

   a. Calibration of analyzer every 8–12 hours.

   b. Blending of air and oxygen to ensure the least amount of oxygen required to maintain desired blood oxygen saturation.

   c. Humidification of all inspired oxygen and air mixtures.

   d. Warming of inspired gases to 34–35°C through a humidification device gives approximately 96% water vapor saturation.

2. **Mean airway pressure (Paw).** Mean airway pressure is an average of the proximal pressure applied to the airway throughout the entire respiratory cycle (see Fig 6–5). The ventilator settings of rate (R), inspiratory time (IT), peak inspiratory pressure (PIP) and peak-end expiratory pressure (PEEP) can be expressed as mean airway pressure by the formula:

$$\frac{(R)(IT)(PIP) + [60-(R)(IT)] \times PEEP}{60} = Paw$$

   a. Maintaining Paw below 10 cm H_2O is associated with lower risk for pneu-

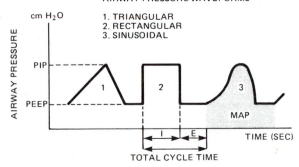

FIGURE 6–5. Graphic representation of ventilator airway pressure waveforms and other ventilator terminology. See Glossary, p 52, for explanations.

mothorax (or other forms of air leakage, such as pulmonary interstitial emphysema).
   b. Paw of high frequency ventilation is *not* equated with the mean airway pressure of conventional mechanical ventilation.
   c. Oxygen index (OI) is a frequently used calculation that incorporates FiO_2, Paw and PaO_2:

$$OI = \frac{FiO_2 \times Paw \times 100}{PaO_2}$$

$$\text{Example: } \frac{0.90 \times 15 \times 100}{50} = 27 \text{ OI}$$

OI values of 30–40 are indicative of severe respiratory distress. If OI is found to increase steadily over a 6 hour period from 30 to 40, profound respiratory failure on CMV is apparent. Mortality may exceed 80%.
3. Pulmonary Functions. New flow sensors (pneumotachographs) allow for frequent or continuous monitoring of mechanical and spontaneous breath mechanics for flow, airway pressure and volume. With flow sensors or pneumotachographs, additional pulmonary function testing is possible. Occluded breath techniques provide passive mechanics for compliance and resistance as well as the determination of time constants.
   a. Flow (V) is the measure of a breath from inspiration, through the point of midinspiration and no flow, to end-expiratory flow. Flow (mL/sec) corresponds to breath volume (see Fig 6–6).
   b. Airway pressure (Paw) is determined in the proximal airway from a differential pressure transducer. Transpulmonary pressure is a measure of the difference between airway pressure and esophageal pressure taken from an indwelling esophageal catheter or balloon.
   c. Tidal volume (V_t), a function of peak inspiratory pressure during mechanical ventilation, is integrated from flow (mL/sec) and measured as ml/breath. By convention, V_t is expressed as breath volume adjusted to body weight as mL/kg. Several devices are now available for continuous bedside tidal volume monitoring. Tidal volume may vary from 5–7 mL/kg for most newborn infants. Infants with birth weights less than 1000 grams require slightly higher measured V_t of 6–7 mL/kg (3.5–5.0 mL/breath for an infant of 600–700 grams birth weight).
   d. Minute ventilation (MV). Respiratory rate and V_t combine to give minute ventilation as:

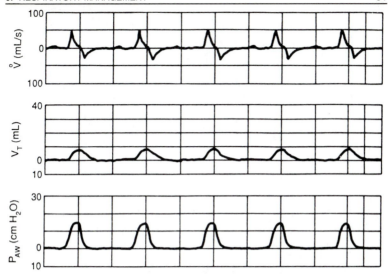

FIGURE 6–6. Waveforms of flow (V), tidal volume (V_T) and airway pressure Paw from an infant on mechanical ventilation.

$$\text{rate} \times V_t = MV(V_E)$$
Example: 40 BPM $\times$ 6.5 mL/kg = 260 mL/kg/min

Normal MV values for newborns are 240–360 ml. Monitoring of V_t and MV simultaneously with Paw provides for graded adjustments of peak inspiratory pressure, positive end expiratory pressure and inspiratory time. Optimal tidal volume should be determined on the basis of adequate MV at the least peak inspiratory pressure and balanced with achieving acceptable blood gases.

e. **Pressure-volume (P-V) and flow-volume (F-V) loops** are a visualization of breath-to-breath dynamics. Flow, volume and pressure signals combine to give P-V and F-V loops (Fig 6–7). Loops give inspiratory and expiratory limits of the breath cycle. F-V loops provide information regarding airway resistance, especially restricted expiratory breath flow (Fig 6–8). P-V loops primarily reflect a changing lung dynamic compliance (Fig 6–9).

f. **Compliance (C_L)** values of less than 1.0 cm H_2O/mL are consistent with interstitial lung disease such as respiratory distress syndrome. Lung compliance of 1.0–2.0 mL/cm H_2O reflects recovery, as in postsurfactant therapy.

g. **Resistance (R_L)** of greater than 100 cm H_2O/L/sec is suggestive of airway disease with restricted airflow as in bronchopulmonary dysplasia.

h. **Time constant (K_t)** is the product of $C_L \times R_L$ in seconds. Normal values are 0.12–0.15 seconds. K_t is a measure of how long it takes for alveolar and proximal airway pressures to equilibrate. At the end of 3 time constants, 95% of the tidal volume is expired from the alveoli. To avoid gas trapping the measured expiratory time should be greater than 3 times K_t (0.36–0.45 seconds).

III. **Ventilatory support.** Infants with respiratory distress may only need supplemental oxygen, whereas those with respiratory failure and apnea require mechanical ven-

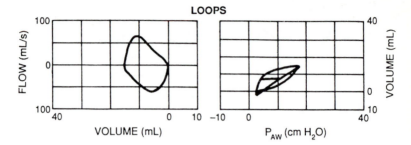

FIGURE 6–7. Typical flow-volume and pressure-volume loops of a premature infant recovering from respiratory distress syndrome on mechanical ventilation.

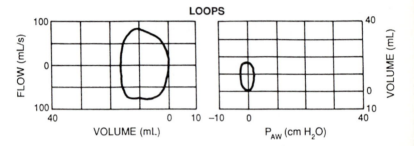

FIGURE 6–8. Normal F-V and P-V loops of preterm infant obtained by face mask study after full recovery and extubation.

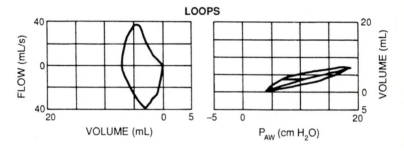

FIGURE 6–9. Typical F-V and P-V loops of infant 10 days old, remaining on mechanical ventilation with increased airway resistance (106 cmH$_2$O/L/sec; note depressed expiratory segment of F-V loop) and marginal compliance (0.95 ml/cmH$_2$O) and rightward displacement of P-V loop.

tilatory support. This section reviews the spectrum of available means for ventilatory support with the exception of high frequency ventilation (see p 62 **VI**).

    A. Oxygen supplementation without mechanical ventilation. Hypoxic infants able to maintain an adequate MV are assisted with free flow oxygen or air-oxygen mixtures.

        1. Oxygen hoods provide an enclosure for blended air-oxygen supply, humidification, and continuous oxygen concentration monitoring. Hoods are easy to use and provide access and visibility to the infant. Pulse oximetry is recommended while hoods are in use.

2. **Mask oxygen** is not suitable for infants because of poor control and lack of monitoring of oxygen supply.

3. **Nasal cannulae** are well-suited for infants needing low concentrations of oxygen. Delivery can be controlled by flow meters delivering as little as 0.025 L/min. Flow rates of 1 L or greater may impart distending airway pressure. Table 6–3 gives approximate percentages of nasal cannula oxygen based on flow rates of 0.25 to 1.0 L/min at blended FiO_2 settings of 40–100%. Pulse oximeter monitoring is recommended while nasal cannulae are in use.

B. **Continuous positive airway pressure (CPAP).** Mask, nasal prongs, or endotracheal tube can be used to apply CPAP. It improves PaO_2 by stabilizing the airway and allowing alveolar recruitment. CO_2 retention may result from excessive distending airway pressure.

1. **Mask CPAP** is used most often as a temporary measure to overcome atelectasis postendotracheal tube suctioning and extubation, or to stabilize spontaneous breathing of an infant after an apneic episode. Pressures may vary from 2–6 cmH_2O.

2. **Nasal CPAP** prongs are the most commonly applied means of measuring CPAP, and are used for assisting respiration in an infant with mild respiratory distress syndrome. They are also used post-extubation to maintain airway distention in the process of weaning from mechanical ventilation and recovery from respiratory diseases. Nasal CPAP is useful when a/A ratios are 0.33 or less. It is also useful in some infants with apnea of infancy. Nasal CPAP stimulates breathing by enhancement of the afferent limb of the Hering-Breuer reflex and spinal-thoracic accessory reflex. CPAP pressures may range from 2–8 cm H_2O, though 2–6 are most often used. Monitoring with pulse oximetry or tCO_2 is required. Over distention of the airway can lead to excessive CO_2 retention and/or air leak (pneumothorax). Gastric distention is a complication of nasal CPAP and a nasogastric tube for decompression should be used. Infants may be fed by nasogastric tube during nasal CPAP therapy with close monitoring of abdominal girth.

3. **Endotracheal tube CPAP** has nearly the same effect as nasal prongs. It is often an intermediate measure after weaning from mechanical ventilation. It is also a means of assisted ventilation when minute ventilation is adequate but secretions are excessive and tracheal suctioning is required. CPAP is usually abandoned for mechanical ventilation when a/A ratios have fallen below 0.22 or the infant develops apneic episodes.

C. **Mechanical ventilation.** Respiratory distress and failure may be defined as either apnea, hypercarbia or hypoxia. These events represent loss of central nervous system control of ventilation or respiratory and metabolic acidosis as CO_2 accumulates and hypoxia persists. Mechanical ventilation reestablishes the loss of tidal volume and minute ventilation and, if effective, removes CO_2

TABLE 6–3. NASAL CANNULA CONVERSION TABLE*

Flow Rate (L/min)	FiO_2			
	100%	80%	60%	40%
0.25	34%	31%	26%	22%
0.5	44%	37%	31%	24%
0.75	60%	42%	35%	25%
1	66%	49%	38%	27%

*General guidelines; numbers are not exact.

and restores alveolar oxygenation. Techniques range from simple hand-held bag and mask to microprocessor-controlled ventilators.

1. **Bag-and-mask or bag-to-endotracheal tube** hand-held assemblies allow for emergency or temporary ventilatory support. Portable manometers are always required for monitoring peak airway pressures during hand-bag ventilation. Bags may be self-inflating or flow-dependent, anesthesia-type bags. All hand-held assemblies must have pop-off valves to avoid excessive pressures to the infant's airway.

2. **Pressure control infant ventilators.** These are the most commonly used ventilators in neonatal care. They are time-cycled for initiating and limiting the inspiratory cycle of ventilation, and pressure-limited to control the flow and volume for each delivered breath. Delivered breath volume and mean airway pressure are determined by ventilator settings. Air-oxygen mixtures are heated and humidified for delivery through the continuous flow circuit attached to the infant's airway. Establishing effective ventilatory settings is the key to successful ventilatory support. Table 6–4 gives basic ventilator setting changes and expected blood gas responses.

   a. **Rate** may vary from 0 to 100, but most commonly support rates are 20 to 60 bpm. Rate is adjusted to combine with tidal volume to provide adequate minute ventilation.

   b. **Inspiratory time (IT)** varies from 0.2 seconds to 1 second, but most commonly IT is 0.28–0.5 seconds. IT must allow for adequate expiratory time (ET) and not violate the time constant for expiration. For example, at a rate of 60 bpm with an IT of 0.35 seconds gives and ET of 0.65. If the time constant proves to be greater than 0.65 ($3 \times K_t = 0.36 - 0.45$ sec) then risk for air trapping and lung over-distention develops.

   c. **Peak inspiratory pressure (PIP).** Delivered tidal volume depends on PIP. Initial choice of PIP is dependent on observation of chest wall movement during hand-bag ventilation, manometer readings during hand-and-bag ventilation and auscultation of breath sounds. Subsequently, PIP should be adjusted to achieve optimal tidal volumes (5–7 mL/kg), minute ventilation and effective gas exchange based on satisfactory blood gas determinations. Optimal tidal volume may vary according to size and gestation of the infant (see p 50 **3.C**).

   d. **Positive end-expiratory pressure** (PEEP). Like CPAP, PEEP is a distending pressure that stabilizes the airway and allows alveolar recruitment and improved alveolar ventilation. Settings for PEEP range from 2–6 cm H_2O pressure, although most commonly, pressures are 2–4 cmH_2O.

   e. Mean airway pressure (Paw). The above ventilator settings determine Paw (see page 49 **I.2**). Paw of 4–20 cm H2O are used with pressure control ventilators. If settings result in Paw above 15 cm H_2O, without improved ventilation, changing to high frequency ventilation should be considered.

TABLE 6–4. CHANGES IN BLOOD GAS LEVELS CAUSED BY CHANGES IN VENTILATOR SETTINGS[a]

	Rate	PIP	PEEP	IT	F_{IO_2}
To increase $PaCO_2$	Decrease	Decrease	NA	NA	NA
To decrease $PaCO_2$	Increase	Increase	NA[b]	NA[c]	NA
To increase PaO_2	NA	Increase	Increase	Increase	Increase
To decrease PaO_2	NA	Decrease	Decrease	NA	Decrease

[a] NA, not applicable.

[b] In severe pulmonary edema and pulmonary hemorrhage, increased PEEP can decrease $PaCO_2$.

[c] Not applicable unless the I:E ratio is excessive.

3. **Volume control infant ventilators.** Previously, volume ventilation was not considered for infants because measurement and monitoring of optimal tidal volumes was not possible. With the development of variable orifice and hot wire continuous flow sensors, volume monitoring and thus volume control ventilation has become available for newborn care.

   a. **Rate** varies as it does for pressure control ventilation. Because volume is preset, monitoring of both mechanical and spontaneous breath tidal volume allows for determination of volume control ventilator-derived minute ventilation versus the infant's own minute ventilation.

   b. **IT** must be set to allow for adequate volume delivery. Exceedingly short IT (< 0.32 sec) reduces volume delivery.

   c. **PIP** varies automatically for the delivery of preset tidal volume in accordance with changing lung compliance. Improving compliance, especially after surfactant therapy, may lead to excessive volume delivery with pressure control ventilators. Volume control ventilation, however, minimizes the risk for lung overdistention.

   d. **PEEP** usage is the same for volume and pressure control ventilation.

   e. **Paw** should be monitored as in pressure control ventilation and the same upper limits (10–15 cm H_2O) suggest high frequency ventilation if Paw increases above 15 cm H_2O.

4. **Synchronized intermittent mechanical ventilation (SIMV).** Mechanical ventilation of the alert, nonsedated, nonparalyzed infant imparts automated breaths irrespective of the infant's own respiratory cycle. The result is repeated bouts of interrupted or "bucked" breaths resulting in patient agitation and poor ventilation (Fig 6–10). Recent technical developments have resulted in synchronized ventilation for both pressure control and volume control ventilators. SIMV is also available with assist control modes for those ventilators that allow for preset rates if an infant becomes apneic on intermittent mechanical ventilation. Advantages of SIMV have been lower PIP settings while achieving optimal tidal volume and maintaining adequate MV at lower mean airway pressures. SIMV also allows for greater patient comfort during mechanical ventilation, less agitation, and much less need for sedation. Four different types of SIMV are now available:

   a. **Synchronizing ventilation with abdominal wall movement** using a Graseby capsule. Abdominal wall movement requires optimal capsule placement (Infant Star/Star Sync, Infasonics, Inc, San Diego, CA).

   b. **Airway flow sensing by hot wire anemometer** allows for flow-synchronized ventilation based on the airway flow signal originating with the first phase of inspiration (Bear Cub/NVM1, Bear Medical, Inc, Riverside, CA). A similar anemometer is also available as a built-in unit with the ventilator. (Baby Log 8000, Draeger, Lubeck, Germany).

   c. **Variable orifice pneumotachometers** for flow-synchronized ventilation use the inspiratory flow signal to synchronize spontaneous breaths with mechanical breaths (VIP Bird, Palm Springs, CA).

   d. **Patient-triggered synchronized ventilation** uses chest wall impedance leads to signal chest wall movement (Sechrist IV/SAVI, Sechrist Inc, Anaheim, CA).

D. **Weaning from mechanical ventilation.** Decreasing mechanical ventilatory support requires clearly defined parameters of ventilatory improvement, monitoring, and documentation that other physical conditions are improved and stable.

   1. **Evaluation for ventilator weaning.**

      a. FiO_2 reduced to 50% with PaO_2 value remaining 50–80 mm Hg. The oxygenation indices of a/A ratio should be improved to greater than 0.40 and the A-a DO_2 gradient less than 250 mm Hg.

      b. Spontaneous breaths should increase in number and spontaneous breath tidal volumes should equal mechanical breath volumes (5–7 mL/kg). The

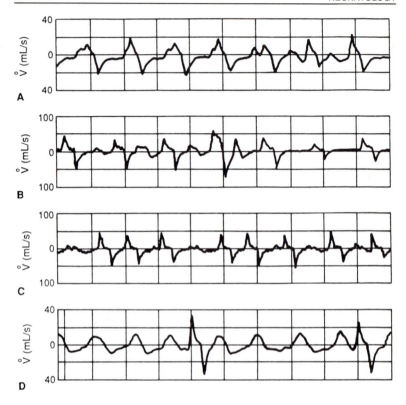

FIGURE 6–10. Waveforms A and B of infants with interrupted breaths on mechanical ventilation without synchronized IMV. Waveforms C are reflective of SIMV at mechanical rates of 40 BPM with infant respiratory rate of 50–60 BPM. Wavefroms D are of SIMV for infant on ventilator rate of 15 BPM and spontaneous infant rate of 55–60 BPM.

decreasing mechanical rate should be matched by infant's increasing rate. A combined MV of spontaneous and mechanical breaths should equal 240–360 mL/min. Monitoring of tidal volume should have shown a progressive decrease of required PIP (eg, 25–18 cm H_2O).

    c. A combined decrease of rate and pressure (ie, MV) must be accompanied by a sustained $Paco_2$ of 40–50 mmHg.

    d. Although controversial, pretreatment of infants with aminophylline is believed by some clinicians to enhance infant response to progressive weaning efforts.

  2. Weaning from mechanical ventilation and extubation

    a. Progressive rate wean. Rate settings should be decreased hourly. Infants ready to be weaned tolerate the rate wean and do not require more FiO_2. An infant should be able to maintain adequate MV without developing hypercarbia or apnea. When the ventilator rate is less than 10 bpm, the infant should be extubated. Some infants may require several hours to wean, whereas others several days to a week or more.

      Disease state, gestational age, and caloric support influence response to weaning process.

      b. CPAP weaning. The rate should be weaned down to 5–10 bpm. If this condition is tolerated for 1 hour, endotracheal CPAP should be set at 3–4 cm water for 2–4 hours. The oxygen concentration should be increased by 5% when the infant is placed on CPAP. If the infant tolerates this step with acceptable blood gases and no respiratory distress, the infant should be started on 5 minutes of CPAP and then given 55 minutes of full ventilatory support. The interval on CPAP should be increased by 5 minutes per hour. Once 60 full minutes of CPAP is tolerated, continuous CPAP can be attempted. Extubation is performed in 2–4 hours if CPAP continues to be well tolerated. This step is controversial for some. Breathing with CPAP requires increased work and some clinicians believe that the potential benefits of CPAP are lost if the infant tires unnecessarily.

   3. Care after extubation. Continued monitoring of blood gases, respiratory effort and vital signs is required. Additional oxygen support is often needed in the immediate postextubation period.

      a. Supplemental oxygen may be given by hood or nasal cannulae. The oxygen concentration should be increased by at least 5% over the last oxygen level obtained while infant was on the ventilator.

      b. Chest physical therapy (q3–4h) after extubation helps to maintain a clear airway. Postural drainage with percussion and suction procedures should be followed routinely. Aerosol treatments with bronchodilators also help to maintain airway patency.

      c. If the infant has had an **increasing oxygen requirement** or has **clinically deteriorated,** an anteroposterior chest x-ray should be obtained at 6 hours postextubation to monitor for atelectasis.

IV. Pharmacologic Respiratory Support and Surfactant. Numerous medications are available for improvement of respiration. They represent a broad range of therapeutics of which the bronchodilators and antiinflammatory drugs are the oldest and most common. The use of mixtures of inhaled gases such as helium and nitric oxide are recent forms of treatment. Sedatives and paralyzing agents remain controversial in neonatal respiratory management. Finally, surfactant replacement therapy has rapidly become a major adjunct to care of preterm infants, and its use has expanded to disease states other than RDS (hyaline membrane disease) for which it was originally intended. All medications are discussed with regard to dosage and side effects elsewhere (see page 467), but are briefly reviewed here for the purpose of incorporating their use into respiratory management strategies.

  A. Bronchodilators (inhaled agents). Most of these drugs are sympathomimetic agents that stimulate beta$_1$, beta$_2$ or alpha-adrenergic receptors. They have both inotropic and chronotropic effects and provide bronchial smooth muscle and vascular relaxation. Albuterol is probably the most commonly used aerosolized bronchodilator. Other bronchodilators are presented in Table 6–5. Two anticholinergic agents (atropine and ipratropium) are also used as inhaled bronchodilators for inhibition of acetylcholine at lung receptor sites and bronchial smooth muscle relaxation. All are used to minimize airway resistance and allow decreased Paw needed for mechanical ventilation.

  B. Bronchodilators (systemic). Aminophylline (parenteral) and theophylline (enteral) are methylxanthines with considerable bronchial dilating action. Neonatal use includes bronchodilatation and stimulation of respiratory effort.

  C. Anti-inflammatory agents

   1. Steroid therapy for anti-inflammatory effect is used to decrease airway edema, leukocyte migration, fibroblast activation and collagen deposition. Various dosage regimens exist for steroid use. Those infants who fail to recover progressively from respiratory disease will have increased airway resistance on mechanical ventilation. Generally, static ventilator settings, minimal improvement of compliance, and increasing resistance (greater than 100 cm H_2O/L/sec) are indicators for steroid therapy for infants 10 days of life or older and who require continued mechanical ventilation.

   2. Cromolyn prevents mast cells from releasing histamine and leukotriene-like

TABLE 6–5. AEROSOL THERAPY IN NEONATES INDICATING DOSING, RECEPTOR EFFECTS AND COMMON SIDE EFFECTS.

Drug	Receptors	Side Effects
Isoproterenol (Isuprel) 0.1–0.25 ml (0.5–1.25 mg) of 0.05% soln. Diluent 1.5–2.0 ml NS or 1/2 NS. Q 3–4 h	β_1 chronotropic inotropic β_2 relax airways and vasculature smooth muscle non-specific	tachycardia arrhythmias tremor hypertension hyperglycemia tolerance excessive smooth muscle relaxation = airway collapse
Albuterol (salbutamol) (Ventolin) 0.02–0.04 ml/kg/dose of 0.5% soln Diluent 1.5–2.0 ml NS or 1/2 NS Q 4–6 h	β_2 long lasting (24 hr, 75% excreted) less side effects of iso-or metaproterenol	tachycardia (potentiated by methylxanthines) hypertension hyperglycemia tremor
Metaproterenol 0.1–0.5 ml (5–12.5 mg) 5% soln Diluent 1.5–2.0 ml 1/2 NS or NS Q 6 h	β_2 less specific for airways than albuterol	same as iso-; cardiac arrhythmias potentiated by hypoxia
Cromolyn (Intal) 20 mg in 2 ml NS Q 6–8 h	anti-inflammatory by stabilizing mast cells	anaphylaxis, caution in patients with liver or renal disease bronchospasm 2° to inflammatory response upper airway irritation
Isoetharine (Bronkosol) 0.1–0.25 (1–2.5 mg) of a 1% soln. Diluent 2.0 ml 1/2 NS or NS Q 4–6 h	β_2, β_1 less specific than metaproterenol or albuterol	some cardiogenic effects
Terbutaline (Brethine) 0.1–0.2 mg/kg in 2 ml NS Q 2–8 h	β_2 peripheral dilatation	hypotension hypoglycemia
Atropine 0.025–0.05 mg/kg in 2–2.5 ml NS or 1/2 NS Q 6–8 h Ipatropium bromide 175 mcg in NS or 1/2 NS	vagolytic	tachycardia arrhythmia low blood pressure ileus airway dryness and thick secretions suggest use in combination with albuterol Am. Rev. Resp. Dis. 1142:1137, 1990
Epinephrine racemic vaponefrin L-epinephrine 0.1–0.3 ml in 2–3 ml NS Q 1/2–2 h × 4	α receptor	tachycardia tremor hypertension L-epinephrine is as effective alone as R-L (racemic) Pediatr. 89:302, 1992

substances. Its actions are slow but progressive over 2–4 weeks. Indications for its use in neonates have not been established. This agent is considered for use in infants with progressive reactive airway disease, prolonged mechanical ventilatory support and minimal response to attempts to wean from the ventilator.

D. Inhaled gas mixtures
  1. **HeliOx** (helium, 78–80% and oxygen, 20–22%) produces an inspired gas less dense than nitrogen-oxygen mixtures or oxygen alone. Use of HeliOx reduces increased resistive load of breathing, improves distribution of ventilation and less turbulence in narrow airways. Limited neonatal use has indicated that HeliOx has been associated with lower inspired oxygen requirements and shorter duration of mechanical ventilatory support.
  2. **Nitric oxide.** Vascular endothelium elaborates a potent vasodilator under normal basal conditions. The factor, known as endothelium-derived relaxing factor (EDRF), is nitric oxide. Many vascular responses to EDRF are known throughout the body. As an inhalant for pulmonary vascular dilatation, it is emerging as a new and potent treatment for persistent pulmonary hypertension and refractory hypoxemia. Nitric oxide is given in concentrations of 20–80 ppm blended with the compressed oxygen of either CMV or high frequency ventilation. Nitric oxide has not been associated with systemic hypotension or other known side effects.

E. Sedatives and paralyzing agents. Agitation is a common problem for infant mechanical ventilation. Infants may have interrupted respiratory cycles and respond by "bucking" or "fighting" the ventilator breaths. The agitation that results is often associated with hypoxic episodes. Sedation or muscle relaxation by paralysis may be required. It should be noted, however, that with the use of ventilators with either flow-sensed or patient-triggered synchronized ventilation (SIMV) much less sedation is required. Paralysis no longer occurs in the author's experience.
  1. **Sedatives** include the use of lorazepam, phenobarbital, fentanyl or morphine. Each agent has advantages and side effects. The author's choice is phenobarbital (10–20 mg/kg/day) with intermittent doses of lorazepam (q6–8h) for episodes of agitation that may break through the background phenobarbital sedation.
  2. **Paralyzing agents** include pancuronium and vercuronium. Muscle relaxation by paralysis results in considerable third-spacing of fluid, requiring added volume expanders to maintain blood pressure and urine output.

F. Surfactant replacement therapy. The availability of surfactant treatment has dramatically changed the care of infants with RDS (HMD). At the time of preparation of the second edition of this manual (1992), only one surfactant preparation was available for general clinical use in the United States (Exosurf Pediatric). Since 1991, two additional preparations have become available, one for general use (Survanta) and one nearing completion of clinical trials (Infasurf). In Europe, two surfactants are widely used, ALEC (a synthetic preparation) and Curosurf (a porcine lung mince extract). A new synthetic surfactant composed of surface active phospholipids and genetically cloned human surfactant SP-B protein peptides is in early FDA monitored clinical trials.
  1. **Composition.** Whether the surfactant material is synthetic or animal-derived, all have DPPC (dipalmatylphosphatidylglycerol) in common. DPPC, or lecithin, is the principal surface tension reducing substance. Other phospholipids are represented and surfactant proteins of SP-A, SP-B and SP-C may be present (Table 6–6).
  2. **Actions.** All surfactant preparations are intended to replace the missing or inactivated natural surfactant of the infant. Surface tension reduction and stabilization of alveolar air-water interface is the basic function of surfactant compounds. Air-water interface stability imparts lower alveolar surface tension and prevents atelectasis, or alternating areas of atelectasis and emphysema.

TABLE 6–6. COMPOSITION OF PULMONARY SURFACTANT (% BY WEIGHT)

Phospholipids		85%
PC	80%	
PG	7%	
PI + PS	5%	
PE	4%	
Sph	2%	
Other	2%	
	100%	
Neutral lipids		7%
(cholesterol, free fatty acids)		
Surfactant-associated proteins		8%
(SP-A, SP-B, SP-C)		
		100%

Note: PC, phosphatidylcholine; PG, phosphatidylglycerol; PI, phosphatidylinositol; PS, phosphatidylserine; PE, phosphatidyl-ethanolamine; Sph, sphingomyelin; SP-A, B, and C, surfactant proteins A, B, and C.

3. **Dosage.** Each preparation has specific dosage and dosing procedures. Direct tracheal instillation is involved in all preparations.
   a. **Prophylactic dosing at birth.** This form of treatment is used less often, and only when resuscitation and surfactant administration can be safely pursued simultaneously.
   b. Administration of surfactant preparations after respiratory distress is established. Currently surfactant therapy occurs at 2–4 hours of life after stabilizing of infant and establishing the diagnosis of RDS (HMD).
   c. Indications for first dose are clinical. Radiographic evidence of RDS (HMD) and a/A ratios of less than 0.22 are necessary. Second dosage may follow at 6–12 hours. Repeat doses should follow failure to improve a/A ratios by 30% or documentation of loss of response after initial 30% improvement of a/A ratio has been seen. Such dosing remains controversial.
4. **Efficacy of surfactant treatment** can be observed for both immediate and long term clinical conditions.
   a. Early effects include a reduction of FiO_2 need and improved PaO_2 and $Paco_2$ (a/A ratio). Likewise, improved tidal volume and compliance should be noted with improved lung function and decreased ventilator peak inspiratory pressures.
   b. Long-term effects should result in decreased necessity for mechanical ventilation and less severe chronic lung disease of infancy. Complications of patent ductus arteriosus (PDA), necrotizing enterocolitis (NEC), and intraventricular hemorrhage (IVH) have not been significantly influenced by surfactant therapy to date.
5. **Side effects.**
   a. A small risk for pulmonary hemorrhage.
   b. Secondary pulmonary infections.
   c. Air leak (pneumothorax) following bolus administration of surfactant compounds. Rapid changes in tidal volume require immediate reduction of peak inspiratory pressures. Failure to do so while also decreasing FiO_2 may lead to air leaks.
6. **Surfactant therapy for diseases other than RDS (HMD).** Encouraging preliminary reports of surfactant therapy have been noted in cases of pneumonia, meconium aspiration syndrome, persistent pulmonary hypertension and adult respiratory distress syndrome (ARDS), but no protocols for treatment are available at this time.
V. **Strategies for respiratory management of certain newborn diseases**
   A. **Respiratory distress syndrome (hyaline membrane disease)**
      1. **Clinical presentation.** Patients are premature with immature lungs and sur-

factant deficiency. Blood gases reflect poor oxygenation, declining a/A ratios (< 0.5) and CO_2 accumulation. Monitoring of lung mechanics reveals poor compliance and diminished tidal volume but near normal airway resistance. Progressive atelectasis due to surfactant deficiency worsens the compliance (lung stiffness), and the work of breathing increases in order to maintain minute ventilation. All of the above results in exhaustion of the infant and ultimately, apnea.

   2. **Management.** Endotracheal intubation and mechanical ventilation follow a decrease of a/A ratio of 0.30. Oxygen supplementation is required to maintain Pao_2 at 50–80 mm Hg. The goal of ventilation is to increase the Pao_2 and decrease the $Paco_2$. Ventilator settings begin with peak inspiratory pressures to allow even movement of the chest wall and provide a tidal volume of 5–7 mL/kg. If tidal volume cannot be measured, chest x-ray for expansion to 8 ribs is an estimate of adequate peak inspiratory pressure. Rates can be determined by decline in CO_2 or by calculating minute ventilation. For the more hypercarbic infants, rates of 50–60 bpm and tidal volumes of 5–6 mL/kg will give minute ventilation of approximately 360. PEEP of 4–6 cm H_2O is most often required. Inspiratory times vary from 0.32–0.38 seconds. As soon as optimal lung expansion, tidal volume, and minute ventilation have been achieved, surfactant therapy by tracheal instillation should begin (2–4 hr of life). A 30% reduction of FiO_2 and 30% increase of a/A ratio should result in decreased PIP while maintaining an adequate tidal volume and minute ventilation.

B. **Group B beta-hemolytic streptococcal (GBS) disease** of newborn with pneumonia and hypotension.

   1. **Clinical presentation.** Infants may be of any gestation but are often nearterm or term. The disease represents interstitial inflammation, atelectasis due to inflammatory debris and surfactant deficiency. Mild respiratory distress with tachypnea rapidly becomes severe, with marked cyanosis and hypoxemia. Ventilatory support is needed as soon as blood gases confirm poor a/A ratio or a-A DO_2. Natural surfactant production is suppressed and alveolar surfactant is inactivated by inflammatory proteins.

   2. **Management.** Following endotracheal intubation, mechanical ventilation should be at a rate that is synchronized with the infant's spontaneous rate (SIMV). Increased peak inspiratory pressures to achieve tidal volumes of 6–8 mL/kg and minute ventilation of 300–360 mL/kg are required in larger infants. Systemic hypotension often accompanies GBS. Excessive PEEP (5–6 cm H_2O) may impede venous return. PEEP of 2–4 cm H_2O is recommended. Inspiratory times are usually 0.35 seconds, although excessive mean airway pressure can be lessened by dropping IT to 0.32–0.33 seconds. Because GBS patients may develop severe hypoxia and persistent pulmonary hypertension, monitoring the oxygen index should begin early. With FiO_2 at 100%, a mean airway pressure falling PaO_2 and calculated OI of 30 or greater ($1.0 \times 15 \times 100/50 = 30$) suggests the need for more advanced respiratory support. High-frequency ventilation (HFV) should be considered along with inhaled nitric oxide therapy. If there is no response to HFV and the OI is greater than 40, extracorporeal membrane oxygenation (ECMO) may also be considered. Surfactant therapy should be performed before ECMO. Additional support includes vasopressors, colloid infusions, antibiotics, intravenous immune globulins, glucose and electrolyte solutions.

C. **Chronic lung disease of infancy (CLDI)**

   1. **Clinical presentation.** Infants are usually two to three weeks old, ventilator dependent, and requiring supplemental oxygen. Lung mechanics reveal marginal compliance of 0.8 to 1.0 mL/cm H_2O and marked increases in resistance to 120–140 cm H_2O/L/sec. Airway resistance is most marked on expiration.

   2. **Management.** Many parameters must be addressed in infants with CLDI. Careful fluid management, sparing use of diuretics, and maximal caloric in-

take are required. Respiratory care includes chest physical therapy and airway humidification. Hypoxia must be avoided by careful pulse oximetry and monitoring of supplemental oxygen to maintain SaO_2 of 92–95%. Bronchodilators, both systemic and aerosol, are helpful. Steroid therapy has been associated with marked improvement in many infants. Cromolyn therapy may be of use but remains controversial. Ventilator management seeks to maintain adequate tidal volume (6–8 mL/kg) delivered over longer inspiratory times (0.38–0.40 sec); however, some infants may require shorter IT. Peak inspiratory pressure is dictated by achieving adequate tidal volume and minute ventilation. Synchronized ventilation is particularly helpful to patients with CLDI. $Paco_2$ may be accepted at higher values (55–60 mm Hg) with adequate renal compensation and acid base balance. Recovery of CLDI infants and extubation requires improved air flow with decreased airway resistance and improved peak end-tidal expiratory flow. Increased ventilator rates with long IT and short expiratory times do not allow for adequate expiratory flow. This represents a violation of the expiratory time constant and resulting air trapping with cystic or bullous changes of the lungs. Maintaining adequate expiratory time at acceptable minute ventilation is essential for ventilatory support and gradual weaning of CLDI patients from mechanical ventilation.

VI. **Overview of high-frequency ventilation (HFV).** HFV refers to a variety of ventilatory strategies and devices designed to provide ventilation at rapid rates and very low tidal volumes. The ability to provide adequate ventilation in spite of reduced tidal volume (equal of less than dead space) may reduce the risk of barotrauma. Rates during HFV are often expressed in Hertz (Hz). A rate of 1 Hz (one cycle/sec) is equivalent to 60 bpm.

   All methods of high frequency ventilation should be administered with the assistance of well-trained respiratory therapists and after comprehensive education of the nursing staff. Furthermore, since rapid changes in ventilation or oxygenation may occur, continuous monitoring is highly recommended. Optimal utilization of these ventilators is evolving and different strategies may be indicated for a particular lung disease.

   A. **Definitive indications for HFV support**
   1. **Pulmonary interstitial emphysema (PIE).** A multicenter trial has demonstrated high-frequency jet ventilation (HFJV) to be superior to conventional ventilation in early PIE as well as in neonates who fail to respond to conventional ventilation.
   2. **Severe bronchopleural fistula.** In severe bronchopleural fistula not responsive to thoracostomy tube evacuation and conventional ventilation, HFJV may provide adequate ventilation and decrease fistula.
   3. **Patients qualifying for ECMO.** Pulmonary hypertension with or without associated parenchymal lung disease (meconium aspiration, pneumonia, hypoplastic lung, diaphragmatic hernia) can result in intractable respiratory failure and high mortality unless treated by ECMO. The prior use of HFV among ECMO candidates has been successful and eliminated the need for ECMO in 25–45% of cases.
   B. **Possible indications.** HFJV has been used with moderate success in infants with other disease processes; it is usually implemented at the point of severe respiratory failure with maximal conventional ventilation (a rescue treatment). Further study is needed to develop clear indications and appropriate ventilatory strategies before HFV can be recommended for routine use in infants with these diseases.
   1. **Pulmonary hypertension.**
   2. **Hyaline membrane disease.**
   3. **Meconium aspiration syndrome.**
   4. **Diaphragmatic hernia with pulmonary hypoplasia.**
   5. **Postoperative Fontan procedures.**
VII. **High-frequency ventilators, techniques and equipment**

Three types of high-frequency ventilators are currently in use: High-frequency jet ventilators (HFJVs), high-frequency flow interrupter (HFFIs) and high-frequency oscillatory ventilators (HFOVs).

A. High-frequency jet ventilator (HFJV). The HFJV injects a high-velocity stream of gas into the endotracheal tube, usually at frequencies between 240–600 bpm and tidal volumes equal to or slightly greater than dead space. During HFJV, expiration is passive. The only FDA-approved HFJV is the Bunnell Life Pulse ventilator, which is discussed here.

1. **Indications.** Mostly used for PIE, the Bunnel ventilator has been used for the other indications described for all types of HFV.

2. **Contraindications.** The only contraindication is an infant too small for intubation with a triple-lumen endotracheal tube (Hi-Lo Jet tracheal tube) necessary for the use of this ventilator. The smallest Hi-Lo tube has a 2.5 mm inside diameter but its outside diameter is equal to a standard 3.0 mm endotracheal tube.

3. **Equipment**
   a. **Bunnell Life Pulse ventilator.** The inspiratory pressure (PIP), jet valve "on time," and respiratory frequency are entered into a digital control panel on the Jet. PIP are servo controlled by the Life Pulse from the distal pressure port. The ventilator has an elaborate alarm system to ensure safety and to help detect changes in pulmonary function. It also has a special humidification system.
   b. **Triple-lumen endotracheal tube.** Intubation with a special lumen endotracheal tube (Hi-Lo Jet tracheal tube) is required. This tube has a distal port for measuring airway pressure, a side port for jet injection, and a standard connection for a conventional ventilator circuit.
   c. **Conventional ventilator.** A conventional ventilator is needed to generate positive end-expiratory pressure (PEEP) and sigh breaths. PEEP and background ventilation are controlled with the conventional ventilator.

4. **Procedure**
   a. **Initiation**
      (1) **Reintubation with a triple-lumen tube**
      (2) **Settings on the jet ventilator** (pressure measurements are obtained through the distal pressure port on the conventional ventilator to help determine the initial jet settings):
         (a) **Default jet valve "on time":** 0.020 seconds.
         (b) **Frequency of jet:** 420/min.
         (c) PIP **on the jet:** Water 2–3 cm below what was on the conventional ventilator. Occasionally infants require considerably less PIP during HFJV.
      (3) **Settings on the conventional ventilator**
         (a) **PEEP:** Maintained at 3–5 cm H_2O.
         (b) **Rate:** As jet ventilator comes up to pressure, rate is decreased to 5–10 bpm.
         (c) **PIP:** Once at pressure, PIP is adjusted to a level 1–3 cm water below that on jet (low enough not to interrupt the jet ventilator).
      (4) **Close observation** is required at all times, especially during initiation.
      (5) Rarely, an infant develops worse air trapping on HFV and require prompt return to CMV.

5. **Management.** Management of HFJV is based on clinical course and radiographic findings.
   a. **Elimination of CO_2.** Alveolar ventilation is much more sensitive to changes in tidal volume than in respiratory frequency during HFV. As a result, the **delta pressure** (PIP minus PEEP) is adjusted to attain adequate elimination of CO_2, while jet valve "on time" and respiratory frequency are usually not readjusted during HFJV.
   b. **Oxygenation.** Oxygenation is often better during HFJV than during conventional mechanical ventilation in neonates with PIE. However, if oxy-

genation is inadequate and if the infant is already on 100% oxygen, an increase in mean airway pressure usually results in improved oxygenation. It can be accomplished by:

(1) Increasing PEEP.

(2) Increasing PIP.

(3) Increasing background conventional ventilator (either rates or pressure).

c. **Positioning of infants.** Positioning infants with the affected side down may speed resolution of PIE. In bilateral air leak, alternating placement on dependent sides may be effective. Diligent observation and frequent radiographs are necessary to avoid hyperinflation of the nondependent side.

6. **Weaning.** When weaning, the following guidelines are used.

a. **PIP is reduced as soon as possible** ($Paco_2 < 35–40$ mm Hg). Because elimination of CO_2 is very sensitive to changes in tidal volume, PIP is weaned 1 cm water at a time.

b. **Oxygen concentration** is weaned if oxygenation remains good ($PaO_2 > 70–80$ mm Hg).

c. Jet valve "on time" and frequency are usually kept constant.

d. Constant attention is paid to the infant's **clinical condition** and radiographs to detect early atelectasis or hyperinflation.

e. **Air leaks** are resolved. Continuation of HFJV occurs until the air leak has been resolved for 24–48 hours, which often corresponds to a dramatic drop in ventilator pressures and oxygen requirement.

f. If no improvement in the condition occurs, a trial of conventional ventilation is used after 6–24 hours on jet ventilation.

7. **Special considerations**

a. **Airway obstruction.** Because of the stiffness of the triple-lumen endotracheal tube, the bevel of the tube may become lodged against the tracheal wall, resulting in airway obstruction. This problem can usually be recognized quickly. Chest wall movement is decreased, although breath sounds may be adequate. The servo pressure (driving pressure) is usually very low. (An obstruction in the endotracheal tube proximal to the distal pressure port results in a high servo pressure alarm). Positioning the tube with the jet port facing anteriorly usually maintains good tube position.

b. **Inadvertent PEEP (air trapping).** In larger infants, the flow of jet gases may result in inadvertent PEEP. Decreasing the background flow on the conventional ventilator may correct the problem, or it may be necessary to decrease the respiratory frequency to allow more time for expiration.

8. **Complications**

a. **Tracheitis.** Necrotizing tracheobronchitis was a frequent complication in the early days of jet ventilation. This problem is much less frequent with the recognition of the critical importance of proper humidification of the jet gases. If tracheitis occurs, emergent bronchoscopy may be indicated. The clinical signs are:

(1) **Increased airway secretions.**

(2) **Evidence of airway obstruction (including air trapping).**

(3) **Acute respiratory acidosis.**

b. **Intraventricular hemorrhage (IVH).** There has been no increase in the incidence or severity of IVH with the use of HFJV.

c. **Bronchopulmonary dysplasia (BPD).** The incidence of BPD appears to be equal (sometimes less) in neonates ventilated with HFJV and as compared with those ventilated with CMV.

B. **High-frequency flow interrupter (HFFI).** The HFFI shares some characteristics with HFOV and HFJV. It operates at frequencies as high as HFOV but does not have active exhalation. Bursts of gas approximate those of HFJV but a standard endotracheal tube can be used. The only FDA-approved HFFI is the Infrasonic Infant Star ventilator, which is discussed here.

1. **Indications.** The indications are the same as those for HFJV. The Infrasonic Infant Star ventilator may not be effective in infants whose birth weight is greater than 1800 g. If an infant of this size qualifies for high-frequency ventilation, HFHV or HFOV may prove to be more effective.

2. **Equipment**
   a. **The Infrasonic Infant Star ventilator.** The manufacturer prefers to call this ventilator a flow oscillator because of the ventilation technique used and its flow characteristics. It can be termed hybrid oscillator, because it has features of both a flow-interrupter (jet) and an oscillator.
      (1) The bursts of gas are 18 milliseconds in duration (preset at the factory). The sudden expansion of gas after the burst creates a rebound negative pressure deflection that closely approximates the active exhalation of oscillatory ventilation.
      (2) The user-defined parameters are frequency (10–20 Hz), mean airway pressure (Paw), and amplitude, which is a function of volume of gas per burst.
   b. **Conventional ventilator.** The high-frequency mode on the Infant Star ventilator must be used in combination with the conventional ventilator. Rate, PEEP, and PAP are set on the conventional ventilator.
   c. **Endotracheal tube.** A regular endotracheal tube is used.

3. **Procedure: Initiation** of Infant Star ventilation
   a. **Conventional ventilator settings**
      (1) **Rate is set at 5 bpm.** It is extremely important to have a conventional rate set during high frequency so that atelectasis does not develop. Tidal volumes are very small during high frequency.
      (2) **PIP and PEEP** are not changed from the original settings.
   b. **HFFI settings**
      (1) **Frequency** is always maintained at 15 Hz (900 bpm). It is not adjusted during HFV.
      (2) **MAP** is determined by the PEEP level and initially should be set to match the MAP prior to the initiation of HVF. That is, if MAP was 15 on conventional ventilatory support, it should be set on the high-frequency ventilator by means of setting the PEEP at 15.
      (3) **Amplitude.** After the frequency and the MAP are set, the amplitude should be adjusted. It should be increased until the chest wall of the infant begins to vibrate visually. This setting is the most difficult and arbitrary to determine. The range is 10–30 mL.
   c. **After the high-frequency device is initially set, arterial blood gas values and chest x-ray studies are used to adjust** settings. Chest x-ray studies are usually done every 6 hours until infant is stabilized.

4. **Management on the Infant Star.** It is important to note that the MAP controls oxygenation and the amplitude controls elimination of CO_2.
   a. **If PaO_2 is low,** MAP should be increased on the Infant Star. PEEP is the main determinant of MAP and lung volume; therefore PEEP levels should be increased until oxygenation is adequate. The conventional rate can be increased, but this is a less effective means of increasing oxygenation.
   b. **If $Paco_2$ is high:**
      (1) Poor oxygenation as well as high $Paco_2$ indicates decreased lung volume; a chest x-ray study at this time often reveals a hypoventilated lung with atelectasis. PEEP should be increased.
      (2) If adequate oxygenation exists, amplitude should be increased until adequate CO_2 removal is achieved.
      (3) Hyperoxygenation may be an indication of air trapping and PEEP should be decreased. A chest x-ray film reveals lung hyperinflation.

5. **Weaning.** Once adequate gas exchange has been achieved and oxygena-

tion is adequate, careful weaning should begin. In general, weaning should follow the pattern described below.

(margin annotations: PaO₂ ✓; "inflat'n" → ↓PEEP; Ⓝ CXR → ↓FiO₂ → ↓PEEP)

a. If PaO_2 is acceptable and a chest x-ray film does not show hyper expansion, wean the FiO_2. (If hyperexpansion is present, PEEP is weaned, follow by c, d, and e below.)

b. When the FiO_2 has been weaned to 60%, wean the PEEP.

c. If $Paco_2$ elimination is good ($Paco_2 < 40$ mm Hg), wean the amplitude.

d. When the amplitude has reached low levels (around 10 mL), conventional breaths may be added to ventilatory strategy.

e. Frequency does not need to be decreased during weaning.

Note: It is necessary to perform serial chest x-ray studies to rule out atelectasis and underinflation while weaning is in progress. The x-ray films may indicate that PEEP has been dropped too low or that amplitude needs to be increased.

6. **Complications.** The main complication is gas trapping resulting in hyperexpansion, which can be prevented by meticulously monitoring serial chest x-ray studies and arterial blood gas values and by appropriate weaning procedures.

C. **High-frequency oscillatory ventilator (HFOV).** The HFOV generates tidal volume less than or equal to dead space by means of an oscillating piston or diaphragm. This mechanism creates active exhalation as well as inspiration. The Sensormedics HFOV is currently FDA-approved for use in neonates.

(margin annotation: Active exhalation!)

1. **Indications.** Respiratory failure: HFOV is indicated when conventional ventilation does not result in adequate oxygenation or ventilation or requires the use of very high airway pressures. Like other forms of HFV, success is more likely when increased airway resistance is not the dominant pulmonary pathophysiology. Best results are seen in cases where parenchymal disease is homogeneous. Some clinicians advocate HFOV as the primary method of assisted ventilation in premature infants with RDS.

2. **Equipment.** The Sensormedics High Frequency Oscillator is a piston oscillator. It is not used in conjunction with a conventional ventilator. The user-defined parameters are frequency, mean airway pressure and power applied for piston displacement.

3. **Procedure: Initiation**
   a. **Conventional ventilator is discontinued.**
   b. **Settings**
      (1) Frequency is usually set at 15 Hz for premature infants with RDS. Larger infants, or those with a significant component of increased airway resistance should be started at 5–10 Hz.
      (2) Paw is set higher (2–5 cm H_2O) than on the previous conventional ventilation. If overdistention or air leaks were present prior to initiation of HFOV, lower Paw should be considered.
      (3) Amplitude (equivalent to PIP on conventional ventilation) is regulated by the power of displacement of the piston. This power is increased until there is visible chest wall vibration.
   c. After HFOV has been initiated, careful and frequent assessment of lung expansion and adequate gas exchange is necessary. Air trapping is a continuous potential threat in HFOV. Signs of overdistention such as descended and flat diaphragms and small heart shadow are monitored with frequent chest x-rays.

4. **Management**
   a. If PaO_2 is low, an increase in Paw may be necessary. Chest radiographs may be helpful in determining the adequacy of lung expansion.
   b. If $Paco_2$ is high:
      (1) If oxygenation is poor the Paw may be too high or too low, resulting in either hyperinflation or widespread collapse, respectively. Again chest x-rays are necessary to differentiate between these two conditions.

(2) If oxygenation is adequate, the amplitude (power) should be increased.

5. Weaning

a. In the absence of hyperinflation FiO_2 is weaned prior to Paw for adequate PaO_2. Below 40% FiO_2, wean Paw exclusively.

b. Paw should be weaned as the lung disease improves with the goal of maintaining optimal lung expansion. Excessively aggressive early weaning of Paw may result in widespread atelectasis and the need for a significant increase in Paw and FiO_2.

c. Amplitude should be weaned for acceptable $Paco_2$.

d. Frequency is usually not adjusted during weaning. A decrease in frequency is necessary when signs of lung overdistention cannot be eliminated by a reduction in Paw.

e. The neonate may be switched to conventional ventilation at low level of support or may be extubated directly from HFOV.

6. Complications. See HFFI.

GLOSSARY OF TERMS USED IN RESPIRATORY SUPPORT

Alveolar to arterial ratio (a/A ratio). See p 44.

Assist. A setting at which the infant initiates the mechanical breath, triggering the ventilator to deliver a preset tidal volume or pressure.

Assist/control. The same as assist, except that if the infant becomes apneic, the ventilator delivers the number of mechanical breaths per minute set on the rate control.

Continuous positive airway pressure (CPAP). A spontaneous mode in which the ambient intrapulmonary pressure that is maintained throughout the respiratory cycle is increased.

Control. A setting at which a certain number of mechanical breaths per minute is delivered. The infant is unable to breathe spontaneously between mechanical breaths.

End-tidal CO_2 ($ETCO_2$). A measure of the pCO_2 of end expiration.

Expiratory time (ET). The amount of time set for the expiratory phase of each mechanical breath.

Flow rate. The amount of gas per minute passing through the ventilator. It must be sufficient to prevent rebreathing (ie, 3 times the minute volume) and to acheive the PIP during inspiratory time. Changes in the flow rate may be necessary if changes in the airway wave form are desired. The normal range is 6–10 L/min; 8 L/min is commonly used.

Fraction of inspired oxygen (FiO_2). The percentage of oxygen concentration of inspired gas expressed as decimals (room air = 0.21).

I:E ratio. Ratio of inspiratory time to expiratory time. The normal values are 1:1, 1:1.5, or 1:2.

Inspiratory time (IT). The amount of time set for the inspiratory phase of each mechanical breath.

Intermittent mechanical ventilation (IMV). Mechanical breaths are delivered at intervals. The infant breathes spontaneously between mechanical breaths.

Mean airway pressure (Paw). Mean airway pressure is the average proximal pressure applied to the airway throughout the entire respiratory cycle. Paw can be calculated by the following formula:

$$\frac{(R)\ (IT)\ (PIP) + [60 - (R)\ (IT)] \times PEEP}{60}$$

Minute ventilation. Tidal volume (proportional to PIP) multiplied by rate.

Oxygen index (OI). See page 50.

Oxyhemoglobin dissociation curve. A curve showing the amount of oxygen that combines with hemoglobin as a function of PaO_2 and $Paco_2$. The curve shifts to the right when oxygen take-up by the blood is less than normal at a given PO_2, and it shifts to the left when oxygen take-up is greater than normal.

PaO$_2$. Partial pressure of arterial oxygen.

PAP. The total airway pressure. In the Siemens Servo 900-C, it is the PIP + PEEP.

Paw. See Mean Airway Pressure.

Pco$_2$. Carbon dioxide partial pressure.

Peak inspiratory pressure (PIP). The highest pressure reached within the proximal airway with each mechanical breath.

Note: In the Siemens Servo 900-C, the PIP is defined as the inspiratory pressure above the PEEP.

PO$_2$. Oxygen partial pressure.

Positive end expiratory pressure (PEEP). The pressure in the airway above ambient pressure during the expiratory phase of mechanical ventilation.

Rate. Number of mechanical breaths per minute delivered by the ventilator.

SaO$_2$. Oxygen saturation of arterial blood.

Tidal volume (V$_t$). The volume of gas inspired or expired during each respiratory cycle.

Total cycle time (Tc). Inspiratory time plus expiratory time.

Wave form. A pattern of change in airway pressure during the entire respiratory cycle. The 3 types of wave forms are square, sine, and triangular. The sine and square forms are the most common. The square wave indicates that the volume is being delivered at a constant rate; the sine wave, at a variable rate (Fig 6–5 p 50).

REFERENCES

Bernstein CT: Synchronous and patient-triggered ventilation in newborns. *Neonatal Respiratory Diseases* 1993; **3**:1–11.

Carter JM, Gertsmann DR, Clark RH, Snyder G, Cornish JD, Null DM. High-frequency oscillatory ventilation for the treatment of acute neonatal respiratory distress failure. *Pediatrics* **85**:159–64, 1990.

Clark RH, Gertsmann DR, Null MN, deLemos A. ospective Randomized comparison of high-frequency oscillatory and conventional ventilation in respiratory distress syndrome. *Journal of Pediatrics.* **122**:609–19, 1993.

Cunningham MD: Assessing pulmonary function in the neonate. In: Pomerance J and Richardson CJ, eds., *Neonataology for the Clinician,* East Norwalk, Appleton & Lange, 1993, pp. 249–255.

Cunningham MD: Intensive care monitoring of pulmonary mechanics for preterm infants undergoing mechanical ventilation. *J Perinatol* 1989; **9**:56.

Cunningham MD, Shook L, Tomazic T: Clinical experience with pulse oximetry in managing oxygen therapy in neonatal intensive care. *J Perinatol* 1988; **8**:333.

Davis JM, Sinkin RA, Aranda JV: Drug therapy for bronchopulmonary dysplasia. *Pediatr Pulmonol* 1990; **8**:117.

Dunn MS, Shennan AT, Zayack D et al: Bovine surfactant replacement therapy in neonates of less than 30 weeks' gestation: A randomized controlled trial of prophylaxis versus treatment. *Pediatrics* 1991; **87**:377.

Ellean C, Galperine R, Guenard H, et al.: Helium-oxygen mixture in respiratory distress syndrome: A double-blind study. *J Pediatr* 1993; **122**:132.

Freeman RK, Poland RL (1992). *Guidelines for Perinatal Care,* 35d edn., American Academy of Pediatrics: Elk Grove, Illinois and American College of Obstetricians and Gynecologists: Washington, D.C.

Flynn JT, Bancalari E, Snyder ES et al.: A cohort study of transcutaneous oxygen tension and the incidence and severity of retinopathy of prematurity. *New Engl J Med* 1992; **326**:1050.

Gerstmann DR, Delemos RA, Clark RH. High-frequency ventilation: Issues of Strategy. (Review) Clinics in Perinatology. **18**:563–80, 1991.

HiFO Study Group, Randomized study of high-frequency oscillatory ventilation in infants with severe respiratory distress syndrome. *Journal of Pediatrics.* **122**:609–19, 1993.

Jobe AH: Pulmonary surfactant therapy. *New Engl J Med* 1993; **328**:861.

Kezler M, Donn SM, Bucciarelli RL, Averson D, Hart M, Lunyong V. Multicenter controlled trial comparing high-frequency jet ventilation and conventional mechanical ventilation in newborn infants with pulmonary interstitial emphysema. *J Pediatr* **119**:85–93, 1991.

Kinsella JP, Neish SR, Ivy DD et al.: Clinical responses to prolonged treatment of persistent pulmonary hypertension of the newborn with low doses of inhaled nitric oxide. *J Pediatr* 1993; **123**:103.

Peris LV, Boix JH, Salom JV et al: Clinical use of arterial/alveolar oxygen tension ratio. *Critical Care Med* 1983; **11:**888.

Primak RA: Factors associated with pulmonary air leak in preterm infants receiving mechanical ventilation. *J Pediatr* 1983; **102:**764.

Spitzer AR et al: Ventilatory response to combined high-frequency jet ventilation and conventional mechanical ventilation for the rescue treatment of severe neonatal lung disease. *Pediat Pulmonol* 1989;**7:**244.

Wilkie RA, Bryan MH: Effect of bronchodilators on airway resistance in ventilator-dependent neonates with chronic lung disease. *J Pediatr* 1987; **111:**278.

7   Fluids and Electrolytes

Fluid and electrolyte therapy is at the center of many management issues of disease in the newborn infant. Therefore, such therapy for neonates must be undertaken with careful planning. The needs of small infants must be met without placing stress on organ systems that are immature or have not yet adapted to extrauterine function. Physiologic principles of fluid and electrolyte balance in newborn infants must be thoroughly understood (Costarino, 1986). For example, excessive fluid administration is associated with bronchopulmonary dysplasia, patent ductus arteriosus, necrotizing enterocolitis, and intraventricular hemorrhage. It is critical that immediate fluid and electrolyte management, with close monitoring, be established to ensure the best outcome for each newborn.

MECHANISMS OF FLUID AND ELECTROLYTE BALANCE

I. **Renal function.** Total body water (TBW) accounts for nearly 75% of the body weight in term newborns and even more in preterm infants. TBW is divided into two large parts: intracellular fluid (ICF) and extracellular fluid (ECF). With increasing gestational age, TBW and ECF volumes both decrease, whereas ICF increases. Both term and preterm infants experience an acute expansion of the ECF by shifts of fluid from the ICF, placental transfusion, and by reabsorption of lung fluid.

Late in gestation and during the first few weeks of life, renal function undergoes changes that influence the balance between salt and water.

A. **Although both term and preterm infants have low glomerular filtration rates** (GFR), the GFR is even lower in preterm infants. The distal nephron can produce dilute urine early in gestation. Therefore, any limitation of the neonatal kidney in excreting excess water results from a low GFR.

B. **In term neonates, the kidneys can only concentrate urine up to 800 mosm/L** compared to an adult kidney, which has a concentration capacity of up to 1500 mosm/L. However, **preterm infants exhibit an even further reduced urine concentrating ability** secondary to a relatively low interstitial urea concentration, an anatomically shortened loop of Henle and distal tubule and collecting system that is less responsive to antidiuretic hormone.

II. **Insensible water loss (IWL).** IWL is evaporation of water through the skin and mucous membranes.

A. **Term infants.** In term infants, maintenance fluid requirements can be expressed as a function of metabolism, as shown in Table 7–1. In newborn infants, one-third of the IWL occurs through the respiratory tract and the remaining two-thirds through the skin.

B. **Preterm infants.** The relationship between metabolism and maintenance fluid requirements does not hold true for infants that weigh less than 800 g at birth or are less than 27 weeks' gestational age.

1. The most important variable influencing IWL is the maturity of the infant. The higher IWL in preterm, low-birth-weight infants results from greater water permeability through a relatively immature epithelial layer, a larger surface-area-to-body-weight ratio, and a relatively greater skin vascularity. The average IWL in preterm infants according to birth weight is listed in Table 7–2.

2. IWL is also influenced by respiratory status and environmental factors such as type of warming unit (radiant warmer versus incubator), phototherapy, room humidity, and ambient temperature. Table 7–3 summarizes the effect ten different factors have on IWL. In general, for healthy premature infants that weigh 800–2000 g and are nursed in closed incubators, IWL increases

TABLE 7-1. THE RELATIONSHIP BETWEEN METABOLISM AND MAINTENANCE FLUIDS

Route	Loss/Gain	Fluid Replacement (mL/100 kcal Metabolized Energy)
Insensible loss		
Skin	Loss	25
Respiration	Loss	15
Urine	Loss	60
Stool	Loss	10
Water of oxidation	Gain	10
Total for maintenance		100

(Modified and reproduced, with permission, from Winters RW: Maintenance fluid therapy. Pages 113–133 In: *The Body Fluids In Pediatrics.* Little, Brown, 1973.)

TABLE 7-2. INSENSIBLE WATER LOSS (IWL) IN PRETERM INFANTS

Birth Weight (g)	Average IWL (mL/kg/d)
> 750–1000	64
1001–1250	56
1251–1500	38
1501–1750	23
1751–2000	20
2001–3250	20

linearly as body weight decreases. However, for sick infants of similar weight nursed on an open radiant warmer and undergoing assisted ventilation, IWL increases exponentially as body weight decreases.

3. When assessing appropriate fluid management in individual cases, birth weight, phototherapy, ambient humidity (ideally 40–50%), type of warmer, and respiratory status must be carefully considered.

III. **Electrolytes.** The principle electrolytes in body fluids are sodium, chloride, potassium, and calcium.

A. **Sodium (Na^+).** Na^+ imbalances are the most common imbalance in neonates. During the first two to four days of life, Na^+ requirements are low, and hyponatremia usually reflects water imbalance. Immature renal function may contribute to continued production of dilute urine in the face of dehydration and hypernatremia.

1. **Hyponatremia.** Predisposing factors include sodium wasting (diuretics, gastrointestinal losses, renal tubular losses), fluid overload (syndrome of inappropriate secretion of anti-diuretic hormone [SIADH]) inatrogenic factors,

TABLE 7-3. FACTORS IN THE NURSERY ENVIRONMENT THAT AFFECT INSENSIBLE WATER LOSS (IWL)

Increases IWL[a]	Decreases IWL[a]
1. Severe prematurity, 100–300%	1. Humidification in incubator, 50–100%
2. Open warmer bed, 50–100%	2. Plastic heat shield in incubator, 30–50%
3. Forced convection, 30–50%	3. Plastic blanket under radiant warmer, 30–50%
4. Phototherapy, 30–50%	4. Tracheal intubation with humidification, 20–30%
5. Hyperthermia, 30–50%	
6. Tachypnea, 20–30%	

[a]Estimates of percent change represent empirical data.

(Modified and reproduced, with permission, from Costarino A, Baumgart S: Modern fluid and electrolyte management of the critically ill premature infant. *Pediatr Clin North Am* 1986;**33**:153.)

sepsis, and hormonal conditions [congenital adrenal hyperplasia]). In addition, a phenomenon known as late hyponatremia of prematurity may occur two to three weeks after the birth of a 26–36-week preterm infant. This condition probably reflects a relative lack of sodium intake to compensate for renal losses and new tissue growth rather than an excess of water intake. Resolution is usually spontaneous as the postconceptual age approaches 40 weeks.

2. **Hypernatremia.** Predisposing factors include dehydration (diabetes insipidus, iatrogenic causes, high output renal failure, and diuretic therapy) and excessive sodium intake.

B. **Potassium (K⁺).** K^+ imbalance, especially hyperkalemia, is most common in very-low-birth-weight infants and in neonates with renal failure.

1. **Hyperkalemia** is also seen with administration of potassium-containing medications (Tromethamine [THAM] and amphotericin B). Low urine output in very-low-birth-weight infants is associated with hyperkalemia and may be life-threatening. Nonoliguric hyperkalemia in such infants is attributed to decreased renal potassium excretion secondary to immature distal tubular function. Increased serum potassium levels in the face of acidosis are indicative of potassium shifts from the intracellular to the extracellular compartment, not necessarily an increase in whole body potassium. ECG changes, including enlarged T waves and increased PR intervals, may accompany hyperkalemia.

2. **Therapy for hyperkalemia** includes discontinuation of potassium administration, alkalinization (eg, with sodium bicarbonate), and calcium administration. Glucose and insulin also shift potassium intracellularly, thus protecting the heart from dysrhythmia. Additional fluids and furosemide may also be given to increase renal excretion of potassium.

C. **Chloride (Cl⁻).** Cl^- imbalance is frequently seen with long-term diuretic therapy (eg, in the treatment of chronic lung disease). Hypochloremia is associated with a metabolic alkalosis and a compensatory respiratory acidosis. This can be corrected by additional Cl^- supplementation and/or discontinuation of the diuretic.

D. **Calcium (Ca⁺⁺).** Ca^{++} imbalances are usually seen with endocrine disturbances and extended diuretic use. Care must be taken in interpreting hypocalcemic levels in the face of hypoalbuminemia. Ionized calcium gives a more true reflection of calcium status in these situations.

FLUID AND ELECTROLYTE REPLACEMENT THERAPY

Fluid replacement in neonates must be carefully calculated to allow for normal loss of ECF and weight while preventing dehydration from insensible water loss, which may lead to hypotension, acidosis, and hypernatremia. It is important to avoid excessive fluid therapy, which has been associated with increased incidence of patent ductus arteriosus, bronchopulmonary dysplasia, intraventricular hemorrhage, and necrotizing enterocolitis in premature infants. Suggested fluid recommendations are based on historically averaged values for healthy infants managed in single-walled incubators (Baumgart, 1982; Bell, 1979; Costarino, 1986; Nash, 1987). For estimated adjustments for environmental variables, see Table 7–3.

I. **Suggested fluids and electrolytes**

A. **Day one**

1. **Term infants.** Give 10% dextrose in water ($D_{10}W$) at a rate of 60–80 mL/kg/d. This amount provides approximately 6–7 mg/kg/min of glucose. Although guidelines for Ca^{++} supplementation in this time frame are variable, it is our practice not to supplement Ca^{++} unless specifically indicated.

2. **Preterm infants.** Preterm infants, particularly those weighing less than 1000 g, require more fluids and are less tolerant of glucose. For infants between 800–1000 g, begin fluids at a rate of 80–100 mL/kg/d, adding the appropriate amount of glucose to provide 5–6 mg/kg/min (approximately

$D_{7.5}W$) and 2 mg calcium gluconate per milliliter. Infants less than 800 g usually require fluids in excess of 120–140 mL/kg/d to compensate for trans-dermal insensible losses and to avoid hyperkalemia, hypovolemia, and hypotension. D_5W provides a more suitable glucose load at these increased rates.

B. Days two to seven. Once tolerance of fluid therapy has been established and urine output is satisfactory (1–2 mL/kg/h), the rate and composition of the solution can be modified. The goals of fluid and electrolyte administration during this period include (1) loss of expected weight during the first 3–5 days (term infants, 10–15% of birth weight; preterm infants, 15–20% of birth weight), (2) maintenance of normal serum electrolytes, and (3) avoidance of oliguria.

   1. **Fluid volume** (range: 80–120 mL/kg/day). Depending on the tolerance of the previous day's fluid therapy, estimations of IWL, and clinical status of the infant (patent ductus arteriosus, congenital heart failure, and pulmonary edema), increases of 10–20 mL/kg/day may be considered. Infants weighing less that 800 g may require additional fluids until the skin becomes more mature (5–7 days). Excessively high fluids (even greater than 160 mL/kg/d) may be required in the face of hyperkalemia.

   2. **Glucose.** Once a glucose load is established and is tolerated, increasing the load by 10–15% per day is appropriate.

   3. **Sodium.** Na^+ requirements range from 2–4 meq/kg/d. However, in some infants, especially the more premature infants with immature kidneys, a larger Na^+ supplement may be necessary to compensate for sodium diuresis. These infants are susceptible to both hypo- and hypernatremia, both of which have been associated with permanent brain injury. Na^+ intake should be adjusted to keep serum sodium levels between 135–145 meq/L.

   4. **Potassium.** K^+ requirements range from 1–2 meq/kg/d. K^+ supplementation is usually not required on the first day of life, and sometimes it is not necessary until the third day. Extreme care should be taken to document renal function before adding K^+ (determination of urine output is usually adequate). Normal serum potassium levels are 3.5–5 meq/L.

   5. **Nutrition.** Enteral feedings should be started as soon as possible. If such feedings supply inadequate caloric intake or a required NPO period is prolonged, total parental nutrition (TPN) may be necessary. TPN may begin as early as 36–48 hours of life if electrolyte and fluid requirements are stable. When enteral feedings are begun, intravenous fluids are progressively decreased as enteral fluid intake is slowly increased. A combined fluid intake of approximately 120 mL/kg/d should be maintained. Enteral feedings supply adequate electrolytes, vitamins, trace elements, and the basic proteins, fats, and carbohydrates when appropriate volumes are given.

II. Monitoring of fluid and electrolyte status. Fluid and electrolyte replacement therapy should be monitored by daily weight measurements, vital signs derminations, and specific urine and serum laboratory studies.

   A. Body weight. The body weight should be recorded daily. The expected weight loss during the first 3–5 days of life is 10–15% of birth weight in term infants (15–20% of birth weight in preterm infants). A loss of more than 20% of birth weight during the first week of life is extreme and suggests uncompensated insensible water loss. If the weight loss is less than 2% per day for the first 4–5 days, fluid administration is probably excessive. A useful tool is an in-bed scale for measuring body weight two or three times per day, especially for sick neonates.

   B. Serum levels. Tests for serum hematocrit, sodium, potassium, blood urea nitrogen, creatinine, osmolality, acidosis, and base deficit should be performed. Increases in any of these parameters may indicate inadequate fluid therapy. Na^+ supplementation of 2–4 meq/kg/d becomes necessary usually no sooner than the second 12 hours of life. The total K^+ balance cannot be effectively measured in the serum because K^+ is mainly an intracellular ion. Hyperkalemia may become a life-threatening problem in infants weighing less than 800 g;

thus electrolytes should be followed frequently (every 4–6 hours) in these infants.
  C. **Fluid intake and output.** Fluid status should be measured by accurate fluid intake and output. Urine output measuring < 1.0 mL/kg/h may indicate a need for increased fluid intake, whereas urine output > 3.0 mL/kg/h may indicate overhydration and the need for restriction. Urine specific gravity, electrolytes, and osmolality may be useful in further assessment of fluid status, although immature kidney function in the preterm infant may make these parameters inaccurate.
  D. **General appearance and vital signs.** Hypotension, poor perfusion, tachycardia, and poor pulses may all be signs of inadequate intake.

FLUID CALCULATIONS

  I. **Environmental factors.** Sick infants under radiant warmers or receiving phototherapy have dramatically increased IWL, and to compensate, additional fluids must be given (Table 7–3).
 II. **Glucose.** The normal glucose requirement is 6–8 mg/kg/min. Intake can be slowly increased to 12–15 mg/kg/min, as tolerated, however, to allow for growth. Glucose intake can be calculated as follows:

$$\frac{\text{Percentage of glucose} \times \text{Rate (mL/h)} \times 0.167}{\text{Weight (kg)}} = \text{Glucose requirement (mg/kg/min)}$$

The alternate method is:

$$\frac{\frac{(\text{Amount of glucose/mL [from Table 7–4]} \times \text{Total fluids})}{\text{Weight (kg)}}}{60 \text{ minutes}} = \frac{\text{Glucose requirement}}{\text{(mg/kg/min)}}$$

III. **Sodium. The normal sodium requirement in infants is 2–3 meq/kg/d.** This value may be higher in premature infants. The following calculations can be used to determine the amount of sodium the infant is receiving.

$$\text{Amount of Na}^+/\text{mL (from Table 7–5)} \times \text{Total fluids/d} = \text{Amount of Na}^+/\text{d}$$

$$\frac{\text{Amount of Na}^+/\text{d}}{\text{Weight (kg)}} = \text{Amount of Na}^+ \text{(kg/d)}$$

TABLE 7–4. GLUCOSE CONCENTRATIONS IN COMMONLY USED INTRAVENOUS FLUIDS

Solution (%)	Glucose Concentration (mg/mL)
D5W	50
D7.5W	75
D10W	100
D12.5W	125
D15W	150

TABLE 7–5. SODIUM CONTENT OF COMMONLY USED INTRAVENOUS FLUIDS

Solution	Sodium Concentration (meq/mL)
3% normal saline	0.500
Normal saline	0.154
$\frac{1}{2}$ normal saline	0.075
$\frac{1}{4}$ normal saline	0.037
$\frac{1}{8}$ normal saline	0.019

IV. Potassium. The normal requirement for potassium in infants is **1–2 meq/kg/d/** The potassium intake can be easily calculated and added to the intravenous fluids as potassium chloride.

MODIFIERS OF FLUID AND ELECTROLYTE REQUIREMENTS

I. IWL. As previously mentioned (see p 70), physiologic and environmental factors influence IWL and thus total fluid requirements.

II. Diabetes insipidus. Either secondary to a central (decreased production) or a nephrogenic (unable to be used by the kidneys) etiology, the activity of antidiuretic hormone (ADH) is decreased. This leads to an increased urine output. Hydration is best maintained by replacement of urine volume and Na^+ loss in addition to IWL. Frequent measurements of body weight (every 12 hours) and Na^+ (every 6–8 hours) are necessary to gauge efficacy of therapy. With diabetes insipidus of central nervous system origin, 1-deamino-8-D-arginine vasopressin (DDAVP) therapy may be helpful.

III. Syndrome of inappropriate antidiuretic hormone (SIADH) secretions. An inappropriate increase in the secretion of ADH results in a decreased urine output with urine osmolality > 100 mosm/L, decreased serum osmolality, and hyponatremia (usually on the basis of volume expansion). SIADH is treated by restriction of fluid to approximately 50–60 mL/kg/d or less.

IV. Renal failure. Renal failure in the neonate is usually secondary to hypoxia or shock. Fluids should be adjusted to compensate only for IWL and replacement of urine volume, if any. K^+ supplementation should be avoided.

REFERENCES

Al-Dahhan J et al: Sodium homeostasis in term and preterm neonates. 1. Renal aspects. *Arch Dis Child* 1983;**58**:335.

Aperia A, Herin P, Zetterstrom R: Sodium chloride and potassium needs in very low birth weight infants. In: *Vitamin and Mineral Requirements in Preterm Infants.* Tsang RC (editor). Marcel Dekker, 1985.

Baumgart S et al: Fluid, electrolyte, and glucose maintenance in the very low birth weight infant. *Clin Pediatr* 1982;**4**:199.

Bell E, Oh W: Fluid and electrolyte balance in very low birth weight infants. *Clin Perinatol* 1979;**6**:139.

Bell Ef et al: Effect of fluid administration on the development of symptomatic patent ductus arteriosus and congestive heart failure in premature infants. *N Engl J Med* 1980;**320**:598.

Cornblath M et al: A controlled study of early fluid administration on survival of low birth weight infants. *Pediatrics* 1966;**38**:547.

Costarino A, Baumgart S: Modern fluid and electrolyte management of the critically ill premature infant. *Pediatr Clin North Am* 1986;**33**:153.

Costarino AT, Baumgart S: Water as Nutrition. In: *Nutritional Needs of the Preterm Infant.* Tsang, RC (editor). Williams & Wilkins, 1993.

Day GM et al: Electrolyte abnormalities in very low birth weight infants. *Pediatr Res* 1976;**10**:522.

Fanaroff A, Klaus M: The gastrointestinal tract: Feeding and selected disorders. In: *Care of the High-Risk Neonate.* Klaus M, Fanaroff A (eds) Saunders, 1986.

Fanaroff A, Martin RJ: Fluid, Electrolytes, and Acid-Base Homeostasis. In: *Neonatal-Perinatal Medicine Diseases of the Fetus and Infant.* Fanaroff A, Martin RJ, (editors). Mosby Year-Book, 1992.

Gruskay J et al: Monoliguric hyperkalemia in the premature infant weighing < 1000 grams. *J Pediatr* 1988;**113**:38.

Lorenz J et al: Water balance in very low birth weight infants: Relationship to water and sodium intake and effect on outcome. *J Pediatr* 1982;**101**:423.

Nash M: Nutrition, body fluids, and acid-base homeostasis. In: *Neonatal-Perinatal Medicine,* Fanaroff A, Martin RJ (eds) 4th ed. Mosby, 1987.

Rees L et al: Hyponatremia in the first week of life in preterm infants. *Arch Dis Child* 1984;**59**:423.

Schrier RW, Gabow P: Hyponatremia and hypernatremia. In: *Textbook of Nephrology.* Massry SG, Glassock RJ (editors). Williams & Wilkins, 1983.

Shaffer S et al: Hyperkalemia in very low birth weight infants. *J Pediatr* 1992;**121**:275.

Zenk K: Calculating dextrose infusion in mg/kg/min. *PeriScope* 1984; Aug 5.

8 Nutritional Management

NUTRITIONAL REQUIREMENTS IN THE NEONATE

I. **Calories**
   A. **To maintain weight,** give 50–60 kcal/kg/d.
   B. **To induce weight gain,** give 100–120 kcal/kg/d to a term infant (gain: 15–30 g/d) and 110–140 kcal/kg/d to a premature infant. Growth in premature infants is assumed to be adequate when it approximates the intrauterine rate (ie, 15 g/kg/d).

II. **Carbohydrates.** Approximately 11–15 g/kg/d are needed (30–60% of total calories).

III. **Proteins.** Adequate protein intake has been estimated at 2.25–4.0 g/kg/d (7–16% of total calories). Protein intake of more than 4.0 g/kg/d should not be exceeded in low birth weight infants.

IV. **Fats.** Fat requirements are 4–6 g/kg/d (limit: less than 55% of total calories, or ketosis may result). To meet essential fatty acid requirements, 2–5% of nonprotein calories should be in the form of linoleic acid and 0.6% in the form of linolenic acid.

V. **Vitamins.** Vitamin requirements are not clearly established. Guidelines are provided in Table 8–1 for low birth weight infants. Vitamin supplementation depends on the type of formula used, as is shown in Table 8–2.

VI. **Fluids.** See Chapter 7 for fluid requirements.

PRINCIPLES OF INFANT FEEDING

I. **Criteria for initiating infant feeding.** Most normal term infants are fed within the first 4 hours. The following criteria should usually be met before initiating infant feedings.
   A. **No** history of excessive **oral secretions,** vomiting, or bilious-stained gastric aspirate.
   B. **Nondistended, soft abdomen,** with normal bowel sounds. If the abdominal examination is abnormal, an abdominal x-ray film should be obtained.
   C. **Clinically stable** infant (intubation permissible).
   D. **Extubation.** At least 6 hours should be allowed to pass after extubation before attempting feeding. The infant should have little respiratory distress and be tolerating extubation well.
   E. **Respiratory rate** less than 60 bpm for oral feeding and less than 80 bpm for gavage feeding. Tachypnea increases the risk of aspiration.
   F. **Prematurity.** Considerable controversy concerns the timing of initial enteral feeding for the preterm infant. No established policies are available. Delays and their duration vary for every institution. In general, enteral feeding is started in the first 3 days of life with the objective of reaching full enteral feeding in 2–3 weeks. Parenteral nutrition, including amino acids and lipids, should be initiated at the same time to provide adequate caloric intake.
      1. For the stable, larger premature neonate (> 1500 g) the first feeding may be given within the first 24 hours of life. Early feeding may allow the release of enteric hormones that exert a trophic effect on the intestinal tract.
      2. On the other hand, apprehension about necrotizing enterocolitis (NEC) (mostly in the very low birth weight infant) has meant that initiation of enteral feeding is often precluded in infants with the following conditions:
         a. Perinatal asphyxia.

TABLE 8–1. DAILY VITAMIN AND MINERAL REQUIREMENTS

Nutrient	Term Infant	Preterm infant
Vitamins		
Vitamin A	500 IU	1400 IU
Vitamin D	400 IU	500–600 IU
Vitamin E	5 IU	5–25 IU
Vitamin C	20 mg	50–60 mg
Vitamin K	15 µg	15 µg
Thiamine	0.2 mg	0.2 mg
Riboflavin	0.4 mg	0.4 mg
Niacin	5 mg	5 mg
Vitamin B_6 (Pyridoxin)	0.4 mg	0.4 mg
Vitamin B_{12}	1.5 µg	1.5 µg
Folic acid	50 µg	50–100 µg
Biotin	6 µg	6 µg
Minerals		
Calcium	60 mg/kg	200 mg/kg
Phosphorus	40 mg/kg	100 mg/kg
Magnesium	8 mg/kg	8 mg/kg
Sodium	1–2 meq/kg	2.5–3.5 meq/kg; < 1.5 kg: 4–8 meq/kg
Potassium	2–3 meq/kg	2–3 meq/kg
Iron	6–10 mg	2 mg/kg (after 6–8 weeks)
Copper	30–40 µg/kg	100–120 µg/kg
Zinc	500 µg/kcal	1200–1500 µg/kg
Manganese	5 µg/100 kcal	10–20 µg/kg
Conditionally Essential Nutrients[a]		
Cystine		225–395 µmol/100 kcal
Taurine		30–60 µmol/100 kcal
Tyrosine		640–800 µmol/100 kcal
Inositol		150–375 µmol/100 kcal
Choline		125–225 µmol/100 kcal

[a]Nutrients that are normally synthesized by humans but for which premature infants may have a reduced synthetic

   b. Mechanical ventilation.
   c. Presence of umbilical vessels catheters.
   d. Patent ductus arteriosus.
   e. Indomethacin treatment.
   f. Sepsis.
   g. Frequent episodes of apnea and bradycardia.
   II. Feeding guidelines and choice of formula. Human milk is recommended for feeding infants whenever possible. If a commercial infant formula is chosen, no special considerations generally apply to normal, full-term newborn infants. Preterm infants may require more careful planning. Many different, highly specialized formulas are available. Table 8–2 outlines indications for various formulas. The composition of commonly used infant formulas and breast milk can be found in Table 8–3.
   A. Formulas
      1. Isoosmolar formulas (270–300 mosm/kg H_2O). The majority of infant formulas are isoosmolar (Similac 20, Enfamil 20, and SMA 20 [with and without iron]). These are the formulas used most often for healthy infants. Premature formulas that contain 24 cal/oz (Similac 24, Enfamil 24, "preemie" SMA 24) are also isoosmolar and are indicated for rapidly growing premature infants.

TABLE 8-2. INFANT FORMULA INDICATIONS AND USES

Formula	Indications	Vitamin and Mineral Supplements[a]
HUMAN MILK		
Donor	Preterm infant < 1200 g.	Multivitamins; iron if > 1500 g; fluoride at 40 weeks' gestation; folic acid until 7000 g.
Maternal	All infants.	
Breast milk fortifiers (see p 88)		
STANDARD FORMULAS		
Isoosmolar		
Enfamil 20	Full-term infants; as supplement to breast milk.	Multivitamins if taking < 32 oz/d.
Similac 20	Preterm infants > 1800–2000 g.	
SMA 20[b]		
Higher Osmolality		
Enfamil 24	Term infants: for infants on fluid restriction or who cannot handle required volumes of 20-cal formula to grow.	
Similac 24 & 27		
SMA 24 & 27		
Low Osmolality		
Similac 13	Preterm and term infants: for conservative initial feeding in infants who have not been fed orally for several days or weeks. *Not for long-term use.*	
SOY FORMULAS		
ProSobee (lactose and sucrose free)	Term infants: milk sensitivity, galactosemia, carbohydrate intolerance. *Do not use in preterm infants. Phytates can bind calcium and cause rickets.*	Multivitamins if taking < 32 oz/d.
Isomil (lactose free)		
Nursoy (lactose free)		
PROTEIN HYDROSYLATE FORMULAS		
Nutramigen	Term infants: Gut sensitivity to proteins, multiple food allergies, persistent diarrhea, galactosemia.	Multivitamins if taking < 32 oz/d.
Pregestimil	Preterm and term infants: disaccharidase deficiency, diarrhea, GI defects, cystic fibrosis, food allergy, celiac disease, transition from TPN to oral feeding.	
Alimentum	Term infants: protein sensitivity, pancreatic insufficiency, diarrhea, allergies, colic carbohydrate and fat malabsorption.	
SPECIAL FORMULAS		
Portagen	Preterm and term infants: pancreatic or bile acid insufficiency, intestinal resection.	Multivitamins if taking < 32 oz/d; calcium needed.
Similac PM 60/40	Preterm and term infants: problem feeders on standard formula; infants with renal, cardiovascular, digestive diseases that require decreased protein and mineral levels, breast-feeding supplement, initial feeding.	Multivitamins and iron if weight > 1500 g.
PREMATURE FORMULAS		
Low Osmolality		
Similac Special Care 20	Premature infants (< 1800–2000 g) who are growing rapidly. These formulas promote growth at intrauterine rates. Vitamin and mineral concentrations are higher to meet the needs of growth. Usually started on 20 cal/oz and advanced to 24 cal/oz as tolerated.	Routine vitamin supplementation not required (*controversial*).
Enfamil Premature 20		
Preemie SMA 20		
Isoosmolar		
Similac Special Care 24	Same as for low-osmolality premature formulas.	Same as for low-osmolality premature formulas.
Enfamil Special Care 24		
Preemie SMA 24		

[a] Such as Polyvisol (Mead Johnson) ½ mL/d.
[b] SMA has decreased sodium content and can be used in patients with congestive heart failure, bronchopulmonary dysplasia, and cardiac disease.

TABLE 8-3. COMPOSITION OF INFANT FORMULAS

Characteristics	Mature Human Breast Milk	Similac 20, Similac with Iron 20	Enfamil 20, Enfamil with Iron 20	SMA, SMA with Iron 20
Calories per liter	747	676	670	676
Osmolality (mosm/kg water)	290	290	278	300
Osmolarity (mosm/liter)	255	270	270	271
Protein				
Grams per liter	10.6	15	15	15
Percent total calories	6	9	9	8.9
Source	Cow's milk	Cow's milk	Reduced minerals, whey, nonfat milk	Nonfat milk, demineralized whey
Fat				
Grams per liter	45	36.3	38	36
Percent total calories	52	48	50	48.2
Source		Oils: soy and coconut	Oils: soy and coconut	Oils[a]
Carbohydrate				
Grams per liter	72	72.3	69	72
Percent total calories	42	43	41	42.9
Source	Lactose	Lactose	Lactose	Lactose
Minerals	mg/L (meq/L)	mg/L (meq/L)	mg/L (meq/L)	mg/L (meq/L)
Calcium	280 (14)	510 (25.4)	460 (23)	420 (20.9)
Chloride	420 (11.9)	450 (12.7)	420 (12)	375 (11)
Iodine	0.06	0.1	0.068	0.06
Iron	0.05	12[b]	12.7[c]	12.0[d]
Magnesium	35	41	52	45
Phosphorus	140	390	310	280
Potassium	525 (13.4)	730 (18.7)	720 (18)	560 (14.3)
Sodium	180 (7.8)	230 (8.3)	181 (8)	150 (6.5)
Zinc	1.2	5.1	5.2	5.0
Vitamins per liter				
Vitamin A (IU)	2230	2030	2100	2000
Vitamin B_1 (mg)	0.21	0.68	0.52	0.67
Vitamin B_2 (mg)	0.35	1.01	1.05	1.0
Vitamin B_6 (mg)	0.20	0.41	0.42	0.42
Vitamin B_{12} (µg)	trace	1.7	1.5	1.3
Vitamin C (mg)	40	60	54	55
Vitamin D (IU)	20	410	420	400
Vitamin E (IU)	2.3 (mg)	20	21	9.5
Vitamin K (µg)	2.1	54	58	55
Folic acid (µg)	24	100	105	50
Niacin (mg)	1.5	7.1	8.4	5.0
Pantothenic acid (mg)	1.8	3.04	3.1	2.1

[a] Oleo, coconut, oleic, and soy oils.
[b] Similac 20 Low Iron contains 1.5 mg iron/liter.
[c] Enfamil 20 Low Iron contains 1.1 mg iron/liter.
[d] SMA LO-IRON contains 1.5 mg iron/liter.
[e] MCT = medium-chain triglycerides.
[f] Special Care 24 Low-Iron 3.0 mg iron/liter.
[g] Low Iron formula.

(continued)

TABLE 8-3. COMPOSITION OF INFANT FORMULAS (continued)

Characteristics	Similac Special Care 20	Enfamil Premature Formula 20	Similac Special Care 24 and with Iron 24	Enfamil Premature Formula 24
Calories per liter	676	670	812	810
Osmolality (mosm/kg water)	250	240	300	300
Osmolarity (mosm/liter)	230	220	260	260
Protein				
Grams per liter	18.3	20	22	24
Percent total calories	11	12	11	12
Source	Cow's milk and whey	Nonfat milk, whey protein concentrate	Cow's milk and whey	Nonfat milk, whey protein concentrate
Fat				
Grams per liter	36.7	34	44.1	41
Percent total calories	47	44	47	44
Source	Oils: MCT* soy, and coconut	Oils: MCT, soy and coconut	Oils: MCT, soy and coconut	Oils: MCT, soy and coconut
Carbohydrate				
Grams per liter	71.7	74	86.1	89
Percent total calories	42	44	42	44
Source	Lactose and polycose glucose polymers	Lactose and corn syrup solids	Lactose and polycose glucose polymers	Lactose and corn syrup solids
Minerals	mg/L · meq/L	mg/L · meq/L	mg/L · meq/L	mg/L · meq/L
Calcium	1220 · 60.8	790 · 40	1460 · 73	1340 · 47
Chloride	640 · 15.5	570 · 16	660 · 18.6	690 · 20
Iodine	0.04	0.05	0.05	0.06
Iron	2.5	1.7	15[f]	2
Magnesium	81	68	100	55
Phosphorus	610	400	730	670
Potassium	870 · 22.3	750 · 19	1050 · 26.9	900 · 21
Sodium	290 · 12.6	260 · 11	350 · 15.2	320 · 14
Zinc	10.1	6.8	12.2	2.6
Vitamins per liter				
Vitamin A (IU)	4600	8100	5520	9700
Vitamin B$_1$ (mg)	1.69	1.69	2.03	2.00
Vitamin B$_2$ (mg)	4.19	2.3	5.03	2.9
Vitamin B$_6$ (mg)	1.69	1.69	2.03	2.0
Vitamin B$_{12}$ (µg)	3.7	2.0	4.5	2.4
Vitamin C (mg)	250	230	300	290
Vitamin D (IU)	1010	2200	1220	2600
Vitamin E (IU)	27	31	32	37
Vitamin K (µg)	81	88	100	106
Folic acid (µg)	250	230	300	290
Niacin (mg)	33.8	27.2	40.6	33.0
Pantothenic acid (mg)	12.8	8.1	15.4	9.7

a Oleo. coconut. oleic. and soy oils.
b Similac 20 Low Iron contains 1.5 mg iron/liter.
c Enfamil 20 Low Iron contains 1.1 mg iron/liter.
d SMA LO-IRON contains 1.5 mg iron/liter.
* MCT = medium-chain triglycerides.
f Special Care 24 Low-Iron 3.0 mg iron/liter.
g Low iron formula.

(continued)

Characteristics	Similac PM 60/40		Similac 27	
Calories per liter	676		913	
Osmolality (mosm/kg water)	280		430	
Osmolarity (mosm/liter)	250		370	
Protein				
Grams per liter	15.8		24.7	
Percent total calories	9		11	
Source	Whey and caseinate		Cow's milk	
Fat				
Grams per liter	37.6		48.1	
Percent total calories	50		47	
Source	Oils: soy and coconut		Oils: soy and coconut	
Carbohydrate				
Grams per liter	69		95.9	
Percent total calories	41		42	
Source	Lactose		Lactose	
Minerals	mg/L	meq/L	mg/L	meq/L
Calcium	380	19	820	41
Chloride	400	11	740	21
Iodine	0.041		0.14	
Iron	1.5		2.0	
Magnesium	41		64	
Phosphorus	190		640	
Potassium	580	14.8	1210	31
Sodium	160	7	310	13.5
Zinc	5.1		6.9	
Vitamins per liter				
Vitamin A (IU)	2030		2740	
Vitamin B$_1$ (mg)	0.68		0.91	
Vitamin B$_2$ (mg)	1.01		1.37	
Vitamin B$_6$ (mg)	0.41		0.55	
Vitamin B$_{12}$ (µg)	1.7		2.3	
Vitamin C (mg)	60		80	
Vitamin D (IU)	410		550	
Vitamin E (IU)	20		27	
Vitamin K (µg)	54		73	
Folic acid (µg)	100		140	
Niacin (mg)	7.1		9.59	
Pantothenic acid (mg)	3.04		4.11	

a Oleo, coconut, oleic, and soy oils.
b Similac 20 Low Iron contains 1.5 mg iron/liter.
c Enfamil 20 Low Iron contains 1.1 mg iron/liter.
d SMA LO-IRON contains 1.5 mg iron/liter.

e MCT = medium-chain triglycerides.
f Special Care 24 Low-Iron 3.0 mg iron/liter.
g Low iron formula.

(continued)

TABLE 8–3. COMPOSITION OF INFANT FORMULAS (continued)

Characteristics	Isomil 20		ProSobee 20		Nutramigen 20		Pregestimil 20	
Calories per liter	676		670		670		670	
Osmolality (mosm/kg water)	250		200		320		320	
Osmolarity (mosm/liter)	220		170		290		290	
Protein								
Grams per liter	20		20		19		19	
Percent total calories	11		12		11		11	
Source	Soy protein isolate		Soy protein isolate		Casein, hydrolysate, cystine, tyrosine, tryptophan		Casein, hydrolysate, cystine, tyrosine, tryptophan	
Fat								
Grams per liter	36.9		36		26		38	
Percent total calories	49		48		35		48	
Source	Oils: soy and coconut		Oils: soy and coconut		Corn oil		Oils: corn and MCT and high oleic safflower	
Carbohydrate								
Grams per liter	68.3		69		91		69	
Percent total calories	40		40		54		41	
Source	Corn syrup and sucrose		Corn syrup solids		Corn syrup and modified corn starch		Corn syrup and modified corn starch	
Minerals	mg/L	meq/L	mg/L	meq/L	mg/L	meq/L	mg/L	meq/L
Calcium	710	35.4	630	31	630	32	630	31
Chloride	420	11.9	560	16	580	16.4	580	16
Iodine	0.1		0.07		0.48		0.48	
Iron	12		12.7		12.7		12.7	
Magnesium	51		74		74		74	
Phosphorus	510		500		420		420	
Potassium	730	18.7	820	20	740	19	740	19
Sodium	300	13.0	240	10	320	14	320	14
Zinc	5.1		5.3		5.3		5.3	
Vitamins per liter								
Vitamin A (IU)	2030		2100		2100		2100	
Vitamin B₁ (mg)	0.41		0.52		0.53		0.53	
Vitamin B₂ (mg)	0.61		0.63		0.63		0.63	
Vitamin B₆ (mg)	0.41		0.42		0.42		0.42	
Vitamin B₁₂ (μg)	3.0		2.1		2.1		2.1	
Vitamin C (mg)	60		55		55		55	
Vitamin D (IU)	410		420		420		420	
Vitamin E (IU)	20		21		21		15.9	
Vitamin K (μg)	100		106		106		106	
Folic acid (μg)	100		106		106		106	
Niacin (mg)	9.13		8.5		85		85	
Pantothenic acid	5.07		3.2		3.2		3.2	

^a Oleo, coconut, oleic, and soy oils
^b Simlac 20 Low Iron contains 1.5 mg iron/liter.
^c Enfamil 20 Low Iron contains 1.1 mg iron/liter
^d SMA LO-IRON contains 1.5 mg iron/liter.
^e MCT = medium-chain triglycerides.
^f Special Care 24 Low-Iron 3.0 mg iron/liter.
^g Low iron formula.

(continued)

Characteristics	Similac, Similac with Iron 24		SMA, SMA with Iron 24		Enfamil, Enfamil with Iron 24		Similac 13	
Calories per liter	812		811		810		440	
Osmolality (mosm/kg water)	380		364		360		200	
Osmolarity (mosm/liter)	340		322		320		190	
Protein								
Grams per liter	22		18		17.8		11.9	
Percent total calories	11		8.9		9		11	
Source	Cow's milk		Nonfat milk, demineralized whey		Nonfat milk, reduced mineral whey		Cow's milk	
Fat								
Grams per liter	42.8		43.2		45		23.2	
Percent total calories	47		48.2		50		47	
Source	Oils: soy and coconut		Oils: soy, coconut, oleo, and oleic		Oils: soy and coconut		Oils: soy and coconut	
Carbohydrate								
Grams per liter	85.3		86.4		83		46.2	
Percent total calories	42		42.9		41		42	
Source	Lactose		Lactose		Lactose		Lactose	
Minerals	mg/L	meq/L	mg/L	meq/L	mg/L	meq/L	mg/L	meq/L
Calcium	730	36.4	504	25.1	560	28	400	20
Chloride	660	18.6	450	12.7	500	14	360	10.2
Iodine	0.12		0.072		0.081		0.066	
Iron	15(1.8)[b]		14.4(1.8)[d]		15.2(1.3)[e]		1.0	
Magnesium	57		54		63		31	
Phosphorus	570		336		380		310	
Potassium	1070	27.4	672	17.2	870	22	580	14.8
Sodium	280	12.2	180	7.8	220	10	150	6.5
Zinc	6.1		6		6.3		3.3	
Vitamins per liter								
Vitamin A (IU)	2240		2400		2500		1320	
Vitamin B$_1$ (mg)	0.81		0.804		0.65		0.440	
Vitamin B$_2$ (mg)	1.22		1.20		1.3		0.66	
Vitamin B$_6$ (mg)	0.42		0.504		0.49		0.26	
Vitamin B$_{12}$ (µg)	2.0		1.6		1.9		1.1	
Vitamin C (mg)	70		66		66		40	
Vitamin D (IU)	490		480		510		260	
Vitamin E (IU)	24		11.4		25		13	
Vitamin K (µg)	65		66		70		35	
Folic acid (µg)	120		60		126		66	
Niacin (mg)	8.53		6.00		10.1		4.62	
Pantothenic acid (mg)	3.65		2.52		3.8		1.98	

[a] Oleo, coconut, oleic, and soy oils.
[b] Similac 20 Low Iron contains 1.5 mg iron/liter.
[c] Enfamil 20 Low Iron contains 1.1 mg iron/liter.
[d] SMA LO-IRON contains 1.5 mg iron/liter.
[e] MCT = medium-chain triglycerides.
[f] Special Care 24 Low-Iron 3.0 mg iron/liter.
[g] Low iron formula.

(continued)

TABLE 8-3. COMPOSITION OF INFANT FORMULAS (continued)

Characteristics	"Preemie" SMA 20		"Preemie" SMA 24		Nursoy 20		Alimentum	
Calories per liter	676		810		676		676	
Osmolality (mosm/kg water)	268		280		296		370	
Osmolarity (mosm/liter)	242		246		266		330	
Protein								
Grams per liter	20		20		21		18.6	
Percent total calories	11.9		9.6		12.3		11	
Source	Nonfat milk, demineralized whey		Nonfat milk, demineralized whey		Soy protein isolate		Casein hydrolysate, cystine, tyrosine, tryptophan	
Fat								
Grams per liter	35		44		36		37.5	
Percent total calories	46.7		48.5		47.4		48	
Source	Oils: soy, coconut, oleic, oleo and MCT		Oils: soy, coconut, oleic, oleo and MCT		Oils: soy, coconut, oleo and oleic		Oils: soy, safflower, MCT	
Carbohydrate								
Grams per liter	70		86		69		46.2	
Percent total calories	41.5		41.9		40.3		42	
Source	Lactose and glucose polymers		Lactose and glucose polymers		Sucrose		Sucrose and modified tapioca starch	
Minerals	mg/L	meq/L	mg/L	meq/L	mg/L	meq/L	mg/L	meq/L
Calcium	750	37.4	750	37.4	600	29.9	710	35.4
Chloride	530	14.9	530	14.9	375	10.6	540	15.3
Iodine	0.083		0.083		0.060		0.100	
Iron	3		3		11.5		12	
Magnesium	70		70		67		51	
Phosphorus	380		400		420		510	
Potassium	750	19.2	750	19.2	700	17.9	800	20.5
Sodium	320	13.9	320	13.9	200	8.7	300	13
Zinc	8		8		5		5.1	
Vitamins per liter								
Vitamin A (IU)	3200		2400		2000		2030	
Vitamin B$_1$ (mg)	0.80		0.800		0.67		0.41	
Vitamin B$_2$ (mg)	1.30		1.30		1.0		0.61	
Vitamin B$_6$ (mg)	0.50		0.410		0.42		0.41	
Vitamin B$_{12}$ (μg)	2.0		2.0		2.0		3.0	
Vitamin C (mg)	70		70		55		60	
Vitamin D (IU)	510		480		400		260	
Vitamin E (IU)	15		15		9.5		20	
Vitamin K (μg)	70		70		100		100	
Folic acid (μg)	100		100		50		100	
Niacin (mg)	6.3		6.3		5.0		9.13	
Pantothenic acid (mg)	3.60		3.60		3.0		5.07	

a Oleo, coconut, oleic, and soy oils.
b Similac 20 Low Iron contains 1.5 mg iron/liter.
c Enfamil 20 Low Iron contains 1.1 mg iron/liter.
d SMA LO-IRON contains 1.5 mg iron/liter.
e MCT = medium-chain triglycerides.
f Special Care 24 Low-Iron 3.0 mg iron/liter.
g Low iron formula.

    2. Hypoosmolar formulas (< 270 mosm/kg H_2O) have a lower osmolality, which can improve feeding tolerance.

        a. Similac 13, with an osmolality of 200 mosm/kg H_2O, was specifically designed as a conservative initial feeding for infants who have not been fed enterally for several days or weeks. It is not suitable for long-term feeding because it does not meet the nutrient needs of most infants.

        b. Other hypoosmolar formulas include most of the premature formulas that contain 20 cal/oz (Similac Special Care 20, Enfamil Premature Formula 20, "preemie" SMA 20), which are designed to be better tolerated by premature infants and satisfy nutritional requirements.

    3. Hyperosmolar formulas (> 300 mosm/kg H_2O) are 24 and 27 cal/oz formulas with the exception of the isoosmolar, 24 cal/oz premature formulas. Formulas such as Similac 24, Enfamil 24, SMA 24, Similac 27, and SMA 27 are hypercaloric formulas designed to provide a greater percentage of the calories as protein and provide increased mineral concentrations. They are used for infants on fluid restriction in order to provide nutritional needs.

B. General guidelines

    1. Initial feedings. Use sterile water or D_5W if the infant is not being breast-fed. $D_{10}W$ should not be used because it is an hypertonic solution.

    2. Subsequent feedings. Controversy surrounds dilution of infant formulas for the next several feedings if the infant tolerates the initial feeding. Some clinicians advocate diluting formulas with sterile water and advance as tolerated (eg, 1/4, 1/2, and then 3/4 strength). Others practitioners believe this is unnecessary and that full-strength formula can be used if the infant tolerates the initial feeding without difficulty. Breast milk is never diluted.

C. Specific guidelines based on **birth weight** and **gestational age** (GA) are presented in this section. For an infant presumed to be at risk for NEC, the rate of enteral feeding advancement should not exceed 20 mL/kg/d and 10 cal/kg/d.

    1. Weight less than 1200 g, GA less than 30 weeks. Gavage feeding through a nasogastric tube is appropriate.

        a. Type of formula

            (1) Initial feeding: Similac 13, diluted premature formulas.

            (2) Maintenance feeding: Premature formulas (20 or 24 cal/oz).

        b. Initial feeding. Give sterile water 0.5–1 mL/h. If tolerated, use initial formula (see above, **1.a**).

        c. Subsequent feedings

            (1) Volume. Give 0.5–1.0 mL/h continuously and increase by 0.5–1.0 mL every other shift. When 10 mL/h is tolerated, change feedings to every 2 hours and advance as tolerated.

            (2) Strength. Use Similac 13 or diluted premature formula for 24–48 hours, and then advance to premature formula. Once full feedings of 20 cal/oz are tolerated, consider advancing to 24 cal/oz feedings.

    2. Weight 1200–1500 g, GA less than 32 weeks. Gavage feeding through a nasogastric tube should be used.

        a. Type of formula. See above **1.a**.

        b. Initial feeding. Give sterile water 2 mL/kg every 2 hours and if tolerated for 4 hours, begin formula.

        c. Subsequent feedings

            (1) Volume. Give 2 mL/kg every 2 hours, and increase by 1 mL every shift up to 20 mL every 2 hours. Then change to feedings every 3 hours.

            (2) Strength. Use Similac 13 or diluted premature formulas for 24 hours and then advance to premature formulas. Once full feedings of 20 cal/oz are tolerated, advance to 24 cal/oz if desired.

    3. Weight 1500–2000 g. Use gavage feeding through a nasogastric tube. A bottle can be attempted if the infant is > 1600 g, > 34 weeks' gestation, and is neurologically intact.

        a. Type of formula. Use premature formulas (usually diluted the first 24 hours). For infants over 1800 g, regular formula may be considered (controversial).

  b. Initial feeding. Give sterile water, 2.5 mL/kg. If tolerated, begin regular formula.

  c. Subsequent feedings. Give 2.5 mL/kg every 3 hours and advance as tolerated.

  4. Weight 2000–2500 g. GA > 36 weeks. Use bottle if infant is neurologically intact.

  a. Type of formula. Use standard formula.

  b. Initial feeding. Give sterile water, 2.5 mL/kg. If tolerated, begin formula or breast milk.

  c. Subsequent feedings. Give 5 mL/kg every 3–4 hours and advance as tolerated.

  5. Weight more than 2500 g. Use bottle if infant is neurologically intact.

  a. Type of formula. Use standard formula.

  b. Initial feeding. See p 86, **4.b.**

  c. Subsequent feedings. Feed every 3–4 hours and advance as tolerated. Use 5 mL/kg; advance 2–5 mL per feeding.

III. Management of feeding intolerance. If feeding is initiated but not tolerated, a complete abdominal examination should be performed. Consider abdominal x-ray studies if physical findings are suspicious. If the abdominal evaluation is normal:

  A. Attempt continuous feedings with a nasogastric or orogastric tube. Check the gastric aspirate and follow the recommendations presented in Chapter 32.

  B. Use a different formula (eg, PM 60/40, Pregestimil) or breast milk, which may be better tolerated. Occasionally, diluting a formula with sterile water is successful (start at 1/4 strength and advance slowly to 1/2 strength, 3/4 strength, and full strength).

IV. Nutritional supplements. Supplements are sometimes added to feedings, primarily to increase caloric intake (Table 8–4). They provide additional energy supplies with no concomitant increase in fluid volume. Some clinicians feel strongly that any necessary caloric supplementation needed should be given as a high-calorie formula (ie, 24 kcal/oz) instead of as a supplement because all nutrients in such a formula are in proportion to one another and allow maximum absorption. Nutritional supplements are often used in infants with bronchopulmonary dysplasia who are not gaining weight and need additional calories with no increase in protein, fat, or water intake.

BREAST-FEEDING

  I. Advantages

  A. Protein quality. The predominance of whey and mixture of amino acids is compatible with the metabolic needs of low-birth-weight infants.

  B. Digestion and absorption are improved with breast milk.

  C. Immunologic benefits. Breast-feeding provides immunologic protection against bacterial and viral infection (particularly upper respiratory tract and gastrointestinal infection). Studies of infants breast-fed more than 6 months show that they have a decreased incidence of cancer.

  D. Promotion of bonding between the mother and infant.

  E. Lower renal solute load, which facilitates better tolerance.

  F. Other advantages. Breast-feeding in preterm infants has been associated with a decreased risk for NEC and a significantly higher intelligence quotient (IQ) at the age of 8 years. The risk of breast and ovarian cancer in the mother also appears to be lower.

  II. Contraindications

  A. Active tuberculosis in the mother.

  B. Certain viral and bacterial infections in the mother. See Appendix G, Isolation Guidelines, for specific recommendations.

  C. Use of medications that are passed in significant amount in the breast milk,

TABLE 8-4. NUTRITIONAL SUPPLEMENTS USED IN INFANTS

Supplement	Nutrient Content	Calories	Indications and Contraindications	Amount to Use
CARBOHYDRATE				
Polycose	Glucose polymers	3.8 kcal/g powder; 2 kcal/mL liquid	Calorie supplementation[a]	**Powder** 0.5 g/oz of 20-cal formula = 22 cal/oz; 1 g/oz of 20-cal formula = 24 cal/oz **Liquid** 1 mL to 1 oz of 20 cal formula = 22 cal/oz
Infant rice cereal	Rice	15 cal/tbs	Thickens feedings	1 tsp/4 oz formula
FAT				
Medium-chain triglyceride (MCT) oil	Lipid fraction of coconut oil	8.3 kcal/g, 7.7 cal/mL	Limit to 50% calories from fat to prevent ketosis; may cause diarrhea; do not use if infant has BPD due to risk of aspiration pneumonia[b]	0.5 mL/4 oz formula = 21 cal/oz; 1 mL/4 oz formula = 22 cal/oz
Vegetable oil	Soy, corn oil	9.0 cal/g (120 cal/tbs)	To increase calories if fat absorption normal[c]	See MCT above
PROTEIN				
Casec	Calcium caseinate	3.4 cal/g (4 g protein/tbs)	Useful in chronic fluid restriction and as breast milk supplement; do not use in premature infants due to high solute load	

[a] Limiting formula intake while increasing calories may compromise protein, vitamin, and mineral intake, which may also lead to hyperglycemia and diarrhea.

[b] Always mix with formula to avoid possibility of lipid aspiration and/or pneumonia.

[c] Vitamin E may need to be increased to at least 1 IU per gram linoleic acid.

which may harm the infant. See Chapter 74 for the effects of medications and substances on lactation and breast-feeding.

III. **Possible contraindications**
   A. Poorly developed sucking reflex in a preterm infant that may not be able to nurse.
   B. A weak or ill infant or one with a cleft lip or palate that may have difficulty. In some cases, the mother can express her milk with a breast pump and it can be bottle-fed to the infant.
   C. Inadequate amounts of protein, sodium, calcium, phosphorus and vitamin D to match intrauterine growth of very low birth weight (< 1500 g) infants. Supplementation may be necessary.
   Note: Temporary problems (eg, sore or cracked nipples, mastitis) resolve with treatment (eg, antibiotics for mastitis) and do not preclude nursing.

IV. **Donor breast milk.** The use of donor breast milk is both regional and controversial. Donor milk is almost always mature breast milk and should be used only until the infant can tolerate formula with adequate vitamin and mineral content. If the mother is unable to provide breast milk for an infant who needs it, breast milk from a donor can be obtained from a human milk bank and bottle-fed to the infant. (The mother's milk is always preferable to donor milk unless contraindicated for one of the reasons given above.)
   A. **Storage.** Breast milk can be stored frozen at –20 °C for up to 6 months and refrigerated at 4 °C for up to 24 hours.
   B. **Screening of breast milk donors.**
      1. Potential donors are screened for chronic disease. The tuberculin skin test must be negative.
         a. The donor's blood must be negative for hepatitis core antibody and surface antigen and HTLV-III antibody.
         b. A history of sexually transmitted disease or infection caused by herpes virus makes the donor unacceptable.
         c. Donors must not be taking any medication, must be nonsmokers, and must limit alcohol intake to 60 mL/d.
      2. Once donors are accepted, they are taught sterile techniques for milk collection.
   C. **Acceptable bacteria levels in donor breast milk.** Samples are tested from each donor for colony-forming units and specific pathogenic organisms. Acceptable standards for raw milk are less than 10,000 colony-forming units per milliliter and no *Staphylococcus aureus* and gram-negative rods. Pasteurization is required if the milk does not meet these standards. Breast milk is not checked for viruses. Cytomegalovirus is destroyed by freezing for more than 7 days.

V. **Breast milk fortifiers (supplements).** The breast milk fortifiers (Table 8–5) are designed as a supplement to be added to mother's milk in rapidly growing premature infants. Preterm human milk beyond the second and third week may contain insufficient amounts of protein, calcium, phosphorus, and, possibly, copper, zinc, and sodium. Clinical experience has shown that the addition of human milk fortifier to a preterm mother's milk resulted in increased somatic growth related to increased protein and energy intake but no regular improvement in mineral retention. Periodic monitoring of urine osmolality, serum blood urea nitrogen, creatinine, and calcium are required. Two fortifiers are currently available.
   A. **Enfamil Human Milk Fortifier**
      1. **Indications.** This is indicated for those premature infants who tolerate unfortified human milk at full feedings, usually at 2–4 weeks of age, up to time of discharge or birth weight 2500–3000 g.
      2. **Composition.** The protein is 60% whey protein and 40% casein, which is similar to breast milk. The carbohydrate is 75% glucose polymers and 25% lactose. The fat is negligible. This fortifier comes in a powder form.
      3. **Calories.** One packet of fortifier added to 50 mL of human milk provides an additional 2 cal/fl oz. The same amount of fortifier added to 25 mL of human milk supplies an additional 4 cal/fl oz.

TABLE 8-5. A COMPARISON OF 2 COMMERCIALLY AVAILABLE BREAST MILK SUPPLEMENTS

	Similac Natural Care (Ross)	Enfamil Human Milk Fortifier (Mead Johnson)
Volume	100 mL (50 mL breast milk plus 50 mL forti-fier)	100 mL (4 packets fortifier plus 100 mL breast milk)
Total calories	73 (24 cal/oz)	81 (24 cal/oz)
Osmolality (mosm/kg water)	300	365
	These supplements add the following to the breast milk	
Calories	9	14
Protein	0.1 g	0.7 g
Fat	0.4 g	0.04 g
Carbohydrate	1.3 g	2.7 g
Minerals		
Calcium	71 mg	60 mg
Chloride	9 mg	17.7
Copper	62 μg	40 μg
Iron	0.1 mg	—
Magnesium	3.4 mg	4 mg
Phosphorus	36 mg	33 mg
Potassium	28 mg	15.6 mg
Sodium	8 mg	7 mg
Vitamins per liter		
Vitamin A (IU)	150	780
Vitamin B_1 (μg)	96	187
Vitamin B_2 (μg)	233	250
Vitamin B_6 (μg)	99	193
Vitamin B_{12} (μg)	0.2	0.21
Vitamin C (mg)	12.8	24
Vitamin D (IU)	58.8	210
Vitamin E (IU)	1.3	3.4
Vitamin K (μg)	4.0	9.1
Folic Acid (μg)	12.8	23
Niacin (μg)	1920	3100
Pantothenic acid (μg)	640	790

Once the powder is added to the milk, the container should be capped and mixed well. It can be covered and stored under refrigeration but should be used within 8 hours.

4. Hypercalcemia has been reported in some extremely low birth weight infants (< 1000 g). For those infants, serum calcium needs to be monitored. Fortification of breast milk should never start below 2 weeks postnatal age at a ratio not exceeding 1 packet of fortifier per 25 mL of breast milk.

B. **Similac Natural Care**
   1. **Indications.** Same as on p 88, **A.1.**
   2. **Composition.** The protein is whey predominant. The carbohydrate is lactose and glucose polymers in equal amounts. The fat is a mixture of 50% medium-chain triglycerides, 30% soy oil, and 20% coconut oil. This fortifier is a ready-to-use liquid formula that can be mixed with human milk.
   3. **Calories.** Similac Natural Care contains 24 cal/fl oz. It is most commonly diluted with human milk in a 1:1 proportion. Storage requirements are the same as on p 88, **3.**

TOTAL PARENTERAL NUTRITION

Total parenteral nutrition (TPN) is intravenous administration of all nutrients (fats, carbohydrates, proteins, vitamins, and minerals) necessary for metabolic requirements and growth. Parenteral nutrition (PN) is supplemental intravenous administration of nutrients. Enteral nutrition (EN) is oral or gavage feedings.

I. Intravenous routes used in PN

A. Central parenteral nutrition. Central parenteral nutrition is usually reserved for patients requiring long-term (> 2 weeks) administration of most calories. Basically, this type of nutrition involves infusion of a hypertonic nutrient solution (15–25% dextrose) into a vessel with rapid flow through an indwelling catheter, the tip of which is in the vena cava just above or beyond the right atrium. Disadvantages include increased risk of infection and complications from placement. Two methods are commonly used for placement.

   1. A percutaneous catheter, positioned in the antecubital or external jugular vein or saphenous vein, is advanced into the superior or inferior vena cava. This technique avoids surgical placement and results in fewer complications. (See Chapter 25 for details of the procedure.)

   2. The catheter (Broviac) can be placed through a surgical cutdown in the internal or external jugular or subclavian vein. The proximal portion of the catheter (which has a polyvinyl cuff to promote fibroblast proliferation for securing the catheter) is tunneled subcutaneously to exit some distance from the insertion site, usually the anterior chest. This protects the catheter from inadvertent dislodgment and reduces the risk of contamination by microorganisms. The anesthesia and surgery needed for placement of the catheter are disadvantages to this method.

B. Peripheral parenteral nutrition. This route [which uses a peripheral vein] is more common in the neonatal intensive care unit (NICU) than central parenteral nutrition and is usually associated with fewer complications. The maximum concentration of dextrose that can be administered using this method is 12.5%.

Note: Parenteral nutrition can be given through an umbilical artery catheter, and this route has been used in some centers. However, the umbilical artery is not a preferred site and should be used with caution.

II. Indications.
PN is used as a supplement to enteral feedings or as a complete substitution (TPN) when adequate nourishment cannot be achieved by the enteral route. Common indications in neonates include congenital malformation of the gastrointestinal tract, gastroschisis, meconium ileus, short bowel syndrome, NEC, paralytic ileus, respiratory distress syndrome, extreme prematurity, sepsis, and malabsorption. PN is usually started on day 3 or 4 of life, depending on the severity of the patient's illness.

III. Caloric concentration.
Caloric densities of various energy sources are as follows:

Dextrose (anhydrous)	3.4 kcal/g
Protein	4 kcal/g
Fat	9 kcal/g
10% fat emulsion	1.1 kcal/mL
20% fat emulsion	2 kcal/mL

IV. Composition of PN solutions

A. Carbohydrates

   1. The only commercially available carbohydrate source is dextrose (glucose). A solution of 5.0–12.5 g/dL is used in peripheral PN and up to 25 g/dL in central PN. Dextrose concentrations should be calculated as milligrams per kilograms per minute.

   2. To allow for an appropriate response of endogenous insulin and to prevent the development of osmotic diuresis secondary to glucosuria, neonates should not routinely be started on more than 6–8 mg/kg/min of dextrose. Frequent testing of urine for the presence of glucose is required. Infusion rates can be increased by 0.5–1 mg/kg/min each day as tolerated to achieve adequate caloric intake. See p 74 for the formula used in calculating the amount of glucose in milligrams per kilogram per minute that an infant is receiving.

B. Proteins. Inadequate protein intake may result in failure to thrive, hypoalbuminemia, and edema. Excessive protein can cause hyperammonemia, serum amino acid imbalance, metabolic acidosis, and cholestatic jaundice.

1. Two kinds of crystalline amino acid solutions are available as nitrogen sources. The standard solutions originally designed for adults are not ideal as they contain high concentrations of amino acids that are potentially neurotoxic in premature infants (glycine, methionine, and phenylalanine). Pediatric crystalline amino acid solutions (TrophAmine and Aminosyn-PF) are available, which contain less of those potentially neurotoxic amino acids as well as additional tyrosine, cystine, and taurine. These pediatric solutions also have a lower pH to allow for the addition of sufficient quantities of calcium (2 meq/dL) and phosphorus (1–2 mm/dL) in order to meet daily requirements.

   Note: It is no longer necessary, except in very low birth weight infants, to gradually increase the protein concentration of PN over several days (Kerner, 1983).

2. Amino acids should not be started unless a minimum of 40 cal/kg/d are given as glucose because the amino acids will be poorly utilized and acidosis and hyperammonemia will develop. Amino acids can be started at a rate of 0.5 g/kg/d in infants weighing less than 1500 g and increased by increments of 0.5 g/kg/d. In term infants, the starting rate can be 1.5 g, with increases of 1 g/kg/d. To avoid hyperammonemia and acidosis, the final concentration should not exceed 3 g/kg/d. At most institutions, amino acid solutions are prepared in 1%, 2%, and 3% concentrations. This works out to the following equivalents:

   100 mL/kg/d of 1% solution = 1 g/kg/d protein
   100 mL/kg/d of 2% solution = 2 g/kg/d protein
   100 mL/kg/d of 3% solution = 3 g/kg/d protein

C. Fats. Because of their high caloric density, intravenous fat solutions (eg, Intralipid, Lyposyn II, Nutralipid, Soyacal) provide a significant portion of daily caloric needs. Most intravenous fat solutions are isotonic (270–300 mosm/L) and are therefore not likely to increase the risk of infiltration of peripheral lines. When administering fat solutions to neonates with unconjugated hyperbilirubinemia, caution may be needed because of the competitive binding of bilirubin and nonesterified fatty acids on albumin, which may increase significantly during infusion.

1. **Concentrations.** Lipid emulsions are supplied either as 10% or 20% solutions providing 10 or 20 grams of triglyceride, respectively. A common regimen is 0.5 g/kg/d on the first day, 1 g/kg/d on the second day, and 2 g/kg/d (maintenance dose) on the third day. The infusion is given continuously over 24 hours, and the rate should not exceed 0.12 g/kg/h. For example, in an infant weighing 2 kg who is to start at an amount of 0.5 g/kg/d:

   2 kg × 0.5 g/kg/d = 1 g/d
   1 mL of 10% Intralipid = 0.1 g
   1 mL/0.1 g = X mL/g
   0.1 X = 1
   X = 10 mL.

   This infant should receive a total of 10 mL of 10% Intralipid in a 24-hour period to equal 0.5 g/kg/d.

   The volume (eg, 10 mL) is divided by 24 hours. It should run at 0.4 mL/h × 24 hours.

   In the very low birth weight infant (< 1000 g) the 20% emulsion is recommended because of the excessive phospholipids liposomes present in the 10% solution.

2. **Complications.** Fat intolerance (hyperlipidemia) may be seen. "Lipidcrits" (checks of the serum for cloudiness caused by excessive fats) are only of value when positive. If negative, blood triglyceride levels should be moni-

TABLE 8-6. RECOMMENDATIONS FOR TRACE ELEMENT SUPPLEMENTATION IN TPN SOLUTIONS FOR NEONATES

Element	Full term	Premature
Zinc (μg)	100–200	400–600
Copper (μg)	10–20	20
Chromium (μg)	0.14–0.2	0.14–0.2
Manganese (μg)	2–10	2–10
Fluoride (μg)	1	1*
Iodine (μg)	3–5	3–5*

* Not well defined in the premature infant.

tored. Such levels should be kept below 150 mg/dL when the child is jaundiced and less than 200 mg/dL otherwise. The infusion of fats should be decreased or stopped when those levels are exceeded.

D. **Vitamins.** Vitamins are added to intravenous solutions in the form of a pediatric multivitamin suspension (MVI Pediatric) based on recommendations by the Nutritional Advisory Committee of American Academy of Pediatrics. The dose of parenteral vitamins for preterm infants should be 2 mL/kg of the 5 mL reconstituted MVI pediatric sterile lyophilized powder.

E. **Trace elements.** Trace elements are added to the solution based on weight and total volume (0.5 mL/kg/wk) for infants on short-term TPN and 0.5 mL/kg/d for long-term TPN. Increased amounts of zinc (1–2 mg/d) are often given to patients who require gastrointestinal surgery to help promote healing. At many institutions, a prepared solution is available. See Table 8–6 for recommended doses of trace elements.

F. **Electrolytes.** Electrolytes can be added according to specific needs, but for low-birth-weight-infants, requirements are usually satisfied by standard amino acid solution formulations that contain electrolytes (Table 8–7).

V. **Monitoring of PN.** Hyperalimentation can cause many alterations in biochemical function. Thus, compulsive anthropometric and laboratory monitoring is essential for all patients. Recommendations are given in Table 8–8.

VI. **Complications of PN.** Most complications of TPN are associated with use of central hyperalimentation and primarily involve infections and catheterization problems. However, metabolic difficulties can occur with both central and peripheral TPN. The major complication of peripheral hyperalimentation is accidental infiltration of the solution, which causes sloughing of the skin.

A. **Infection.** Sepsis can occur in infants receiving central hyperalimentation. The most common organisms include coagulase-positive and coagulase-negative

TABLE 8-7. COMPOSITION OF AMINO ACID SOLUTIONS FOR LOW BIRTH WEIGHT INFANTS—STANDARD FORMULATIONS

Electrolytes (meq/L)	Amino Acid Concentration					
	1.0%		2.0%		3.0%	
	A[a]	T[b]	A	T	A	T
Na$^+$	20	20	20	20	20	20
Cl$^-$	20	20	20	20	20	20
K$^+$	15	15	15	15	15	15
Mg^{++}	11	11	11	11	11	11
Ca^{++}	15	15	15	15	15	15
Acetate	7.6	9.3	15.3	18.6	22.8	27.9
Phosphorus (mmol/L)	10	10	10	10	10	10

[a] A = Aminosyn PF.
[b] T = TrophAmine.

TABLE 8-8. MONITORING SCHEDULE FOR NEONATES RECEIVING PARENTERAL NUTRITION

Measurement	Baseline Study	Frequency of Measurement
Anthropometric		
Weight	Yes	Daily
Length	Yes	Weekly
Head circumference	Yes	Daily
Metabolic		
Glucose	Yes	Daily
(Dextrostix when changing detrose concentrations)		
Calcium and phosphorus	Yes	Twice per week initially, then weekly
Electrolytes (Na, Cl, K, CO_2)	Yes	Once a day for 3 days, then twice a week
Magnesium	Yes	Weekly
Hematocrit	Yes	Every other day for 1 week, then weekly
BUN and creatinine	Yes	Twice a week, then weekly
Bilirubin	Yes	Weekly
Ammonia	Yes	Weekly if using high protein
Total protein and albumin	Yes	Weekly
SGOT or SGPT	Yes	Weekly
Triglycerides	Yes	Weekly for patients on intravenous fat
Urine		
Specific gravity and glucose	Yes	For first week, test each urine sample; then once/shift

Staphylococcus, Streptococcus viridans, Escherichia coli, Pseudomonas spp, *Klebsiella* spp, and *Candida albicans.* Contamination of the central line can occur as a result of infection at the insertion site or use of the line for blood sampling or administration of blood. It is best not to open the line.

B. Catheterization-associated problems. Complications associated with placement of central catheters (specifically in the subclavian vein) occur in approximately 4–9% of patients. Complications include pneumothorax, pneumomediastinum, hemorrhage, and chylothorax (caused by injury to the thoracic duct). Thrombosis of the vein adjacent to the catheter tip, resulting in "superior vena cava syndrome" (edema of the face, neck, and eyes), may be seen. Pulmonary embolism can also occur secondary to thrombosis. Malpositioned catheters may result in collection of fluid in the pleural cavity, causing hydrothorax, or in the pericardial space, causing tamponade.

C. Metabolic complications

1. **Hyperglycemia:** resulting from excessive intake or change in metabolic rate such as infection.
2. **Hypoglycemia** from sudden cessation of infusion (secondary to intravenous infiltration).
3. **Azotemia** from excessive protein (nitrogen) uptake.
4. **Hyperammonemia.** All currently available amino acid mixtures contain adequate arginine (> 0.05 mmol/kg/d) so that if an increase in blood ammonia can be seen, symptomatic hyperammonemia does not occur.
5. **Abnormal serum and tissue amino acid pattern.**
6. **Mild metabolic alkalosis.**
7. **Cholestatic liver disease.** With prolonged administration of intravenous dextrose and protein and absence of enteral feeding, cholestasis usually occurs. The incidence ranges from as high as 80% in very low birth weight infants receiving TPN for more than 30 days (with no enteral feeding) to 15% or lower in neonates weighing more than 1500 g receiving TPN for 14 days or less. Monitoring for abnormalities in liver function and the development of direct hyperbilirubinemia is important in long-term TPN.

   a. Bacterial infection may play a significant role in its occurrence.

   b. The use of amino acid mixtures designed to maintain normal plasma amino acid patterns and early starting (as soon as possible) of enteral feedings in small amounts may help alleviate this problem.

8. **Complications of fat administration.** Infusion of fat emulsion has been associated with several metabolic disturbances, hyperlipidemia, platelet dysfunction, acute allergic reactions, deposition of pigment in the liver, and lipid deposition in the blood vessels of the lung. Most metabolic problems apparently occur with rapid rates of infusion and are not seen at infusion rates of less than 0.12 g/kg/h.

9. **Fatty acid deficiencies.**

   a. If PN is administered without adding fat emulsion, deficiency of essential fatty acids may occur. This deficiency is associated with decreased platelet aggregation (thromboxane A_2 deficiency), poor weight gain, scaly rash, sparse hair growth, and thrombocytopenia. These problems usually occur after 10 days in full-term infants and after 2 days in preterm infants.

   b. The absence of long-chain polyunsaturated fatty acids (omega-3 and omega-6 fatty acids) in the available lipid emulsions is of concern. These fatty acids may be essential to the developing eyes and brain of the human neonate.

10. **Mineral deficiency.** Most minerals are transferred to the fetus during the last trimester of pregnancy. The following problems may occur.

    a. Osteopenia, rickets, and pathologic fractures (see Chapter 70).

    b. Zinc deficiency occurs if zinc is not added to TPN after 4 weeks. Infants with this deficiency can present with poor growth, diarrhea, alopecia, increased susceptibility to infection, and skin desquamation surrounding the mouth and anus (acrodermatitis enteropathica). Zinc losses are increased in patients with an ileostomy or colostomy.

    c. Infants with copper deficiency presents with osteoporosis, hemolytic anemia, neutropenia, and depigmentation of the skin.

CALORIC CALCULATIONS

An infant should receive 100–120 kcal/kg/d for growth. (Infants require fewer calories [80–90 cal/kg/d] if receiving TPN only.) Some hypermetabolic infants may require more than 120 kcal/kg/d. For maintenance of a positive nitrogen balance, 60–80 kcal/kg/d by oral intake are necessary. Equations for calculation of caloric intake for oral formula and TPN follow:

I. **Infant formulas.** Most standard infant formulas contain 0.67 kcal/mL. Specific caloric concentrations of formulas are given in Table 8–3. To calculate total daily calories, use the following equation:

$$\text{kcal/kg/d} = \frac{\text{kcal/mL} \times \text{Total mL of formula}}{\text{Weight (kg)}}$$

II. **Carbohydrates.** If only dextrose infusion is given, the total daily caloric intake is calculated as shown below. (See Table 8–9 for caloric concentration of common solutions.)

$$\text{kcal/kg/d} = \frac{\text{mL solution/h} \times 24\text{ h} \times \text{kcal in solution}}{\text{Weight (kg)}}$$

III. **Proteins.** Use the same formula given for carbohydrates (see above) and the caloric concentrations given in Table 8–9.

IV. **Fat emulsions.** A 10% fat emulsion (Intralipid) contains 1.1 kcal/mL; a 20% emulsion, 2 kcal/mL. Use the following formula to calculate daily caloric intake supplied by Intralipid 10%.

$$\text{kcal/kg/d} = \frac{\text{Total mL/d of solution} \times 1.1\text{ kcal/mL}}{\text{Weight (kg)}}$$

TABLE 8–9. CALORIC CONCENTRATIONS OF VARIOUS PARENTERAL SOLUTIONS

Dextrose Solutions (Anhydrous) in kcal/mL	
D5 = 0.17	D15 = 0.51
D7.5 = 0.255	D20 = 0.68
D10 = 0.34	D25 = 0.85
D12.5 = 0.425	

Protein Solutions (g/d)	Percent Concentration	Caloric Concentration (kcal/mL)
0.5 g	0.5%	0.02
1.0 g	1%	0.04
1.5 g	1.5%	0.06
2.0 g	2.0%	0.08
2.5 g	2.5%	0.10
3.0 g	3.0%	0.12
(0.5% solution, if given 100 mL/d = 0.5 g protein/d)		

REFERENCES

Barnes LA (editor): *Pediatric Nutrition Handbook,* 3rd ed. American Academy of Pediatrics, 1993.

Fitzgerald KA, MacKay MW: Calcium and phosphate solubility in neonatal parenteral nutrient solutions containing TrophAmine. *Am J Hosp Pharm* 1986:**43:**88.

Hartge P, et al: A case control study of epithelial ovarian cancer. *Am J Obstet Gynecol* 1989:**161:**10.

Kerner JA Jr (editor): *Manual of Pediatric Parenteral Nutrition.* Wiley, 1983.

Merritt RJ: Cholestasis associated with total parenteral nutrition. *J Pediatr Gastroenterol Nutr* 1986;**5:**9.

Moore MC et al: Evaluation of pediatric multiple vitamin preparation for total parenteral nutrition in infants and children. 1. Blood levels of water-soluble vitamins. *Pediatrics* 1986:**77:**530.

Lucas A: Enteral Nutrition. In: *Nutritional Needs of the Preterm Infant. Scientific Basis and Practical Guidelines.* Tsang RC et al (editors). In: Williams & Wilkins, 1993.

Heird WC, Gomez MC: Parenteral Nutrition. *Nutritional Needs of the Preterm Infant. Scientific Basis and Practical Guidelines.* Tsang RC (editor). Williams & Wilkins, 1993.

9 Neonatal Radiology

COMMON RADIOLOGIC TECHNIQUES

I. **X-ray studies.** The need for x-rays must always be weighed against the risks of neonatal exposure to radiation (3–5 mrem per x-ray). No studies on infant exposure to radiation in neonatal intensive care units (NICUs) have been performed. However, 1000 rem delivered to the mother causes abortion of the fetus. The infant's gonads should be shielded as much as possible, and any person holding the infant during the x-ray procedure should also wear a protective shield. Individuals standing 6–10 feet from the x-ray machine receive negligible radiation, as 10 feet is the maximum "scatter" area for x-rays.

A. **Chest x-rays**

1. **The anteroposterior (AP) view** is the single best view for identification of heart or lung disease or verification of endotracheal tube placement. It also is the best view to obtain in an emergency if an air leak is suspected.

2. **The cross-table lateral view** can be used to diagnose pneumothorax in conjunction with an AP view. It does not show which side the pneumothorax is on, however.

3. **The lateral decubitus view** is best for ruling out a small pneumothorax or one that is difficult to assess on the AP view. In a newborn infant the denser tissue of the lung tends to collapse posteriorly. For example, if a pneumothorax is on the left side, a right lateral decubitus view of the chest should be obtained, with the infant placed on the right side with the left side up. An air pocket is visible on the side on which the pneumothorax is present. The only disadvantages of the lateral decubitus view are (1) that it is sometimes difficult to perform in unstable infants and (2) that it takes more time than a regular AP view.

4. **The upright view,** which is rarely used in the NICU, can identify abdominal perforation by showing free air under the diaphragm.

B. **Abdominal x-rays**

1. **AP view** is the single best view for diagnosis of abdominal disorders and checking placement of umbilical artery and vein catheters.

2. **The cross-table lateral view** helps diagnose abdominal perforation, but the left lateral decubitus view is better for this purpose. Abdominal perforations may be missed.

3. **The left lateral decubitus view** (infant placed on the left side with the right side up) is best for diagnosis of perforation. Free intra-abdominal air, which is visible as an air pocket above the liver, is associated with perforation or recent abdominal surgery.

C. **Barium contrast studies (barium swallow, barium enema).** Barium sulfate, an inert compound, is not absorbed from the gastrointestinal tract. It does not cause fluid shifts except in infants in whom the possibility of barium retention in the colon, where water may be absorbed, is high.

1. **Indications.** The use of barium as a contrast agent is recommended for:

a. **Gastrointestinal (GI) tract imaging.** Barium enema is used to rule out lower abdominal obstruction.

b. **Suspected esophageal atresia** with or without tracheoesophageal fistula. Barium swallow is rarely used. However, most esophageal atresias can be diagnosed by inserting a radiopaque nasogastric tube; the tube will be seen curled up in the blind esophageal pouch. If additional confirmation is required, air can be injected under fluoroscopy to distend the pouch.

   c. Suspected esophageal perforation. Barium swallow is used if previous studies with water-soluble agents have been negative.

   d. Suspected gastroesophageal reflux. Barium swallow is used as the first-line study.

   2. **Contraindications.** Barium-contrast studies are not recommended in infants with **suspected abdominal perforation,** because barium is irritating to the peritoneum and can result in "barium peritonitis."

D. High-osmolality water-soluble contrast studies

   1. **Advantages** of these agents (Hypaque or Gastrograffin) over barium

      a. These materials are not toxic to the peritoneum if they leak from the GI tract, and they are absorbed and cleared from the body.

      b. Because these agents draw water into the bowel lumen, they may be used therapeutically to relieve some cases of bowel obstruction or treat meconium ileus.

   2. **Disadvantages**

      a. Severe fluid shifts may occur. Thus fluid and electrolyte status must be followed closely if these agents are used.

      b. These materials are extremely toxic if they are aspirated into the lungs.

      c. Necrotizing enterocolitis resulting in death has been reported. Bowel necrosis has rarely occurred following the use of these agents for meconium ileus.

   3. **Indications**

      a. Evaluation of the bowel if perforation is suspected.

      b. Differentiation of ileus from obstruction.

      c. Treatment of meconium obstruction syndromes.

E. Low-osmolality water-soluble contrast agents. These agents (metrizamide, iohexol iopamidol, and ioxaglate) have many advantages over barium and the high-osmolality contrast agents.

   1. **Advantages**

      a. These agents do not cause fluid shifts.

      b. If bowel perforation is present, these substances are nontoxic to the peritoneal cavity. In addition, they do not damage the bowel mucosa.

      c. If aspiration occurs, severe pulmonary complications do not result.

   2. **Disadvantages** include a much higher cost than barium or other water-soluble agents.

   3. **Indications**

      a. Suspected tracheoesophageal fistula.

      b. Suspected gastroesophageal reflux.

      c. Suspected esophageal obstruction.

      d. Evaluation of the bowel if perforation is suspected.

      e. Unexplained pneumoperitoneum.

      f. Suspected intussusception or distal small bowel or colon obstruction.

      g. Evaluation of "gasless abdomen" in neonate more than 12 hours of age.

F. Radionuclide studies. Radionuclide studies provide more physiologic than anatomic information and usually involve a lower radiation dose to the patient when compared to x-rays.

   1. **Reflux Scintiscan** is used for documentation and quantitation of gastroesophageal reflux. This procedure is comparable to the pH probe examination and superior to the barium swallow. Technetium-99m pertechnitate in a water-based solution is instilled into the stomach. The patient is then scanned in the supine position for 1–2 hours with a gamma camera.

   2. **Radionuclide cystogram** is used for documentation and quantitation of vesicoureteric reflux. Advantages over the radiographic voiding cystourethragram (VCUG) is much lower radiation dose (50–100 times) and a longer monitoring period (1–2 hours). Disadvantages include much poorer

anatomic detail; bladder diverticula, posterior urethral valves, or mild reflux, cannot be reliably identified. This technique should not be the focus of the initial examination for vesicoureteric reflux in a boy.

3. **Radionuclide bone scan** is used for evaluation of possible osteomyelitis. This procedure involves a three-phase study (blood flow, blood pool, and bone uptake) following intravenous injection of technetium-99m methylene diphosphate (MDP).

   a. **Advantages** include a sensitivity to bony changes earlier than with the radiograph.

   b. **Disadvantages** are several. Such a bone scan (1) may not identify the acute phase of osteomyelitis (ie, first 24–48 hours); (2) it requires absence of patient motion; (3) it gives poorer anatomic detail than radiographs; and (4) resultant areas of positive uptake ("hot spots") are nonspecific.

II. **Ultrasonography**

A. **Ultrasonography of the head** is performed to rule out intraventricular hemorrhage and to grade the size of ventricles. It can be performed in most NICUs with a portable ultrasound unit. No special preparation is needed. However, an open anterior fontanelle must be present and no intravenous lines should be placed in the scalp. The classification of intraventricular hemorrhage based on ultrasonographic findings (developed by Papile) is given below. Examples are shown in Figures 9–1, 9–2, 9–3, and 9–4.

   • **Grade I.** Subependymal, germinal matrix hemorrhage.
   • **Grade II.** Intraventricular extension without ventricular dilatation.
   • **Grade III.** Intraventricular extension with ventricular dilatation.
   • **Grade IV.** Intraventricular and intraparenchymal hemorrhage.

B. **Abdominal ultrasonography** is useful in the evaluation of abdominal distention, abdominal masses, and renal failure.

III. **Computed tomographic (CT) scanning.**

A. **CT scanning of the head** is more complicated than ultrasonography, because the patient must be moved to the CT unit and be adequately sedated. CT scanning provides more information than ultrasonography of the head, however.

B. This technique can be used to diagnose intraventricular, subdural or subarachnoid bleeding and cerebral edema or infarction. To diagnose cerebral infarction infusion of contrast medium is necessary. If infusion is used, blood urea nitrogen and creatinine determinations must be obtained before the CT test to rule out renal impairment, which may be a contraindication to the use of intravenous contrast media. An intravenous line must be placed, preferably not in the head.

IV. **Magnetic resonance imaging (MRI).** Use of MRI in the neonate is now an acceptable mode of imaging and its use is expanding. MRI is superior to CT for imaging the brain stem, spinal cord, soft tissues, and areas of high bony CT artifact.

A. **Advantages** are the absence of ionizing radiation and visualization of vascular anatomy without contrast agents.

B. Major **disadvantages** are (1) that it cannot be performed on critically ill infants requiring ventilator support, (2) the scanning time is longer, and (3) sedation is usually required for infants.

RADIOGRAPHIC EXAMPLES

Invasive life support and monitoring techniques depend on proper positioning of the device being used. Caution is necessary when identifying ribs in the newborn and correlating vertebrae as a means for determining the proper position of a line or tube. Occasional errors are made because it is assumed that infants have 12 ribs as do older children and adults. In fact, it is not uncommon for infants to have a noncalcified

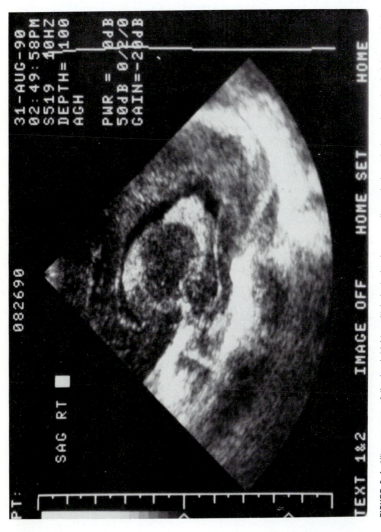

FIGURE 9–1. Ultrasonogram of the head (right sagittal view) showing a small germinal matrix hemorrhage (grade I intraventricular hemorrhage).

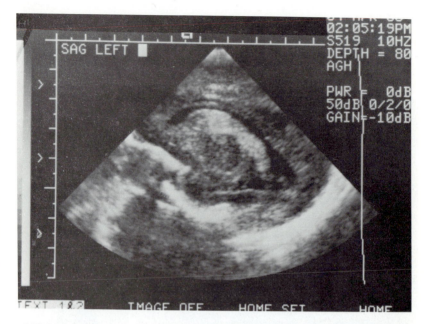

FIGURE 9–2. Ultrasonogram of the head (left sagittal view) showing germinal matrix and intraventricular hemorrhage but minimal ventricular enlargement. Same patient as in Figure 9–3.

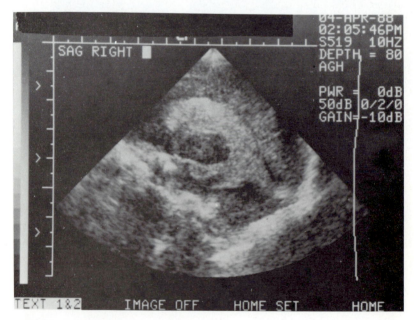

FIGURE 9–3. Ultrasonogram for same patient as in Figure 9–2, right sagittal view, demonstrating a large intraventricular hemorrhage with enlarged ventricle (grade III).

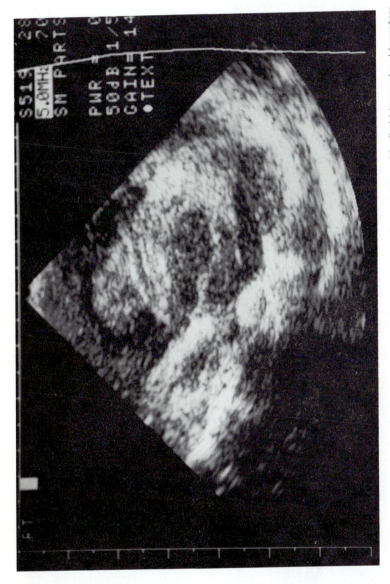

FIGURE 9-4. Ultrasonogram of the head (left sagittal view) demonstrating intraventricular hemorrhage and localized intraparenchymal hemorrhage (Grade IV).

12th rib; thus the 11th rib is mistaken for the 12th rib and an incorrect count of the lumbar vertebrae follows.

I. **Endotracheal intubation.**

 A. The tip of the endotracheal tube should be halfway between the thoracic inlet (medial ends of the clavicles) and the carina. Correct tube placement is shown in Figure 9–5.

 B. If the tube has been placed in the right main-stem bronchus, a chest x-ray film shows asymmetrical aeration with hyperinflation and atelectasis. If the tube is directed toward the left main-stem bronchus, suspect esophageal intubation first and not left main-stem bronchus intubation. With the tube placed in the esophagus, x-ray studies may show gaseous distention of the esophagus below the carina. An endotracheal tube placed too high will have the tip above the clavicle and the x-ray film may show diffuse atelectasis. If correct placement cannot be verified by x-ray film, direct laryngoscopy should be performed.

II. **Umbilical vein catheterization (UVC).** The catheter should be in the inferior vena cava, just above the diaphragm. The catheter appears to the right of the vertebrae on an x-ray film and follows the ductus venosus. Figure 9–6 shows correct placement.

III. **Umbilical artery catheterization (UAC).** The use of high versus low umbilical artery catheterization depends on institutional preference. Some clinicians feel that high catheters are associated with a higher risk of hypertension and that low catheters have a higher risk of vasospasms, but this has not been proved.

 A. If **high placement** is desired, the tip should be between thoracic vertebrae six and nine (above the origin of the celiac axis) (Fig 9–7).

 B. For **low placement,** the tip should be below the lumbar vertebrae (L3) and optimally between L3 and L4 (Fig 9–8). A catheter placed below L5 usually

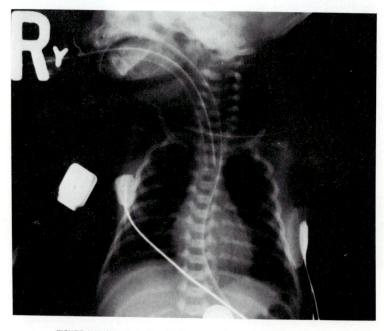

FIGURE 9–5. Chest x-ray film showing proper placement of endotracheal tube.

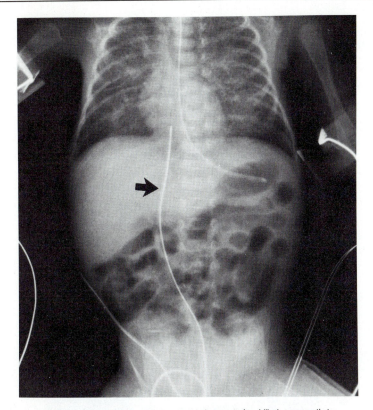

FIGURE 9–6. Abdominal x-ray showing correct placement of umbilical venous catheter.

does not function well and carries a risk of severe vasospasm in small arteries. Note that the catheter turns downward and then upward on an abdominal x-ray film. The upward turn is the point at which the catheter passes through the internal iliac artery (hypogastric artery).

Note: If both a UAC and UVC are positioned and an x-ray study is performed, it is necessary to differentiate the two in order that proper line placement can be assessed. The UAC turns downward and then upward on the x-ray film, whereas the UVC appears to the right of the vertebrae and does not turn.

RADIOGRAPHIC PEARLS

I. Pulmonary diseases

A. Hyaline membrane disease. A fine, diffuse reticulogranular pattern is seen secondary to microatelectasis of the alveoli. An x-ray film of the bronchi reveals radiolucent areas known as air bronchograms caused by air in the major airways.

B. Meconium aspiration. Bilateral, patchy, coarse infiltrates and hyperinflation of the airways are evident.

C. Pneumonia. Diffuse alveolar or interstitial disease is usually asymmetric and localized. Group B streptococcal pneumonia can appear much the same as hyaline membrane disease. Pneumatocele can be seen with staphyloccal

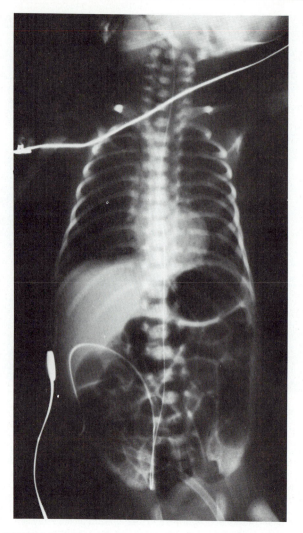

FIGURE 9–7. X-ray film showing correct positioning of high umbilical artery catheter.

pneumonia. Pleural effusions and empyema are apparent with any bacterial pneumonia.
D. Transient tachypnea of the newborn. Hyperaeration with symmetrical perihilar infiltrates is evident. Pleural fluid may be seen as prominence of the minor fissure.
E. Bronchopulmonary dysplasia. Many centers no longer rely on the following grading system for this condition, but it is included for historical purposes.
  • **Grade I:** X-ray findings are similar to those of severe hyaline membrane disease.
  • **Grade II:** Dense parenchymal opacification is seen.
  • **Grade III:** A bubbly fibrocytic pattern is evident.

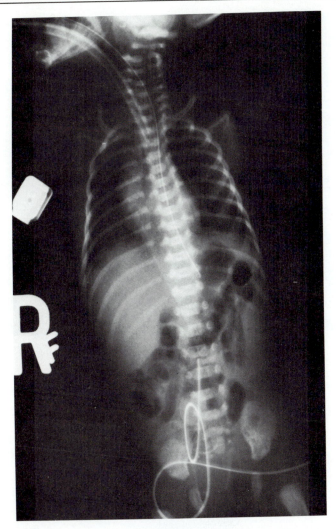

FIGURE 9–8. Abdominal x-ray film showing correct positioning of low umbilical artery catheter.

- **Grade IV:** Hyperinflation is present, with multiple fine, lacy densities spreading to the periphery and with areas of lucency extending to the bullae.
- F. **Wilson-Mikity syndrome.** Hyperaeration and a bubblelike appearance of the lung are apparent (cystic lesions with thickening of interstitial structures).
- G. **Air leak syndromes**
    1. **Pneumopericardium.** Air completely surrounds the heart, including the inferior border (Fig 9–9).
    2. **Pneumomediastinum**
        a. **AP view.** A hyperlucent rim of air is present lateral to the cardiac border and thymus. This rim may displace the thymus superiorly away from the cardiac silhouette (angel wing sign) (Fig 9–10).

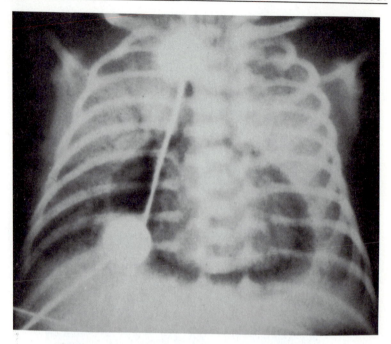

FIGURE 9–9. Chest x-ray film showing pneumopericardium in a 2-day-old infant.

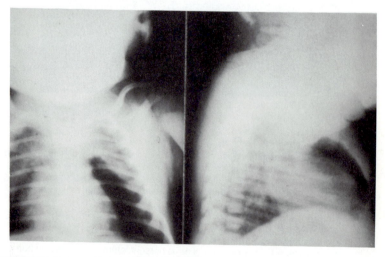

FIGURE 9–10. Pneumomediastinum. **Right:** Cross-table lateral chest x-ray. **Left:** Anteroposterior chest x-ray film.

      b. **Lateral view.** An air collection is seen either substernally (anterior pneu-
momediastinum) or in the retrocardiac area (posterior pneumomediastinum) (Fig 9–10).
3. **Pneumothorax.** The lung is displaced away from the chest wall by a radiolucent band of air. The affected lung is collapsed (Fig 9–11). The pneumothorax is often not obvious, and in some cases, it is very difficult to see (only
a subtle rim of air) and requires careful inspection of the x-ray films.
4. **Tension pneumothorax.** The diaphragm on the affected side is depressed,
the mediastinum is shifted to the contralateral hemithorax, and collapse of
the ipsilateral lobes is evident.
5. **Pulmonary interstitial emphysema.** Single or multiple circular radiolucencies with well-demarcated walls are seen in a localized or duffuse pattern. The volume of the involved portion of the lung is markedly increased
(Fig 9–12).
H. **Atelectasis.** A decrease in lung volume or collapse of part or all of a lung is
apparent. The mediastinum is shifted toward the affected side of collapse.
Compensatory hyperinflation of the involved lung is seen.

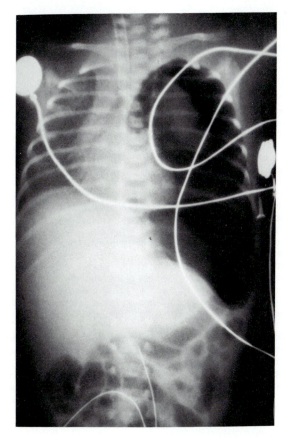

FIGURE 9–11. Left pneumothorax as shown on an anteroposterior chest x-ray film in a ventilated infant on day
2 of life.

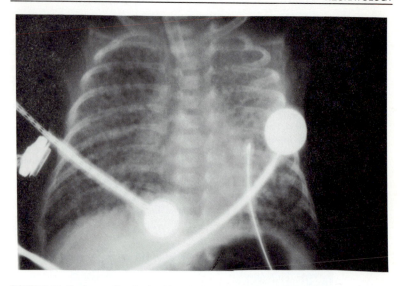

FIGURE 9–12. Chest x-ray film showing bilateral pulmonary interstitial emphysema (PIE) in a 7-day-old ventilated infant.

1. **Microatelectasis.** See p 103 (hyaline membrane disease).
2. **Generalized atelectasis.** An area of "white-out" is visible on the x-ray film. It may be seen in severe respiratory distress syndrome or airway obstruction or if the endotracheal tube is not in the trachea. This condition may also be seen in hypoventilation.
3. **Lobar atelectasis.** Lobar atelectasis is atelectasis of one lobe. The most common site is the right upper lobe, which appears as an area of "white-out" on the x-ray film. In addition, the right minor fissure may be elevated. This type of atelectasis commonly occurs after extubation.
  I. **Pulmonary hypoplasia.** Small lungs and a bell-shaped thorax are seen. The lungs appear radiolucent.
  J. **Pulmonary edema.** The lungs appear diffuse and hazy with an area of greatest density around the hilum of each lung. Heart size is usually increased.
II. **Cardiac diseases.** The cardiac/thoracic index, which normally should be less than 0.6, is the ratio of the length of the base of the heart divided by the length of the thorax. An index greater than 0.6 suggests cardiomegaly. The pulmonary vascularity is increased if more than 2 or 3 end-on vessels are present and if the diameter of the descending branch of the right pulmonary artery exceeds that of the trachea.
  A. **Cardiac dextroversion.** The cardiac apex is on the right and the aortic arch and stomach bubble on the left. The incidence of congenital heart disease associated with this finding is high.
  B. **Congestive heart failure.** Cardiomegaly, pulmonary venous congestion (engorgement and increased diameter of the pulmonary veins), diffuse opacification in the perihilar regions, and pleural effusions (sometimes) are seen.
  C. **Patent ductus arteriosus.** Cardiomegaly, pulmonary edema, ductal haze (pulmonary edema with a patent ductus arteriosus), and increased pulmonary vascular markings are evident.
  D. **Ventricular septal defect.** Findings include cardiomegaly, increase in pulmo-

nary vessels, enlargement of the left ventricle and left atrium, and enlargement of the main pulmonary artery.

  E. **Coarctation of the aorta**

    1. **Preductal coarctation.** Generalized cardiomegaly, with normal pulmonary vascularity, is seen.

    2. **Postductal coarctation.** An enlarged left ventricle and left atrium and a dilated ascending aorta are found.

  F. **Tetralogy of Fallot.** The heart is boot-shaped. Associated with an enlarged right atrium, right ventricle, and small pulmonary artery is a normal left atrium and left ventricle. There is decreased pulmonary vascularity.

  G. **Transposition of the great arteries.** The x-ray film may show cardiomegaly, with an enlarged right atrium and right ventricle, narrow mediastinum, and increased pulmonary vascular markings, but in most cases the x-ray appears normal.

  H. **Total anomalous pulmonary venous return.** Pulmonary venous markings are increased. Cardiomegaly is minimal or absent. Congestive heart failure and pulmonary edema may be present.

  I. **Hypoplastic left heart syndrome.** The chest x-ray can be normal at first but then may show cardiomegaly, pulmonary vascular congestion, and have an enlarged right atrium and ventricle.

  J. **Tricuspid atresia.** Cardiac enlargement, enlargement of the left ventricle, small pulmonary arteries, and decreased pulmonary vascularity are seen.

  K. **Truncus arteriosus.** Characteristic findings include biventricular cardiomegaly, increased pulmonary vascularity, and straightening of the left cardiac border.

  L. **Atrial septal defect.** Varying degrees of enlargement of the right atrium and ventricle are seen. The aorta and left ventricle are small, and the pulmonary artery is large. Increased pulmonary vascularity is also evident.

  M. **Ebstein's anomaly.** Gross cardiomegaly and decreased pulmonary vascularity are apparent.

  N. **Pulmonary stenosis.** Cardiomegaly and decreased pulmonary markings are seen.

III. **Abdominal disorders.**

  A. **Changes in the following normal patterns** should raise suspicion of gastrointestinal tract disease.

    1. Air in the stomach should occur within 30 minutes after delivery.

    2. Air in the small bowel should be seen by 3–4 hours of age.

    3. Air in the colon and rectum should be seen by 6–8 hours of age.

  B. **Intestinal obstruction.** Air-fluid levels are seen proximal to the obstruction. Gaseous intestinal distention is present. Gas may be decreased or absent distal to the obstruction.

  C. **Ascites.** Gas-filled loops of bowel, if present, are located in the center of the abdomen. The abdomen may be distended, with relatively small amounts of gas **("ground glass" appearance).** A uniform increase in the density of the abdomen, particularly in the flank areas, may be evident.

  D. **Calcification** in the abdomen is most often seen secondary to meconium peritonitis, which may also cause calcifications in the scrotum in male infants. Calcifications in the abdomen may also be seen in infants with neuroblastoma or teratoma or may signify calcification of the adrenals following adrenal hemorrhage.

  E. **Pneumoperitoneum**

    1. **Supine view.** Free air is seen as a central lucency (Fig 9–13).

    2. **Upright view.** Free air is present in a subdiaphragmatic location.

    3. **Left lateral decubitus view.** Air collects over the lateral border of the liver, separating it from the abdominal wall.

  F. **Pneumatosis intestinalis.** Intraluminal gas in the bowel wall (produced by bacteria that have invaded the bowel wall) appears as a string of submucosal

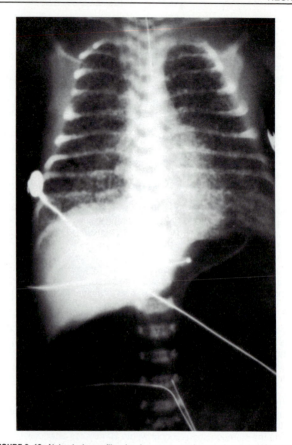

FIGURE 9–13. Abdominal x-ray film showing pneumoperitoneum in a 3-day-old infant.

bubbles. It is most frequently seen in infants with necrotizing enterocolitis (Fig 9–14).

G. Situs inversus. The stomach, aortic arch, and cardiac apex appear on the right. This finding is not associated with an increased incidence of intrinsic heart disease.

H. Ileus. Distended loops of bowel are present. Air-fluid levels may be seen on the upright or cross-table lateral x-ray film.

I. Absence of gas in the abdomen. Absence of gas in the abdomen may be seen in patients taking muscle-paralyzing medications (eg, pancuronium) because they do not swallow air. It may also be evident in infants with esophageal atresia without tracheoesophageal fistula.

J. Intraportal air. Air is demonstrated in the portal veins (often best seen on a lateral view). This finding may indicate bowel necrosis, such as that which occurs in advanced stages of necrotizing enterocolitis; intestinal infarction secondary to mesenteric vessel occlusion; or iatrogenically introduced gas into the portal vein, which can occur during umbilical vein catheterization or exchange transfusion.

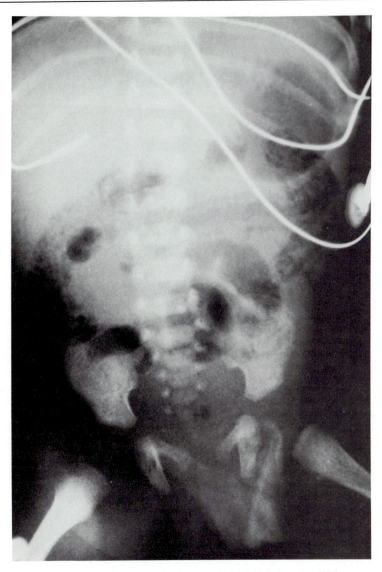

FIGURE 9–14. Abdominal x-ray film showing pneumatosis intestinalis in a 4-day-old infant.

10 Management of the Extremely Low Birth Weight Infant During the First Week of Life

This chapter addresses the initial care of premature infants of less than 1000 g birth weight, also known as "extremely low birth weight infants." Many aspects of this care are *controversial,* and each institution has developed its own philosophy, style, and techniques for managing these infants, especially those weighing less than 750 g at birth. Therefore, it is of utmost importance to learn and follow the practices of your own institution. This chapter presents guidelines we have found useful for stabilizing and caring for extremely small infants.

I. **Temperature and humidity control.** Because the tiny baby has little subcutaneous tissue, relatively large skin surface area and minimal energy reserves, a **neutral thermal environment** is essential for its survival. Such an environment is defined as the environmental temperature that minimizes heat loss so that oxygen consumption is not increased and metabolic stress is not incurred. To maintain minimal evaporative heat loss, it is best if the environmental humidity is at least 40–50%.

A. **Incubators or radiant warmers.** Extremely low birth weight infants may initially be managed either in **double-walled incubators or under radiant heaters with protective plastic sheeting or covers.** Hypothermia must be avoided. The definition of hypothermia is not readily agreed upon, however. Some centers strive for core temperatures of 37.0 °C, whereas others allow the infants to be maintained at temperatures as low as 35.5 °C. Guidelines for Perinatal Care, of the American College of Obstetrics and Gynecology and the American Academy of Pediatrics, recommend maintaining either a skin temperature of 36.0–36.5 °C or a core body temperature of 36.0–37.5 °C.

B. **Humidification.** Tiny infants have increased insensible water loss due largely to evaporation. In particular, the ratio of their body surface area to body weight is greatly increased. They also have a greater proportion of body water relative to body mass. Furthermore, transcutaneous water loss is enhanced by their thin epidermis and underdeveloped stratum corneum. These evaporative losses are minimized by increased environmental humidity. **Humidification within the incubator or the area beneath the plastic protective cover of a radiant warmer is recommended.**

1. Use a **respiratory care humidification unit,** the same as that used with oxygen hoods. The fluids utilized for the humidification in these systems should be changed every 24 hours. (If the manufactured humidity reservoirs of the incubators are used, special attention to infection control is needed, especially to prevent skin infections.)

2. Maintain a surrounding **humidity of at least 40–50%.** Use of a hand-held humidistat or hygrometer allows hourly checking of ambient humidity.

C. **Monitoring and maintenance of body temperature.** Infants weighing less than 1000 g have poor mechanisms for regulation of temperature and depend on environmental support.

1. Maintain skin temperature of 36–37.0 °C. Rectal temperatures in tiny babies are discouraged.

2. Using a servocontrol skin probe, record skin temperature and environmental

temperature every hour until skin temperature is stable (36–36.5 °C) and follow thereafter with recordings at 2-hour intervals.

3. Check axillary temperature only if skin temperature is outside the range of 36–36.5 °C. Periodically check axillary temperature. You may need to change from servo- to non-servocontrol (manual) to warm the smallest infants.

4. Record incubator humidity every hour until it is stable (40–50%) and then every 2 hours for maintenance.

5. If minor surgical procedures are required, convert the overhead radiant warmer to servocontrol set at 37–38 °C. Use prewarmed sterile drapes and instruments.

6. Low birth weight infants must be weighed at least once daily for management of fluids and electrolytes. The incubator should have an **in-bed scale for continuous weighing of infant to minimize handling and removal from a controlled environment,** thus maximizing temperature control. The **scale should be preheated** with the incubator before admission and should be calibrated after optimal air temperature and humidity have been established.

7. **Other heat conserving practices** include utilizing of hats, fetal positioning, port-sleeves on incubators, and sheepskin-covered heating pads (infants should not lie directly on the heating pad as thermal burns may result).

8. **Accessory items for infant care must be prewarmed.** These items include all new linens, blood pressure cuffs, x-ray cassettes, sterile towels, intravenous fluids, stethoscope, saline lavages, diapers, invasive tubes, and any items that come in direct contact with the infant. Placement of these items in the infant's incubator 30 minutes before use warms these items to the infant's neutral thermal requirement. (Take care not to place these items next to the infant.)

D. **Rewarming hypothermic infants.** Rewarming of infants who become hypothermic must be gradual. Radiant warming heat sources may be used in addition to the double-walled incubator. Manual control of the incubator may be necessary if the response to rewarming is too slow. In general, the rewarming rate should not exceed 0.6 °C per hour. Continual observation of environmental and skin temperatures is essential to evaluate rewarming efforts. Frequent monitoring and observation of the infant is necessary to assess tolerance. When skin temperature of 36.5 °C is achieved, rewarming efforts should be gradually discontinued and temperature maintenance by servocontrol should be followed. Excessive warming of these infants must be avoided, as core body temperatures greater than 37.5 °C cause increased insensible water losses, increased oxygen consumption, and deviations in vital signs.

E. **Infants on mechanical ventilation**

1. For all infants receiving mechanical ventilation, especially those weighing less than 1000 g, **humidification and warming of administered respiratory gases** is important to minimize insensible fluid losses.

2. **In-line warming of respiratory gas circuits** minimizes "rain out" of the hu-

TABLE 10–1. GUIDELINES FOR INTRAVENOUS FLUIDS IN THE VERY LOW BIRTH WEIGHT INFANT THE FIRST DAY OF LIFE

Weight (g)	Type of Fluid	SGA*	AGA*
500–599	D_5W	140	200 mL/kg/d
600–699	D_5W	120	180 mL/kg/d
700–799	D_5W	100	160 mL/kg/d
800–899	D_5W	80	120 mL/kg/d
900–999	$D_{10}W$	70	100 mL/kg/d

* SGA = small for gestational age; AGA = appropriate for gestational age.

midified air and oxygen and maintains airway temperature, which should be 32–35 °C.

II. **Fluids and electrolytes.** Because of increased insensible water loss and immature renal function, these infants have increased fluid requirements, necessitating **intravenous fluid therapy** or, in some cases, infusion of fluids through the umbilical artery. (See Chap 7.)

A. **Intravenous fluid therapy (fluid volume and type of fluid)**

1. **First day of life.** Guidelines for the type of fluid and volume per kilogram of body weight are given in Table 10–1 for the first day of life. The table gives suggested volumes (including line flushes and medications) for infants in double-walled incubators with a constant humidity of 40–50% and stable skin temperatures of 36–36.5 °C. For babies of the same weight, small-for-gestational-age infants require lesser amounts of fluid.

a. **Additional fluid is required if phototherapy is used** (see p 121 **C.2**); the fluid volume should be increased by 10–20 mL/kg/d.

b. **Additional fluid is required if the infant is exposed to direct overhead radiant heat.** Extreme insensible body fluid losses occur in tiny babies under direct radiant heat if not shielded by protective plastic sheeting or enclosed in protective plastic hoods or other types of enclosures. However, be aware that excessive fluid intake may contribute to the development of a hemodynamically significant patent ductus arteriosus and should be avoided.

2. **Second and subsequent days of life.** Fluid management on the second and subsequent days depends on changes in body weight, renal function (blood urea nitrogen [BUN], creatinine and urine output), and serum electrolyte concentrations (see Chap 7).

B. **Infusion of fluids through umbilical catheters.** Add **heparin,** 1 unit/mL, to fluids infused through umbilical catheters. For the fluid volume and type, see Table 10–1.

C. **For line flushing, use the same fluids as those being infused as intravenous fluids.** Avoid normal saline as a flush solution because of excessive sodium. In addition, avoid hypotonic solutions (less than 0.45 normal saline or less than 5% dextrose); these solutions may cause red cell hemolysis.

D. **Monitoring of fluid therapy.** The infant's fluid status should be evaluated at least twice daily and the fluid intake should be adjusted accordingly. Monitoring of fluid status is done by measurements of body weight, urine output, urine specific gravity, hemodynamic measurements, serum sodium, and other less reliable parameters such as hematocrit and physical examination.

1. **Body weight.** The most important way of monitoring fluid therapy is by measurement of body weight. If an in-bed scale is used, weigh the baby every 12 hours. If an in-bed scale is not available, weighing may have to be delayed to every 24 to 48 hours, depending on the stability of the tiny infant, to prevent excessive handling and cold stress. A weight loss of up to 15% of birth weight may be experienced by the end of the first week of life. Greater weight loss is considered excessive, and environmental controls for insensible fluid losses and fluid management must be carefully reviewed.

2. **Urine output and specific gravity.** Monitoring urine output is the second most important method of monitoring fluid therapy. For greatest accuracy, diapers should be weighed before use and immediately following void. In addition to urine volume, urine specific gravity should be determined to check renal function and the state of hydration.

a. **First 12 hours:** Any amount of urine output is acceptable.

b. **Twelve to 24 hours:** The minimum acceptable urine output is 0.5 mL/kg/h, with urine specific gravity of 1.008–1.015.

c. **Second day and after:** Normal urine output for the second day is 1–2 mL/kg/h. After the second day of life, urine output may increase to 3.0–3.5 mL/kg/h; 4–5 mL/kg/h is excessive and indicates early fluid overload, which may lead to electrolyte loss. Urine specific gravity should fluctuate between 1.008 and 1.015. Values outside this range warrant reevaluation of fluid management or environmental humidity control.

3. **Hemodynamic monitoring** is a valuable tool in assessing fluid status in the infant.

   a. **Heart rate.** The accelerated heart rate of the tiny baby, which averages 140–160 bpm, is generally considered within normal limits. Tachycardia, with a heart rate in excess of 160 bpm, may be a sign of hypovolemia.

   b. **Arterial blood pressure.** The most accurate measurement of arterial blood pressure is via indwelling arterial line and transducer. Cuff pressures may be difficult to obtain due to infants small size and lower systemic pressures. (See Appendix C for normal blood pressure values.)

   c. **Central venous pressure (CVP).** CVP monitoring may be done via high umbilical venous line and transducer. Parameters are not well established for infants of this size. In our experience, deviations from the infant's baseline can provide valuable information; lower CVP values may indicate hypovolemia, whereas higher values may indicate fluid overload.

4. **Electrolyte values.** Serum electrolyte levels should be monitored at least twice daily, or every 4–8 hours for the most immature infants.

   a. **Sodium.** Initially, tiny infants have a sufficient sodium level (132–138 meq/L) and require no sodium intake. However, when the serum sodium level begins to decrease (usually on the third to fifth day of life), sodium should be added to the intravenous fluids (3–8 meq/kg/d of sodium). In subsequent monitoring of the serum sodium levels:

      (1) If sodium is greater than 142 meq/L, consider that the sodium intake is too high or the infant is dehydrated.

      (2) If sodium is less than 133 meq/L, more sodium may be needed, or the infant may have fluid overload. If the decrease in the serum sodium level is believed to be due to fluid overload, the total daily fluids should be reduced.

      Note: Hypernatremia in the first few days of life may be due to dehydration or to inadvertent sodium administration from normal saline catheter flushes. Flush catheters only with the intravenous fluids being used for maintenance fluid therapy. If infusion is being done through an umbilical artery catheter, heparinized intravenous fluid must be used for flushing.

   b. **Potassium**

      (1) **During the first 48 hours after birth,** tiny babies are prone to the development of increased serum potassium levels of 5 meq/L or more (range 4.0–8.0 meq/L). The increase is due mostly to immature renal tubular function. Most clinicians recommend that no potassium be given during this time. Electrocardiographic changes are not usually seen until the serum potassium level is greater than 9.0 meq/L. The following clinical guidelines are offered.

         (a) **Serum potassium 7–8 meq/L.** Accept the value as the upper limit and observe the infant and the ECG. Repeat serum studies every 4–6 hours.

         (b) **Serum potassium 8–9 meq/L.** Check urine output. The minimal acceptable output is 1–2 mL/kg/h (2–3 mL/kg/h is preferred) with urine specific gravity of 1.006 to 1.012). Observe for elevated or peaked T wave changes on the bedside heart rate monitor. Monitor BUN and creatinine.

         (c) **Serum potassium levels greater than 9 meq/L** are usually pathologic and are associated with decreasing renal function, cardiac irregularities, or both. Consider administration of sodium bicarbonate, calcium solutions, or glucose/insulin infusions (consultation required) (see Chap 37 for details on the management of hyperkalemia). Kayexalate enemas and exchange transfusion have had little effect and may further complicate the infant's condition.

(2) **Third to sixth day after birth.** Usually by the third to the sixth day, the initially elevated serum potassium level begins to decrease. As potassium levels approach 4 meq/L, add supplemental potassium to intravenous fluids. Begin with 1–2 meq/kg/d. Measure serum potassium every 6–12 hours until the level is stabilized at 4.1–4.8 meq/L.

III. **Blood glucose.** As with larger high-risk infants, extremely low birth weight infants should be supported with 4–6 mg/kg/min glucose infusion. This support can usually be achieved by starting with a 5% dextrose solution. (Use of a 10% dextrose solution may result in hyperglycemia.) Meter testing of blood glucose should be performed every 2 hours until a stable blood glucose level (50–90 mg/dL) has been established. All urine samples should be checked for glucosuria. Trace glucosuria is acceptable and may occur with a blood glucose level as low as 120 mg/dL, but higher levels of serum glucose and glycosuria require recalculation of glucose administration and total fluid administration.

IV. **Calcium.** Serum calcium should be monitored once or twice daily. When the serum calcium decreases below 7.5 mg/dL, we institute treatment with calcium gluconate (for dosage, see p 473). This decrease usually happens on the second day of life. Although a few infants may not require calcium therapy, some centers routinely institute daily maintenance calcium supplementation in their intravenous solutions (eg, 2 mg calcium gluconate per milliliter of intravenous solution).

V. **Hyperalimentation.** Hyperalimentation should be started as soon as the infant's fluid and electrolyte (sodium and potassium) and glucose have stabilized, usually late in the first week of life.

VI. **Respiratory support.** Virtually all of these infants initially require **mechanical ventilation.** Although some centers prefer a trial of nasal continuous positive airway pressure (CPAP) prior to intubation, we have found that it is often prudent to electively intubate these infants in the delivery room.

   A. **Endotracheal intubation**

      1. **Type of endotracheal tube.** When possible, use an endotracheal tube with 1-cm markings on the side. The internal diameter (ID) of the tube should routinely be 2.5 mm or 3.0 mm, according to body weight:

         (a) 500–1000 g: 2.5 mm ID
         (b) 1000–1250 g: 3.0 mm ID

      2. **Endotracheal tube placement.** (The procedure for endotracheal tube placement is described in detail in Chapter 18.) Proper placement should be confirmed by a chest x-ray study, performed with the infant's head in the midline position. After correct placement has been confirmed, the numbers (or letters) on the tube that are at the infant's gum line should be noted. As a means of subsequently checking proper tube position, every shift the nurse responsible for the infant should check and record the numbers or letters at the gum line. Any adjustment of the endotracheal tube requires a subsequent chest x-ray study to confirm the tube position.

   B. **Mechanical ventilation.** Initial ventilator settings vary from institution to institution. Tiny infants respond to a wide range of ventilator settings. Some do relatively well on 20–30 cycles/min; others require 50–60 cycles/min, with inspiratory times ranging from 0.28 to 0.50 second. The minimum airway pressure possible should be used. Seek to maintain mechanical breath tidal volumes of 5–7 mL/kg; often this may be achieved with as little as 8–12 cm inspiratory pressure and 2–3 cm positive end-expiratory pressure. Higher pressures increase the risk of barotrauma and the development of chronic lung disease and must be avoided. We have found that pressures can be kept to a minimum by allowing a mild to moderate respiratory acidosis (pH 7.25–7.32 and Pco_2 45–58 mm Hg). The following ventilatory support guidelines are offered for the initiation of respiratory care. Each tiny infant requires frequent reassessment and revision of settings and parameters. **Recommended initial settings for pressure-limited time-cycled ventilators are:**

      1. **Rate:** 20–60 breaths/min (usually 30).
      2. **Inspiratory time (IT):** 0.3–0.5 second (usually 0.33).

3. **Peak inspiratory pressure:** 12–20 cm water (select peak inspiratory pressure on the basis of tidal volume if it can be measured; usually 5.0–7.0 mL/kg).
4. **Mean airway pressure (MAP):** Less than 8 cm water.
5. **F$_{IO_2}$:** As required per initial P$_{O_2}$ values.
6. **Flow rate:** 6–8 L/min.

C. **Monitoring of ventilatory status**
  1. **Oxygenation**
    a. **Blood gas sampling.** Arterial catheterization (see Chap 14 for details) should be performed for frequent blood gas sampling. Routinely, these infants require blood gas sampling every 2–4 hours. Sampling may need to be done more frequently, possibly as often as every 20 minutes, but less frequent sampling is desirable as soon as possible to minimize stress and blood loss and the need for blood replacement.
      (1) **Desirable arterial blood gas values**
        (a) **Pa$_{O_2}$:** 45–60 mm Hg.
        (b) **Pa$_{CO_2}$:** 45–55 mm Hg. A slightly higher Pa$_{CO_2}$ is acceptable if the pH remains acceptable.
        (c) **pH:** 7.25–7.32 is acceptable.
      (2) **Abnormal blood gas values** indicate the need for immediate chest x-ray (see **3,** below), chest wall transillumination (see p 238), and repeat blood gas determinations.
    b. **Continuous oxygen monitoring** should also be performed, preferably by pulse oximetry. Transcutaneous electrode monitoring of oxygen and carbon dioxide is discouraged because of possible skin damage in tiny babies. The air/oxygen mixture should be adjusted to maintain the pulse oximeter reading between 88 and 92% hemoglobin oxygen saturation. Excess oxygenation must be avoided in this grouping of infants. Failure to regulate the administation of oxygen can contribute to the development of retinopathy of prematurity (ROP) and bronchopulmonary dysplasia (BPD).
  2. **Infant's appearance.** Abrupt changes in the infant's color or the appearance of cyanosis indicate the need for immediate assessment by chest wall transilluminaton, chest x-ray study, and blood gas sampling.
  3. **Chest x-ray study**
    a. **Indications**
      (1) Abnormal or sudden change in blood gas values.
      (2) Adjustment of the endotracheal tube (to confirm proper positioning).
      (3) Sudden change in infant's status.
    b. **Technique.** Chest x-ray should be performed with the infant's head in the midline position to check for endotracheal tube placement.
    c. **X-ray evaluation.** Check chest x-ray film for expansion of the lung, chest wall, and diaphragm. Overexpansion (hyperlucent lungs and diaphragms below ninth rib) must be avoided. If overexpansion is present, consider decreasing the peak airway pressure. Some tiny babies do very well with peak inspiratory pressures as low as 8 cm water.

D. **Suctioning.** Suctioning should be done only as needed and not more frequently than every 4 hours.
  1. **Assessment of the need for suctioning.** To assess need for suction, the nurse and/or physician should consider:
    a. **Breath sounds.** Wet or diminished breath sounds may indicate secretions obstructing the airways and the need for suctioning.
    b. **Blood gas values.** If the Pa$_{CO_2}$ is increasing above 50 mm Hg, suctioning should be considered to clean the airways and avoid the "ball-valve" effect of thick secretions.
  2. **Technique**
    a. Suctioning should be done only to the depth of the endotracheal tube. Use suctioning guide or marked (1-cm increments) suction catheter.

      b. Lavage fluid for suctioning should be sterile normal saline. Use 1–2 drops for each suctioning procedure. Lavage solution should be warmed to 36–37 °C.

      c. Suction should be regulated at 60–80 mm Hg.

      d. Minimize the effects of suctioning by: preoxygenating with a 5–15% increase in oxygen, increasing the baseline ventilatory rate, and using in-line suctioning devices.

  E. Extubation

    1. Indications. Occasionally extremely low birth weight infants may be extubated by the end of the first week of life. Many require maintenance mechanical ventilation beyond the first month of life. Indications for extubation include:

      a. Ventilator rate less than 10 bpm.

      b. Oxygen requirements less than 30% FIo$_2$.

      c. Regular spontaneous respiratory rate.

      d. Adequate spontaneous tidal volume (3.8–5.0 mL/kg).

      e. Pulmonary function tests (if available) revealing a compliance of 0.9–1.1 mL/cm water.

      f. Stable blood gas values (within normal ranges).

      g. Stable chest x-ray findings on serial examinations.

    2. Technique. Apnea is usually not a problem for tiny babies in the first few days of life, perhaps because of the use of mechanical ventilation. To prevent apnea, we start treatment with **theophylline before extubation** (see p 510). The procedure for tube removal is the same as for larger infants.

VII. Surfactant. (See Chap 6.) Most centers administer surfactant replacement to these infants. It should be administered according to the protocol provided with the specific surfactant replacement product.

VIII. Patent ductus arteriosus. (See p 288.) Efforts should be made to minimize the risk of patent ductus arteriosus (PDA). Overhydration must be avoided. If the infant shows any sign of a hemodynamically significant PDA, medical treatment should commence. Some centers institute prophylactic indomethacin therapy, although this is somewhat *controversial.*

IX. Transfusion. These infants are usually born anemic, with hematocrits less than 40 and they require frequent specimen draws and numerous transfusions. We try to keep the hematocrit between 35 and 40%. Lower values may be acceptable if the infant is asymptomatic. A cumulative record of blood drawn is also a useful indicator in the decision to transfuse. The pulic is increasingly aware of transfusion issues, and parents should be encouraged to participate in a directed-donor program.

X. Skin care. Meticulous skin care is advised. Maintenance of intact skin is the tiny baby's most effective barrier against infection, insensible fluid loss, protein loss, blood loss and provides for more effective body temperature control. Minimal use of tape is recommended because the infant's skin is fragile and tears may result in removal. Alternatives to tape include the use of Hollihesive (a skin barrier) or hydrogel adhesive, which removes easily with water. Hydrogel adhesive infant care products include electrodes, temp-probe covers and bili-masks. In addition, the very thin skin of the tiny baby allows absorption of many substances. Skin care must focus on maintaining skin integrity and minimizing exposure to topical agents.

  A. Cut servocontrol skin probe covers to the smallest size possible (try a 2-cm diameter circle) to reduce skin damage due to the adhesive.

  B. Monitoring of oxygen therapy is best accomplished by use of a pulse oximeter for hemoglobin oxygen saturations. The probe must be placed carefully to prevent pressure sores. The site should be rotated at a minimum of every 12 hours. Alternative means of oxygen monitoring include umbilical catheter blood sampling. The use of transcutaneous oxygen and carbon dioxide gel electrodes is discouraged. Heated gel electrodes have caused serious skin burns in extremely low birth weight infants.

C. **Urine bags and blood pressure cuffs should not routinely be used** because of adhesives and sharp plastic edge cuts. For urine collection, turn diaper plastic side up. Bladder aspirations are discouraged.

D. **Prophylactic eye ointment should be applied** per routine admission plan. If the eyelids are fused, apply along the lash line.

E. **When the physician prepares the skin for a procedure (eg, placement of UAC, UVC, chest tube) 1 mL of warm half-strength Betadine solution should be measured out.** (One milliliter is sufficient to effectively disinfect 50–60 cm^2 of skin area.) After the procedure is completed, the solution should be sponged off immediately with warm sterile water.

F. **Attach ECG electrodes using as little adhesive as possible.** Options are:
   1. Consider using electrode jacket.
   2. Consider stretch gauze to strap the ECG leads to the extremities if limb leads are used.
   3. Trim the adhesive electrode patch to minimize adhesive on the skin.

G. **Bathing is not appropriate for the tiny baby.** Soiled areas can be gently cleansed with cotton balls and warm water.

H. **Avoid the use of anything that dries out the skin,** such as soaps and alcohol.

 I. **Medium-chain triglyceride (MCT) oil is useful for helping remove adhesive tape, probe covers, and electrode patches.**
   Note: **When skin appears dry, thickened, and no longer shiny or translucent** (usually 10–14 days), these skin care recommendations and procedures may be modified or discontinued.

XI. **Other special considerations for the extremely low birth weight infant**
   A. **Infection**
      1. **Cultures.** Many of these infants are born infected or from an infected environment. Blood and urine cultures should be obtained. Unless there is a strong suspicion of meningitis, lumbar puncture should not be performed.
      2. **Antibiotics.** After obtaining cultures, these infants should be started on **ampicillin** and an **aminoglycoside.** The aminoglycoside is usually started at a dosing interval of once a day. The peak and trough serum levels of the aminoglycoside must be monitored and the dosage should be adjusted appropriately. (See Chap 73.)
      3. **Intravenous gamma globulin therapy.** Preliminary studies suggest that prophylactic treatment with intravenous gamma globulin may prevent infections in these small infants. This therapy depends on the practice of your individual institution (see p 485).
   B. **Central nervous system hemorrhage**
      1. **Pharmacologic prevention.** Although many prophylactic therapies have been proposed—phenobarbital, indomethacin, ethamsylate, pancuronium, vitamin K, and vitamin E—none has received widespread acceptance and none can be recommended at this time. As much as possible, these infants should be maintained with normal blood pressures, blood volumes, acid-base status, and oxygenation. Transfusions should be given slowly (over at least 30 minutes, preferably slower). The use of sodium bicarbonate should be kept to a minimum. Hemodynamic stability is essential, as the fragile capillaries of the germinal matrix are especially vulnerable to deviations in cerebral blood flow.
      2. **Monitoring.** Initial **cranial ultrasonography** is usually performed as soon after birth as practical. It should always be performed within the first 4 to 7 days of life.
      3. **Minimal stimulation.** These tiny infants tolerate handling and procedures poorly. Other stressors include noise, light, and activity. Routine tasks should be clustered to allow the infant undisturbed periods of rest.
      4. **Positioning.** The fetus is maintained in a flexed position. Care should be taken to simulate this positioning in the extremely premature infant. A flexed side-lying or prone posture with supportive boundaries is pre-

ferred. Change in position is recommended every 4 hours or at the infant's cue.

C. **Hyperbilirubinemia**

  1. **Risk.** There appears to be little risk from mild or moderate hyperbilirubinemia in these infants. Still, efforts should be made to keep the serum bilirubin below 10 mg/dL. Serum bilirubin may be monitored at least twice daily, and an exchange transfusion should be considered when the bilirubin approaches 12 mg/dL (see Chap 35).

  2. **Phototherapy.** Phototherapy to reduce the serum bilirubin level appears to have little or no risk in these infants and can be used to prevent the need for exchange transfusion. The additional use of the fiber optic phototherapy blanket is useful when it is necessary to rapidly reduce bilirubin levels. Many centers start phototherapy immediately after birth. If the infant is treated with phototherapy, the fluid intake should be increased by 10–20 mL/kg/d.

D. **Social problems.** Many of these families have unexpected problems at the time of the birth. Nearly all have numerous social problems prior to the infant's discharge. A social service consultation is mandatory for all of these families. Parent conferences involving the physician, social worker and primary nurse help the family understand the complex, extended care of their infant. Parent-infant bonding should be promoted, and parents should be encouraged to assist in caring for their child.

REFERENCES

Brown C: Using bedscales in the neonatal intensive care unit. *Neonatal Network* 1991:**9**:37.

Cabal LA, Larrazabal C, Siassi B: Hemodynamic variables in infants weighing less than 1000 grams. *Clin Perinatol* 1986;**13**:327.

Costarino AT Jr et al: Sodium restriction versus daily maintenance replacement in very low birth weight premature neonate: A randomized, blind therapeutic trial. *J Pediatr* 1992;**129**:99.

Cunningham MD, Desai NS: Methods of assessment and findings regarding pulmonary function in infants less than 1000 grams. *Clin Perinatol* 1986;**13**:299.

Dietch JS: Periventricular-intraventricular hemorrhage in the very low birth weight infant. *Neonatal Network* 1993;**12**:7.

Evans JC: Incidence of hypoxemia associated with caregiving in preterm infants. *Neonatal Network* 1991;**10**:17.

Evans N, Moorcraft J: Effect of patency of the ductus arteriosus on blood pressure in very preterm infants. *Arch Dis Child* 1992;**67**:1169.

Holtrop PC, Ruedisueli K, Maisels MJ: Double verses single phototherapy in low birth weight newborns. *Pediatrics* 1992;**90**:674.

Shaffer SG et al: Hyperkalemia in very low birth weight infants. *J Pediatr* 1991;**121**:275.

Shah AR et al: Fluctuations in cerebral oxygenation and blood volume during endotracheal suctioning in premature infants. *J Pediatr* 1992;**120**:769.

11 Extracorporeal Membrane Oxygenation (ECMO)

I. **Introduction.** Extracorporeal membrane oxygenation (ECMO) is a technique in which an infant's venous blood is pumped through a membrane oxygenator (artificial lung) whereby oxygen is added and carbon dioxide is removed. The blood is then pumped back into the patient's venous (venovenous ECMO) or arterial circulation (venoarterial ECMO). The procedure allows the lungs to rest and averts continuous high-pressure mechanical ventilation in severe respiratory failure (Zwischenberger, 1986). During ECMO, the lungs continue to function at a low volume and low pressure to prevent atelectasis and to maintain minimal alveolar ventilation. The patient is entirely dependent on the membrane for oxygenation and removal of carbon dioxide.

II. **Indications.** ECMO is currently used primarily for critically ill term newborns with reversible respiratory failure who have failed maximal medical management. Each ECMO center must establish its own specific criteria for both reversible respiratory failure *and* maximal medical management. These criteria should identify infants who would have at least an 80% mortality and significant morbidity without ECMO. Infants should be identified in time to institute ECMO before it's too late.

Diseases that have been treated by ECMO include meconium aspiration syndrome, congenital diaphragmatic hernia, sepsis, persistent pulmonary hypertension (usually secondary to meconium aspiration or severe asphyxia), cardiac failure following open heart surgery, respiratory distress syndrome and sepsis/pneumonia.

A. **ECMO entry criteria.** The following criteria should be applied only after failure of maximal medical therapy (100% F_{IO_2}, induction and maintenance of alkalosis, tolazoline).

1. Weight greater than 2 kg; gestational age $\geq$ 34 weeks.
2. No more than 7–10 days of assisted ventilation.
3. Reversible lung disease.
4. No major bleeding disorder or major intracranial hemorrhage.
5. The patient must have been screened with echocardiography to rule out cyanotic congenital heart disease.
6. **PLUS** one of the following:
   a. Alveolar-to-arterial oxygen gradient ($A-aDO_2$) is greater than 610 for 8 hours (80% mortality). (Normal $A-aDO_2$ is less than 20 mm Hg.)

$$A-aDO_2 = \left[(F_{IO_2})(Pb - 47) - \frac{(Paco_2)}{R} \right] - Pao_2$$

   Pb = barometric pressure (760 mm Hg); 47 = water vapor pressure; $Paco_2$ = alveolar CO_2 (approximately equivalent to the $Paco_2$); R = respiratory quotient (0.8).
   b. PIP is greater than or equal to 38 and $A-aDO_2$ is equal to or less than 605 for 4 hours (84% mortality).

   Note: Some centers use oxygen index (OI) rather than $A-aDO_2$.

$$OI = \frac{F_{IO_2} \times MAP \times 100}{Pao_2}$$

   a. OI is greater than 40 in 3 ABGs (80% mortality).
   b. OI is greater than 25 (50% mortality).
III. Contraindications. See Table 11–1.
IV. Procedure. Uniform guidelines should be established to describe essential equipment, procedures, personnel, and training required for neonatal ECMO. A multidisciplinary team approach is necessary because of the variety of diseases treated by ECMO as well as the variety of resulting complications. Venoarterial ECMO is usually preferred for neonatal patients because it provides both cardiac and respiratory support and because it is easier to oxygenate the blood. (See Figure 11–1.)
   A. Catheters are placed in the right internal jugular vein and right common carotid artery, with the venous catheter advanced so that it rests in the right atrium. The arterial catheter is advanced to the entrance of the aortic arch.
   B. During an ECMO "run," the infant's blood must be heparinized to avoid clotting the circuit. Usually a loading dose of 100–150 units heparin/kg is required during the cannulation procedure, with a heparin drip of 20–70 units/kg/h.
   C. As bypass is achieved, ventilator settings are reduced to final settings: FIO_2, 0.21; ventilator rate, 10–15 breaths/min; pressure limit, 15 cm water and positive end-expiratory pressure (PEEP), 5–10 cm water. An average ECMO "run" is 5 days but may be as long as 21 days.
   D. Some ECMO centers are successfully re-anastomosing the carotid artery after the procedure, but long-term evaluation of these infants is just beginning.
V. Complications
   A. Infant
      1. Intracranial hemorrhage (incidence varies between 7 and 42%).
      2. Pulmonary hemorrhage.
      3. Nasal bleeding.
      4. Hypertension.
      5. GI hemorrhage.
      6. Cardiac arrhythmias.
      7. Electrolyte abnormalities.
      8. Hemolysis.
      9. Thrombocytopenia.
     10. Acute renal failure.
     11. Seizures.
   B. Mechanical
      1. Oxygenator failure.
      2. Tubing rupture.
      3. Pump failure.
      4. Heat exchanger failure.
      5. Air embolization.
      6. Membrane lung failure.
      7. Cannulation difficulties.

TABLE 11–1. CONTRAINDICATIONS TO EXTRACORPOREAL MEMBRANE OXYGENATION (ECMO)

Contraindications	Reason
Gestational age < 34 weeks	Risk of intracranial hemorrhage
Birth weight < 2000 g	Surgical difficulties with vessel cannulation
Mechanical ventilation > 7–10 days	Irreversible lung disease likely
Intracranial hemorrhage > grade I	High risk of progression of hemorrhage
Coagulopathy	Higher risk of bleeding
Severe perinatal asphyxia with evidence of severe brain damage	Poor neurologic outcome
Severe congenital anomalies	Poor outcome despite ECMO
Cyanotic congenital heart disease without cardiopulmonary failure	Other interventions are indicated

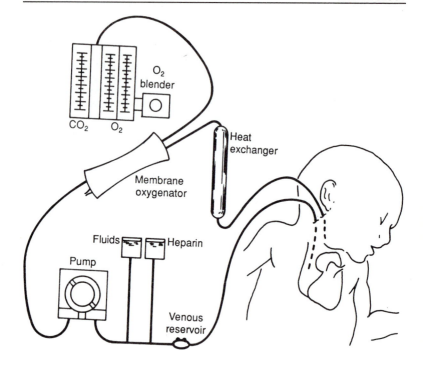

FIGURE 11–1. The veno-arterial extracorporeal membrane oxygenation circuit. Blood is withdrawn from the right atrium through a catheter entering the internal jugular vein. Heparin, medications and fluids are added. The membrane removes CO_2 and adds oxygen. The blood is then warmed and returned to the ascending aorta through a catheter in the internal carotid artery. *(Reproduced with permission from Short BL and Pearson GD. Journal of Intensive Care Medicine, Volume 1, Number 1, 1986)*

VI. Prognosis. The Neonatal ECMO Registry was established in 1985 and currently has over 7500 neonatal patients, the first of whom was treated in 1975. As of this writing (1993), overall neonatal survival is 81%. The registry also keeps track of survival rates for specific diseases, and these data are as follows. For meconium aspiration syndrome, the survival rate is 94%; for pulmonary hypertension, 84%; for hyaline membrane disease, 83%; for sepsis/pneumonia, 77%; and for congenital diaphragmatic hernia, 59%.

Long-term follow-up of these high-risk babies has fortunately been an integral part of most ECMO programs. In general, the survivors do well, particularly when consideration is given to how sick they were before they went on ECMO. The majority are neurodevelopmentally normal. Factors associated with developmental delay and/or handicaps are major intracranial hemorrhage, chronic lung disease, and gestational age < 37 weeks (Glass, 1993). Continued comprehensive long-term follow-up is essential before we can be reassured about the outcome of survivors of this high-technology procedure.

REFERENCES

Glass P: Patient neurodevelopmental outcomes after neonatal ECMO. Chapter 16 in: *Extracorporeal Life Support.* Arensman RM, Cornish JD (eds). Blackwell Scientific Publications, 1993.

Klein MD: Neonatal ECMO. *ASAIO Trans* 1988;**34(1):**39.

Marsh TD, Wilkerson SA, Cook LN: Extracorporeal membrane oxygenation selection criteria:

Partial pressure of arterial oxygen versus alveolar-arterial oxygen gradient. *Pediatrics* 1988; **82(2):**162.

The Neonatal ECMO Registry of the Extracorporeal Life Support Organization. Ann Arbor, Michigan, April 1993.

Short BL, Miller MK, Anderson KD: Extracorporeal membrane oxygenation in the management of respiratory failure in the newborn. *Clin Perinatol* 1987;**14:**737.

Stolar CJ, Dillow PW: Extracorporeal membrane oxygenation for neonatal respiratory failure. *Surg Ann* 1987;**19:**111.

Toomasian JM et al: National experience with extracorporeal membrane oxygenation for newborn respiratory failure. Data from 715 cases. *ASAIO Trans* 1988;**34:**140.

12 Infant Transport

As regionalization and specialization of care for newborn infants have developed, a new type of team has been created especially for transport of these infants from a referring hospital to a level III center (neonatal intensive care unit [NICU]). A great deal of planning must take place in order for these teams to function effectively, and clear guidelines must be set up regarding personnel, procedures, and equipment needed (Guidelines for Perinatal Care, 1992). Policies and procedures will reflect the unique characteristics of each region (eg, size, geography, economics, sophistication of medical services). Lines of communication must always be open between the referring hospital and the NICU at all levels (administrators, physicians, nurses) and with ambulance or air services. Ideally, the mother would be transferred to the level III center before delivery of a high-risk infant, but this is not always possible.

I. **Transport team.** The team may include physicians, nurses, respiratory therapists, and/or emergency medical technicians (Bose, 1984). Special training must be provided in the care of sick infants. A specific medical protocol is set up. The team should be able to contact the attending neonatologist at any time during transport. Appropriate insurance coverage is necessary for team members, and questions of liability must be worked out with legal consultation between hospitals, ambulance services, and aircraft services.

At the referring hospital, team members should conduct themselves as professional representatives of the NICU, avoiding conflict with or criticism of the referring hospital staff. Questions about transport protocol should be worked out directly between the referring physician and the attending neonatologist.

II. **Equipment.** Each transport team should be self-sufficient. Medications and equipment can be chosen according to published lists (Ferrara, 1980). Special emphasis is placed on maintaining thermal neutrality (eg, plastic swaddling; heated, humidified inspired air mixtures). Noise and vibration often compromise auditory and visual monitoring, and well-calibrated indwelling blood pressure and oxygen tension monitors (or transcutaneous oximetry) may be useful. An instant camera is a "must" because pictures of the infant may be the mother's only psychological support for days.

III. **Protocol for stabilization and transfer.** The goal of stabilization is to make the transfer uneventful.

   A. **General procedures.** *Attention to the details of stabilization is important!* Unless active resuscitation is under way, the team's first task at the referring hospital is to *listen* to the history and assessment of the infant's status. The vital signs are then obtained. At this point, a precise diagnosis of all the infant's problems may be less important than predicting what the infant will need during transport. It is prudent to initiate anticipated interventions before leaving the referring hospital. For example, an infant with increasing work of breathing and increasing needs for inspired oxygen who faces a 2-hour journey probably should be placed on mechanical ventilation and have an intravenous line in place before transfer begins. In most cases, an infant is not ready for transport until basic neonatal needs are met: **thermoneutrality, acceptable cardiac and respiratory function, and blood glucose levels in the normal range.** Vital signs must be stable and catheters and tubes appropriately placed. Problems that may occur during transport should be anticipated. The NICU should be given an expected arrival time. The parents should be allowed to see and touch the infant before transport. During transport, vigilant monitoring should continue for unexpected changes in the infant's status. The respiratory rate, heart rate, blood pressure, and oxygen saturation levels should be followed. Transcutaneous oximetry should be used if available. After transfer is completed, the team should talk with the parents and, if possible, with the referring physician.

B. Prophylactic antibiotic therapy. Infants at risk for sepsis and those with indwelling catheters should probably receive antibiotic therapy. Culture of blood samples may be performed at the referring hospital or at the NICU. Antibiotic dosages are given in Chapter 73.

C. Gastric intubation. If the infant has a gastrointestinal disorder (including ileus accompanying critical illness) or diaphragmatic hernia or if continuous positive airway pressure is administered through the nose or a mask, venting of the stomach with a nasogastric or orogastric tube is indicated, especially if airplane or helicopter transport will be used. Venting should be done prior to transport, because the air trapped in the gastrointestinal tract will expand in volume as atmospheric pressure decreases (see below, **V.B, Dysbarism**).

D. Temperature control and fluid balance. Special attention to temperature and fluid balance is required for infants with open lesions (eg, myelomeningocele, omphalocele). A dry or moist protective dressing over the lesion can be covered by thin plastic wrap to reduce radiant heat loss.

IV. Evaluation of transport. Each transport should have a scoring system that reflects the "before" and "after" status of the infant (Hermansen, 1988). For example, vital signs and glucose oxidase measurements taken when the team first arrives at the referring hospital should be compared to the same measurements taken on admission to the NICU. This system provides quality control of transports and is useful in outreach education to convey constructive criticism to referring hospitals.

V. Special considerations in air transport. Each region should develop protocols for choosing ground or air transport, based on distance, nature of terrain, location of landing sites, and availability of aircraft and ambulances (American Academy of Pediatrics, 1986).

A. Safety guidelines. Clear guidelines should be established regarding air transport. Decisions regarding flight safety should be made according to weather and other flight conditions (ie, the pilot should not be given information on the age of the patient or the severity of the illness before making decisions on flight safety). Controlled landing sites familiar to the pilot should be used. Loading and unloading of the aircraft should not take place while engines are running; an idling helicopter is dangerous.

B. Dysbarism. In helicopters and unpressurized aircraft, dysbarism (imbalance between air pressure in the atmosphere and the pressure of gases within the body) causes predictable problems. Partial pressures of inspired gases decrease as altitude increases, so infants will require an increased concentration of inspired oxygen (Ferrara, 1980). Trapped free air in the thorax or intestines will expand in volume and may cause significant pulmonary embarrassment. A cuffed tube or catheter should be evacuated before takeoff.

Note: Because blood pressure varies with changing gravitational force, fluctuations noted during climbing or descent should not be cause for alarm.

REFERENCES

American Academy of Pediatrics Committee on Hospital Care: Guidelines for air and ground transportation of pediatric patients. *Pediatrics* 1986;**78:**943.

Bose CL, Jung AL, Thornton JW: Neonatal transport. *Perinatol Neonatal* 1984;**8:**61.

Ferrara A, Harin A: *Emergency Transfer of the High-Risk Neonate.* Mosby, 1980.

Hermansen MC et al: A validation of a scoring system to evaluate the condition of transported very low birth weight neonates. *Am J Perinatol* 1988;**5:**74.

Interhospital care of the perinatal patient. Chapter 2 in: *Guidelines for Perinatal Care,* 3rd ed. American Academy of Pediatrics, 1992.

13 Follow-Up of High-Risk Infants

As neonatal intensive care continues to develop as a medical specialty, concern has grown regarding the quality of life of high-risk infants. Follow-up clinics are a valuable, and even necessary, adjunct to neonatal intensive care in that they provide both service to infants and families and feedback to neonatologists and obstetricians.

I. **Goals of neonatal follow-up clinic**
   A. **Early identification of developmental disability.** Some infants will be referred for further diagnostic evaluation and/or community services.
   B. **Parent counseling.** Parents of children who do well can be reassured by positive feedback. Parents of children with disabilities will need help in coping with their child's problems. Physical and occupational therapists can provide valuable suggestions regarding positioning, handling, and feeding infants.
   C. **Identification and treatment of medical complications.** Some disorders may not be anticipated at the time of discharge from the neonatal intensive care unit (NICU).
   D. **Feedback for neonatologists, pediatricians, obstetricians, and pediatric surgeons** regarding developmental progress, medical status, and unusual or unforeseen complications in these infants is essential.

II. **Staff of neonatal follow-up clinic.** Pediatricians, developmental pediatricians, and neonatologists make up the regular staff of the clinic. Special consultation may be needed from audiologists, ophthalmologists, psychologists, physical therapists, occupational therapists, speech and language specialists, social workers, respiratory therapists, nutritionists, pediatric surgeons, and orthopedic surgeons.

III. **Risk factors for developmental disability.** It is virtually impossible to diagnose developmental disability with certainty in the neonatal period, but a number of perinatal risk factors have been identified.
   A. **Prematurity.** Although the majority of preterm infants are not significantly handicapped, they do have a higher incidence of cerebral palsy and mental retardation than the general population (5–10% of preterm infants with birth weight below 1500 g, 10–40% with birth weight below 750 g). Preterm infants also have a higher risk of minimal cerebral dysfunction, including language disorders, visual perception problems, attention deficits, and learning disabilities. Preterm infants with slow head growth (especially in the postnatal period), asphyxia, sepsis (especially meningitis), chronic lung disease, abnormal neonatal neurodevelopmental examinations, and abnormalities on cranial ultrasonography or CT scanning have an increased risk of developmental disability. Cranial abnormalities, including intraventricular hemorrhage (especially grades III and IV), ventricular dilatation (with or without hemorrhage), cortical atrophy and periventricular echodensities (periventricular leukomalacia), are all associated with a poor prognosis. The incidence of handicaps is very high with periventricular echodensities, especially if they are bilateral and large.
   B. **Intrauterine growth retardation (IUGR).** Although full-term infants who are small for gestational age (SGA) appear to have no (or only slightly higher) risk of cerebral palsy and mental retardation, they have a high incidence of minimal cerebral dysfunction, especially learning disability. Preterm SGA infants have a high incidence of cerebral palsy and mental retardation (Pena, 1988). The risk of developmental disability in SGA infants is usually determined by the cause of IUGR, timing of the insult, and subsequent perinatal complications (eg, asphyxia, hypoglycemia, polycythemia) (Allen, 1984).
   C. **Asphyxia.** Perinatal asphyxia is associated with later developmental disability

but is frequently difficult to define. Apgar scores are useful in predicting the outcome only when they are very low (score of 0–3) for extended periods of time (> 10 minutes) in full-term newborns (Nelson, 1981). Most outcome studies have focused on severely asphyxiated infants who required prolonged resuscitation or who were symptomatic as newborns. The mortality rate for this group is high (50%); however, 75% of the survivors are free of major handicaps. Those with handicaps usually have multiple handicaps, including severe mental retardation, spastic quadriplegia, microcephaly, seizures, and sensory impairment. The number and type of neonatal symptoms correlate with the degree of later disability, as do abnormalities on EEG and CT scan (Brown, 1974; Samat, 1976; Robertson, 1985; Fitzhardinge, 1982).

D. Other risk factors. Other perinatal factors are less common but are associated with a high risk of handicap.

  1. TORCH infections. Infants with congenital cytomegalovirus infection, toxoplasmosis, or rubella who are symptomatic at birth have a high incidence (60–90%) of developmental disability. Even if asymptomatic as neonates, they are at risk for sensory impairment and learning disability.

  2. Infection, especially meningitis, carries a risk of later developmental disability.

  3. Hypoglycemia and polycythemia. The presence of symptomatic hypoglycemia or polycythemia (hyperviscosity) at birth is associated with handicap.

  4. In Utero exposure to drugs. Maternal use of heroin or methadone during pregnancy can lead to neonatal withdrawal syndrome and a higher rate of attention deficits and behavior problems in preschool and school age children. Fetal alcohol syndrome includes growth deficiency, dysmorphic features, congenital anomalies, mental retardation, hyperactivity, and fine motor dysfunction. Maternal use of cocaine has been associated with lower birthweights, microcephaly, cerebral infarction, abruption placenta, fetal distress, and behavioral and EEG abnormalities in the newborns, but the long-term effects of cocaine use during pregnancy are unknown. Other drugs that appear to affect fetal development include dilantin, trimethadione, valproate, warfarin, aminopterin, and retinoic acid.

IV. Parameters requiring follow-up

A. Growth. Growth parameters and trends should be carefully monitored at each follow-up visit. These include **length, weight, and head circumference** (see also Appendix F). Although most preterm infants "catch up" in growth during the first year, some SGA infants, extremely immature infants, and infants with severe chronic lung disease may always remain small. Slow head growth may be an early indication of developmental disability.

B. Blood pressure. A silent sequela of neonatal intensive care that may have serious long-term consequences is high blood pressure. Blood pressure measurements should be performed for all infants on a periodic basis.

C. Breathing disorders

  1. Apnea. Infants requiring home apnea monitors and/or those receiving theophylline for apnea require close follow-up, with special attention paid to whether or not resuscitation has been required. When to discontinue monitoring is a matter of debate and is usually decided by the physician and the family. (See also Apnea and Periodic Breathing, p 177)

  2. Chronic lung disease. Infants with chronic lung disease require specialized medical and developmental follow-up. The decision to discontinue administration of supplemental oxygen or to taper the amount should be based on pulse oximeter studies during periods of sleep, wakefulness, and feeding and on clinical criteria (ie, growth, exercise intolerance). Poor growth, sleeping or feeding difficulties, rising hematocrit, increasing abnormalities on ECG and echocardiogram, and plateauing or loss of developmental progress after discontinuing oxygen all suggest intermittent hypoxia; oxygen administration should be resumed, and the infant should be restudied. Some infants with chronic lung disease who have done well breathing room air for some time may have problems if they develop upper or lower respiratory tract infections.

D. Hearing. Infants with a family history of childhood hearing impairment, congenital perinatal hearing (eg, TORCH) infection, congenital malformations of the head or neck, birth weight less than 1500 g, hyperbilirubinemia requiring exchange transfusion, bacterial meningitis, or severe perinatal asphyxia or who were exposed to ototoxic drugs (eg, furosemide, gentamicin, vancomycin) are at risk for hearing impairment and should be referred for evaluation. Because hearing is essential for the acquisition of language, it is important to diagnose hearing impairment as early as possible. Some NICUs screen for hearing loss with **brain-stem auditory evoked potentials** or more recently, transient evoked otoacoustic emissions. This test can identify infants with a high risk of hearing impairment who need careful audiologic follow-up. However, because of the high false-positive results, it is difficult to diagnose hearing loss with certainty in the neonatal period.

E. Vision. Preterm infants who were given oxygen in the neonatal period are at risk for developing **retinopathy of prematurity.** An indirect ophthalmoscopic examination should be performed at 5–7 weeks by a pediatric ophthalmologist for all oxygen-exposed premature infants who weigh less than 1800 g or are delivered at less than 35 weeks gestation. Infants less than 1300 g or 30 weeks gestation require examination regardless of oxygen exposure. Until the retina is fully vascularized, follow-up ophthalmologic examinations should be performed every 2 weeks (or every week if active disease is progressing). Infants with congenital infection and asphyxia should also have ophthalmologic examinations and follow-up. All high-risk infants should have an assessment of visual acuity at 1–5 years.

F. Language and motor skills. For each infant, a history of language and motor milestones should be obtained and compared to norms for the age (Caputo, 1980). Infants with persistent delay, dissociation, or deviance should be carefully assessed for disability by a developmental pediatrician or multidisciplinary team.

1. Delay is late acquisition of milestones.

2. Dissociation is delay in one area of development compared to other areas and can help diagnose disability (eg, delay in gross and fine motor development with normal language development suggests cerebral palsy, whereas delay in language acquisition with normal motor development suggests mental retardation, language disorder, or hearing impairment).

3. Deviance is acquisition of milestones out of normal sequence (eg, the child is able to stand but does not sit well).

G. Neurologic development is a dynamic process, and what is normal at a certain age may be abnormal at another. The examiner must know what is normal at each age and must decide if deviations from normal are significant. Preterm infants are often hypotonic at birth but develop flexor tone in a caudocephalad direction. Preterm infants at term and full-term newborns have flexor hypertonia and lose this flexor tone in a caudocephalad direction (ie, at 1–2 months from term there is more flexor tone in the arms than the legs). By 4 months from term, muscle tone should be the same in the upper and lower extremities.

1. Neurodevelopmental examination of high-risk infants should include assessment of:

  a. Posture.

  b. Muscle tone in the extremities.

  c. Axial (neck and trunk) muscle tone.

  d. Deep tendon reflexes.

  e. Pathologic reflexes (eg, Babinski reflex).

  f. Primitive reflexes (eg, Moro reflex, asymmetric tonic neck reflex).

  g. Postural reactions (eg, righting or equilibrium response).

2. Abnormalities in high-risk infants. Many high-risk infants have some abnormalities during the first year of life that may resolve by age 1 year, even if they disappear or do not cause significant functional impairment. These early neuromotor abnormalities may signal late fine motor dysfunctory problems with balance, attention deficit, behavior problems, and/or learning disability. The presence of multiple persistent abnormalities in conjunction with motor delay suggests cerebral palsy. These infants should be referred for multidisciplinary evaluation. Because damage to the central nervous system is seldom focal, infants with motor impairment are likely to have associated deficits (eg, mental retardation, learning disability, sensory impairment) that eventually may be more debilitating. The following developmental abnormalities are commonly seen in high-risk infants during the first year of life.

  a. **Hypotonia** (generalized or axial) is especially common in preterm infants and infants with chronic lung disease.
  b. **Hypertonia** is seen most often in the lower extremities (hips and ankles) in preterm infants.
  c. **Asymmetry** of function, tone, posture, or reflexes may be seen.
  d. **Neck extensor hypertonia and shoulder retraction** is common in infants with chronic lung disease, tracheostomy, or prolonged intubation and may interfere with head control, hand use, rolling, sitting, and getting in and out of sitting.
  e. **Involuntary movements, grimacing, and poor coordination** are indicative of extrapyramidal involvement.
  f. **Feeding problems** may occur.

H. **Cognitive development.** Language development is one of the most reliable predictors of intelligence and can help identify children with cognitive impairment. Cognitive evaluation may be difficult in infants. High-risk children should have a psychological evaluation at age 1–3 years and before starting school because of the risk of learning disability. An audiologic evaluation should be performed by 6–9 months to rule out hearing impairment.

V. **Correction for prematurity.** Correcting for prematurity when assessing physical or psychological development continues to be *controversial*. Recent data suggest that motor milestone development proceeds according to age from conception and that one should correct for the degree of prematurity. Recommendations regarding correction for cognitive abilities varies widely: some correct completely throughout childhood; some correct only to age 1 or 2; some use partial correction. We recommend calculating both the child's chronologic age and age corrected for degree of prematurity (term age equivalent, or adjusted age). A child's language and problem-solving abilities should fall between these 2 ages. The older a child becomes the less important this issue is: By the time a child is 5, arithmetically 3 months' difference (eg, 60 vs 57 months) matters little.

VI. **Multidisciplinary evaluation.** The presence of one disability is an indication for careful evaluation in other areas. Brain damage is seldom focal and often diffuse. These infants should be referred for complete multidisciplinary evaluation to identify areas of strength and weakness and to formulate an appropriate rehabilitation program. A comprehensive overview allows for a more realistic determination of prognosis. Appropriate counseling can then be given to the parents.

REFERENCES

Allen MC: The high risk infant. *Pediatr Clin North Am* 1993;**40:**479–90.

Allen MC: Developmental implication of intrauterine growth retardation. *Inf Young Children* 1992;**5:**13–28.

Allen MC, Alexander GR: Gross motor milestones in preterm infants: Correction for degree of prematurity. *J Pediatr* 1990;**116:**955.

Allen MC, Alexander GR: Using gross motor milestones to identify very preterm infants at risk for cerebral palsy. *Dev Med Child Neurol.* 1992;**34:**226–32.

Allen MC, Jones MD: Medical complications of prematurity. *Obstet Gynecol* 1986;**67:**427.

Bandstra ES, Bunkett G: Maternal-fetal and neonatal effects of in utero cocaine exposure. *Semin Perinatol* 1991;**15:**288–301.

Brown JK et al: Neurological aspects of perinatal asphyxia. *Dev Med Child Neurol* 1974;**16:**567.

Capute AJ, Palmer FB: A pediatric overview of the spectrum of developmental disabilities. *J Dev Behav Pediatr* 1980;**1**:66.

Capute AJ et al: Normal gross motor development: The influence of race, sex and socioeconomic status. *Dev Med Child Neurol* 1985;**27**:635.

Capute AJ et al: Clinical linguistic and auditory milestone scale: Prediction of cognition in infancy. *Dev Med Child Neurol* 1986;**28**:762.

Dipietro JA, Allen MC: Estimation of gestational age: Implications for developmental research. *Child Dev* 1991;**62**:1184–99.

Fitzhardinge PM, Flodmark D, Ashby S: The prognostic value of computed tomography of the brain in asphyxiated premature infants. *J Pediatr* 1982;**100**:476.

Hack M, Fanaroff AA: Outcomes of extremely low birth weight infants between 1982 and 1988. *N Engl J Med* 1989;**24**:1262.

Nelson KB, Ellenberg JH: Apgar scores as predictors of chronic neurologic disability. *Pediatrics* 1981;**68**:36.

Pena IC, Teberg AJ, Finello KM: The premature small for gestational age infant during the first year of life: Comparison by birthweight and gestational age. *J Pediatr* 1988;**113**:1066.

Robertson C, Finer N: Term infants with hypoxic-ischemic encephalopathy: Outcome at 3–5 years. *Dev Med Child Neurol* 1985;**27**:473–84.

Samat HB, Samat MS: Neonatal encephalopathy following fetal distress: A clinical and electroencephalographic study. *Arch Neurol* 1976;**33**:696.

14 Arterial Access

All procedures involving blood or secretions should be performed with gloves.

ARTERIAL PUNCTURE (RADIAL ARTERY PUNCTURE)

I. **Indications.** Arterial puncture is performed (1) to obtain blood for blood gas measurements or (2) when blood is needed and venous or capillary blood samples cannot be obtained.

II. **Equipment.** A 23- or 25-gauge scalp vein needle, a 1- or 3-mL syringe, povidone-iodine and alcohol swabs, a 4 × 4 gauze pad, gloves, and 1:1000 heparin.

III. **Procedure**

A. If submitting a blood gas sample, most hospitals already have 1-mL syringes coated with heparin. If this is not available, draw a small amount of heparin (concentration, 1:1000) into the syringe to be used for submitting the blood gas sample and then discard the excess heparin from the syringe. The small amount of heparin coating the syringe is sufficient to prevent coagulation of the sample. Excessive amounts of heparin may interfere with laboratory results, causing a falsely low pH and $PaCO_2$. If any other laboratory test is to be performed, do not use heparin.

B. The radial artery is the most frequently used puncture site and will be described here. An alternative site is the posterior tibial artery . Use of femoral arteries should be reserved for emergency situations. Brachial arteries should not be used because there is minimal collateral circulation and a risk of median nerve damage.

C. Check for collateral circulation and patency of the ulnar artery by means of the **Allen test.** First elevate the arm and simultaneously occlude the radial and ulnar arteries at the wrist, and then rub the palm to cause blanching. Release pressure on the ulnar artery. If normal color returns in the palm in less than 10 seconds, adequate collateral circulation from the ulnar artery is present. If normal color does not return for 15 seconds or longer or does not return at all, the collateral circulation is poor and it is best not to use the radial artery in this arm. The radial and ulnar arteries in the other arm should then be tested for collateral circulation.

D. To obtain the blood sample, take the patient's hand in your left hand (for a right-handed operator) and extend the wrist. Palpate the radial artery with the index finger of your left hand (Fig 14–1). Marking the puncture site with a fingernail imprint may be helpful.

E. Clean the puncture site first with a povidone-iodine swab and then with an alcohol swab.

F. Puncture the skin at about a 30-degree angle, and slowly advance the needle with the bevel up until blood appears in the tubing (Fig 14–1). With arterial blood samples, little aspiration is needed to fill the syringe.

G. Collect the least amount of blood needed for this and any other test in a neonate. The volume of blood taken should not exceed 3–5% of the total blood volume (the total blood volume in a neonate is approximately 80 mL/kg). As an example, if 4 mL of blood is drawn from an infant weighing 1 kg, this represents 5% of the total blood volume.

H. Withdraw the needle and apply firm, but not occlusive, pressure to the site for at least 5 minutes with a 4 × 4 gauze pad to ensure adequate hemostasis.

I. Before submitting an arterial blood gas sample, **expel air bubbles** from the

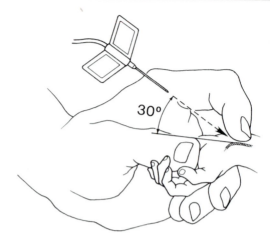

FIGURE 14–1. Technique of arterial puncture in the neonate.

sample and tightly cap the syringe. Failure to do this can lead to errors in testing. (See **IV.D**, below).

J. Place the syringe in ice and take it to the laboratory immediately. Note the collection time, the patient's temperature, and hemoglobin on the laboratory slip.

IV. Complications

A. Hematoma. To minimize the risk of hematoma, use the smallest-gauge needle possible, and immediately after withdrawing the needle, apply pressure for approximately 5 minutes. Hematomas will usually resolve spontaneously.

B. Arteriospasm, thrombosis, and embolism. These complications can be minimized by using the smallest-gauge needle possible. With thrombosis, the vessel will usually recanalize over a period of time. Arteriospasm will usually resolve spontaneously.

C. Infection. The risk of infection is rare and can be minimized by using strict sterile technique. Infection is commonly caused by gram-positive organisms such as *Staphylococcus epidermis,* which should be treated with nafcillin or vancomycin and gentamicin (see Chap 73). Drug sensitivities at the specific hospital should be checked.

D. Inaccuracy of blood gas results. Too much heparin in the syringe may result in a falsely low pH and $PaCO_2$. Remove excess heparin before obtaining the blood sample. Air bubbles caused by failure to cap the syringe may falsely elevate the PaO_2 and falsely lower the $PaCO_2$.

PERCUTANEOUS ARTERIAL CATHETERIZATION

I. Indications

A. When frequent arterial blood samples are required and an umbilical arterial catheter cannot be placed or has been removed because of complications, percutaneous arterial catheterization is required.

B. This procedure is also indicated when intra-arterial blood pressure monitoring is required.

II. Equipment.
Use a 22- or 24-gauge needle with a 1-inch catheter encasement (Jelco or Angiocath). A 24-gauge needle is recommended for infants weighing less than 1500 g. Also needed are an armboard (or 2 tongue blades taped together), adhesive tape, sterile drapes, povidone-iodine and alcohol swabs, gloves, antisep-

tic ointment, a needle holder, suture scissors, 4–0 or 5–0 silk sutures, normal saline or 1/2 normal saline solution (latter preferred in premature infants to decrease incidence of hypernatremia) in a 1-mL or 3-mL syringe heparinized saline solution (1 unit of heparin per mL saline) in a pressure bag, and connecting tubing.

III. Procedure. Two methods are described here, both using the radial artery, which is the most commonly used site. An alternative site is the posterior tibial artery. Transillumination may be helpful in locating the artery in premature infants. Arterial catheterization requires a great deal of patience.

A. Method 1

1. Verify adequate collateral circulation using the Allen test described previously (see p 000).
2. Place the infant's wrist on an armboard (some prefer to use an intravenous bag), and hyperextend the wrist by placing gauze underneath it. Tape the arm and hand securely to the board (Fig 14–2). Put on gloves, and place sterile drapes around the puncture site. Cleanse the site, first with povidone-iodine swabs and then with alcohol swabs.
3. Puncture both the anterior and posterior walls of the artery at a 30- to 45-degree angle. Remove the stylet. There should be little or no backflow of blood.
4. Pull the catheter back slowly until blood is seen; this signifies that the arterial lumen has been entered.
5. Advance the catheter after attaching the syringe and flush the catheter. Never use hypertonic solutions to flush an arterial line.
6. Secure the catheter with 4–0 or 5–0 silk sutures in 2 or 3 places. Occasionally, it is not possible to suture the catheter, and it should be securely taped instead.
7. Connect the tubing from the heparinized saline pressure bag to the catheter.
8. Place povidone-iodine ointment on the area where the catheter enters the skin, and cover the area with gauze taped securely in place.

B. Method 2 (alternative method)

1. Perform steps 1 and 2 as above.
2. Puncture the anterior wall of the artery until blood return is seen. At this point, the catheter should be in the lumen of the artery.
3. Advance the catheter into the artery while simultaneously withdrawing the

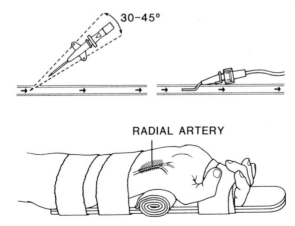

FIGURE 14–2. When placing an indwelling arterial catheter, the wrist should be secured as shown. The catheter assembly is introduced at a 30- to 45-degree angle.

needle. The blood should be flowing freely from the catheter if the catheter is properly positioned.

4. Attach the syringe and flush the catheter.

5. Secure the line as in method 1.

IV. Complications

    A. Arteriospasm. The risk of arteriospasm can be minimized by using the smallest-gauge catheter possible and performing as few punctures as possible. If arteriospasm occurs, the catheter must be removed until the spasm resolves.

    B. Embolism or thrombosis. To prevent these complications, make certain that air is not introduced into the catheter and that the catheter is flushed with heparinized saline.

    C. Skin ischemia or gangrene. Adequate collateral circulation decreases the risk of this complication. Always perform the Allen test to verify collateral flow (see p 133, **III.C**).

    D. Hematoma. See p 134, **IV.A**.

    E. Blood loss. Accidental loss of catheter position, resulting in hemorrhage, can occur.

    F. Infection.

UMBILICAL ARTERY CATHETERIZATION

  I. Indications

    A. Umbilical artery catheterization is indicated when frequent measurements of arterial blood gases are required.

    B. This procedure is also used for continuous arterial blood pressure monitoring.

    C. To provide exchange transfusion.

  II. Equipment. Prepackaged umbilical artery catheterization trays usually include sterile drapes, tape measure, needle holder, suture scissors, hemostat, forceps, scalpel, and a blunt needle. Also needed are a 3-way stopcock, an umbilical artery catheter (3.5F for an infant weighing < 1.2 kg, 5F for an infant weighing > 1.2 kg), umbilical tape, silk tape (eg Dermicel), 3–0 silk suture, gauze pads, antiseptic solution, gloves, mask and hat, a 10-mL syringe, normal or 1/2 normal saline solution, and a 22-gauge needle.

  III. Procedure

    A. Place the patient supine. Wrap a diaper around both legs and tape the diaper to the bed. This stabilizes the patient for the procedure and allows observation of the feet for vasospasm.

    B. Put on sterile gloves, mask, hat, and a sterile gown.

    C. Prepare the umbilical catheter tray by attaching the stopcock to the blunt needle and then attaching the catheter to the blunt needle. Fill the 10-mL syringe with flush solution, and inject through the catheter.

    D. Clean the umbilical cord area with antiseptic solution. Place sterile drapes around the umbilicus, leaving the feet and head exposed. Observe the infant closely during the procedure for vasospasm in the legs or signs of distress.

    E. Tie a piece of umbilical tape around the base of the umbilical cord tight enough to minimize blood loss but loosely enough so that the catheter can be passed easily through the vessel (snug but not tight). Cut off the excess umbilical cord with scissors or a scalpel, leaving a 1-cm stump. A scalpel usually makes a cleaner cut, so that the vessels are more easily seen. There are *usually* 2 umbilical arteries and one umbilical vein. The arteries are smaller and are usually located at 4 and 7 o'clock. The vein usually has a floppy wall (Fig 14–3A and B).

    F. Using the curved hemostat, grasp the end of the umbilicus to hold it upright and steady.

    G. Use the forceps to open and dilate the umbilical artery. First, place one arm of the forceps in the artery, and then use both arms to gently dilate the vessel (Fig 14–3C and D).

    H. Once the artery is sufficiently dilated, insert the catheter.

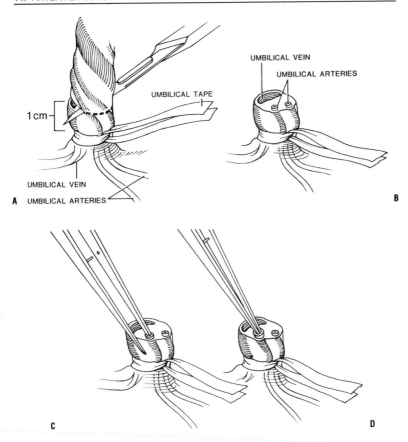

FIGURE 14–3. A: The umbilical cord should be amputated, leaving a 1-cm stump. **B:** Identification of the umbilical vessels. **C and D:** A forceps is used to gently dilate the umbilical artery.

I. Be certain you know the correct length of catheter to be inserted. The catheter is positioned in one of 2 ways. In so-called **"low catheterization,"** the tip of the catheter lies below the level of L3 or L4. In **"high catheterization,"** the tip lies above the diaphragm at the level of T6 to T9. Positioning is usually determined by the routine at a given institution. High positioning is associated with hypertension and an increased risk of intraventricular hemorrhage. Low positioning has been associated with more episodes of vasospasm of the lower extremities. The length of catheter needed can be obtained from the **Umbilical Catheter Measurements** (Appendix J, page 565). A rapid method for determining the length needed for low catheterization is to measure two-thirds of the distance from the umbilicus to the midportion of the clavicle.

J. Once the catheter is in position, aspirate to verify blood return.

K. Secure the catheter as shown in Fig 14–4. The silk tape is folded over part way, the catheter is placed, and the remaining portion of the tape is folded over. Suture the silk tape to the skin at the base of the umbilicus as shown, using 3–0 silk sutures. Connect the tubing to the monitor and flush it. No special dressing is needed. The umbilical stump with the catheter in place is left open to the air.

L. Obtain an abdominal x-ray film to verify the position of a low catheter. To check

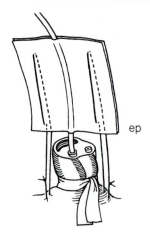

FIGURE 14–4. The umbilical artery catheter is secured with silk tape, which is attached to the base of the umbilicus with 000 silk sutures.

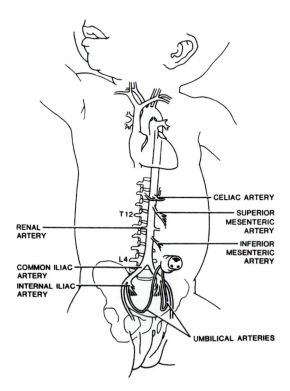

FIGURE 14–5. Important landmarks, related vessels, and path of the umbilical artery. The internal iliac artery is also called the *hypogastric artery.*

the position of a high catheter, obtain a chest x-ray film. Figure 14–5 shows landmarks and the relationship of umbilical arteries to the other major abdominal arteries. X-ray films showing positioning can be found in Chapter 9.

IV. Complications

A. Infection. Infection can be minimized by using strict sterile technique. No attempt should be made to advance a catheter once it has been placed and sutured into position; instead, the catheter should be replaced.

B. Vascular accidents. Thrombosis or infarction may occur. Vasospasm may lead to loss of an extremity. Hypertension is a long-term complication caused by stenosis of the renal artery as a result of improper catheter placement near the renal arteries.

C. Hemorrhage. Hemorrhage may occur if the catheter or tubing becomes disconnected. The tubing stopcocks must be securely fastened. If hemorrhage occurs, blood volume replacement may be necessary.

D. Vessel perforation. The catheter should never be forced into position. If the catheter cannot be easily advanced, use of another vessel should be attempted. If perforation occurs, surgical intervention may be necessary.

15 Bladder Aspiration (Suprapubic Urine Collection)

I. **Indications.** Bladder aspiration is performed to obtain urine for culture when less invasive technique is not possible.

II. **Equipment.** Sterile gloves, povidone-iodine solution, a 23- or 25-gauge 1-inch needle with a 3-mL syringe attached, 4 × 4 gauze pads, gloves, and a sterile container.

III. **Procedure**

A. Be certain that voiding has not occurred within the previous hour so that there will be enough urine in the bladder to make collection worthwhile.

B. An assistant should hold the infant's legs in the frog-leg position.

C. Locate the site of bladder puncture, which is approximately 0.5–1 cm above the pubic symphysis, in the midline of the lower abdomen.

D. Put on sterile gloves, and clean the skin at the puncture site with antiseptic solution.

E. Palpate the pubic symphysis. Insert the needle approximately 0.5–1 cm above the pubic symphysis at a 90-degree angle (Fig 15–1).

F. Advance the needle while aspirating at the same time. Do not advance the needle once urine is seen in the syringe. This precaution helps prevent perforation of the posterior wall of the bladder.

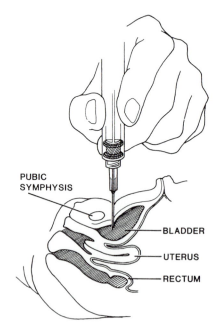

PUBIC
SYMPHYSIS

BLADDER

UTERUS

RECTUM

FIGURE 15–1. Technique of suprapubic bladder aspiration.

G. Withdraw the needle, and maintain pressure over the site of puncture.

H. Place a sterile cap on the syringe or transfer the specimen to a sterile urine cup, and submit the specimen to the laboratory.

IV. Complications

A. Bleeding. Microscopic hematuria may occur after bladder aspiration but is usually transient and rarely causes concern. Hemorrhage may occur if there is a bleeding disorder. The platelet count should be checked before aspiration is performed and if low, the procedure should not be performed.

B. Infection. Infection is not likely to occur if strict sterile technique is used.

C. Perforation of bowel. With careful identification of the landmarks described above, this complication is rare. If the bowel is perforated (indicated by aspiration of bowel contents), close observation is recommended, and intravenous antibiotics should be considered.

16 Bladder Catheterization

I. Indications
A. Bladder catheterization is performed when a urine specimen is needed and a clean-catch specimen cannot be obtained or suprapubic aspiration cannot be performed.

B. The procedure is performed to monitor urinary output, to relieve urinary retention, or to obtain a cystogram or voiding cystourethrogram.

II. Equipment.
Sterile gloves, cotton balls, povidone-iodine solution, sterile drapes, lubricant, a sterile collection bottle, and urethral catheters (3.5F umbilical artery catheter for infants weighing < 1000 g; 5F feeding tube for infants weighing 1000–1800 g; 8F feeding tube for infants weighing > 1800 g).

III. Procedure
A. Males
1. Place the infant supine, with the thighs abducted (frog-leg position).
2. Cleanse the penis with povidone-iodine solution, starting with the meatus and moving in a proximal direction.
3. Put on sterile gloves, and drape the area with sterile towels.
4. Place the tip of the catheter in sterile lubricant.
5. Hold the penis approximately perpendicular to the body to straighten the penile urethra and help prevent false passage. Advance the catheter until urine appears. A slight resistance may be felt as the catheter passes the external sphincter, and steady, gentle pressure is usually needed to advance past this area. Never force the catheter (Fig 16–1).
6. Collect the urine specimen. If the catheter is to remain in place, some feel it should be taped to the lower abdomen rather than the leg in males to help decrease stricture formation caused by pressure on the posterior urethra.

B. Females
1. Place the infant supine, with the thighs abducted (frog-leg position).
2. Separate the labia, and cleanse the area around the meatus with povidone-

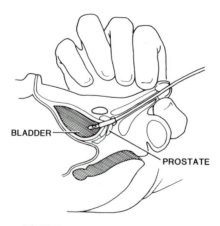

BLADDER

PROSTATE

FIGURE 16–1. Bladder catheterization in the male.

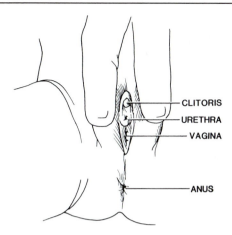

FIGURE 16–2. Landmarks used in catheterization of the bladder in females.

iodine solution. Use anterior-to-posterior strokes to prevent fecal contamination.

3. Put on sterile gloves, and drape sterile towels around the labia.

4. Spread the labia with 2 fingers. See Figure 16–2 for landmarks used in the catheterization of the bladder in females. Lubricate the catheter, and advance it in the urethra until urine appears. Tape the catheter to the leg if it is to remain in position.

IV. Complications

    A. Infection. Strict sterile technique is necessary to help prevent infection. "In and-out" catheterization carries a small risk of urinary tract infection. The longer a catheter is left in place, the greater the chance of infection.

    B. Trauma to the urethra ("false passage") or bladder. Trauma to the urethra or bladder is more common in males. It can be prevented by adequately lubricating the catheter and stretching the penis to straighten the urethra. The catheter should never be forced if resistance is felt.

    C. Hematuria. Hematuria is usually transient but may require irrigation with normal saline solution.

    D. Stricture. Stricture is more common in males. It is usually caused by using a catheter that is too large or by prolonged or traumatic catheterization. In males, taping the catheter to the anterior abdominal wall will help decrease the pressure on the posterior urethra.

17 Chest Tube Placement

I. Indications
  A. Tension pneumothorax causing respiratory compromise and decreased venous return to the heart, resulting in decreased cardiac output and hypotension.
  B. Pneumothorax compromising ventilation and causing increased work of breathing, hypoxia, and increased $PaCO_2$.
  C. Drainage of a pleural effusion or to obtain fluid for diagnosis.

II. Equipment.
Prepackaged chest tube trays typically consist of sterile towels, 4×4 gauze pads, 3–0 silk suture, curved hemostats, a No. 15 or 11 scalpel, scissors, needle holder, antiseptic solution, antibiotic ointment, 1% lidocaine, 3-mL syringe, and 25-gauge needle. The chest tube should be a 10F catheter for infants weighing less than 2000 g and a 12F catheter for infants weighing more than 2000 g. Sterile gloves, mask, hat, and gown, and a suction-drainage system (eg, Pleurevac system) are also needed.

III. Procedure
  A. The site of chest tube insertion is determined by examining the AP and cross-table lateral or lateral decubitus chest films. Air collects in the uppermost areas of the chest and fluid in the most dependent areas. For air collections, place the tube anteriorly. For fluid collections, place the tube posteriorly and laterally. **Transillumination** of the chest may help detect pneumothorax. With the lights in the room turned down, a strong light source is placed on the anterior chest wall above the nipple and in the axilla. The affected side will usually appear hyperlucent and will "light up" when compared to the unaffected side. Transillumination may not reveal a small pneumothorax. Unless the infant's status is rapidly deteriorating, a chest x-ray film should be obtained to confirm pneumothorax before the chest tube is inserted.
  B. Position the patient so that the site of insertion is accessible. The most common position is supine, with the arm at a 90-degree angle on the affected side.
  C. Select the appropriate site (Fig 17–1). For anterior placement, the site should be the second or third intercostal space at the midclavicular line. For posterior placement, use the fourth, fifth, or sixth intercostal space at the anterior axillary line. The nipple is a landmark for the fourth intercostal space.
  D. Put on a sterile gown, mask, hat, and gloves. Cleanse the area of insertion with povidone-iodine solution, and drape.
  E. Infiltrate the area superficially with 0.5–1.0% lidocaine and then down to the rib. Infiltrate into the intercostal muscles and along the parietal pleura. Make a small incision (approximately the width of the tube, usually no greater than 0.75 cm) in the skin over the rib just below the intercostal space where the tube is to be inserted (Fig 17–2A).
  F. Insert a closed, curved hemostat into the incision, and spread the tissues down to the rib. Using the tip of the hemostat, puncture the pleura just above the rib and spread gently. Remember that the intercostal nerves, arteries, and veins lie below the ribs (Fig 17–2A). This maneuver helps create a subcutaneous tunnel that aids in closing the tract when the tube is removed.
  G. When the pleura has been penetrated, a rush of air will often be heard.
  H. Insert the chest tube through the opened hemostat (Fig 17–2B). Be certain that the side holes of the tube are within the pleural cavity. The presence of moisture in the tube usually confirms proper placement in the intrapleural cavity. Use of a trocar guide is usually unnecessary and may increase the risk of com-

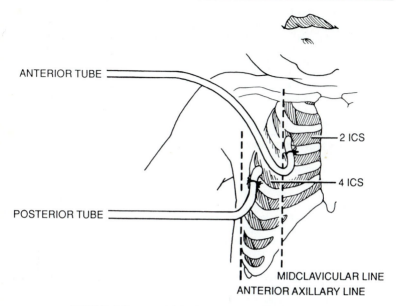

FIGURE 17–1. Recommended sites for chest tube insertion in the neonate.

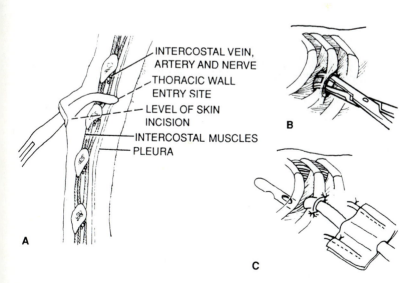

FIGURE 17–2. Procedures of chest tube insertion. **A:** Level of skin incision and thoracic wall entry site in relation to the rib and neurovascular bundle. **B:** Opened hemostat through which chest tube is inserted. **C:** Chest tube secured to skin with silk sutures.

plications. The chest tube should be inserted 2–3 cm for a small preterm infant and 3–4 cm for a term infant. (These are guidelines only; the length of tube to be inserted will vary based on the size of the infant.) An alternative approach to tube insertion is to measure the length from the insertion site to the apex of the lung and tie a silk suture around the tube the same distance from the tip. Position the tube until the silk suture is just outside the skin.

I. Hold the tube steady first and then allow an assistant to connect the tube to a water-seal vacuum drainage system (eg, Pleur-evac system). Five to 10 cm of suction pressure is usually used. Start at the lower level of suction and increase as needed if the pneumothorax or effusion does not resolve. Systems such as the Pleur-evac provide continuous suction and water seal. Water seal prevents air from being drawn back into the pleural space.

J. Secure the chest tube with 000 silk sutures and silk tape (Fig 17–2C). Close the skin opening with sutures if necessary. Obtain a chest x-ray to verify placement and check for residual fluid or pneumothorax. Positioning of the tube must always be verified by a chest x-ray film.

IV. Complications

A. **Infection.** Strict sterile technique will help minimize the risk of infection. Many institutions recommend prophylactic antibiotics (eg, nafcillin, see p 495) when a chest tube is placed (*controversial*).

B. **Bleeding.** Bleeding may occur if one of the major vessels (intercostal, axillary, pulmonary, or mammary) is perforated or the lung is damaged during the procedure. This complication can be avoided if landmarks are properly identified. Bleeding is less likely if a trocar is *not* used. Bleeding may stop during suctioning, however if significant bleeding continues, immediate surgical consultation is usually necessary.

C. **Nerve damage.** Passing the tube over the top of the rib will help avoid injury to the intercostal nerve running under the rib.

D. **Lung trauma.** Can be minimized by never forcing the tube into position.

18 Endotracheal Intubation

I. Indications.
  A. To provide mechanical respiratory support.
  B. Obtain aspirates for culture.
  C. Assist in bronchopulmonary hygeine ("pulmonary toilet").
  D. Alleviate subglottic stenosis.
  E. Clear the trachea of meconium.

II. Equipment.
Correct endotracheal tube, using the guidelines in Table 18–1. Pediatric laryngoscope handle with blade (No. 0 blade for infants weighing < 3000 g, No. 1 Miller blade for infants weighing > 3000 g), a bag-and-mask apparatus, an endotracheal tube adapter, oxygen source with tubing, suction apparatus, tape, scissors, a stylet (*optional*), gloves, and tincture of benzoin.

III. Procedure
  A. The endotracheal tube should be precut to eliminate dead space. Some newer tubes are marked "oral" or "nasal" and should be cut appropriately.
  B. Be certain that the light source on the laryngoscope is working before beginning the procedure. A bag-and-mask apparatus with 100% oxygen should be available at the bedside. Place the stylet (if used) in the endotracheal tube. Flexible stylets are optional but may help guide the tube into position more efficiently.
  C. Place the infant in the "sniffing position" (neck slightly extended). Hyperextension of the neck in infants may cause the trachea to collapse.
  D. Cautiously suction the oropharynx as needed to make the landmarks clearly visible.
  E. Monitor the infant's heart rate and color.
  F. Hold the laryngoscope with the left hand. Insert the scope into the right side of the mouth, and sweep the tongue to the left side.
  G. Advance the blade a few millimeters, passing it beneath the epiglottis.
  H. Lift the blade vertically to elevate the epiglottis and visualize the glottis (Fig 18–1). Remember, **the purpose of the laryngoscope is to vertically lift the epiglottis, not to pry it open.**
  I. To better visualize the vocal cords, gentle external pressure can be placed on the thyroid cartilage by an assistant.
  J. Pass the endotracheal tube along the right side of the mouth and down past the vocal cords during inspiration. It is best to advance the tube *only* 2–2.5 cm into the trachea to avoid placement in the right mainstem bronchus. It may be helpful to tape the tube at the lip when the tube has been advanced 7 cm in a 1-kg

TABLE 18–1. RECOMMENDED SIZE OF ENDOTRACHEAL TUBE BASED ON INFANT'S WEIGHT OR GESTATIONAL AGE*

Tube Size (ID mm)	Weight	Gestational Age
2.5	Below 1000 g	Below 28 weeks
3.0	1000–2000 g	28–34 weeks
3.5	2000–3000 g	34–38 weeks
4.0	Above 3000 g	Above 38 weeks

*Based on recommendations by the American Heart Association and American Academy of Pediatrics.
Reproduced, with permission, from *Textbook of Neonatal Resuscitation*, 1987. Copyright American Heart Association.

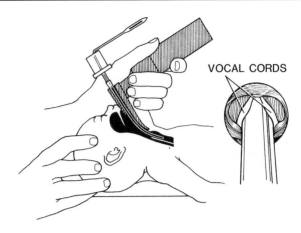

VOCAL CORDS

FIGURE 18–1. Endotracheal intubation in the neonate.

infant, 8 cm in a 2-kg infant, or 9 cm in a 3-kg infant. (Rule of "1, 2, 3/7, 8, 9"). The stylet should be gently removed while the tube is held in position.

   K. Confirm the position of the tube. The resuscitation bag is attached to the tube, and an assistant provides mechanical breaths while the physician listens for equal breath sounds on both sides of the chest. Auscultate the stomach to be certain that the esophagus was not inadvertently entered.
   L. Paint the skin with tincture of benzoin. Tape the tube securely in place.
   M. Obtain a chest x-ray film to confirm proper placement of the tube.
IV. Complications
   A. Tracheal perforation. Tracheal perforation is a rare complication requiring surgical intervention. It can be prevented by careful use of the laryngoscope and endotracheal tube.
   B. Esophageal perforation. Esophageal perforation is usually caused by traumatic intubation. Treatment depends on the degree of perforation. Most injuries can be managed by use of parenteral nutrition until the leak seals, use of broad-spectrum antibiotics, and observation for signs of infection. A barium swallow contrast study may be necessary after several weeks to evaluate healing or rule out stricture formation.
   C. Laryngeal edema. Laryngeal edema is usually seen after extubation and may cause respiratory distress. A short course of steroids (eg, dexamethasone) can be given intravenously before and just after extubation. However, systemic dexamethasone has no effect in reducing acute post extubation stridor in neonates.
   D. Palatal grooves. Palatal grooves are usually seen in cases of long-term intubation and typically resolve with time.
   E. Subglottic stenosis. Subglottic stenosis is most often associated with long-term endotracheal intubation (> 3–4 weeks). Surgical correction is usually necessary. With prolonged intubation, consideration may be given to formal surgical tracheostomy to help prevent stenosis.

19 Exchange Transfusion

Exchange transfusions are a technique used most often to maintain serum bilirubin at levels below neurotoxicity. A level of bilirubin at which to begin an exchange transfusion is currently under considerable debate (see Chapter 58 for more details). Exchange transfusions are also used to control other conditions such as polycythemia or anemia. Three types of exchange transfusion are commonly used: (1) 2-volume exchange, (2) isovolumetric 2-volume exchange, and (3) partial exchange (< 2 volumes) with normal saline, 5% albumin in saline or plasma protein fraction (Plasmanate). These procedures are used primarily in sick newborn infants but may also be used for intrauterine exchanges in fetuses at high risk for central nervous system toxicity (eg, erythroblastosis fetalis) by percutaneous umbilical blood sampling (PUBS) and umbilical vein catheterization under ultrasound guidance.

I. Indications

A. **Hyperbilirubinemia.** Exchange transfusions are used in infants with hyperbilirubinemia of any origin when the serum bilirubin level may reach or exceeds a level that puts the infant at risk for central nervous system toxicity (eg, kernicterus) if left untreated (see Appendix H). Two-volume exchange transfusions over 50–70 minutes are usually recommended for removal and reduction of serum bilirubin. Efficiency of bilirubin removal is increased in slower exchanges because of extravascular and intravascular bilirubin equilibration.

B. **Hemolytic disease of the newborn.** This results from destruction of fetal red blood cells (RBC) by passively acquired maternal antibodies. Exchange transfusion aids in removing antibody-coated RBCs, thereby prolonging intravascular RBC survival. It also removes potentially toxic bilirubin from an increased bilirubin load resulting from RBC breakdown, and provides plasma volume and albumin for bilirubin binding. Repeated 2-volume exchange transfusions may be needed when RBC destruction is rapid.

C. **Sepsis.** Neonatal sepsis may be associated with shock caused by bacterial endotoxins. A 2-volume exchange may help remove bacteria, toxins, fibrin split products, and accumulated lactic acid. It may also provide immunoglobulins, complement, and coagulating factors.

D. **Disseminated intravascular coagulation (DIC)** from multiple causes. A 2-volume exchange transfusion is preferred, but depending on the sick infant's condition, any one of the exchange methods may help provide necessary coagulation factors and help reduce the underlying etiology for the abnormal coagulation. Repletion of clotting factors by transfusion of fresh frozen plasma (10–15 mL/kg) may be all that is necessary in less severe cases of DIC.

E. **Metabolic disorders causing severe acidosis** (eg, aminoaciduria with associated hyperammonemia). Partial exchanges are usually acceptable. Peritoneal dialysis may also be useful for treating some progressive metabolic disorders.

F. **Severe fluid or electrolyte imbalance** (eg, hyperkalemia, hypernatremia, fluid overload). Isovolumetric partial exchanges are recommended to prevent large electrolyte fluctuations with each aliquot of blood exchanged. Transfusions with blood products may bind calcium; therefore, calcium gluconate should be handy. Fresh blood products should be used to prevent contribution of the by-products of older blood, such as excess potassium.

G. **Polycythemia.** It is usually best to give a partial exchange transfusion using normal saline. Plasma protein fraction (eg, Plasmanate) or 5% albumin in saline may also be used; however, normal saline is preferred because it reduces both the polycythemia and the hyperviscosity of the infant's circulating blood volume. Either plasma protein fraction or 5% albumin may leave viscosity unchanged despite reductions in circulating red cell mass.

  H. Severe anemia (normovolemic or hypervolemic) causing cardiac failure, as in hydrops fetalis, is best treated with a partial exchange transfusion using packed red blood cells.

  I. Any disorder requiring complement, opsonins, or gamma globulin. These infants may require frequent exchanges, and their fluid status must be carefully managed. Partial exchanges are recommended.

II. Equipment
  A. Radiant warmer.
  B. Equipment for respiratory support and resuscitation (eg, oxygen, suctioning device). This equipment and medications used in resuscitation should be immediately available.
  C. Equipment for monitoring the heart rate, blood pressure, respiratory rate, temperature, Pao_2, $Paco_2$, and Sao_2.
  D. Equipment for umbilical artery and umbilical vein catheterization (see Chaps 14 and 25).
  E. Disposable exchange transfusion tray.
  F. Nasogastric tube for evacuating the stomach before beginning the transfusion.
  G. A temperature-controlled device must be used for warming of the blood before and during the transfusion. The device should have an internal disposable coil and connectors to the donor blood bag and the exchange transfusion circuit. The blood should be warmed to a temperature of 37 °C. Use of makeshift water baths or heaters is not advised, because blood that is too warm may hemolyze.
  H. An assistant to help maintain a sterile field, monitor and assess the infant, and record the procedure and exchanged volumes.

III. Blood transfusion
  A. Blood collection
    1. Homologous blood. Blood donated by an anonymous donor with a compatible blood type is most commonly used. Donor-directed blood (blood donated by a selected blood type compatible person) is another option.
    2. CMV-negative blood is recommended, and blood may be freshly washed to remove accumulated metabolites and acids if greater than 72 hours old.
  B. Blood typing and cross matching
    1. Infants with Rh incompatibility. The blood must be type O, Rh negative, low titer anti-A, anti-B blood. It must be cross-matched with the mother's plasma and red blood cells.
    2. Infants with ABO incompatibility. The blood must be type O, Rh compatible (with the mother and the infant) or Rh negative, low titer anti-A, anti-B blood. It must be cross-matched with the infant's and with the mother's blood.
    3. Other blood group incompatibilities. For other hemolytic diseases (eg, anti-Rh-c, anti-Kell, anti-Duffy), blood must be cross-matched to the mother's blood to avoid offending antigens.
    4. Hyperbilirubinemia, metabolic imbalance, or hemolysis not caused by isoimmune disorders. The blood must be cross-matched against the infant's plasma and red blood cells.
  C. Freshness and preservation of blood. In newborn infants, it is preferable to use blood or plasma that has been collected in citrate-phosphate-dextrose (CPD). The blood should be less than 72 hours old. These 2 factors will ensure that the blood pH is above 7.0. For disorders associated with hydrops fetalis or fetal asphyxia, it is best to use blood that is less than 24 hours old. The pH of the donor blood should be determined: if it is less than 7.25, consider buffering blood with tromethamine (THAM), 10 mL of 0.3 molar solution per 500 mL of blood.
  D. Hematocrit. Most blood banks can reconstitute a unit of blood to a desired

hematocrit (Hct) of 50–70%. The blood should be agitated periodically during the transfusion to maintain an even hematocrit.

E. **Potassium levels in donor blood.** Potassium levels in the donor blood should be determined if the infant is asphyxiated or in shock and renal impairment is suspected. If potassium levels are higher than 7 meq/L, consider using a unit of blood that has been collected more recently or a unit of washed red blood cells.

F. **Temperature of the blood.** Warming of blood is especially important in low birth weight and sick newborn infants.

IV. Procedure

A. **Simple 2-volume exchange transfusion is used for uncomplicated hyperbilirubinemia**

1. The normal blood volume in a full-term newborn infant is 80 mL/kg. In an infant weighing 2 kg, the volume would be 160 mL. Twice this volume of blood is exchanged in a 2-volume transfusion. Therefore, the amount of blood needed for a 2-kg infant would be 320 mL. Low birth weight and the blood volume of extremely premature newborns (may be up to 95 mL/kg) should be taken into account when calculating exchange volumes.

2. Allow adequate time for **blood typing and cross matching** at the blood bank. The infant's bilirubin level will increase during this time, and this increase must be taken into account when ordering the blood.

3. Perform the transfusion in an **intensive care setting.** Place the infant in the supine position. Restraints must be snug but not tight. A nasogastric tube should be passed to **evacuate the stomach** and should be left in place to maintain gastric decompression and prevent regurgitation and aspiration of gastric juices.

4. Scrub and put on a sterile gown and gloves.

5. Perform **umbilical vein catheterization** and confirm the position by x-ray (see p 103). If an isovolumetric exchange is to be performed, then an umbilical artery catheter must also be placed and confirmed by x-ray (see p 104).

6. Have the unit of blood prepared.
   a. Check the **blood types** of the donor and the infant.
   b. Check the **temperature** of the blood and warming procedures.
   c. Check the **hematocrit.** The blood should be agitated regularly to maintain a constant hematocrit.

7. Attach the bag of blood to the tubing and stopcocks according to the directions on the transfusion tray. The orientation of the stopcocks for infusion and withdrawal must be double-checked by the assistant.

8. Establish the volume of each aliquot (Table 19–1).

B. **Isovolumetric 2-volume exchange transfusion.** Isovolumetric 2-volume exchange transfusion is performed using a double setup, with infusion via the umbilical vein and withdrawal via the umbilical artery. This method is preferred when volume shifts during simple exchange might cause or aggravate myocardial insufficiency (eg, hydrops fetalis). Two operators are usually needed—one to perform the infusion and one the withdrawal.

1. Perform **steps 1–6** as in simple 2-volume exchange transfusion. In addition, perform umbilical artery catheterization.

TABLE 19–1. ALIQUOTS USUALLY USED IN NEONATAL EXCHANGE TRANSFUSION

Infant Weight	Aliquot (mL)
More than 3 kg	20
2–3 kg	15
1–2 kg	10
850 g–1 kg	5
Less than 850 g	1–3

2. Attach the unit of blood to the tubing and stopcocks attached to the umbilical vein catheter. If the catheter is to be left in place after the exchange transfusion (usually, to monitor central venous pressure), it should be placed above the diaphragm, with placement confirmed by chest x-ray film.

3. The tubing and the stopcocks of the second setup are attached to the umbilical artery catheter and to a sterile plastic bag for discarding the exchanged blood.

4. If isovolumetric exchange is being performed because of cardiac failure, the central venous pressure can be determined via the umbilical vein catheter; it should be placed above the diaphragm, in the inferior vena cava.

C. **Partial exchange transfusion.** A partial exchange transfusion is performed in the same manner as 2-volume exchange transfusion. If a partial exchange is for polycythemia (using normal saline or other blood product) or anemia (packed red blood cells), the following formula can be used to determine the volume of the transfusion:

$$\text{Volume of exchange (mL)} = \frac{\text{Estimated blood volume (mL} \times \text{Weight (kg)} \times \text{(Observed Hct} - \text{Desired Hct)}}{\text{Observed Hct}}$$

D. **Isovolumetric partial exchange transfusion** with packed red blood cells is the best procedure in cases of severe hydrops fetalis.

E. **Ancillary procedures**
   1. **Laboratory studies.** Blood should be obtained for laboratory studies before and after exchange transfusion.
      a. **Blood chemistry studies** include total calcium, sodium, potassium, chloride, pH, $Paco_2$, acid-base status, bicarbonate, and serum glucose.
      b. **Hematologic studies** include hemoglobin, hematocrit, platelet count, white blood cell count, and differential count. Blood for retyping and cross-matching following exchange is often requested by the blood bank to verify typing and re-cross-matching, and for study of transfusion reaction, if needed.
      c. **Blood culture** is recommended following exchange transfusion (*controversial*).
   2. **Administration of calcium gluconate.** The citrate buffer binds calcium and transiently lowers ionized calcium levels. Treatment of suspected hypocalcemia in patients receiving transfusions is controversial. Some physicians routinely administer 1–2 mL of calcium gluconate 10% by slow infusion after each 100 mL of exchange donor blood. Others maintain that this treatment has no therapeutic effect unless hypocalcemia is documented by ECG showing a change in the QT interval.
   3. **Phototherapy.** Begin or resume phototherapy following exchange transfusion for disorders involving a high bilirubin level.
   4. **Monitoring of serum bilirubin levels.** Continue to monitor serum bilirubin levels following transfusion at 2, 4, and 6 hours and then at 6-hour intervals. A rebound of bilirubin levels is to be expected 2–4 hours after the transfusion.
   5. **Remedication.** Patients receiving antibiotics or anticonvulsants will need to be remedicated. Unless the cardiac status is deteriorating or serum digoxin levels are too low, patients receiving digoxin should not be remedicated.
   6. **Antibiotic prophylaxis** following the transfusion should be considered on an individual basis. Infection is uncommon but is the most frequent complication.

V. **Complications**
   A. **Infection.** Bacteremia (usually due to a *Staphylococcus* organism), hepatitis, cytomegalovirus infection, malaria, and acquired immune deficiency syndrome (AIDS) have been reported.
   B. **Vascular complications.** Clot or air embolism, arteriospasm of the lower limbs, thrombosis, and infarction of major organs may occur.
   C. **Coagulopathies.** Coagulopathies may be due to thrombocytopenia or dimin-

ished coagulation factors. Platelets may decrease by more than 50% after a 2-volume exchange transfusion.

D. Electrolyte abnormalities. Hyperkalemia and hypocalcemia can occur.

E. Hypoglycemia. Hypoglycemia is especially likely in infants of diabetic mothers and those with erythroblastosis fetalis.

F. Metabolic acidosis. Metabolic acidosis from stored donor blood (due to the acid load) occurs less often in citrate phosphate dextrose (CPD) blood.

G. Metabolic alkalosis. Metabolic alkalosis may occur because of delayed clearing of citrate preservative from the donated blood by the liver.

H. Necrotizing enterocolitis. An increased incidence of necrotizing enterocolitis following exchange transfusion has been suggested. For this reason, the umbilical vein catheter should be removed after the procedure unless central venous pressure monitoring is required. Also, we recommend that feedings should be delayed for at least 24 hours to observe the infant for the possibility of post-exchange ileus.

20 Gastric Intubation

I. Indications

  A. Enteric feeding. Gastric intubation is needed for enteric feeding in the following situations.

  1. **High respiratory rate.** At some institutions, the infant is given enteric feedings if the respiratory rate is greater than 60 breaths/min in order to decrease the risk of aspiration pneumonia.

  2. **Neurologic disease.** If neurologic disease impairs the sucking reflex or ability to feed, enteric feeding is needed.

  3. **Premature infants.** Many premature infants with immature suck and swallow mechanisms tire before they can take in enough calories with normal feeding to maintain growth.

  B. Gastric decompression. Gastric decompression may be required in infants with necrotizing enterocolitis, bowel obstruction, or ileus.

  C. Administration of medications.

  D. Analysis of gastric contents.

II. Equipment.
Infant feeding tube (5F or 8F), stethoscope, sterile water (to lubricate the tube), a syringe (5–10 ml), 2-inch adhesive tape, gloves, and suctioning equipment.

III. Procedure

  A. Monitor the patient's heart rate and respiratory function throughout this procedure.

  B. Place the infant in the supine position, with the head of the bed elevated.

  C. The length of tubing needed is determined by measuring the distance from the nose to the xiphoid process. Mark the length on the tube.

  D. Moisten the end of the tube with sterile water.

  E. The tube can be placed in one of two positions.

  1. **Nasal insertion.** Flex the neck, push the nose up, and insert the tube, directing it straight back. Advance the tube the desired distance.

  2. **Oral insertion.** Push the tongue down with a tongue depressor and pass the tube into the oropharynx. Advance the tube slowly the desired distance.

  F. Continue to observe the infant for respiratory distress or bradycardia.

  G. Determine the location of the tube. One method is to inject air into the tube with a syringe and listen for a rush of air in the stomach. One study found this method unreliable because a rush of air can occur when the tip is in the distal esophagus. They recommended either palpating the tube in the abdomen, or aspirating the contents to determine the acidity by pH tape. If the location is still uncertain, obtain an x-ray film. If feedings are to be initiated, the position should also be verified by plain x-ray.

  H. Aspirate the gastric contents.

  I. Secure the tube to the face with benzoin and 2-inch tape.

IV. Complications

  A. Apnea and bradycardia. Apnea and bradycardia are usually mediated by a vagal response and will usually resolve without specific treatment.

  B. Perforation of the esophagus, posterior pharynx, stomach, or duodenum. The tube should never be forced during insertion.

  C. Hypoxia. Always have bag-and-mask ventilation with 100% oxygen available to treat this problem.

  D. Aspiration. Aspiration can occur if feeding has been initiated in a tube that is accidentally inserted into the lung or if the GI tract is not passing the feedings out of the stomach. Periodically check the residual volumes in the stomach to prevent over-distension and aspiration.

21 Heelstick (Capillary Blood Sampling)

I. Indications
  A. Collection of blood samples when only a small amount of blood is needed or when there is difficulty obtaining samples by venipuncture.
  B. Capillary blood gas sampling.
  C. Blood cultures when venous access is not possible.

II. Equipment.
A sterile lancet (2-mm lancet if infant weighs < 1500 g or if only a small amount of blood is needed, 4-mm lancet in larger infants or if more blood is required). Also needed are alcohol swabs, 4 × 4 sterile gauze pads, a capillary tube (for hematocrit and bilirubin tests) or a caraway tube (if more blood is needed [eg, for blood chemistry determinations]), clay to seal the end of the tube, a warm washcloth, gloves, and a diaper.

III. Procedure
  A. Wrap the foot in a warm washcloth and then a diaper for 5 minutes. Although this is not mandatory, it will produce hyperemia, which increases vascularity, making blood collection easier.
  B. Choose the area of puncture (Fig 21–1). Do not use the center of the heel, because there is an increased incidence of osteomyelitis if this area is used.
  C. Wipe the area with an alcohol swab, and let it dry. If the area is wet with alcohol, hemolysis may occur, altering the results of blood testing.
  D. Encircle the heel with the palm of the hand and the index finger (Fig 21–1).
  E. Make a quick, deep (not greater than 2.5-mm) puncture with a lancet. Wipe off the first drop of blood. Gently squeeze the heel, and place the collection tube at the site of the puncture. The tube should automatically fill by capillary action. It may be necessary to gently "pump" the heel to continue the blood flow. Allow enough time for capillary refill of the heel. Avoid excessive squeezing which may cause hemolysis and give inaccurate results. Seal the end of the tube with clay.
  F. Maintain pressure on the puncture site with a dry sterile gauze pad until the bleeding stops. A 4 × 4 gauze pad can be wrapped around the heel and left on to provide hemostasis.

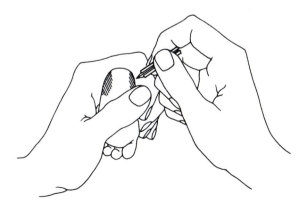

FIGURE 21–1. Use the shaded area when performing a heelstick in an infant.

IV. **Complications**

    A. Cellulitis. Cellulitis risk can be minimized with the proper use of sterile technique. A culture of tissue from the affected area should be obtained, and use of broad-spectrum antibiotics should be considered.

    B. Osteomyelitis. This complication usually occurs in the calcaneus bone. Avoid the center area of the heel and do not make the puncture opening too deep. If osteomyelitis occurs, tissue should be obtained for culture and broad-spectrum antibiotics started until a specific organism is identified. Consultation with specialists in infectious disease and orthopedics is usually obtained.

    C. Scarring of the heel. Scarring occurs when there have been multiple punctures in the same area. If extensive scarring is present, consider another technique of blood collection such as central venous sampling.

    D. Pain. Pain caused by routine heelsticks in premature infants can cause marked declines in hemoglobin oxygen saturation as measured by pulse oximetry. Some institutions advocate topical lidocaine (0.5–1.0%) prior to the procedure.

    E. Calcified nodules. These usually disappear by 30 months of age.

    F. Inaccurate results. Falsely elevated dextrostix, hematocrit, and inaccurate blood gas values can all occur with heelstick sampling.

22 Lumbar Puncture (Spinal Tap)

I. Indications
   A. Obtain cerebrospinal fluid (CSF) for the diagnosis of central nervous system disorders such as meningitis or subarachnoid hemorrhage.
   B. Drain cerebrospinal fluid in communicating hydrocephalus associated with intraventricular hemorrhage. (Serial lumbar punctures for this are *controversial.*)
   C. Administration of intrathecal medications.
   D. Monitor efficacy of antibiotics used to treat CNS infections.
II. Materials required. Lumbar puncture kit (usually contains 3 sterile specimen tubes, sterile drapes, sterile gauze, 22-gauge 1-inch spinal needle with stylet, 1% lidocaine), gloves, povidone-iodine solution, 1-mL syringe.
III. Procedure. (Normal CSF values are listed in Appendix D.)
   A. An assistant should restrain the infant in a sitting or lateral decubitus position. The position to use depends on personal preference. An intubated, critically ill infant must be treated in the lateral decubitus position. Some clinicians feel that if CSF cannot be obtained in the lateral decubitus position, the sitting position should be used. In the lateral decubitus position, the head and legs must be flexed (knee-chest position). The neck does not have to be fully flexed. Make sure airway patency is maintained.
   B. Once the infant is in position, check for landmarks (Fig 22–1). Palpate the iliac crest and slide your finger down to the L4 vertebral body. Then use the L4–L5 interspace as the site of the lumbar puncture. It is sometimes easier to make a nail imprint at the exact location to mark the site.
   C. Prepare the materials (open sterile containers, pour antiseptic [Betadine solution] solution into the well located in the plastic lumbar puncture kit).
   D. Put gloves on and clean the lumbar area with antiseptic solution, starting at the

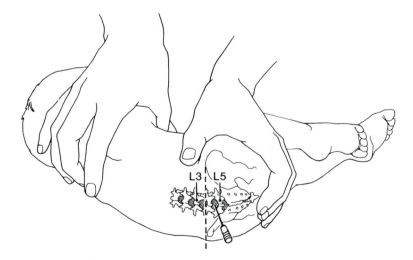

FIGURE 22–1. Positioning and landmarks used for lumbar puncture. The iliac crest (dotted line) marks the approximate level of L4.

interspace selected. Prep in a widening circle from that interspace up and over the iliac crest.

E. Drape the area with one towel under the infant and one towel covering everything but the selected interspace.

F. Palpate again to find the selected interspace. At this time, 0.1–0.2 mL of 1% lidocaine can be injected subcutaneously for pain relief (*optional*). (**Note:** Physiologic instability is not reduced with lidocaine use during the procedure.)

G. Insert the needle in the midline with steady force aimed toward the umbilicus.

H. Advance the needle slowly and then remove the stylet to check for appearance of fluid. One usually does not feel a "pop" as the ligamentum flavum and dura are penetrated, as is the case with older children and adults. It is therefore necessary to remove the stylet frequently to keep from going too far and getting a bloody specimen.

I. Collect about 1 mL of CSF in each of the 3 sterile specimen tubes by allowing the fluid to drip into the tubes.

J. Replace the stylet and withdraw the needle.

K. Maintain pressure on the area, and clean off the antiseptic solution.

L. For routine CSF examination, send 3 tubes of CSF to the laboratory in the following recommended order:
Tube 1: For Gram stain, culture, and sensitivity testing.
Tube 2: For glucose and protein levels.
Tube 3: For cell count and differential.

M. If a bloody specimen is obtained in the first tube, observe for clearing in the second and third tubes.
1. If bleeding clears, the tap was traumatic.
2. If blood does not clear but forms clots, a blood vessel has probably been punctured. Since CSF has not been obtained, a repeat tap must be done.
3. If blood does not clear and does not clot, the infant probably has had intraventricular bleeding.

IV. Complications

A. Infection. Use of sterile technique will reduce the chance that bacteria may be introduced into the CSF and cause infection. Bacteremia may result if a blood vessel is punctured after the needle has passed through contaminated CSF.

B. Intraspinal epidermoid tumor. This occurs as a result of performing a lumbar puncture with a needle that does not have a stylet. It is caused by a "plug" of epithelial tissue being displaced into the dura. Note, however that the incidence of traumatic LP is not reduced by use of a needle without a stylet.

C. Herniation of cerebral tissue through the foramen magnum. This is not a common problem in neonatal intensive care units because of the open fontanelle in infants.

D. Spinal cord and nerve damage. To avoid this complication, use only interspaces below L4.

E. Apnea and bradycardia sometimes occur from respiratory compromise caused by the infant being held too tightly during the procedure.

F. Hypoxia. Increasing the oxygen during the procedure may help to prevent transient hypoxia.

23 Abdominal Paracentesis

I. Indications
    A. Obtain peritoneal fluid for diagnostic tests to determine the cause of ascites.
    B. Therapeutic procedure such as removal of peritoneal fluid to aid in ventilation.

II. Materials required.
Sterile drapes, sterile gloves, povidone-iodine solution, sterile gauze pads, sterile tubes for fluid, 10-mL syringe, 22- or 24-gauge catheter over-needle assembly. (22-gauge for infants < 2000 g, 24-gauge for infants > 2000 g).

III. Procedure
    A. The infant should be supine with both legs restrained. To restrict all movements of the legs, a diaper can be wrapped around the legs and secured in place.
    B. Choose the site for paracentesis. The area between the umbilicus and the pubic bone is not generally used in neonates because of the danger of perforating the bladder or bowel wall. The sites most frequently used are the right and left flanks. A good rule is to draw a horizontal line passing through the umbilicus and select a site between this line and the inguinal ligament (Fig 23–1).
    C. Prepare the area with povidone-iodine in a circular fashion, starting at the puncture site.
    D. Put on sterile gloves, and drape the area.

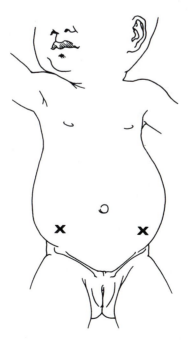

FIGURE 23–1. Recommended sites for abdominal paracentesis.

E. Insert the needle at the selected site. A "Z-track" technique is usually used to prevent persistent leakage of fluid after the tap. Insert the needle perpendicular to the skin. When the needle is just under the skin, move it 0.5 cm before puncturing the abdominal wall.

F. Advance the needle, aspirating until fluid appears in the barrel of the syringe. Then remove the needle and aspirate the contents slowly with the catheter. It may be necessary to reposition the catheter to obtain an adequate amount of fluid. Once the necessary amount of fluid is taken (usually 3–5 mL for specific tests, or enough to aid ventilation), remove the catheter. If too much fluid is removed or if it is removed too rapidly, hypotension may result.

G. Cover with a sterile gauze pad until leakage has stopped.

IV. Complications

A. Hypotension. Hypotension is caused by removing too much fluid or removing fluid too rapidly. To minimize this possibility, take only the amount needed for studies or what is needed to improve ventilation. Always remove fluid slowly.

B. Infection. The risk of peritonitis is minimized by using strict sterile technique.

C. Perforation of the intestine. To help prevent perforation, use the shortest needle possible and take careful note of landmarks (see **III.B**, p 159). If perforation occurs, broad-spectrum antibiotics may be indicated with close observation for signs of infection.

D. Perforation of the bladder. Perforation of the bladder is normally self-limited and requires no specific treatment.

E. Persistent fluid leak. The "Z-track" technique, as described above in **III.E**, usually prevents the problem of persistent leakage of fluid. Persistent fluid leaks may have to be bagged to quantify the volume .

24 Pericardiocentesis

I. Indications
A. Treatment of cardiac tamponade caused by pneumopericardium or pericardial effusion.

B. To obtain pericardial fluid for diagnostic studies in infants with pericardial effusion.

II. Materials required.
Povidone-iodine solution, sterile gloves and gown, 22- or 24-gauge 1-inch catheter-over-needle assembly, sterile drapes, 10-mL syringe, connecting tube, and underwater seal for use if the catheter is to be left indwelling.

III. Procedure *
A. Prepare the area (xiphoid and precordium) with antiseptic solution. Put on sterile gloves and gown.

B. Drape the area, leaving the xiphoid and a 2-cm circular area around it exposed.

C. Prepare the needle by attaching the syringe to it. If you want to leave an indwelling catheter, a 3-way stopcock and tubing should be attached to the needle in addition to the syringe.

D. Identify the area where the needle is to be inserted. The area most commonly used is approximately 0.5 cm to the left of and just below the infant's xiphoid (Fig 24–1).

E. Insert the needle at about a 30-degree angle, aiming toward the midclavicular line on the left (Fig 24–1).

F. Apply constant suction on the syringe while advancing the needle.

G. Once air or fluid is obtained (depending on which is to be evacuated), remove the needle from the catheter. Withdraw the necessary amount of air or fluid, ie, enough to relieve symptoms or obtain sufficient fluid for laboratory studies.

H. If an indwelling catheter is to be left in place, secure it with tape and attach the tubing to continuous suction.

I. Obtain a chest x-ray film to confirm the position of the catheter and the effectiveness of drainage.

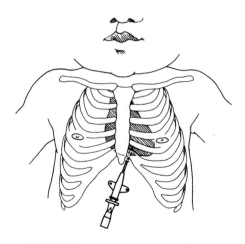

FIGURE 24–1. Recommended sites for pericardiocentesis.

IV. Complications

A. Puncturing the heart. Avoid this complication by advancing the needle only far enough to obtain fluid or air. Another technique to avoid puncturing the heart is to attach the ECG anterior chest lead to the needle with an alligator clip. If changes are seen on the ECG (eg, ectopic beats, changes in the ST segment, or increase in the QRS voltage), the needle has contacted the myocardium and should be withdrawn. Avoid leaving a metal needle indwelling for continuous drainage.

B. Pneumothorax or hemothorax. This can occur if landmarks are not used and "blind" punctures are done. If this complication has occurred, a chest tube on the affected side is usually needed.

C. Infection. Strict sterile technique will minimize the risk of infection.

25 Venous Access

PERCUTANEOUS VENOUS CATHETERIZATION

I. Indications
  A. Administration of intravenous medications and fluids.
  B. Administration of parenteral nutrition.
II. Materials required. Arm board, adhesive tape, tourniquet, alcohol swabs, normal saline for flush (1/2 normal saline if concerned about hypernatremia), povidone-iodine ointment, needle (23- or 25-gauge scalp vein needle or 22- to 24- gauge catheter-over-needle [Angiocath]).
III. Procedure
  A. Scalp vein needle
    1. **Select the vein to use.** The following can be used in the neonate (Fig 25–1). It is useful to select the "Y" region of the vein, where 2 veins join together. The needle can be inserted in the crotch of the veins.
      a. Scalp. Supratrochlear, superficial temporal, or posterior auricular vein.
      b. Back of hand. Dorsal arch vein.
      c. Forearm. Median antebrachial or accessory cephalic vein.
      d. Foot. Dorsal arch vein.
      e. Antecubital fossa. Basilic or cubital vein.
      f. Ankle. Greater saphenous vein.
    2. **Shave the area if a scalp vein is to be used.**
    3. **Restrain the extremity** on an armboard or have an assistant help hold the extremity or the head.
    4. **Apply a tourniquet** proximal to the puncture site. If a scalp vein is to be used, a rubber band can be placed around the head, just above the eyebrows.
    5. **Clean the area with alcohol swabs.**
    6. **Fill the tubing with flush.** Detach the syringe from the needle.
    7. **Grasp the plastic wings** and, using your free index finger, **pull the skin taut** to help stabilize the vein.
    8. **Insert the needle** through the skin and advance approximately 0.5 cm prior to entry of the side of the vessel. Alternatively, the vessel can be entered directly after puncture of the skin, but this often results in the vessel being punctured "through and through" (Fig 25–2).
    9. **Advance the needle** until blood appears in the tubing.
    10. **Gently inject some of the flush** to assure patency and proper positioning of the needle.
    11. **Connect the intravenous tubing and fluid and tape the needle in position.**
  B. Catheter-over-needle assembly (Angiocath)
    1. **Steps 1–5 above,** as for scalp vein needle.
    2. **Fill the needle and hub with flush** via syringe; then remove the syringe.
    3. **Pull the skin taut** to stabilize the vein.
    4. **Puncture the skin;** then enter the side of the vein in a separate motion. Alternately, the skin and the vein can be entered in one motion.
    5. **Carefully advance the needle** until blood appears in the hub.
    6. **Withdraw the needle** while advancing the catheter.
    7. **Remove the tourniquet** and gently inject some normal saline into the catheter to verify patency and position.

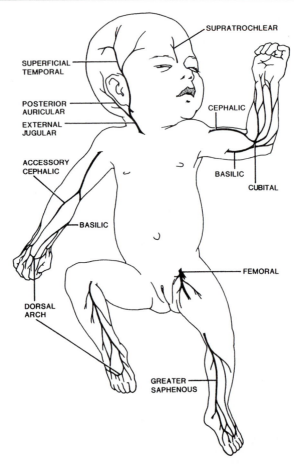

FIGURE 25–1. Sites for venous access frequently used in the neonate.

    8. Connect the intravenous tubing and fluid and tape securely in place.
IV. Complications
    A. Infection. The risk of infection can be minimized by using sterile technique including antiseptic prep.
    B. Phlebitis. The risk of phlebitis is increased the longer a catheter is left in place, especially if left in greater than 72 hours.
    C. Vasospasm. Vasospasm rarely occurs when veins are accessed and usually resolves spontaneously.
    D. Hematoma. Hematoma at the site can often be managed effectively by gentle manual pressure.
    E. Embolus air or clot. Never allow the end of the catheter to be open to the air, and make sure that the intravenous line is flushed free of air bubbles before it is connected.
    F. Infiltration of subcutaneous tissue. Intravenous solution may leak out into the subcutaneous tissue as a result of improper catheter placement or damage to the vessel. To help prevent this, confirm placement of the catheter with the flush solution before the catheter is connected to the intravenous solution. Infiltration often means that the catheter needs to be removed.

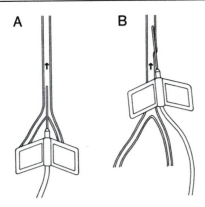

FIGURE 25–2. Two techniques for entering the vein for intravenous access. **A:** Direct puncture. **B:** Side entry.

VENIPUNCTURE (Phlebotomy)

I. Indications
  A. To obtain a blood sample for analysis or culture.
  B. To give medications.
II. Materials required. A 23- or 25-gauge scalp vein needle, alcohol and povidone-iodine swabs, specimen containers (eg, red-topped tube), tourniquet or rubber band (for scalp), 4 × 4 sterile gauze pads, syringe.
III. Procedure
  A. Have an assistant restrain the infant.
  B. Decide which vein to use (see Fig 25–1 to help with vein selection).
  C. If an assistant is not available, **restrain the specific area selected** for venipuncture. For example, tape the extremity on an armboard.
  D. "Tourniquet" the extremity to occlude the vein. Use either a rubber band (for the head), a tourniquet, or an assistant's hand to encircle the area proximal to the vein.
  E. Prepare the site with antiseptic solution.
  F. With the bevel up, puncture the skin, and then **direct the needle into the vein at a 45-degree angle.**
  G. Once blood enters the tubing, **attach the syringe and collect the blood slowly** (or administer the medication).
  H. Remove the tourniquet.
  I. Remove the needle and apply gentle pressure on the area until hemostasis has occurred. If blood has been collected, distribute it to the appropriate containers to send to the laboratory.
IV. Complications
  A. Infection is a rare complication that can be minimized by using sterile technique.
  B. Venous thrombosis is often unavoidable, especially when multiple punctures are performed on the same vein.
  C. Hematoma or hemorrhage is avoided by applying pressure to the site long enough after the needle is removed to assure hemostasis.

UMBILICAL VEIN CATHETERIZATION

I. Indications
  A. Central venous pressure monitoring.
  B. Immediate access for intravenous fluids, emergency medications.
  C. Exchange transfusion, partial exchange transfusion.

D. Long-term central venous access in extremely low birth weight infants.

II. Materials required. Same as for umbilical artery catheterization (see p 136), except that a 5F catheter should be used for infants weighing less than 3.5 kg and an 8F catheter for infants over 3.5 kg.

III. Procedure

    A. Place the infant supine with a diaper wrapped around both legs to help stabilize the infant.

    B. Prep the area around the umbilicus with povidone-iodine solution. Put gown and gloves on.

    C. Prepare the tray as you would for the umbilical artery catheterization procedure (see p 136).

    D. Put sterile drapes on, leaving the umbilical area exposed.

    E. Tie a piece of umbilical tape around the base of the umbilicus.

    F. Cut the excess umbilical cord with a scalpel or scissor, leaving a stump of about 0.5–1.0 cm. Identify the umbilical vein. The umbilical vein is thin-walled, larger than the 2 arteries, and is close to the periphery of the stump (Fig 14–3B).

    G. Grasp the end of the umbilicus with the curved hemostat to hold it upright and steady (Fig 25–3A).

    H. Open and dilate the umbilical vein with the forceps.

    I. Once the vein is sufficiently dilated, insert the catheter (Fig 25–3B).

    J. To determine the specific length of catheter needed, see Appendix J.

    K. Another method is to measure the length from the xiphoid to the umbilicus and add 0.5–1.0 cm. This number is how far the venous line should be inserted.

    L. Connect the catheter to the fluid and tubing. Place a piece of silk tape on the catheter, and secure it to the base of the umbilicus with silk sutures (see Fig 14–4).

    M. Obtain an x-ray film to confirm the position (see Fig 9–6). The correct position for a central venous pressure line is with the catheter tip 0.5–1.0 cm above the diaphragm.

    N. Never advance a catheter once it is secured in place.

    O. Occasionally, a catheter will enter the portal vein. (Fig 25–4.) You should suspect that you have entered the portal vein if you meet resistance and can-

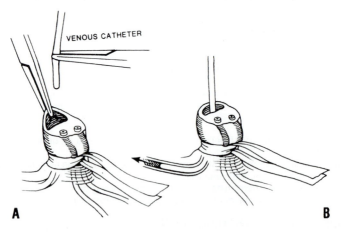

FIGURE 25–3. Umbilical vein catheterization. **A:** The umbilical stump is held upright before the catheter is inserted. **B:** The catheter is passed into the umbilical vein.

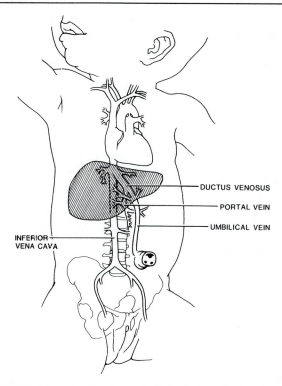

FIGURE 25–4. Anatomic relationships used in placement of umbilical venous catheter.

not advance the catheter the desired distance or if you detect a "bobbing" motion of the catheter. To correct this, you can do several things.

1. Try injecting flush as you advance the catheter. Sometimes this makes it easier to pass the catheter through the ductus venosus.
2. Pass another catheter (smaller size, usually 3.5F) through the same opening. Sometimes this allows one catheter to go through the ductus venosus while the other enters the portal system. The one in the portal system can then be removed.

IV. **Complications**

A. **Infection.** Minimize the risk through the use of strict sterile technique, and never advance a catheter that has already been positioned.

B. **Thrombolic or embolic phenomenon.** Never allow air to enter the end of the catheter. A nonfunctioning catheter should be removed. Never try to flush clots from the end of the catheter.

C. **Hepatic necrosis.** Do not allow a catheter to remain in the portal system. In case of emergency placement, the catheter should be advanced only 3 cm (just until blood returns) to avoid hepatic infusion.

D. **Cardiac arrhythmias.** Arrhythmias are usually caused by a catheter that is inserted too far and is irritating the heart.

E. **Portal hypertension.** Portal hypertension is caused by a catheter that is positioned in the portal system.

F. **Necrotizing enterocolitis.** NEC is thought to be a complication of umbilical vein catheters, especially if left in place over 24 hours.

INTRAOSSEOUS INFUSION

I. **Indications.** Immediate vascular access (for administration of fluids and medications) in management of emergencies when other methods of vascular access have been attempted and have failed. Many agents have been infused by this technique in the literature including IV solutions (ringers lactate, normal saline, etc), blood and blood products and a wide variety of medications.

II. **Materials required.** Povidone-iodine solution, 4 × 4 sterile gauze pads, syringe, sterile towels, gloves, 18-gauge disposable iliac bone marrow aspiration needle (preferred needle) or 18- to 20-gauge short spinal needle with stylet, short hypodermic needle (20-gauge), or butterfly needle (16- to 19- gauge), sterile drape, syringe with saline flush.

III. **Procedure.** The **proximal tibia** is the preferred site and will be described here. (See Fig 25–5.) Other sites are the distal tibia and distal femur.

   A. **Restrain the lower leg.**

   B. **Place a small sandbag or intravenous bag behind the knee** for support.

   C. **Select the area** in the midline on the flat surface of the anterior tibia, 1–3 cm below the tibial tuberosity.

   D. **Clean the area** with betadine. Sterile drapes can be placed around the area that is going to be used.

   E. **Insert the needle** at an angle of 10–15 degrees toward the foot to avoid the growth plate.

   F. **Advance the needle** until a lack of resistance is felt (usually no more than 1 cm is necessary), at which point entry into the marrow space should have occurred.

   G. **Remove the stylet.** (**Note:** At this point, aspiration of bone marrow for laboratory studies can be done, if needed. Bone marrow aspirates can be sent for blood chemistry values, carbon dioxide level, pH, hemoglobin level, culture and sensitivity, and blood type and cross-match.) Secure the needle to the skin with tape to prevent it from dislodging.

   H. **Attach the needle to intravenous fluids.** Hypertonic and alkaline solutions should be diluted 1:2 with normal saline.

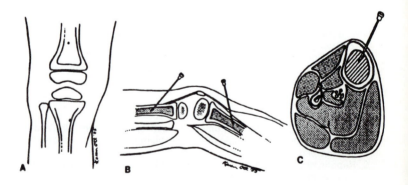

FIGURE 25–5. Technique of intraosseous infusion. **A.** Anterior view of sites on the tibia and fibula. **B.** Sagittal view. **C.** Cross section through the tibia. (Reproduced with permission from Hodge D. Intraosseous Infusion: A review. Pediatric Emergency Care.1:215, 1985.)

   I. Withdraw the needle and apply pressure over the puncture site.
   J. To avoid the risk of infectious complications, **this method of vascular access should optimally be used for less than 2 hours.**
IV. Complications
   A. **Fluid infiltration** of subcutaneous tissue (most common).
   B. **Subperiosteal infiltration** of fluid.
   C. **Localized cellulitis.**
   D. **Formation of subcutaneous abscesses.**
   E. **Clotting of bone marrow,** resulting in loss of vascular access.
   F. **Osteomyelitis** (rare).
   G. **Fracture** of the bone. X-ray confirmation of the needle should be done to confirm position and rule out fracture.
   H. **Compartment syndrome.**
   I. **Blasts in the peripheral blood.** Blasts in the peripheral blood have been noted in two patients following intraosseous infusions, who have no malignant, infectious, or infiltrative disease of the bone marrow.

This section outlines common problems encountered in the neonatal intensive care unit (NICU) or newborn nursery. Guidelines for rapid diagnosis and treatment are given. Clinical situations and institutional guidelines may vary extensively, and recommendations for treatment should be modified based on these factors. If a treatment approach is designated "controversial," it signifies that the approach has been useful at some institutions but may not have been confirmed in randomized trials.

26 Arrhythmia

I. Problem. An infant has an abnormal tracing on the heart rate monitor.

II. Immediate questions

A. What is the heart rate? Heart rate in newborns varies from 70 to 190 beats/min (bpm). It is normally 120–140 bpm but may decrease to 70–90 bpm during sleep and increase to 170–190 bpm with increased activity such as crying. See Table 26–1 for normal heart rate values.

B. Is the abnormality continuous or transient? Transient episodes of sinus bradycardia, tachycardia, or arrhythmias (usually lasting less than 15 seconds) are benign and do not require further workup. Episodes lasting longer than 15 seconds usually require full electrocardiographic assessment.

C. Is the infant symptomatic? A symptomatic infant may need immediate treatment. Signs and symptoms of some pathologic arrhythmias include tachypnea, poor skin perfusion, lethargy, hepatomegaly, and rales on pulmonary examination. All of these signs and symptoms may signify congestive heart failure, which may accompany arrhythmias. Congestive heart failure because of rapid cardiac rhythms is unusual with heart rates less than 240 bpm.

III. Differential diagnosis

A. Heart rate abnormalities

1. Tachycardia. Tachycardia is a heart rate greater than 2 standard deviations above the mean for age (Table 26–1).

a. Benign causes

(1) Postdelivery.

(2) Heat or cold stress.

(3) Painful stimuli.

(4) Medications (eg, atropine, theophylline (aminophylline), epinephrine, intravenous glucagon, pancuronium bromide [Pavulon], tolazoline, and isoproterenol) can cause tachycardia.

b. Pathologic causes

(1) More common: Fever, shock, hypoxia, anemia, sepsis, patent ductus arteriosus, congestive heart failure.

(2) Less common: Hyperthyroidism, metabolic disorders, cardiac arrhythmias, hyperammonemia.

2. Bradycardia. Bradycardia is a heart rate greater than 2 standard deviations below the mean for age (Table 26–1). Transient bradycardia is fairly common in newborns, with rates in the range of 60–70 bpm.

TABLE 26–1. MINIMUM AND MAXIMUM HEART RATES IN NORMAL NEWBORNS

Age	Minimum	Mean	Maximum	SD[a]
0–24 hrs	85	119	145	16.1
1–7 days	100	133	175	22.3
8–30 days	115	163	190	19.9

[a]Standard deviation

Reproduced, with permission from Hastreiter AR, Abella JE: The electrocardiogram in the newborn period. I The normal infant, *J Pediatr* 1971;**78**:146.

    a. Benign causes
        (1) Defecation.
        (2) Vomiting.
        (3) Micturition.
        (4) Gavage feedings.
        (5) Suctioning.
        (6) Medications: propranolol, digitalis, atropine, and infusion of calcium.
    b. Pathologic causes
        (1) More common: Hypoxia, apnea, convulsions, airway obstruction, air leak (eg, pneumothorax), congestive heart failure, intracranial bleeding, severe acidosis, severe hypothermia.
        (2) Less common: hyperkalemia, cardiac arrhythmias, pulmonary hemorrhage, diaphragmatic hernia, hypothyroidism, hydrocephalus.
B. Arrhythmias
    1. Benign arrhythmias include any transient episode (less than 15 seconds) of sinus bradycardia and tachycardia and any of the benign causes of sinus tachycardia and bradycardia noted above in A.1, 2. Sinus arrhythmia, which is a phasic variation in the heart rate often associated with respiration, is also benign.
    2. Pathologic
        a. Supraventricular tachycardia, the most common type of cardiac arrhythmia seen in the neonate (Fig 26–1A).
        b. Atrial flutter, difficult to distinguish from other supraventricular tachycardias, unless the block is greater than 2:1.
        c. Atrial fibrillation, less common than supraventricular tachycardia or atrial flutter.
        d. Wolff-Parkinson-White syndrome (short PR interval and delta wave, slow upstroke of the QRS complex), difficult to identify when the rate is fast (Fig 26–1B).
        e. Ectopic beats.
        f. Ventricular tachycardia.
        g. Atrioventricular block, with symptoms occurring in newborns with complete AV block and ventricular rates less than 55/min.
    3. Secondary to extracardiac disease
        a. Sepsis (usually tachycardia).
        b. Diseases of the central nervous system (usually bradycardia).
        c. Hypoglycemia.
        d. Drug toxicity.
            (1) Digoxin. The effect of this drug is potentiated by hypokalemia, alkalosis, hypercalcemia, and hypomagnesemia.
            (2) Quinidine.
            (3) Theophylline.
        e. Adrenal insufficiency.
        f. Electrolyte (potassium, sodium, magnesium, calcium) abnormalities.
        g. Metabolic acidosis or alkalosis.

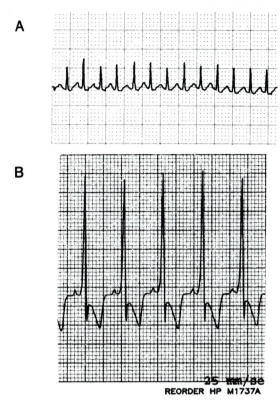

FIGURE 26–1. A. Supraventricular, narrow QRS tachycardia with a rate of 300 beats per minute. The PR interval is long for this rate. **B.** Wolff-Parkinson-White (WPW) with a short PR interval and a delta upstroke on the QRS complex. The T waves are often discordant.

IV. Data base

A. Physical examination. Perform a complete physical examination. Check for signs of congestive heart failure (tachypnea, rales on pulmonary examination, enlarged liver, and cardiomegaly). Vomiting and lethargy may be seen in patients with digoxin toxicity. Hypokalemia can cause ileus.

B. Laboratory studies

1. **Electrolyte, calcium, and magnesium levels.**
2. **Blood gas levels** may reveal acidosis or hypoxia.
3. **Drug levels** to evaluate for toxicity:
   a. **Digoxin.** Normal serum levels are 0.5–2.0 ng/mL (sometimes up to 4 ng/mL). Elevated levels of digoxin alone are not diagnostic of toxicity; clinical and ECG findings consistent with toxicity are also needed and many neonates have naturally occurring substances which interfere with the RIA test for digoxin.
   b. **Quinidine.** Normal serum levels are 3–7 mg/mL. Toxicity is associated with levels greater than 7 mg/mL.
   c. **Theophylline.** Normal levels are 4–12 μg/mL. Toxicity is associated with levels greater than 15–20 μg/mL.

C. Radiologic and other studies

1. Electrocardiography. Full electrocardiographic evaluation should be performed in all infants who have an abnormal ECG tracing that lasts longer than 15 seconds or is not related to a benign condition. Diagnostic features of the common arrhythmias are listed below.

  a. Supraventricular tachycardia
    (1) Ventricular rate of 180–300/min.
    (2) No change in heart rate with activity or crying.
    (3) Abnormal P wave or PR interval.
    (4) Fixed RR interval.

  b. Atrial flutter
    (1) Atrial rate is 220–400/min.
    (2) Sawtooth configuration seen best in leads V1, 2, 3, but often difficult to identify when a 2:1 block or rapid ventricular rate is present.
    (3) QRS complex is usually normal.

  c. Atrial fibrillation
    (1) Irregular atrial waves that vary in size and shape from beat to beat.
    (2) Atrial rate is 350–600/min.
    (3) QRS complex is normal, but ventricular response is irregular.

  d. Wolff-Parkinson-White syndrome
    (1) Short PR interval.
    (2) Widened QRS complex.
    (3) Presence of delta wave.

  e. Ventricular tachycardia
    (1) Ventricular premature beats at a rate of 120–200/min.
    (2) Widened QRS complex.

  f. Ectopic beats
    (1) Abnormal P wave.
    (2) Widened QRS complex.

  g. Atrioventricular block
    (1) First-degree block
      (a) Prolonged PR interval (normal 0.08–0.12).
      (b) Normal sinus rhythm.
      (c) Normal QRS complex.
    (2) Second-degree block
      (a) Mobitz type 1
        (i) Prolonged PR interval with a dropped ventricular beat.
        (ii) Normal QRS complex.
      (b) Mobitz type II. Constant PR interval with dropped ventricular beats.
    (3) Third-degree block
      (a) Regular atrial beat.
      (b) Slower ventricular rate.
      (c) Independent atrial and ventricular beat.
      (d) Atrial rate increases with crying or level of activity. Ventricular rate usually stays the same.

  h. Hyperkalemia
    (1) Tall, tented T waves.
    (2) Widened QRS complex.
    (3) Flat and wide P wave.
    (4) Ventricular fibrillation and late asystole.

  i. Hypokalemia
    (1) Prolonged QT and PR interval.
    (2) Depressed ST segment.
    (3) Flat T wave.

  j. Hypocalcemia. Prolonged QT interval.

  k. Hypercalcemia. Shortened QT interval.

  l. Hypomagnesemia. Same as hyperkalemia.

  m. Hyponatremia

          (1) Short QT interval.

          (2) Increased duration of QRS complex.

    n. Hypernatremia

          (1) Prolonged QT interval.

          (2) Decreased duration of QRS complex.

    o. Metabolic acidosis

          (1) Prolonged PR and QRS interval.

          (2) Increased amplitude of P wave.

          (3) Tall, peaked T waves.

    p. Metabolic alkalosis. Inverted T wave.

    q. Digoxin

          (1) Therapeutic levels: prolonged PR interval, short QT interval.

          (2) Toxic levels: most common are sinoatrial (SA) block, second- degree atrioventricular (AV) block, multiple ectopic beats; also, atrioventricular block, bradycardia.

    r. Quinidine

          (1) Therapeutic levels: prolonged PR and QT intervals, decreased amplitude of P wave, widened QRS complex.

          (2) Toxic levels: prolonged PR interval, prolonged QRS complex; AV block, multifocal ventricular premature beats.

    s. Theophylline

          (1) Therapeutic levels: no effect.

          (2) Toxic levels: tachycardia, conduction abnormality.

  2. Chest x-ray studies should be obtained in all infants with suspected heart failure or air leak.

V. Plan

  A. General management. First decide if the arrhythmia is benign or pathologic as noted above. If it is pathologic, full electrocardiographic evaluation must be performed. Any acid-base disorder, hypoxia, or electrolyte abnormality needs to be corrected.

  B. Specific management

    1. Heart rate abnormalities

      a. Tachycardia

        (1) Benign. No treatment is necessary, as the tachycardia is usually secondary to a self-limited event.

        (2) Medications. With certain medications, such as theophylline, you can order a serum drug level to determine if it is in the toxic range. If it is, lowering the dosage may restore normal rhythm. Otherwise, a decision needs to be made to accept the tachycardia if the medication is needed or to discontinue the drug.

        (3) Pathologic conditions. The underlying disease should be treated.

      b. Bradycardia

        (1) Benign. No treatment is usually necessary.

        (2) Drug-related. Check serum drug level if possible; then consider lowering the dosage or discontinuing the drug unless it is necessary.

        (3) Pathologic

          (a) Treat the underlying disease.

          (b) In severe hypotension or cardiac arrest, check the airway and initiate breathing and cardiac compressions.

          (c) Administer atropine, epinephrine, or isoproterenol to restore normal rhythm (see Chap 73 for dosages and other pharmacologic information).

    2. Arrhythmias. (See Chap 73 for dosages of drugs mentioned below and for other pharmacologic information; see p 176 for technique of cardioversion.)

      a. Benign. Only observation is indicated (no other treatment).

      b. Pathologic. Treat any underlying acid-base disorders, hypoxia, or electrolyte abnormalities.

        (1) Supraventricular tachycardia

       (a) If the infant's condition is critical, electrical cardioversion is indicated, with digoxin started for maintenance therapy.

       (b) If the infant's condition is stable, vagal stimulation (ice cold washcloth applied to the infant's face for a few seconds) can be tried. If this is ineffective, digoxin should be started. Other drugs that may be used instead of digoxin are propranolol and quinidine.

    (2) Atrial flutter

       (a) If the infant's condition is critical (severe CHF or unstable hemodynamic state), perform electrical cardioversion, with digoxin started for maintenance therapy.

       (b) If the infant is stable, start digoxin, which slows the ventricular rate. A combination of digoxin and quinidine may be used instead of digoxin alone.

    (3) Recurrent atrial flutter: Management is the same as that for atrial flutter.

    (4) Atrial fibrillation. Management is the same as that for atrial flutter.

    (5) Wolff-Parkinson-White syndrome. Treat any symptomatic arrhythmias that may occur. (High incidence of supraventricular tachycardia.)

    (6) Ventricular tachycardia. Perform electrical cardioversion (except in digitalis toxicity), with lidocaine started for maintenance therapy. Although lidocaine is the drug of choice, other drugs that may be used are procainamide, phenytoin, or bretylium.

3. Ectopic beats

  a. Asymptomatic. No treatment is necessary.

  b. Symptomatic. Underlying heart disease with ectopic beats that are compromising cardiac output: suppress with phenytoin, propranolol, or quinidine.

4. Atrioventricular block

  a. First degree. No specific treatment is usually necessary.

  b. Second degree. Treat underlying cause.

  c. Third degree (complete). If the infant is asymptomatic, only observation is necessary. Occasionally, the rate is low enough that transvenous pacing is necessary on an urgent basis, with the need for subsequent permanent pacing. Check the mother for anti-rho antibodies since there is an association with complete heart block.

5. Arrhythmias secondary to extracardiac cause

  a. Pathologic conditions. Treat underlying disease.

  b. Digoxin toxicity. Check PR interval before each dose, obtain stat serum digoxin level, and hold dose. Consider digoxin immune fab (ovine) (Digibind) (see p 480).

  c. Quinidine toxicity. Discontinue medication.

  d. Theophylline toxicity. Reduce dosage or discontinue medication.

6. Electrolyte abnormalities

  a. Check serum electrolyte levels with repeat determinations.

  b. Treat electrolyte abnormalities accordingly (see Chap 7).

VI. Technique of cardioversion. Place the paddles at the apex (left lower chest in fifth intercostal space in the anterior axillary line) and base of the heart (right of midline below clavicle). Remember to place a saline-soaked gauze pad beneath each paddle to ensure good electrical conduction. The dose is 1–4 joules/kg, which should be increased 50–100% each time an electrical charge is delivered. When cardioversion is used for infants with ventricular fibrillation, the synch switch should be off.

27 Apnea and Bradycardia ("A's and B's")

I. **Problem.** An infant has just had an apneic episode with bradycardia. Apnea is the absence of breathing for greater than 20 seconds with or without a decrease in heart rate. Bradycardia is a heart rate less than 100/min.

II. **Immediate questions**

A. **What is the gestational age of the infant?** Apnea and bradycardia are common in premature infants. In term infants, they are uncommon and are usually associated with a serious disorder. Apnea in a term infant is never physiologic; it usually requires a full workup to determine the cause.

B. **Was significant stimulation needed to return the heart rate to normal?** An infant requiring significant stimulation (eg, oxygen by bag-and-mask ventilation) needs immediate evaluation and treatment. An infant who has had one episode of apnea and bradycardia not requiring oxygen supplementation may not need a full evaluation unless the infant is term.

C. **If the patient is already receiving medication (eg, theophylline) for apnea and bradycardia, is the dosage adequate?** Determining the serum drug level is helpful.

D. **Did the episode occur during or after feeding?** Insertion of a nasogastric tube may cause a vagal reflex, resulting in apnea and bradycardia. Gastroesophageal reflux may cause apnea and bradycardia during or shortly after feeding. Consider aspiration in an infant who has been doing well and feeding.

E. **How old is the infant?** Apnea and bradycardia in the first 24 hours is usually pathologic, whereas if the infant is more than 3 days old, apnea of prematurity is high on the list of differential diagnoses.

III. **Differential diagnosis.** Causes of apnea and bradycardia can be classified according to diseases and disorders of various organ systems, gestational age, or postnatal age.

A. **Diseases and disorders of various organ systems**

1. **Head and central nervous system**
   a. Perinatal asphyxia.
   b. Intraventricular or subarachnoid hemorrhage.
   c. Meningitis.
   d. Hydrocephalus with increased intracranial pressure.
   e. Cerebral infarct with seizures.
   f. Seizures.

2. **Respiratory system**
   a. Hypoxia.
   b. Airway obstruction.
   c. Lung disease.
   d. Inadequate ventilation or performing extubation too early.

3. **Cardiovascular system**
   a. Congestive heart failure.
   b. Patent ductus arteriosus.
   c. Cardiac disorders such as congenital heart block, hypoplastic left heart syndrome, and transposition of the great vessels.

4. **Gastrointestinal tract**
   a. Necrotizing enterocolitis (NEC).
   b. Gastroesophageal reflux.

      c. Feeding intolerance.
- **5. Hematologic system**
  - **a. Anemia.** There is no specific hematocrit at which apnea and bradycardia will occur. They have been seen in infants with anemia of prematurity. These infants have significant relief after transfusion.
  - **b. Polycythemia.** This disorder is more common in term infants.
- **6. Other diseases and disorders**
  - **a. Temperature instability.** Apnea and bradycardia may occur in patients with temperature instability, especially hyperthermia but also hypothermia. Note the incubator temperature. An infant may have a normal body temperature but have a rise in incubator temperature (meaning that the infant is hypothermic) or require a lower incubator temperature (meaning that the infant is hyperthermic). Any rapid fluctuation of temperature can cause apnea. Cold stress can occur after birth, during transport, or a procedure and produce apnea.
  - **b. Infection (sepsis).**
  - **c. Electrolyte imbalance.** Hypoglycemia, hyponatremia, hypernatremia, hypermagnesemia, hyperkalemia, hyperammonemia, and hypocalcemia can cause apnea and bradycardia.
  - **d. Vagal reflex.** This may occur secondary to nasogastric tube insertion, feeding, or suctioning.
  - **e. Drugs.** High levels of phenobarbital or other sedatives such as diazepam and chloral hydrate may cause apnea and bradycardia. Oversedation from maternal drugs such as magnesium sulfate, opiates, and general anesthesia can all cause apnea in the newborn.
- **B. Gestational age.** See Table 27–1.
  - **1. Full-term infants.** In full-term infants of any neonatal age, apnea and bradycardia are usually not due to physiologic causes. The disease or disorder causing apnea and bradycardia must be identified.
  - **2. Preterm infants.** More common causes of apnea and bradycardia in preterm infants are listed in Table 27–1. The most common cause is apnea of prematurity. It occurs in infants that are usually < 34 weeks gestation, weigh < 1800 g, and have no other identifiable cause of the apnea and bradycardia.
- **C. Postnatal age.** Certain types of conditions produce apnea at varying postnatal ages.
  - **1. Onset within hours after birth:** oversedation from maternal drugs, asphyxia, seizures, hypermagnesemia, hyaline membrane disease.
  - **2. Onset less than 1 week:** patent ductus arteriosus, periventricular-intraventricular hemorrhage.
  - **3. Onset greater than 1 week of age:** posthemorrhagic hydrocephalus, seizures.

TABLE 27–1. MORE COMMON CAUSES OF APNEA AND BRADYCARDIA ACCORDING TO GESTATIONAL AGE.

Premature infant	Full-Term infant	All Ages
Apnea of Prematurity	Cerebral infarction	Sepsis
PDA	Polycythemia	NEC
HMD		Meningitis
Respiratory insufficiency of prematurity		Aspiration
		GE reflux
Posthemorrhagic hydrocephalus		Pneumonia
PV-IVH		Cardiac disorder
		Postextubation atelectasis
		Seizures
		Cold stress
		Asphyxia

    4. Onset between 6–10 weeks: anemia of prematurity

    5. Variable onset: sepsis, necrotizing enterocolitis, meningitis, aspiration, gastroesophageal reflux, cardiac disorder, pneumonia, cold stress, fluctuations in temperatures.

IV. Data base. Determine whether there has been any prenatal risk of sepsis. The cord pH should be obtained to rule out birth asphyxia. A history of feeding intolerance will increase the suspicion of necrotizing enterocolitis.

   A. Physical examination. Perform a complete physical examination, paying careful attention to the following signs.

     1. Head. Look for signs of increased intracranial pressure.

     2. Heart. Listen for a murmur or gallop.

     3. Lungs. Check for adequate movement of the chest if mechanical ventilation is being used.

     4. Abdomen. Check for abdominal distention, one of the earliest signs of NEC. Other signs of NEC are decreased bowel sounds and visible bowel loops.

     5. Skin. An infant with polycythemia has a ruddy appearance. Pallor is associated with anemia.

   B. Laboratory studies

     1. Complete blood count and differential. Findings may suggest infection, possible anemia, or polycythemia.

     2. Serum electrolyte, calcium, and glucose levels help rule out metabolic abnormality.

     3. Serum phenobarbital and/or theophylline levels are obtained if indicated.

     4. Arterial blood gas levels should be obtained to rule out hypoxia and acidosis.

   C. Radiologic and other studies

     1. Chest x-ray study. A chest x-ray study should be performed immediately if there is any suspicion of heart or lung disease.

     2. Electrocardiography. If cardiac disease is suspected, electrocardiography should be performed.

     3. Abdominal x-ray study. An abdominal x-ray study should be performed immediately if indicated. It may detect signs of NEC (see p 177).

     4. Ultrasonography of the head is performed to rule out periventricular-intraventricular hemorrhage or hydrocephalus.

     5. CT scanning of the head will detect cerebral infarction and subarachnoid hemorrhage if present.

     6. Barium swallow is performed to rule out gastroesophageal reflux only in cases of apnea and bradycardia associated with feeding.

     7. Lumbar puncture. Lumbar puncture and CSF examination should be performed if meningitis is suspected or if increased intracranial pressure from hydrocephalus is causing apnea and bradycardia.

     8. Esophageal-pH probe testing (acid reflux test of Tuttle and Grossman) is useful in determining whether gastroesophageal reflux is present. A small-caliber tube (to which a pH electrode is attached) is passed into the distal esophagus. Continuous monitoring can be carried out over 4–24 hours. If the pH is acidic, gastroesophageal reflux is occurring.

     9. Electroencephalography. Because apnea and bradycardia may be a manifestation of seizure activity, an electroencephalogram (EEG) is obtained in any infant who may be having seizures.

    10. Pneumography, thermistor pneumography, and polysomnography. See p 415 for a detailed discussion of these procedures.

V. Plan

   A. Determine the cause of apnea and bradycardia and treat if possible.

   B. Apnea of prematurity

     1. General measures

      a. Provide tactile stimulation.

      b. Place the infant on a water bed or an oscillating bed if it is the practice of your institution. Randomized controlled studies have shown this measure not to be effective, but it is still used in some institutions.

2. Specific treatment

  a. Theophylline or caffeine is used initially. Caffeine seems to have fewer side effects than theophylline, but the choice of drug depends on institutional preference and availability. Therapy can usually be discontinued by 37 weeks' postconceptional age. (See Chap 73 for dosages, side effects, and other pharmacologic information.)

  b. If the above drug trial fails, use **continuous positive airway pressure (CPAP)** via nasal prongs at a rate of 2–4 cm of water and continue administration of the drug.

  c. If apnea persists, begin **doxapram.** Doxapram has had limited clinical use but appears to be efficacious. One concern regarding doxapram is that it contains benzyl alcohol as a preservative. (See Chap 73 for drug dosage, side effects, and other pharmacologic information.)

  d. Mechanical ventilation should be used if apnea and bradycardia cannot be controlled by drug therapy and/or nasal CPAP. Low pressures are used at the rate necessary to prevent apnea. (See p 49.)

3. Long-term monitoring of respiratory function. See p 417.

C. Anemia. Most institutions do not treat anemia if the infant is asymptomatic and is feeding and growing and the reticulocyte count indicates that red cells are being made (> 5–6%). If the hematocrit is low ("low" is usually < 21–25%, based on your institution) and if the infant is symptomatic and not feeding well and the reticulocyte count is not appropriate for the low hematocrit (ie, reticulocyte is < 2–3%), transfusion is indicated (*controversial*).

D. Gastroesophageal reflux. Keep the infant in the prone position as much as possible; use small-volume, thickened feedings. Reglan may also be tried (see Chap 73 for dosage and other pharmacologic information).

28 Bloody Stool

I. Problem. A newborn infant has passed a bloody stool.

II. Immediate questions

A. Is it grossly bloody? This finding is usually an ominous sign; an exception is swallowed maternal blood, which is a benign condition. A grossly bloody stool usually occurs in infants with a lesion in the ileum or colon or with massive upper gastrointestinal tract bleeding. Necrotizing enterocolitis is the most common cause of bloody stool in premature infants and should be strongly suspected in the differential diagnosis.

B. Is the stool otherwise normal in color but with streaks of blood? This description is more characteristic of a lesion in the anal canal, such as anal fissure.

C. Is the stool positive only for occult blood? Occult blood often signifies that the blood is from the upper gastrointestinal tract (proximal to the ligament of Treitz). Nasogastric trauma and swallowed maternal blood are common causes. Microscopic blood as an isolated finding is usually not significant.

D. Was the infant given vitamin K at birth? Hemorrhagic disease of the newborn may present with bloody stools, as may any coagulopathy.

III. Differential diagnosis

A. Occult blood only, no visible blood
1. Swallowing of maternal blood during delivery or breast-feeding (secondary to cracked nipples) may be the cause.
2. Nasogastric tube trauma.
3. Necrotizing enterocolitis.
4. Formula intolerance. Milk protein sensitivity is secondary to cow's milk or soybean formula and symptoms of blood in the stool usually occur in the 2nd or 3rd week of life.
5. Gastritis or ulcer. Stress ulcers may occur in the stomach or duodenum and are associated with prolonged, severe illness. Steroid therapy, especially prolonged, is associated with ulcers. Hemorrhagic gastritis can occur from tolazoline and theophylline therapy.
6. Unknown etiology.

B. Streaks of visible blood in the stool
1. Anal fissure.
2. Rectal trauma. This is often secondary to temperature probes.

C. Grossly bloody stool
1. Necrotizing enterocolitis.
2. Disseminated intravascular coagulation. There may be bleeding from other sites.
3. Hemorrhagic disease of the newborn. This entity occurs from Vitamin K deficiency and can be prevented if it is administered at birth. Bloody stools typically appear on the second or third day of life.
4. Other surgical diseases such as malrotation with midgut volvulus, Meckel's diverticulum, Hirshsprung enterocolitis, intestinal duplications, and intussusception (rare in the neonatal period).
5. Intestinal infections such as *Shigella, Salmonella, Campylobacter, Yersinia,* and enteropathogenic strains of *E coli.*
6. Severe liver disease.
7. Other infections such as CMV, TOXO, syphilis, and bacterial sepsis.

IV. DATA BASE. The age of the infant is important. If the infant is less than 7 days old, swallowing of maternal blood is a possible cause; in older infants, it is an unlikely cause.

  A. Physical examination
    1. **Examination of peripheral perfusion.** Evaluate the infant's peripheral perfusion. An infant with necrotizing enterocolitis can be poorly perfused and may appear to be in early or impending shock.
    2. **Abdominal examination.** Check for bowel sounds and tenderness. If the abdomen is soft, nontender, and there is no erythema, a pathologic process is probably not occurring. If the abdomen is distended, rigid, or tender, a pathologic process is likely to be present. Abdominal distention is the most common sign of necrotizing enterocolitis. If there are red streaks and erythema on the abdominal wall, suspect necrotizing enterocolitis with peritonitis.
    3. **Anal examination.** If the infant's condition is stable, perform a visual examination of the anus to check for anal fissure or tear.
  B. Laboratory studies
    1. **Apt test.** If swallowed maternal blood is suspected, perform the **Apt test,** which differentiates maternal from fetal blood. The test is performed as follows: Mix equal parts of the bloody material with water and centrifuge it. Add 1 part 0.25-molar sodium hydroxide to 5 parts of the pink supernatant. If the fluid remains pink, the blood is fetal in origin because hemoglobin F stays pink. Hemoglobin A from maternal blood is hydrolyzed and changes color from pink to yellow brown.
    2. **Stool culture.** Obtain a stool culture. Certain pathogens cause bloody stools, but they are rare in the neonatal nursery.
    3. **Coagulation studies.** Coagulation studies should be performed to rule out disseminated intravascular coagulation or a bleeding disorder. The usual studies are partial thromboplastin time (PTT), prothrombin time (PT), fibrinogen level, and platelet count. Thrombocytopenia can also be seen with cow's milk protein allergy.
    4. **If necrotizing enterocolitis (NEC) is suspected, the following studies should be performed.**
      a. **Complete blood count with differential.** This test is done to establish an inflammatory response and to check for thrombocytopenia and anemia.
      b. **Serum potassium levels.** Hyperkalemia due to hemolysis may occur.
      c. **Blood gas levels.** Blood gases should be measured to rule out metabolic acidosis, which is often associated with sepsis or necrotizing enterocolitis.
  C. Radiologic and other studies. A **plain x-ray film of the abdomen** is useful if necrotizing enterocolitis or a surgical abdomen is suspected. Look for an abnormal gas pattern, thickened bowel wall, or pneumatosis intestinalis. Pneumatosis can appear as a "soap bubble" area. If a suspicious area appears on the abdominal x-ray film in the right upper quadrant, it is usually not stool. A left lateral decubitus view of the abdomen may show free air if perforation has occurred. Surgical conditions usually show signs of intestinal obstruction.
V. Plan
  A. Swallowed maternal blood. Only observation is necessary.
  B. Anal fissure and rectal trauma. Observation is indicated. Petroleum jelly applied to the anus may promote healing.
  C. Necrotizing enterocolitis. (See Chap 64.)
  D. Nasogastric trauma. In most cases of bloody stool involving nasogastric tubes, trauma is mild and requires only observation. If the tube is too large, replacing it with a smaller one may resolve the problem. If there has been significant bleeding, gastric lavages are helpful; it is *controversial* whether tepid water or normal saline is best. Then, if possible, removal of the nasogastric tube is recommended.

E. **Formula intolerance.** This diagnosis is difficult to document, so it is usually made if the patient has remission of symptoms when the formula is eliminated.

F. **Gastritis or ulcers.** Treatment usually consists of ranitidine or cimetidine (see Chap 73 for dosages and other pharmacologic information). Use of antacids is *controversial,* as some clinicians feel concretions may result from the use of antacids.

G. **Unknown etiology.** If no cause is found, the infant is usually closely followed, and in the majority of the cases, the bleeding will subside.

H. **Intestinal infections.** Antibiotic treatment and isolation are standard treatment. (See Chap 73 and Appendix G).

I. **Hemorrhagic disease of the newborn.** Intravenous vitamin K is usually adequate therapy (see Chap 73).

J. **Surgical conditions.** These all require immediate surgical evaluation.

29 Abnormal Blood Gas

I. Problem. An abnormal blood gas value is reported by the laboratory for a neonate.

II. Immediate questions

A. What component of the blood gas is abnormal? Accepted normal values for an arterial blood gas sample are pH between 7.35 and 7.45, $Paco_2$ between 35 and 45 (slightly higher values may be accepted if the blood pH remains normal), and Pao_2 between 55 and 65 on room air.

B. Is this blood gas value very different from the patient's previous blood gas determination? This is a key question. If the patient has had metabolic acidosis on the last 5 blood gas measurements and now has metabolic alkalosis, it might be best to repeat the blood gas measurements before initiating treatment. Do not treat the infant on the basis of one abnormal gas value, especially if the infant's clinical status has not changed.

C. How was the sample collected? Blood gas measurements can be reported on arterial, venous, or capillary blood samples. Arterial blood samples are the best indicator of pH, $Paco_2$, and Pao_2. Venous blood samples will give a lower pH value and a higher Pco_2 than arterial samples. Capillary samples will give a fair assessment of the infant's pH, Pco_2. Capillary samples give a lower pH value (but not as low as the venous pH) and a slightly higher Pco_2 than arterial samples. An accurate capillary blood gas measurement cannot be obtained on an infant who is hypotensive or in shock.

D. Is the infant on ventilatory support? Management of abnormal blood gas levels is approached differently in an intubated infant than in a patient breathing room air.

III. Differential diagnosis

A. Metabolic acidosis. This is defined as a pH value < 7.35 with a normal carbon dioxide value and a base deficit > 5.

   1. Common causes
     a. Sepsis.
     b. Necrotizing enterocolitis.
     c. Hypothermia or cold stress.
     d. Asphyxia
     e. Periventricular-intraventricular hemorrhage.
     f. Patent ductus arteriosus.
     g. Shock.
     h. Factitious acidosis (too much heparin in the syringe).
     i. Drugs (eg, acetazolamide [Diamox]).

   2. Less common causes
     a. Renal tubular acidosis. This involves a defect in the reabsorption of bicarbonate or secretion of hydrogen ion and can present in 3 forms: proximal, distal, or mixed.
     b. Inborn errors of metabolism. See Table 59–4 for those diseases that present with metabolic acidosis.
     c. Maternal use of salicylates and maternal acidosis.
     d. Renal failure.
     e. Congenital lactic acidosis.
     f. GI losses such as frequent loose stools.

B. Metabolic alkalosis. This is defined as a pH value > 7.45 with a base excess of > 5.

   1. Common causes

      a. Excess alkali administration (eg, sodium bicarbonate, citrate, acetate, or lactate infusion).

      b. Potassium depletion.

      c. Prolonged nasogastric suction.

      d. Diuretic therapy (such as in patients with bronchopulmonary dysplasia [BPD]).

    2. Less common causes

      a. Bartter's syndrome.

      b. Primary hyperaldosteronism.

C. Low CO_2 high O_2

    1. Overventilation.

    2. Air bubble in the syringe.

    3. Hyperventilation therapy as in persistent pulmonary hypertension.

D. High CO_2, normal or high O_2

    1. Obstructed endotracheal tube (eg, mucous plug).

    2. Endotracheal tube down the right main stem bronchus or at the carina.

    3. Pneumothorax.

    4. Patent ductus arteriosus. Clinical signs and symptoms include metabolic acidosis, congestive heart failure, bounding pulses, active precordium, deteriorating blood gases with an increase in the ventilator settings, and a large heart with increased pulmonary vascularity on chest x-ray film.

    5. Ventilator malfunction.

E. High CO_2, low O_2

    1. Pneumothorax.

    2. Improper endotracheal tube position. An endotracheal tube positioned in the oropharynx will cause this type of blood gas result.

    3. Increasing respiratory failure.

    4. Patent ductus arteriosus (PDA).

    5. Insufficient respiratory support.

    6. Atelectasis.

F. Normal CO_2, low O_2

    1. Agitation.

    2. Pneumothorax.

    3. Improper endotracheal tube position.

    4. Atelectasis.

    5. Pulmonary hypertension.

    6. Pulmonary edema.

IV. Data base

  A. Physical examination. Evaluate for signs of sepsis (eg, hypotension, poor perfusion). Check for equal breath sounds; asymmetric breath sounds suggest pneumothorax. Observe for chest wall movement. Listen for breath sounds over the chest vs the epigastric region, which may help determine if the endotracheal tube is malpositioned. Listen to the heart for any murmur and palpate for cardiac displacement.

  B. Laboratory studies

    1. Repeat blood gas measurement. Especially if the result is unexpected or if a major clinical decision is to be made on the basis of venous or capillary blood gas values, an arterial blood sample should be obtained and sent to the laboratory for blood gas values.

    2. Complete blood count and differential are helpful if sepsis is being considered.

    3. Serum potassium level. Severe metabolic alkalosis can cause hypokalemia.

  C. Radiologic and other studies

    1. Transillumination of the chest should be done if pneumothorax is suspected (see p 238 for details on this procedure).

    2. Chest x-ray study. A chest x-ray study should be performed if an abnormal blood gas value is reported by the laboratory unless there is an obvious cause. An anteroposterior x-ray view should be obtained to check endotracheal tube placement, to rule out air leak (eg, pneumothorax), to check heart size and pulmonary vascularity (increased or decreased), and to determine if the infant is being hypoventilated or hyperventilated.

3. **Abdominal x-ray study.** An abdominal x-ray study should be done if necrotizing enterocolitis is suspected in a patient with **severe metabolic acidosis.**

4. **Ultrasonography of the head** will diagnose intraventricular hemorrhage if present.

5. **Echocardiography.** Patient ductus arteriosus or other cardiac abnormality may be detected with echocardiography.

V. Plan

A. **Overall plan.** Verify the blood gas result, find the cause of the problem, and provide appropriate treatment for the specific cause. The first step is to examine the infant. If the infant's clinical status has not changed, repeat blood gas measurements to verify the report. If the clinical status has changed, the abnormal report is probably correct; repeat blood gas measurements can be obtained, but further evaluation of the infant should begin.

B. **Specific management**

1. **Metabolic acidosis**

   a. **General measures.** Most institutions treat acidosis with an alkali infusion if the base excess is greater than −5 to −10 or if the pH is equal to or less than 7.25. The alkali can be given as 1 dose over 20 to 30 minutes or it can be given as an 8- to 12-hour correction. If the acidosis is mild, usually only 1 dose is given and repeat blood gas measurements are obtained. If the acidosis is severe, a dose is given and correction is started at the same time. One of 3 medications is used.

   (1) **Sodium bicarbonate** can be used if the infant's serum sodium and Pco_2 are not high. If given as a one-time dose, it should be 1–2 meq/kg diluted 1:1 with sterile water. It should be given over 20–30 minutes unless the infant is unstable, in which case an intravenous push dose can be given at a rate of 1 mL/min. To calculate how much to give as an 8- to 12-hour correction:

   Bicarbonate dose (meq) = Base deficit × Body weight (kg) × 0.3

   is the total dose required to correct the base deficit. It should be added to the intravenous fluids, and the correction should be given over 8–12 hours.

   (2) **Tromethamine (THAM)** can be used in infants who have metabolic acidosis but have a high serum sodium or high Pco_2. *It should be used only in infants who have a good urine output.* (See Chap 73 for dosage and other pharmacologic information.)

   (3) **Polycitrate (Polycitra).** This alkali is especially useful in patients receiving acetazolamide (Diamox). It consists of 1 meq sodium, 1 meq potassium, and 2 meq citrate. Each meq of citrate equals 1 meq bicarbonate. The dose is 2–3 meq/kg/d polycitrate in 3–4 divided doses. Adjust the dosage to maintain a normal pH.

   b. **The underlying cause should be treated** as outlined below.

   (1) **Sepsis.** Initiate a septic workup and consider broad- spectrum antibiotics. (See Chap 73 for specific antibiotic agents, dosages, and other pharmacologic information.)

   (2) **Necrotizing enterocolitis.** (See Chap 64.)

   (3) **Hypothermia or cold stress.** See section on treatment of hypothermia. (p 38).

   (4) **Periventricular-Intraventricular hemorrhage.** Weekly ultrasonographic examinations of the head and daily head circumferences are indicated. If hydrocephalus occurs, neurosurgical consultation should be obtained to detect possible shunting.

    (5) Patent ductus arteriosus. The patient who has a clinically symptomatic PDA should be treated. Treatment includes furosemide, decreasing fluid intake, and a course of indomethacin (See Chap 73 for drug dosages and other pharmacologic information.)

    (6) Renal tubular acidosis. Treatment consists of sodium bicarbonate therapy (see p 184).

    (7) Inborn errors of metabolism. (See Chap 59.)

    (8) Maternal use of salicylates. Acidosis usually resolves without treatment.

    (9) Renal failure. (See p 432).

  (10) Congenital lactic acidosis. Correction of the metabolic acidosis (see p 184) and megavitamin therapy are indicated.

2. Metabolic alkalosis. The treatment of metabolic alkalosis depends on the cause.

  a. Excess alkali. Adjust or discontinue the dose of THAM, sodium bicarbonate, or polycitrate.

  b. Hypokalemia. If the serum potassium level is low, metabolic alkalosis can occur because potassium is exchanged for hydrogen. The infant's potassium level should be corrected (see Chap 40).

  c. Prolonged nasogastric suction is treated with intravenous fluid replacement, usually with 1/2 normal saline containing 20 meq potassium chloride, replaced milliliter for milliliter each shift.

  d. Diuretics. Mild alkalosis is sometimes seen; no specific treatment is usually necessary.

  e. Bartter's syndrome is treated with potassium replacement and adequate nutrition.

  f. Primary hyperaldosteronism is treated with dexamethasone. (See Chap 73 for dosage and other pharmacologic information.)

3. Other causes of abnormal blood gases

  a. Pneumothorax. (see p 000.)

  b. Mucous plug. If an infant has decreased breath sounds on both sides of the chest and has retractions, a plugged endotracheal tube is probably responsible. The infant can be suctioned and, if clinically stable, repeat blood gas measurements are obtained. If the infant is in extreme distress, the tube should be replaced.

  c. Overventilation. If the blood gas levels reveal overventilation, the ventilation parameters need to be adjusted. If the oxygen level is high, the following parameters can be decreased: oxygen, positive end-expiratory pressure (PEEP), peak inspiratory pressure (PIP), or inspiratory time (IT). If the patient's carbon dioxide level is low, the following parameters can be decreased: rate, positive inspiratory pressure (PIP), or expiratory time (ET). Deciding which parameter to wean depends on the patient's lung disease and the disease course. Ventilator changes are discussed on p 000.

  d. Agitation. An agitated infant may have a drop in oxygenation and may need to be sedated or have ventilator settings changed. One may have to sit by the bedside and try different rates to see if he or she fights less. If sedation is chosen, phenobarbital, diazepam, chloral hydrate, meperidine, or morphine may be used. (See Chap 73 for dosages and other pharmacologic information.) Use the agent with which your institution has experience. **Remember, agitation can be a sign of hypoxia, so a blood gas level should be obtained prior to ordering sedation.** If there is documented hypoxia, attempts to increase oxygenation should be used.

  e. Problem with endotracheal tube placement. An infant who has a tube down his right main-stem bronchus will have breath sounds on the right only. An infant with a tube that has dislodged or become plugged will have decreased or no breath sounds on chest auscultation. The patient needs to be reintubated.

f. **Ventilator malfunction.** Respiratory Therapy should be notified to check the ventilator and replace it if necessary.

g. **Increasing respiratory failure.** Ventilator settings need to be adjusted.

h. **Insufficient respiratory support.** If the infant's chest is not moving, the PIP is not high enough, and adjustment of the ventilator setting is needed.

i. **Atelectasis.** Treatment consists of percussion and postural drainage and possibly increased PIP or PEEP.

j. **Pulmonary edema.** Diuretics (eg, furosemide) (see Chap 73) and mechanical ventilation are indicated.

k. **Pulmonary hypertension.** (See p 290.)

30 Cyanosis

I. **Problem.** During a physical examination, an infant appears blue.
II. **Immediate questions**
   A. **Does the infant have respiratory distress?** If the infant has increased respiratory effort with increased rate, retractions, and nasal flaring, respiratory disease should be high on the list of differential diagnoses. Cyanotic heart disease usually presents without respiratory symptoms but can have effortless tachypnea (rapid respiratory rate without retractions). Blood disorders usually present without respiratory or cardiac symptoms.
   B. **Does the infant have a murmur?** A murmur usually implies heart disease. Transposition of the great vessels can present without a murmur.
   C. **Is the cyanosis continuous, intermittent, sudden in onset, or occurring only with feeding?** Intermittent cyanosis is more common with neurologic disorders, as these infants may have apneic spells alternating with periods of normal breathing. Continuous cyanosis is usually associated with intrinsic lung disease or heart disease. Cyanosis with feeding may occur with esophageal atresia and severe esophageal reflux. Sudden onset of cyanosis may occur with an air leak, such as pneumothorax. Cyanosis that disappears with crying may signify choanal atresia.
   D. **Is there differential cyanosis?** If there is cyanosis of the upper or lower part of the body only, it usually signifies serious heart disease. The more common pattern is cyanosis restricted to the lower half of the body, which is seen in patients with patent ductus arteriosus. Cyanosis restricted to the upper half of the body is seen occasionally in patients with pulmonary hypertension, patent ductus arteriosus, coarctation of the aorta, and D-transposition of the great arteries.
   E. **What is the prenatal and delivery history?** An infant of a diabetic mother has increased risk for hypoglycemia, polycythemia, respiratory distress syndrome (RDS), and heart disease. Infection, such as that which can occur with premature rupture of the membranes, may cause shock and hypotension with resultant cyanosis. Amniotic fluid abnormalities, such as oligohydramnios (associated with hypoplastic lungs) or polyhydramnios (associated with esophageal atresia), may suggest a cause for the cyanosis. Cesarean section is associated with increased respiratory distress.
III. **Differential diagnosis.** The causes of cyanosis can be classified as respiratory, cardiac, central nervous system, or other disorders.
   A. **Respiratory diseases**
      1. **Lung diseases**
         a. Hyaline membrane disease.
         b. Transient tachypnea of the newborn.
         c. Pneumonia.
         d. Meconium aspiration.
      2. **Air leak syndrome.**
      3. **Congenital defects** (eg, diaphragmatic hernia and hypoplastic lungs).
   B. **Cardiac diseases**
      1. **All cyanotic heart diseases,** including transposition of the great arteries, total anomalous pulmonary venous return, Ebstein's anomaly, tricuspid atresia, pulmonary atresia, pulmonary stenosis, tetralogy of Fallot, patent ductus arteriosus, and ventricular septal defect.
      2. **Persistent pulmonary hypertension.**

3. Severe congestive heart failure.
C. Central nervous system (CNS) diseases. Periventricular-intraventricular hemorrhage, meningitis, and primary seizure disorder can all cause cyanosis. Neuromuscular disorders such as Werdnig-Hoffman and congenital myotonic dystrophy can cause cyanosis.
D. Other disorders
   1. Methemoglobinemia. May be familial.
   2. Polycythemia/Hyperviscosity syndrome.
   3. Hypothermia, hypoglycemia, sepsis, pseudocyanosis caused by fluorescent lighting.
   4. Respiratory depression secondary to maternal medications (eg, magnesium sulfate and narcotics).
   5. Shock.
   6. Choanal atresia. Nasal passage obstruction caused most commonly by a bony abnormality.
IV. Data base. Obtain a prenatal and delivery history (see p 189).
   A. Physical examination
      1. Assess the infant for central vs peripheral cyanosis. In central cyanosis, the skin, lips, and tongue will appear blue. In central cyanosis, the PaO_2 is less than 50 torr. In peripheral cyanosis, the skin is bluish but the oral mucous membranes will be pink. Check the nasal passage for choanal atresia.
      2. Assess the heart. Check for any murmurs. Assess heart rate and blood pressure.
      3. Assess the lungs. Is there retraction, flaring of nose, grunting?
      4. Assess the abdomen for an enlarged liver. The liver can be enlarged in congestive heart failure and hyperexpansion of the lungs. Absence of bowel sounds may suggest a diaphragmatic hernia.
      5. Check the pulses. In coarctation of the aorta, the femoral pulses will be decreased. In patent ductus arteriosus, the pulses will be bounding.
      6. Consider neurologic problems. Check for apnea and periodic breathing, which may be associated with immaturity of the nervous system. Observe the infant for seizures, which can cause cyanosis if the infant is not breathing during seizures.
   B. Laboratory studies
      1. Arterial blood gas measurements on room air. If the patient is not hypoxic, it suggests methemoglobinemia, polycythemia, or CNS disease. If the patient is hypoxic, perform the 100% hyperoxic test, described below.
      2. Hyperoxic test. Measure arterial oxygen on room air. Then place the infant on 100% oxygen for 10–20 minutes. With cyanotic heart disease the PaO_2 will not increase significantly. If the PaO_2 rises above 150mm Hg, cardiac disease can generally be excluded. Whereas in lung disease the arterial oxygen saturation should improve and go above 150 mm.
      3. Right to left shunt test. This test should be done to rule out persistent pulmonary hypertension. Draw a simultaneous sample of blood from the right radial artery (preductal) and the descending aorta (postductal). If there is a difference of greater than 15% (preductal > postductal), then the shunt is significant.
      4. Complete blood count and differential may reveal an infection process. A central hematocrit of more than 65% confirms polycythemia.
      5. Serum glucose level will detect hypoglycemia.
      6. Methemoglobin level. A drop of blood exposed to air has a chocolate hue. To confirm the diagnosis, a spectrophotometric determination should be done by the lab.
   C. Radiologic and other studies
      1. Transillumination of the chest (see p 238) should be done on an emergent basis if pneumothorax is suspected.
      2. Chest x-ray may be normal, suggesting CNS disease or another cause for the cyanosis (see **III.D,** above). It can verify lung disease, air leak, or dia-

phragmatic hernia. It can help diagnose heart disease by evaluating the heart size and pulmonary vascularity. The heart size may be normal or enlarged in hypoglycemia, polycythemia, shock, and sepsis.

3. **Electrocardiography** should be done to help determine the cause of the cyanosis. The ECG is usually normal in patients with methemoglobinemia or hypoglycemia; it is normal but may show right ventricular hypertrophy in patients with polycythemia, pulmonary hypertension, or primary lung disease. It is very helpful in identifying patients with tricuspid atresia; it will show left axis deviation and left ventricular hypertrophy.

4. **Echocardiography** should be performed if cardiac disease is suspected or if the diagnosis is unclear.

V. Plan

A. **General management.** Act quickly and accomplish many of the diagnostic tasks at once.

1. **Perform a rapid physical examination.** Transilluminate the chest (see p 238), and if a tension pneumothorax is present, rapid needle decompression may be needed (see p 239).
2. **Order stat laboratory tests (eg, blood gas levels, complete blood count, and chest x-ray film).**
3. **Perform the hyperoxic test.** (See above.)

B. **Specific management**

1. **Lung disease.** (See Chap 67) Respiratory depression caused by narcotics is treated with naloxone (Narcan) (see Chap 73 for dosage and other pharmacologic information).
2. **Air leak (pneumothorax).** (See p 238)
3. **Congenital defects.** Surgery is indicated for diaphragmatic hernia.
4. **Cardiac disease.** The use of prostaglandin E_1 (PGE_1) is indicated for right heart outflow obstruction (tricuspid atresia, pulmonic stenosis, and pulmonary atresia), left heart outflow obstruction (hypoplastic left heart syndrome, critical aortic valve stenosis, preductal coarctation of the aorta, and interrupted aortic arch), and transposition of the great arteries. PGE_1 is contraindicated for hyaline membrane disease, persistent pulmonary hypertension, and dominant left-to-right shunt (patent ductus arteriosus, truncus arteriosus, or ventricular septal defect). **If the diagnosis is uncertain, a trial of PGE_1 can be given over 30 minutes in an effort to improve blood gas values.**
5. **CNS disorders.** Treat the underlying disease (see Chap 65).
6. **Methemoglobinemia.** Treat the infant with methylene blue only if the methemoglobin level is markedly increased and the infant is in cardiopulmonary distress (tachypnea and tachycardia). Administer intravenously 1 mg/kg of a 1% solution of **methylene blue** in normal saline. The cyanosis should clear within 1–2 hours.
7. **Shock.** (See Chap 42.)
8. **Polycythemia.** (See Chap 47.)
9. **Choanal atresia.** The infant usually requires surgery.
10. **Hypothermia.** Rewarming is necessary and the technique is described on p 38.
11. **Hypoglycemia.** (See Chap 39.)

31 Eye Discharge (Conjunctivitis)

I. **Problem.** Eye discharge is noted.

II. **Immediate questions**

A. **How old is the infant?** Age is an important factor in determining the cause of eye discharge. Within the first 24–48 hours of life, the most likely cause is conjunctivitis secondary to use of ocular silver nitrate drops immediately after birth to prevent gonococcal ophthalmia. At 2–5 days, a bacterial infection is most likely. The organisms that most commonly cause conjunctivitis in the neonatal period are *Neisseria gonorrhoeae* and *Staphylococcus aureus*. *Chlamydia trachomatis* conjunctivitis is usually seen after the first week of life; it often presents as late as the third week. *Pseudomonas aeruginosa* infections are typically seen between the 5th and 18th days of life. Herpes conjunctivitis is seen 2 to 14 days after birth.

B. **Is the discharge unilateral or bilateral?** Bilateral conjunctivitis is seen with infection due to *C trachomatis* or *N gonorrhoeae* or use of silver nitrate. Unilateral conjunctivitis is seen with *S aureus* and *P aeruginosa*.

C. **What are the characteristics of the discharge?** It is important to distinguish between purulent and watery discharge. Purulent discharge is more common with bacterial infection. Infection due to *Chlamydia* may be watery early in the course and purulent later on. A greenish discharge is more characteristic of *P aeruginosa*.

III. **Differential diagnosis**

A. **Chemical conjunctivitis** is usually secondary to the use of silver nitrate ocular drops. It is not seen as frequently as in the past because many nurseries are using erythromycin ophthalmic ointment, which causes less ocular irritation and offers protection against chlamydial and gonococcal infections. Silver nitrate drops are recommended over erythromycin ophthalmic ointment if the patient population has a high number of penicillinase producing *Neisseria gonorrhoeae*.

B. **Gonococcal conjunctivitis** is most commonly transmitted from the mother. The incidence is low because of prophylactic treatment immediately after birth.

C. **Staphylococcal conjunctivitis** is usually a nosocomial infection.

D. **Chlamydial conjunctivitis** is transmitted from the mother. Approximately 30–35% of infants delivered vaginally to mothers with chlamydia will develop conjunctivitis.

E. **Pseudomonal conjunctivitis** is usually a nosocomial infection and is becoming more common in neonatal nurseries. The organism thrives in moisture-filled environments such as respiratory equipment.

F. **Lacrimal duct obstruction (dacryostenosis).** In this disorder, the nasolacrimal duct may fail to canalize completely at birth. The obstruction is usually at the nasal end of the duct. The symptoms are persistent tearing and a mucoid discharge in the inner corner of the eye. The disorder is usually unilateral.

G. **Other bacterial infections** include infections due to *Haemophilus* species, streptococci, and pneumococci.

H. **Herpes simplex keratoconjunctivitis.** Herpes simplex Type 2 can cause unilateral or bilateral conjunctivitis, optic neuritis, and chorioretinitis. Herpes should be suspected if the conjunctiva is not responding to antibiotic therapy.

IV. **Data base**

A. **Physical examination**

1. **Ophthalmic exam.** Examine both eyes for swelling and edema of the eye-

lids and check the conjunctiva for injection (congestion of blood vessels). A purulent discharge, edema, and erythema of the lids as well as injection of the conjunctiva are suggestive of bacterial conjunctivitis.

    2. Perform a complete physical examination to rule out signs of systemic infection.

B. Laboratory studies

    1. Always obtain a gram-stained smear of the discharge to check for white blood cells (a sign of infection) and bacteria to identify the specific organism. **A sample of the discharge should also be submitted for culture and sensitivity testing.** It will verify the specific organism seen on gram-stained smear and will indicate antibiotic sensitivities.

        a. *N gonorrhoeae* **conjunctivitis:** Gram-negative intracellular diplococci and white blood cells are seen.

        b. *S aureus* **conjunctivitis:** Gram-positive cocci in clusters and white blood cells are seen.

        c. *P aeruginosa* **conjunctivitis:** Gram-negative bacilli and white blood cells are found.

        d. Chemical conjunctivitis, lacrimal duct obstruction, herpes simplex, and *C trachomatis* **conjunctivitis:** The gram-stained smear will be negative.

        e. Conjunctivitis caused by *Haemophilus* **species:** Gram-negative coccoid rods are seen.

        f. Streptococcal or pneumococcal conjunctivitis: Streptococci are gram-positive spherical cocci and pneumococci are gram-positive lancet-shaped encapsulated diplococci.

    2. If a chlamydial infection is suspected, material is gathered for Giemsa staining by scraping (*not swabbing*) the lower conjunctiva with a wire loop or blunt spatula to obtain epithelial cells. If chlamydial infection is present, **inclusion bodies** will be seen within the epithelial cells.

    3. If herpes is suspected, a conjunctival scraping will show multinucleated giant cells with intracytoplasmic inclusions. Also, the conjunctiva should be swabbed and transported on special viral transport media for culture.

C. Radiologic and other studies. None are usually needed.

V. Plan. Based on the results of Gram's stain and Giemsa's stain, empiric treatment should be started after a specimen of the discharge is sent to the laboratory for culture rather than waiting for the results.

A. Chemical conjunctivitis. Observation only is needed. This disorder usually resolves within 48–72 hours.

B. Gonococcal conjunctivitis

    1. Isolate the infant during the first 24 hours of parenteral antibiotic therapy.

    2. Evaluate for disseminated disease. Blood and CSF cultures must be obtained.

    3. For gonococcal conjunctivitis without dissemination and infants born to mothers with active gonorrhea, single dose therapy of Ceftriaxone sodium 50 mg/kg IM or IV (up to maximum of 125 mg) is recommended. For disseminated disease, Ceftriaxone 25–50 mg/kg IV or IM every 12 hours for 7 days. It should be given for 14 days if meningitis is present.

    4. Irrigate the eyes with sterile isotonic saline solution every 1–2 hours until clear. Topical gentamicin eye drops 4 times a day for 7 days is recommended.

    5. Because gonococcal ophthalmia can lead to blindness, an ophthalmologic consultation is usually requested.

C. Staphylococcal conjunctivitis

    1. Isolate the infant to prevent spread of infection.

    2. Treat the infant with either topical Neosporin ophthalmic ointment or erythromycin ointment, 4 times per day for 7–10 days.

    3. Observe for local or systemic spread of infection.

D. Chlamydial conjunctivitis

1. Treat the infant with erythromycin ophthalmic ointment 4 times per day for 2–3 weeks.
2. Erythromycin suspension, 40 mg/kg/d orally for 2–3 weeks, is recommended because it is more effective in eradicating the conjunctivitis than with just topical therapy and oral therapy increases the chances of eradicating nasopharyngeal infection. Systemic treatment is also recommended because of the high risk of associated pneumonitis.

E. Pseudomonal conjunctivitis
1. Isolate the patient.
2. Treat the conjunctivitis with gentamicin ophthalmic ointment 4 times per day for 2 weeks.
3. Gentamicin or Tobramycin (see Chap 73) should also be given intravenously because sepsis may follow pseudomonal conjunctivitis.
4. Because this infection may be devastating, an ophthalmologist should be consulted.

F. Lacrimal duct obstruction
1. Most obstructions clear spontaneously without treatment.
2. Massaging the inside corner of the eye over the lacrimal sac, with expression toward the nose, may help to establish patency.
3. If the problem does not resolve in the first few months of life, the infant should be evaluated by an ophthalmologist.

G. Other bacterial infections.
1. Local saline irrigation.
2. Neosporin ophthalmic ointment or Erythromycin 0.5% ophthalmic ointment applied every 6 hours is usually adequate.

H. Herpes simplex conjunctivitis.
1. Isolate the patient.
2. Obtain a complete set of viral cultures (blood, CSF, oropharynx, and any lesions).
3. Topical therapy with 3% vidarabine ointment or 1% idoxuridine ointment 5 times a day for 10 days.
4. Systemic acyclovir therapy is indicated. See dosage p 467.
5. Ophthalmologic evaluation and follow-up is necessary as these infants may develop chorioretinitis, cataracts, and retinopathy.

32 Gastric Aspirate (Residuals)

I. **Problem.** The nurse alerts you that a gastric aspirate has been obtained in an infant. Gastric aspiration is a procedure by which the stomach is aspirated with an oral or nasogastric tube. The procedure is usually performed before each feeding to determine whether the feedings are being tolerated and digested.

II. **Immediate questions**

A. **What is the volume of the aspirate?** A volume of more than 30% of the total formula given at the last feeding may be abnormal and requires more extensive evaluation. A gastric aspirate of more than 10–15 mL is considered excessive.

B. **What is the character of the aspirate (ie, bilious, bloody, undigested, digested)?** This is important in the differential diagnosis (see **III.A**).

C. **Are the vital signs normal?** Abnormal vital signs may indicate a pathologic process, possibly an intra-abdominal process.

D. **Is the abdomen soft, with good bowel sounds, or distended, with visible bowel loops?** Absence of bowel sounds, distention, tenderness, and erythema are signs of peritonitis. Absence of bowel sounds may also indicate ileus.

E. **When was the last stool passed?** Constipation resulting in abdominal distention may cause feeding intolerance and increased gastric aspirates.

III. **Differential diagnosis.** The characteristics of the aspirate can provide important clinical clues to the cause of the problem and are outlined below.

A. **Bilious in color.** This type of aspirate is usually a serious problem especially if it occurs in the first 72 hours of life.

1. **Bowel obstruction.** One study found that 31% of infants with bilious vomiting in the first 72 hours of life had obstruction, of which 20% required surgery.

2. **NEC.**

3. **Meconium plug.**

4. **Meconium ileus.**

5. **Hirshsprung's disease.**

6. **Malrotation of the intestine.**

7. **Volvulus.**

8. **Ileus.**

9. **Factitious.** Passage of the feeding tube into the duodenum instead of the stomach can cause a bilious aspirate.

B. **Nonbilious in color.**

1. **Problems with feeding regimen.** Undigested or digested formula may be seen in the aspirate if the feeding regimen is too aggressive. This problem is especially likely in small premature infants who are given a small amount of formula initially and then are given larger volumes too rapidly.

a. **Aspirate containing undigested formula** may be seen if the interval between feedings is too short.

b. **Aspirate containing digested formula** may be a sign of delayed gastric emptying or overfeeding. Also, if the osmolarity of the formula is increased by the addition of vitamins, retained digested formula may be seen.

2. **Other.**

a. **NEC.**

b. **Pyloric stenosis.**

c. **Post NEC stricture.**

   d. **Infections.**
   e. **Inborn errors of metabolism.**
   f. **Constipation.** Especially if the abdomen is full but soft and no stool has passed in 48–72 hours.
   g. **Adrenogenital syndrome.**
   h. **Adrenal hypoplasia.**
   i. **Formula intolerance.** Formula intolerance is an uncommon cause of aspirate but should nonetheless be considered. Some infants do not tolerate the carbohydrate source in some formulas. If the infant is receiving a lactose-containing formula (eg., Similac, Enfamil), a stool pH should be performed to rule out **lactose intolerance.** If the stool pH is acidic (< 5.0), lactose intolerance may be present. In these cases, there is usually a strong family history of milk intolerance. It is more common to see diarrhea than gastric aspirates with lactose intolerance.
C. **Bloody in color.**
   1. **Trauma from nasogastric intubation.**
   2. **Swallowed maternal blood.**
   3. **Bleeding disorder.** Vitamin K deficiency, disseminated intravascular coagulation, and any congenital coagulopathy can all cause a bloody aspirate.
   4. **Stress ulcer.**
   5. **Severe fetal asphyxia.**
   6. **NEC.**
   7. **Gastric volvulus or duplication.** These are rare.
   8. **Medications. The following medications can cause a bloody aspirate: Tolazoline, theophylline, indomethacin, and corticosteriods.** It is important to note that theophylline is a rare cause of bloody gastric aspirate. Tolazoline administration, especially by continuous infusion, can cause a massive gastric hemorrhage.
IV. **Data base**
A. **Physical examination.** Perform a complete physical examination, paying particular attention to the abdomen. Check for bowel sounds (absent bowel sounds may indicate ileus or peritonitis), abdominal distention, tenderness to palpation and erythema of the abdomen (this may signify peritonitis), or visible bowel loops. Check for hernias, as they may cause obstruction.
B. **Laboratory studies**
   1. **A complete blood count with differential** is performed to evaluate for sepsis if suspected. The hematocrit and platelet count may be checked if bleeding has occurred.
   2. **Blood culture** is performed if sepsis is suspected and before antibiotics are started.
   3. **Serum potassium level.** If ileus is present, a serum potassium level should be obtained to rule out hypokalemia.
   4. **Stool pH.** If there is a family history of milk intolerance, a stool pH should be obtained to rule out lactose intolerance (stool pH will usually be < 5.0).
   5. **Coagulation profile (prothrombin time [PT], partial thromboplastin time [PTT], fibrinogen, and platelets).** A bloody aspirate may signify the presence of a coagulopathy, and in this case, coagulation studies should be obtained.
C. **Radiologic and other studies**
   1. **Plain x-ray film (flatplate) of the abdomen.** A plain x- ray film of the abdomen should be obtained if the aspirate is bilious, if there is any abnormality on physical examination, or if aspirates continue. The x-ray film will show whether the nasogastric tube is in the correct position and will define the bowel gas pattern. Look for an unusual gas pattern, pneumatosis intestinalis, ileus, or evidence of bowel obstruction.
   2. **Upright x-ray film of the abdomen.** If bowel obstruction is suspected on the film, obtain an upright x-ray film of the abdomen and look for air-fluid levels.

V. Plan. The approach to management of the neonate with increased gastric aspirates is usually initially based on the nature of the aspirate.
- **A. Bilious aspirate**
  1. **Surgical problem, eg, bowel obstruction, malrotation, volvulus, meconium plug.** A nasogastric tube should be placed for decompression of the stomach. Consultation with a pediatric surgeon should be obtained immediately.
  2. **NEC.** A nasogastric tube should be placed to rest the gut, the infant should be NPO. Further management see Chap 64.
  3. **Ileus.** If ileus is diagnosed, the patient is fed nothing orally and a nasogastric tube is placed for decompression of the stomach. Ileus in the neonate may be secondary to the following underlying causes, which should be treated if possible.
     - a. **Sepsis.**
     - b. **Necrotizing enterocolitis.**
     - c. **Prematurity.**
     - d. **Hypokalemia.**
     - e. **Effects of maternal drugs** (especially magnesium sulfate).
     - g. **Pneumonia.**
     - h. **Hypothyroidism.**
  4. **Factitious.** An x-ray will confirm the position of the nasogastric tube distally in the duodenum. Replace or reposition the tube in the stomach.
- **B. Nonbilious aspirate.**
  1. **Aspirate containing undigested formula.** If the volume of undigested formula in the aspirate does not exceed 30% of the previous feeding or 10–15 mL total, and the physical examination and vital signs are normal, the volume can be replaced. The time interval between feedings may not be long enough for digestion to take place. If the infant is being fed every 2 hours and aspirates continue, the feeding interval may be increased to 3 hours. If aspirates still continue, the patient must be reevaluated. An abdominal x-ray should be obtained. The patient may have to be fed intravenously to allow the gut to rest.
  2. **Aspirate containing digested formula.** The aspirate is usually discarded, especially if it contains a large amount of mucus. If the physical examination and vital signs are normal, continue feedings and aspiration of stomach contents. If reflux continues, the patient must be reassessed. An abdominal film must be taken, and oral feedings should be discontinued for a time to let the gut rest. The number of calories given should be calculated to make certain that overfeeding (usually > 130 kcal/kg/d) is not occurring.
  3. **Other.**
     - a. **NEC.** See Chap 64.
     - b. **Pyloric stenosis.**
     - c. **Post NEC stricture.**
     - d. **Infections.** If sepsis is likely, broad spectrum antibiotics are started after a laboratory workup is performed. A penicillin (usually ampicillin) and an aminoglycoside (usually gentamicin) are given initially, until culture results are obtained (see Chap 73 for drug dosages and other pharmacological information). The patient is usually not fed orally if this diagnosis is entertained; an infant with sepsis usually does not tolerate oral feedings.
     - e. **Inborn errors of metabolism.**
     - f. **Constipation.** Anal stimulation can be attemped. If this fails, a glycerin suppository can be given. (See also Chap 43.)
     - g. **Adrenogenital syndrome**
     - h. **Adrenal hypoplasia.**
     - i. **Formula intolerance.** A trial of lactose-free formula (eg, Prosobee, Isomil) can be instituted if lactose intolerance is verified.
- **C. Bloody aspirate**
  1. **Nasogastric trauma.** (See p 200.)

2. Gastrointestinal hemorrhage
a. Stress ulcer
(1) Stress ulcer is treated with gastric lavages of tepid water, 1/2 **normal saline, or normal saline**—5 mL/kg given by nasogastric tube until the bleeding has subsided. (*Note:* There is *controversy about which fluid to use.* Some clinicians feel that if water is used, hyponatremia may occur, and if normal saline is used, hypernatremia may occur. Follow your institution's guidelines. *Never use cold water lavages,* because they lower the infant's core temperature too rapidly.)

(2) If the above lavages do not stop the bleeding, a **lavage of 0.1 mL of 1:10,000 epinephrine solution in 10 mL of sterile water** can be used. This recommendation is also *controversial.*

(3) The infant is usually started on **ranitidine or cimetidine.** (See Chap 73 for dosages and other pharmacologic information.) Ranitidine is usually preferred because it has fewer side effects.

(4) **Antacids** may be used (eg, Maalox 2–5 mL, depending on the size of the infant, placed in the nasogastric tube every 4 hours until bleeding has subsided), but this recommendation is also *controversial;* some clinicians feel that it may cause concretions in the gastrointestinal tract.

b. Disseminated intravascular coagulation (DIC).
If clotting studies are abnormal and if gastrointestinal hemorrhage and hemorrhage at other sites are occurring, the cause of the coagulopathy must be identified and treated. Immediate transfusion of blood or fresh-frozen plasma, or both, may be needed, depending on the amount of blood loss and blood pressure levels. Platelets may be needed, depending on the platelet count.

c. Vitamin K deficiency.
Hemorrhage may occur if vitamin K injection was not given at birth. Vitamin K_1 (1 mg intramuscularly or intravenously) needs to be given.

d. Necrotizing enterocolitis.
See Chap 64.

D. Aspirate containing undigested formula.
If the volume of undigested formula in the aspirate does not exceed 30% of the previous feeding and the physical examination and vital signs are normal, the volume can be replaced. The time interval between feedings may not be long enough for digestion to take place. If the infant is being fed every 2 hours and aspirates continue, the feeding interval may be increased to 3 hours. If aspirates still continue, the patient must be reevaluated. An abdominal x-ray film should be obtained. The patient may have to be fed intravenously to allow the gut to rest.

E. Aspirate containing digested formula.
This aspirate is usually discarded, especially if it contains a large amount of mucus. If the physical examination and vital signs are normal, continue feedings and aspiration of stomach contents. If reflux continues, the patient must be reassessed. An abdominal film must be taken, and oral feedings should be discontinued for a time to let the gut rest. The number of calories given should be calculated to make certain that overfeeding (usually > 130 kcal/kg/d) is not occurring.

F. Sepsis.
If sepsis is likely, broad-spectrum antibiotics are started after a laboratory workup is performed. A penicillin (usually ampicillin) and an aminoglycoside (usually gentamicin) are given initially, until culture results are obtained (see Chap 73 for drug dosages and other pharmacologic information). The patient is usually not fed orally if this diagnosis is entertained because an infant with sepsis usually does not tolerate oral feedings.

G. Formula intolerance.
A trial of lactose-free formula (eg, ProSobee, Isomil) can be instituted if lactose intolerance is verified.

H. Constipation.
Anal stimulation can be attempted. If this fails, a glycerin suppository can be given. (See also Chap 43.)

33 Gastrointestinal Bleeding from the Upper Tract

I. **Problem.** Vomiting of bright red blood or active bleeding from the nasogastric tube is seen.
II. **Immediate questions**
  A. **What are the vital signs?** If the blood pressure is dropping and there is active bleeding from the nasogastric tube, urgent colloid replacement is necessary.
  B. **What is the hematocrit?** A spun hematocrit should be done as soon as possible. The result is used as a baseline value and to determine if blood replacement should be done immediately. Remember, with an acute episode of bleeding, the hematocrit may not reflect the blood loss for several hours.
  C. **Is blood available in the blood bank should transfusion be necessary?** Verify that the infant has been typed and cross-matched so that blood will be quickly available if necessary.
  D. **Is there bleeding from other sites?** Bleeding from other sites suggests disseminated intravascular coagulation or another coagulopathy. If bleeding is coming only from the nasogastric tube, disorders such as stress ulcer, nasogastric trauma, and swallowing of maternal blood are likely causes to consider in the differential diagnosis.
  E. **How old is the infant?** During the first day of life, vomiting of bright red blood or the presence of bright red blood in the nasogastric tube is frequently secondary to swallowing of maternal blood during delivery. Infants with this problem are clinically stable, with normal vital signs.
  F. **What medications are being given?** Certain medications are associated with an increased incidence of gastrointestinal bleeding. The most common of these medications are indomethacin (Indocin), tolazoline (Priscoline), and corticosteroids.
  G. **Was vitamin K given at birth?** Failure to give vitamin K at birth may result in a bleeding disorder, usually at 3–4 days of life.
III. **Differential diagnosis**
  A. **Idiopathic etiology.** More than 50% of cases have no clear diagnosis.
  B. **Swallowing of maternal blood.** This accounts for about 10% of cases. Typically blood is swallowed during cesarean section delivery.
  C. **Stress ulcer.**
  D. **Nasogastric trauma.**
  E. **Necrotizing enterocolitis.** This is a rare cause of upper GI tract bleeding and indicates extensive disease.
  F. **Coagulopathy.** Hemorrhagic disease of the newborn and disseminated intravascular coagulation account for approximately 20% of cases. Also congenital coagulopathies (most commonly factor 8 deficiency (hemophilia A) and factor 9 deficiency (hemophilia B) can cause GI bleeding from the upper tract.
  G. **Drug-induced bleeding.** Indomethacin, corticosteroids, tolazoline, and other drugs may cause upper GI tract bleeding. Theophylline is a rare cause.
  H. **Gastric volvulus and gastric duplication** are rare causes of GI bleeding.
  I. **Severe fetal asphyxia.**
IV. **Data base**
  A. **Physical examination.** A complete physical examination should be performed, paying particular attention to observation of other possible bleeding sites.

B. Laboratory studies

1. **Apt test.** The Apt test should be performed if swallowing of maternal blood is a possible cause (see p 000).
2. **Hematocrit** should be checked as a baseline and serially to gauge the extent of blood loss.
3. **Coagulation studies (prothrombin time [PT], partial thromboplastin time [PTT], fibrinogen, and platelets).** These studies should be done to rule out disseminated intravascular coagulation and other coagulopathies.

C. Radiologic and other studies.
An **abdominal x-ray film** should be obtained to assess the bowel gas pattern and to rule out necrotizing enterocolitis. The x-ray film will also show the position of the nasogastric tube and rule out any surgical problem.

V. Plan

A. General measures.
The most important goal is to stop the bleeding. This measure should be taken in every case except in infants who have swallowed maternal blood. (Infants with this problem are usually only a few hours old, are not sick, and have a positive Apt test result. Once stomach aspiration is performed, no more blood is obtained.) To help stop an acute episode of gastrointestinal bleeding, the following measures can be used.

1. **Gastric lavage.** The technique for gastric lavage is explained on p 198.
2. **Epinephrine lavage** (1:10,000 solution), 0.1 mL diluted in 10 mL of sterile water, can be used if tepid water lavages do not stop the bleeding (*controversial*).
3. **Colloid replacement.** If the blood pressure is low or dropping, colloid (usually Plasmanate or albumin) can be given immediately.
4. **Blood replacement** may be indicated, depending on the result of hematocrit values obtained from the laboratory.

B. Specific measures

1. **Idiopathic.** In cases in which no cause is determined, the bleeding usually subsides and no other treatment is necessary.
2. **Swallowing of maternal blood.** Perform the Apt test to confirm maternal hemoglobin (see p 000). No treatment is necessary.
3. **Stress ulcer.** Stress ulcer is commonly diagnosed following an episode of gastrointestinal bleeding. This disorder is difficult to confirm by radiologic studies, and they are not often obtained. Remission usually occurs; recurrence is rare. Antacids (eg, Maalox) may be given, but it is considered a controversial treatment because of the possibility of concretion formation. If used, the dosage for Maalox is 2–5 mL given by nasogastric tube every 4 hours. Ranitidine (now preferred because of less central nervous system, hepatic, and platelet side effects) or cimetidine is often used during the period of bleeding (see Chap 73 for dosages and other pharmacologic information).
4. **Nasogastric trauma.** This may occur if the nasogastric tube is too large or insertion is traumatic. Use the smallest nasogastric tube possible. Observation is indicated.
5. **Necrotizing enterocolitis.** Severe cases of necrotizing enterocolitis will cause upper gastrointestinal bleeding. Treatment is discussed in Chapter 64.
6. **Coagulopathy**
   a. **Hemorrhagic disease of the newborn.** This is more common in infants who have not received vitamin K at birth, ie home deliveries. If the history of vitamin K administration is unknown, give 1 mg vitamin K, intramuscularly. Administer it intravenously if active bleeding is occurring.
   b. **Disseminated intravascular coagulation (DIC).** If DIC is present, bleeding from other sites is usually seen. Coagulation studies will be abnormal (increased PT and PTT and decreased fibrinogen levels). Treat the underlying condition and support blood pressure with multiple transfusions of colloid, as needed. Platelets may need to be given. The cause

of DIC (eg, hypoxia, acidosis, bacterial or viral disease, toxoplasmosis, necrotizing enterocolitis, shock, erythroblastosis fetalis) must be investigated. Several obstetric disorders, including abruptio placentae, chorioangioma, eclampsia, and fetal death associated with twin gestation, may give rise to DIC.

   c. **Congenital coagulopathies.** The most common that present with bleeding are due to factor 8 deficiency (hemophilia A) and factor 9 deficiency (hemophilia B). Specific lab testing and appropriate consultation with a pediatric hematologist is appropriate.

7. **Drug-induced bleeding.** The drug responsible for the bleeding should be stopped if possible.

8. **Gastric volvulus and duplication.** Urgent surgical consultation is recommended.

9. **Severe fetal asphyxia.** See Chap 66.

34 Conjugated (Direct) Hyperbilirubinemia

I. **Problem.** An infant's direct (conjugated) serum bilirubin level is 3 mg/dL. (A value greater than 1.5 or 2.0 mg/dL [or a fraction greater than 15–20% of the total serum bilirubin] is considered abnormal at any age.) A persistent or increasing high direct bilirubin is always pathologic and must be evaluated promptly to minimize long-term sequelae.

II. **Immediate questions**

A. **Is the infant receiving total parenteral nutrition (TPN)?** TPN may cause direct hyperbilirubinemia by an unknown mechanism. It usually does not occur until the infant has been on TPN for greater than 2 weeks. It occurs in greater than 50% of infants weighing less than 1000 grams and in less than 10% of term infants.

B. **Is a bacterial or viral infection present?** Infection may cause hepatocellular damage, leading to increased direct bilirubin levels.

C. **Did direct hyperbilirubinemia occur only after feedings had been established?** If this is the case, a metabolic disorder such as galactosemia may be present.

III. **Differential diagnosis.** (See also Chap 58.)

A. **More common causes of direct hyperbilirubinemia**

1. **Biliary atresia** is the most common cause, occurring in approximately 1:10,000 live births.
2. **Idiopathic neonatal hepatitis** is the second most common cause and it occurs in approximately 1:5000 live births. This diagnosis is made after all other known causes have been excluded.
3. **Alpha$_1$-antitrypsin deficiency** is the third most common cause and occurs in approximately 1:20,000 live births.
4. **Hyperalimentation.**
5. **Bacterial infection** (sepsis or urinary tract infection).
6. **Intrauterine infection** (TORCH, Hepatitis B and C).
7. **Inspissated bile** from hemolytic disease.
8. **Choledochal cyst.**
9. **Galactosemia.**

B. **Less common causes of direct hyperbilirubinemia**

1. **Bile-duct stenosis.**
2. **Neoplasm.**
3. **Cholelithiasis.**
4. **Dubin-Johnson syndrome.**
5. **Cystic fibrosis.**
6. **Hypothyroidism.**
7. **Rotor's syndrome.**
8. **Storage disease (Niemann-Pick disease, Gaucher's disease).**
9. **Hereditary fructose intolerance.**
10. **Trisomy 21, 18.**
11. **Other infections** such as varicella, Coxsackie, ECHO, listeria.
12. **Drug induced.**
13. **Tyrosinemia.**
14. **Shock.**
15. **Alagille syndrome.**

   16. Zellweger syndrome.
IV. Data base. A detailed history, including prenatal (to evaluate for intrauterine infection or hemolytic disease) and postnatal (feeding history as well as the presence of any acholic stools) should be obtained. The clinical hallmarks of the disease include **icterus, acholic stools, and dark urine.**

   A. Physical examination. Particular attention should be given to examination of the abdomen. Palpate for an enlarged liver or spleen. Splenomegaly is more common in neonatal hepatitis but can be a late sign in biliary atresia. Check carefully for signs of sepsis. Know the characteristics of the syndromes and look for any unusual features.

   B. Laboratory studies
   1. For the common causes, the workup should be as follows:
      a. Complete blood count and differential may help to determine if infection is present.
      b. Coombs' test may indicate the possibility of hemolytic disease.
      c. Prothrombin time (PT), partial thromboplastin time (PTT), and serum albumin level will help evaluate hepatic function.
      d. Reticulocyte count may be elevated (ie, > 4–5%) if bleeding has occurred.
      e. Liver function tests should include AST (SGOT) ALT (SGPT), and alkaline phosphatase. Elevated levels of AST and ALT signify hepatocellular damage. Elevated alkaline phosphatase levels may signify biliary obstruction.
      f. Blood and urine culture. If sepsis is considered, blood and urine samples must be obtained for culture.
      g. Testing for viral disease. Determine the serum IgM level. If high, test for TORCH infections (see page 345). Urine is tested for cytomegalovirus and a serum hepatitis profile is obtained (hepatitis surface antigen and IgM hepatitis A antibody). Hepatitis B markers need to be tested in mother and infant.
      h. Serum alpha$_1$-antitrypsin levels. These levels are obtained to rule out alpha$_1$-antitrypsin deficiency.
      i. Urine-reducing substance should be determined if galactosemia is suspected.
   2. For the less common causes, perform the following additional studies.
      a. Serum thyroxine (T4) and thyroid stimulating hormone (TSH) levels should be obtained if hypothyroidism is suspected.
      b. Sweat chloride test. A quantitative sweat chloride test should be done to rule out cystic fibrosis.
      c. Urine metabolic screen.

   C. Radiologic and other studies
   1. Ultrasonography. Ultrasound examination of the liver and biliary tract will rule out choledochal cyst, stones, and tumor and will also provide information on the gallbladder. The absence of the gallbladder may suggest biliary atresia.
   2. Radionuclide scans allow evaluation of the biliary anatomy.
   3. Operative cholangiogram should be done if biliary atresia is suspected.
   4. Liver biopsy is usually performed after all other tests have been performed and a definitive diagnosis is still needed.

V. Plan. The cause of direct hyperbilirubinemia is determined. This section will just discuss the treatment plans of the more common causes of cholestatic jaundice. Supportive care is indicated. More detailed management information is presented in Chapter 58.

   A. Biliary atresia. Operative exploratory surgery with intraoperative cholangiography is usually the initial step. Hepatic portoenterostomy (**Kasai Procedure**) is currently the initial procedure of choice, with the possibility of liver transplantation in the future.

   B. Idiopathic neonatal hepatitis. Supportive care with a fair prognosis exists.

C. **Alpha₁-antitrypsin.** The only curative therapy is liver transplantation.

D. **Hyperalimentation.** Consider stopping the TPN. Most infants recover with clearing of cholestasis in 1–3 months after normal feedings have begun. The use of phenobarbital therapy is *controversial.*

E. **Bacterial infection.** If there are signs of sepsis, appropriate cultures should be sent and empiric antibiotic therapy should be initiated.

F. **Intrauterine infection.** Appropriate antiviral agents or other medications should be started if indicated.

G. **Inspissated bile** secondary to hemolytic disease is treated with supportive management. The use of phenobarbital is *controversial.*

H. **Choledochal cyst.** The treatment is surgical removal.

I. **Galactosemia.** Immediate elimination of lactose and galactose containing products.

35 Unconjugated (Indirect) Hyperbilirubinemia

I. **Problem.** An infant's indirect (unconjugated) serum bilirubin level is 10 mg/dL.

II. **Immediate questions**

  A. **How old is the infant?** High indirect serum bilirubin levels during the first 24 hours of life are *never* physiologic. Hemolytic disease (Rh isoimmunization or ABO incompatibility) or congenital infection is a likely cause. The age of the infant helps to determine the bilirubin level at which phototherapy should be initiated.

  B. **Is the infant dehydrated?** If the infant is dehydrated, fluid administration may lower the serum bilirubin level. Fluids can be given orally if tolerated, otherwise, intravenous fluids should be given. An example is an infant who is being totally breast-fed, and at 3 days of age the mother's milk has not come in, so the infant becomes dehydrated. Remember, babies have to be very dehydrated for fluid replacement to lower the bilirubin.

  C. **Is the infant being breast-fed?** Breast milk jaundice may be present; the cause is unknown.

III. **Differential diagnosis.** (See also Chap 58.)

  A. **More common causes of indirect hyperbilirubinemia**
    1. Physiologic hyperbilirubinemia.
    2. ABO incompatibility.
    3. Breast milk jaundice.
    4. Rh isoimmunization.
    5. Infection. (congenital syphilis, viral, or protozoal infections). Jaundice as the only sign of underlying sepsis is rare. In one study of 171 newborns readmitted for a mean bilirubin of 18.8, not one case of sepsis was identified.
    6. Subdural hematoma or cephalohematoma.
    7. Excessive bruising.
    8. Infant of diabetic mother.
    9. Polycythemia/Hyperviscosity.

  B. **Less common causes of indirect hyperbilirubinemia**
    1. Glucose-6-phosphate dehydrogenase (G6PD) deficiency.
    2. Pyruvate kinase deficiency.
    3. Congenital spherocytosis.
    4. Lucey-Driscoll syndrome (familial neonatal jaundice).
    5. Crigler-Najjar disease.
    6. Hypothyroidism.
    7. Hemoglobinopathy. Alpha and Beta thallesemia are examples of this.

IV. **Data base.**

  A. **Physical examination.** Particular attention should be paid to signs of bruising, cephalohematoma, or intracranial bleeding.

  B. **Laboratory studies.** Recent studies have questioned the validity of ordering extensive tests on any infant with a question of hyperbilirubinemia. Recent recommendations suggest that in normal and healthy term infants less tests are necessary.

    1. **Normal, otherwise healthy term newborn:**
      a. **Blood type and group** of mother and infant (cord blood).
      b. **Direct Coombs' test on the infant** (cord blood) if there is incompatibility with the mother.

      c. Serum bilirubin level if there is jaundice in the first 24 hours or moderate jaundice associated with a positive Coombs' test, parental anxiety, or other signs of illness.
   2. Any other infant:
      a. Total and direct serum bilirubin levels. In term infants, direct bilirubin is indicated only if the jaundice is persistent or the infant ill.
      b. Complete blood count and differential. This test is indicated if hemolytic disease or anemia is suspected.
      c. Mother's blood type with Rh determination.
      d. Infant's blood type with Rh determination.
      e. Direct and indirect Coombs' tests.
      f. Reticulocyte count. Consider this test if the infant is anemic or there is suspicion of hemolytic disease.
      g. Red blood cell smear. Fragmented red blood cells should be present in hemolysis.
      h. G6PD screen. Consider sending this if the infant is Mediterranean, the jaundice is late onset, and there is evidence of hemolysis (low hematocrit, high reticulocyte count, and a peripheral smear shows nucleated RBCs and other fragmented cells).
  C. Radiologic and other studies. None are usually necessary.
V. Plan (See also Chap 58).
  A. Phototherapy. Phototherapy should be initiated according to the guidelines in Appendix H. If phototherapy is used, perform the following additional procedures.
    1. Increase the maintenance infusion of intravenous fluids by 0.5 mL/kg/h if the infant weighs less than 1500 g and by 1 mL/kg/h if the infant weighs more than 1500 g. (**Note:** Water supplements to breast-fed infants do not reduce serum bilirubin.)
    2. Perform total bilirubin testing every 6–8 hours.
    3. Attempt regular feedings, if possible and feed frequently. Feeding increases bilirubin excretion by stooling which decreases the enterohepatic cycle. One study revealed that mothers who nursed on average more than eight times per 24 hours in the first three days of life had significantly lower serum bilirubin levels (6.5 vs 9.3).
    4. Phototherapy can be safely discontinued once serum bilirubin levels have fallen 2 mg/dL or more below the level at which phototherapy was initiated. Once phototherapy is stopped, a rebound increase in the serum bilirubin level of approximately 2 mg/dL will occur.
  B. Drug therapy. Phenobarbital has been shown to be effective in reducing the serum bilirubin level by increasing hepatic glucuronyl transferase activity and conjugation of bilirubin. It is usually used in severe cases of prolonged hyperbilirubinemia only. (See Chap 73 for dosage and other pharmacologic information.)
  C. Exchange Transfusion. (See Table 35–1.) The procedure for exchange transfusion is discussed in Chapter 19. There is considerable controversy concerning the exact level to initiate exchange transfusion. The overall status, (sick or well) birth weight, gestational age, and age of the infant are all important con-

TABLE 35–1. GENERAL GUIDELINES FOR EXCHANGE TRANSFUSION (SEE TEXT FOR EXPLANATION).

Clinical Setting	Indirect Bilirubin mg/dL
Full-term well infant without hemolysis	25–29
Full-term sick infant or with hemolysis	17.5–23.4
Premature infant (no hemolysis or illness)	= or > 15
500–800 g sick infant or with hemolysis	10–12
> 1800 g and healthy	18

siderations. In many cases, institutional guidelines are established and should be followed. Some general guidelines are listed in Table 35–1. Remember, these are guidelines only and each individual patient must be considered. If the infant is sick (signs of hemolysis, sepsis, etc), has a lower gestational age, is on day 1 or 2 of life, or if the birth weight is low, would tend to lower the number that is used for exchange transfusion.

36 Hyperglycemia

I. Problem. The nurse reports that an infant has a blood glucose of 240 mg/dL. (Hyperglycemia is defined as a serum blood glucose level > 125 mg/dL in term infants, and > 150 mg/dL in premature infants.)

II. Immediate questions

A. What is the serum glucose value on laboratory testing? Dextrostix values are often inaccurate because the procedure is performed incorrectly or the Dextrostix strips are old and no longer reliable. Chemstrip-bG values are thought to be more reliable by some, but it is best to obtain a serum glucose level from the laboratory before initiating treatment.

B. Is glucose being spilled in the urine? A trace amount of glucose in the urine is accepted as normal. If the urinary glucose level is +1, +2, or greater, the renal threshold has been reached and there is an increased chance of osmotic diuresis. Some institutions accept a urinary glucose level of +1 without treating the patient (*controversial*).

C. How much glucose is the patient receiving? Normal maintenance glucose therapy in infants not being fed orally is 6 mg/kg/min. To determine this, see p 74.

D. Are there signs of sepsis? Sepsis may cause hyperglycemia by inducing a stress response.

III. Differential diagnosis. Hyperglycemia occurs more often in premature infants. The main concern with hyperglycemia is it can cause hyperosmolarity, osmotic diuresis, and subsequent dehydration. There may be a risk of intracranial hemorrhage with hyperosmolarity.

A. Excess glucose administration. Incorrect calculation of glucose levels or errors in formulation of intravenous fluids may cause hyperglycemia.

B. Inability to metabolize glucose may occur with prematurity or secondary to sepsis or stress.

C. Hypoxia can cause hyperglycemia.

D. Ingestion of hyperosmolar formula. Hyperosmolar formula can cause a transient hyperglycemia.

E. Transient neonatal diabetes mellitus is a rare disorder. Most patients with the disorder are term infants with evidence of intrauterine malnutrition. The disorder may present at any time from 2 days up to 6 weeks of age. The most common findings are hyperglycemia, dehydration, glycosuria, and acidosis.

F. Medications such as maternal use of diazoxide can cause hyperglycemia in the infant. Drugs used in infants that have been associated with hyperglycemia include caffeine, theophylline, corticosteroids, and phenytoin.

IV. Data base

A. Physical examination. Perform a complete physical examination. Look for subtle signs of sepsis (eg, temperature instability, changes in peripheral perfusion, or any changes in gastric aspirates if the infant is feeding). Determine maternal and infant medications.

B. Laboratory studies

1. **Serum glucose level.** Confirm the rapid paper-strip test result with a serum glucose level.

2. **Urine dipstick testing for glucose level.**

3. **Complete blood count and differential** are performed as screening tests for sepsis.

4. **Blood and urine cultures** are indicated if sepsis is suspected and if antibiotics are to be started.

5. **Serum electrolytes.** Hyperglycemia may cause osmotic diuresis, which may lead to electrolyte losses and dehydration. Therefore it is important to follow serum electrolyte levels in hyperglycemic patients.

6. **Serum insulin level** is obtained if concerned about transient neonatal diabetes mellitus. The levels are usually low, in view of the hyperglycemia.

C. **Radiologic and other studies.** None are usually required; however, a chest x-ray study may be useful in the evaluation of sepsis.

V. **Plan**

A. **Excess glucose administration**

1. **Positive urinary glucose level.** Decrease the amount of glucose being given by decreasing the concentration of dextrose in intravenous fluids or by decreasing the infusion rate. Most infants who are not feeding require approximately 6 mg/kg/min of glucose to maintain normal glucose levels. Use Dextrostix or Chemstrip-bG testing every 4–6 hours and check for glucose in the urine with each voiding.

2. **Negative urinary glucose level.** If glucose is being given to increase the caloric intake, it is acceptable to have a higher serum glucose level as long as glucose is not being spilled in the urine. Perform Dextrostix and urinary glucose testing every 4–6 hours.

B. **Inability to metabolize glucose.** Sepsis should always be considered in an infant with hyperglycemia. If the blood count looks suspicious or if there are clinical signs of sepsis, it is acceptable to treat the infant for 3 days with antibiotics and then stop if cultures are negative. Ampicillin and an aminoglycoside are usually given initially (see Chap 73 for dosages and other pharmacologic information). Treatment of infants unable to metabolize glucose for any reason is described below.

1. **Decrease the concentration of glucose or the rate of infusion until a normal serum glucose level is present.** Do not use a solution that has a dextrose concentration of less than 4.7%. Such a solution is hypo-osmolar and could cause hemolysis, with resulting hyperkalemia. If a glucose concentration of less than 4.7% is used, electrolytes should be added.

2. **Insulin.** Insulin administration is usually not recommended in neonates because of their erratic response and because studies to date have been conflicting. Potassium levels need to be followed when giving insulin therapy. If insulin is used, it can be given in one of 2 ways.

   a. **An insulin infusion** may be given at a rate of 0.02–0.1/unit/kg/h. Albumin, which used to be added to the bag to prevent adherence of the insulin to the plastic tubing, is now considered unnecessary. It is currently thought that by simply flushing the solution with an adequate amount of the insulin-containing solution, all binding sites and the tubing will be saturated satisfactorily prior to beginning the insulin infusion. Dextrostix testing must be performed every 30 minutes until the level of glucose is stable.

   b. **Insulin may be given subcutaneously,** 0.1 unit/kg every 6 hours. Chemistrip-bG testing (or Dextrostix testing) must be performed every 30 minutes to 1 hour until the glucose level is stable.

C. **Hypoxia.** Treat the hypoxia, and if needed, insulin therapy can be used as above in **V.B.2.**

D. **Hyperosmolar formula use.** This usually occurs with inappropriate formula dilution. The formula needs to be discontinued and the infant rehydrated. Specific instructions should be given to prevent mistakes in mixing concentrated formulas.

E. **Transient neonatal diabetes mellitus**

1. **Give intravenous (or oral) fluids** and follow the urine output, blood pH, and serum electrolyte levels.

2. **Give insulin,** either by constant infusion or subcutaneously, 1–2 units/kg/d. Follow glucose levels with Chemstrip-bG testing (or Dextrostix testing) every 4–6 hours. This disease usually resolves in a period of days to months.

3. **Repeat serum insulin values** to rule out permanent diabetes mellitus.

F. **Medications**

1. **If the infant is receiving theophylline,** the serum theophylline level should be checked to detect possible toxicity, with resulting hyperglycemia. Other signs of **theophylline toxicity** include tachycardia, jitteriness, feeding intolerance, and seizures. If the level is high, the dosage must be altered or the drug discontinued.

2. With maternal use of **diazoxide,** the infant may have tachycardia and hypotension as well as hyperglycemia. Toxicity in the infant is usually self-limited, and only observation is usually necessary.

3. **Caffeine, steroids, and phenytoin.** If possible, the medication should be discontinued.

37 Hyperkalemia

I. **Problem.** The serum potassium level is greater than 5.5 meq/dL. Normal potassium levels are 3.5–5.5 meq/dL.

II. **Immediate questions**

A. **How was the specimen collected and what is the central serum potassium level?** Blood obtained by heelstick may yield falsely elevated potassium levels secondary to hemolysis. Blood drawn through a tiny needle may cause hemolysis and falsely elevated potassium levels.

B. **How much potassium is the infant receiving?** Normal amounts of potassium given for maintenance are 1–3 meq/kg/d.

C. **Does the ECG show cardiac changes characteristic of hyperkalemia?** Early cardiac changes include tall, "tented" T waves. Other signs include a wide QRS complex; prolonged PR interval; wide, flat P waves; ventricular tachycardia; ventricular fibrillation; and cardiac arrest.

D. **What are the blood urea nitrogen and creatinine levels? What is the urine output and weight?** Elevated blood urea nitrogen and creatinine measurements indicate renal insufficiency. Another indication of renal failure is decreasing or inadequate urine output with weight gain.

III. **Differential diagnosis**

A. **Falsely elevated potassium level.** This is usually caused by hemolysis during phlebotomy or heelstick or by drawing of blood proximal to an intravenous site that contains potassium.

B. **Excess potassium administration.** This can occur from giving too much potassium in the intravenous fluids. Potassium suplements are not usually necessary on the first day of life and often not necessary until day 3, with the typical requirement of 1–2 meq/kg/d.

C. **Pathologic hemolysis of red blood cells.** This may be secondary to intraventricular hemorrhage, use of a hypotonic glucose solution (< 4.7% dextrose), Pseudomonas sepsis, or Rh incompatibility.

D. **Renal failure.** Acute renal failure or renal immaturity can lead to hyperkalemia.

E. **Metabolic or respiratory acidosis.** Systemic acidosis causes potassium to move out of cells, resulting in hyperkalemia. For every 0.1 unit decrease in pH, the serum potassium will increase approximately 0.3–1.3 meq/L.

F. **Tissue necrosis.** In certain disease states, such as necrotizing enterocolitis (NEC), tissue necrosis can occur and hyperkalemia may result.

G. **Medications.** Certain medications contain potassium and will elevate the serum potassium level. Digoxin therapy can lead to hyperkalemia secondary to redistribution of potassium. K^+ sparing diurectics cause decreased potassium losses. Both propanolol and phenylephrine are associated with hyperkalemia. High glucose load can lead to hyperkalemia secondary to increases in plasma osmolality. Hyperkalemia occurs with THAM administration.

H. **Adrenal insufficiency.** In salt-losing congenital adrenal hyperplasia, the infants will have low serum sodium and chloride and elevated levels of potassium.

I. **Decreased insulin levels** is associated with hyperkalemia.

IV. **Data base**

A. **Physical examination.** Perform a complete physical examination, paying special attention to the abdomen for signs of NEC (abdominal distention, decreased bowel sounds, visible bowel loops).

B. **Laboratory studies**

1. **Serum potassium level.**
2. **Serum ionized and total calcium levels.** Because hypocalcemia may potentiate the effects of hyperkalemia, maintain normal serum calcium concentrations.
3. **Serum pH.** The serum pH is obtained to rule out acidosis, which may potentiate hyperkalemia.
4. **Blood urea nitrogen and serum creatinine levels** may reveal renal insufficiency.
5. **Urine specific gravity** is obtained to assess renal status.

C. **Radiologic studies**
1. **Abdominal x-ray study.** If necrotizing enterocolitis is suspected, an abdominal x-ray film should be obtained.
2. **Electrocardiography.** ECG may reveal the cardiac changes characteristic of hyperkalemia and will provide a baseline study (see **II.C**, p 211).

V. **Plan.** Treat specific etiology. Check calculation of potassium in the intravenous fluids and make sure excess is not being given. Stop any potassium containing medications. Renal failure can be treated with fluid restriction. If adrenal insufficiency exists, hormonal therapy is indicated. With the following plan, it is important to monitor EKG changes during therapy.

A. **Hyperkalemia without ECG changes**
1. **Stop administration of potassium** in intravenous fluids; also consider stopping any potassium-containing medications.
2. **Check the serum potassium level frequently** (every 4–6 hours).
3. **Furosemide (Lasix)** can be given if renal function is adequate; the usual dose is 1 mg/kg given intravenously (*controversial*). (See Chap 73).
4. **Sodium polystyrene sulfonate (Kayexalate),** a potassium-exchange resin, can be given. One gram of resin removes approximately 1 meq of potassium. The usual dose is 1 g/kg/dose orally every 6 hours or rectally every 2–6 hours. (See Chap 73.)
5. **Insulin and glucose** can be used (see **B.4,** below).

B. **Hyperkalemia with ECG changes** (see p 211, **II.C.**)
1. **Stop administration of potassium** in intravenous fluids. Verify that ventilation is adequate to correct respiratory acidosis.
2. **Give sodium bicarbonate;** the usual dose is 1 meq/kg intravenously. Inducing alkalosis will drive potassium ions into the cells.
3. **Give calcium gluconate;** the usual dose is 50 mg/kg/dose intravenously. Calcium provides some protection for the heart from the effects of hyperkalemia.
4. **Glucose and insulin** may be given to drive potassium into the cells. The usual dose is 250–500 mg/kg/dose of dextrose intravenously, followed by regular insulin, 0.2 unit/kg/dose intravenously over 1 hour. Monitor the infant for hypoglycemia.
5. Start administration of sodium polystyrene sulfonate (see **A.4,** above). It will lower the potassium level slowly and is therefore of limited value acutely.

C. **Refractory hyperkalemia.** If all of the above measures fail to lower the potassium level, other measures, such as exchange transfusion with freshly washed red blood cells, hemofiltration, and renal dialysis, must be considered.

38 Hypertension

I. Problem. An infant has a systolic blood pressure greater than 90 mm Hg. Hypertension is defined as a blood pressure greater than two standard deviations above normal values for age and weight. The values for normal blood pressure are given in Appendix C, p 547. It can also be defined as a systolic BP > 90 torr and a diastolic > 60 in full-term infants, and a systolic > 80 torr and a diastolic > 50 torr in premature infants.

II. Immediate questions

A. How was the blood pressure taken? Doppler flow ultrasonography is the most reliable noninvasive method of measurement. The size of the cuff is important. The cuff should encircle two-thirds of the length of the upper extremity. If the cuff is too narrow, the blood pressure will be falsely elevated. If measurements are taken by means of an umbilical artery catheter, be certain the catheter is free of bubbles or clots and the transducer is calibrated or erroneous results will occur.

B. Is an umbilical artery catheter in place, or has one been in place in the past? Umbilical artery catheters are associated with an increased incidence of renovascular hypertension. There is no relation between the time the catheter is in and the development of hypertension. A catheter-related aortic thrombosis can also produce hypertension. The following conditions are risk factors to thrombus formation in the aorta: BPD, PDA, hypervolemia, and certain CNS disorders.

C. Are symptoms of hypertension present? Infants with hypertension may be asymptomatic or may have the following symptoms: tachypnea, cyanosis, seizures, lethargy, increased tone, apnea, abdominal distention, fever, and mottling. They may also present with congestive heart failure and respiratory distress.

D. What is the blood pressure in the extremities? The blood pressure in a normal infant should be higher in the legs than in the arms. If the pressure is lower in the legs, coarctation of the aorta may be the cause of the hypertension.

E. What is the birth weight and postnatal age of the infant? The normal blood pressure values increase with increasing birth weight and age. Values rise approximately 1–2 mm Hg per day during the first week of life and then approximately 1–2 mm Hg per week over the next 6 weeks.

F. Is the infant in pain or agitated? Pain (such as that from a surgical procedure), crying, agitation, or suctioning can all cause a transient rise in blood pressure.

III. Differential diagnosis

A. More common causes of hypertension

1. **Renal artery thrombosis.**
2. **Aortic thrombosis.**
3. **Obstructive uropathy.**
4. **Infantile polycystic kidneys.**
5. **Renal failure.**
6. **Medications** such as theophylline and corticosteroids.
7. **Fluid overload.**
8. **Pain, agitation.**
9. **Bronchopulmonary dysplasia (BPD).** Approximately 40% of patients with BPD have hypertension. The etiology is probably multifactorial (increased renin activity and catecholamine secretion may be associated with chronic lung disease).

      10. Coarctation of the aorta.
   B. Less Common Causes
      1. Renal artery stenosis. The infant will be hypertensive from birth.
      2. Renal vein thrombosis.
      3. Hypoplasia or dysplasia of the kidneys.
      4. Pyelonephritis.
      5. Medications such as ocular phenylephrine, pancuronium, dopamine, DOCA, and epinephrine.
      6. Primary hyperaldosteronism.
      7. Neuroblastoma or pheochromocytoma.
      8. Hyperthyroidism.
      9. Adrenogenital syndrome.
      10. Increased intracranial pressure secondary to intracranial hemorrhage, hydrocephalus, meningitis, or subdural hemorrhage.
      11. Closure of abdominal wall defects.
      12. Seizures.
IV. Data base
   A. Physical examination
      1. Check the femoral pulse, which is absent or decreased in coarctation of the aorta.
      2. Examine the abdomen carefully for masses and to determine the size of the kidneys. An enlarged kidney may indicate tumor, polycystic kidneys, obstruction, or renal vein thrombosis.
   B. Laboratory studies. Figure 38–1 is an overview of a complete evaluation.
      1. Assessment of renal function. To assess renal function, perform the following tests.
         a. Serum creatinine and blood urea nitrogen levels. Elevated serum creatinine and blood urea nitrogen levels may indicate renal insufficiency, which may be associated with hypertension.
         b. Urinalysis. Red cells in the urine suggest obstruction, infection, or renal vein thrombosis.
         c. Urine culture. To rule out pyelonephritis.
         d. Serum electrolytes and carbon dioxide. A low serum potassium level and high carbon dioxide level will be seen in primary hyperaldosteronism.
      2. Plasma renin levels may be elevated in patients with renovascular disease. Levels will be low in patients with primary hyperaldosteronism.
   C. Radiologic and other studies
      1. Abdominal ultrasonography. The preferred screening test in neonates to detect abdominal masses as well as kidney obstruction. Doppler flow ultrasonography can screen for arterial or venous problems.
      2. Cranial ultrasonography. To rule out intraventricular hemorrhage.
      3. Echocardiography. If a disease such as coarctation is suspected.
      4. Intravenous pyelography. Usually of limited value in the newborn due to poor renal concentrating ability.
      5. Further studies. The following invasive procedures and laboratory studies are sometimes necessary to further evaluate the infant with hypertension.
         a. Arteriography to evaluate renovascular disease **or venacavography** to evaluate renal vein thrombosis.
         b. Renal vein renin level to further evaluate renovascular disease.
         c. Renal biopsy to rule out any intrinsic renal disease.
         d. 24-hour urinary catecholamines to evaluate for pheochromocytoma.
         e. Urinary 17-hydroxysteroid and 17-ketosteroid levels to evaluate for Cushing's syndrome and congenital adrenal hyperplasia.
V. Plan
   A. General. Treat any obvious underlying condition. Stop medications if they are causing hypertension. Correct fluid overload by decreasing fluids and administering diuretics.
   B. Drug therapy. To guide drug therapy, decide if the hypertension is mild, mod-

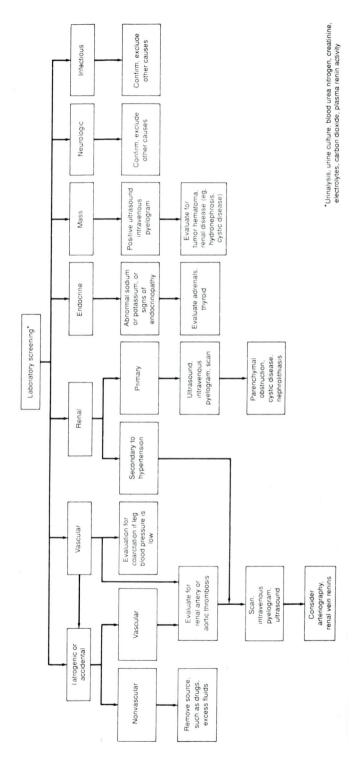

FIGURE 38-1. Evaluation of hypertension in the newborn. (Modified and reproduced, with permission, from Adelman RD: Hypertension in infants. Pediatr Ann [Sept] 1989; **18**:568.)

*Urinalysis, urine culture, blood urea nitrogen, creatinine, electrolytes, carbon dioxide, plasma renin activity

erate, or life-threatening. (Dosages and other pharmacologic information for the following drugs are given in Chapter 73.)

1. **Life-threatening hypertension** (blood pressure extremely high and symptoms present). Give nitroprusside (Nipride) or diazoxide (Hyperstat).
2. **Moderate hypertension**
   a. **Give hydralazine alone.**
   b. **Give hydralazine in combination with a diuretic or a beta blocker** (propranolol).
   c. **Give captopril alone.** This drug is contraindicated in infants with bilateral renovascular disease.
   d. **Either furosemide or chlorothiazide can be used in combination with hydralazine and/or captopril.** Propranolol and methyldopa are other drugs that can be used in combination with hydralazine and/or captopril.
3. **Mild hypertension**
   a. **Simple observation** is required for asymptomatic patients.
   b. **Diuretics** are necessary if nonpharmacologic measures fail.
   c. **Hydralazine,** a vasodilator, may be used if the above measures fail.

39 Hypoglycemia

I. **Problem.** An infant has a low blood glucose level on Dextrostix or Chemstrip-bG testing. Hypoglycemia is defined as a blood sugar less than 40 mg/dL in a term or premature infant.

II. **Immediate questions**

    A. **Has the value been repeated, and has a serum blood sugar been sent to the laboratory?** Dextrostix or Chemstrip-bG strips can sometimes give incorrect values if the test is not done properly or if the strips used are too old. Send a serum sample to the laboratory before starting treatment.

    B. **Is the infant symptomatic?** Symptoms of hypoglycemia include apnea, hypotonia, inadequate sucking reflex, cyanosis, tremors, pallor, high-pitched cry, jitteriness, eye rolling, seizures, lethargy, and temperature instability. Some infants can have hypoglycemia and no symptoms.

    C. **Is the mother a diabetic?** Infants of diabetic mothers have approximately a 40% chance of having hypoglycemia. Diabetic mothers have fluctuating hyperglycemia that causes fetal hyperglycemia. This fetal hyperglycemia causes pancreatic B cell hyperplasia, which in turn causes hyperinsulinism. After delivery, hyperinsulinism persists and hypoglycemia results.

    D. **How much glucose is the infant receiving?** The normal glucose requirement is 6 mg/kg/min. If the glucose order was written arbitrarily and not calculated on the basis of the body weight, the infant may not be getting enough glucose. (See p 74, for glucose calculations.)

III. **Differential diagnosis**

    A. **Decreased glycogen stores**

        1. **Intrauterine growth retardation (IUGR) or small for gestational age (SGA).**

        2. **Premature infants.**

        3. **Postmature infants.**

    B. **Increased circulating insulin**

        1. **Infant of diabetic mother (IODM).**

        2. **Beckwith-Wiedemann syndrome** (visceromegaly, macroglossia, and hypoglycemia).

        3. **Maternal drugs** such as beta-sympathomimetic agents (eg, terbutaline, ritodrine) or chlorpropamide.

        4. **Islet cell dysplasias** such as beta cell hyperplasia.

        5. **Insulin-producing tumors** such as nesidioblastoma.

    C. **Insufficient amount of glucose administered.** See II.D, above.

    D. **Endocrine disorders**

        1. **Panhypopituitarism.**

        2. **Growth hormone deficiency.**

        3. **Hypothyroidism.**

        4. **Cortisol deficiency.**

        5. **Defects in metabolism.**

            a. Amino-acid metabolism (maple syrup urine disease, methylmalonic acidemia, hereditary tyrosinemia, and propionicacidemia).

            b. Carbohydrate metabolism (galactosemia, fructose intolerance, and type 1 glycogen storage disease).

        6. **Adrenogenital syndrome.**

        7. **Adrenal hemorrhage.**

    E. **Other causes**

1. **Sepsis.**
2. **Asphyxia.**
3. **Hypothermia.**
4. **Polycythemia.**
5. **Shock.**
6. **Maternal use of propranolol.**

IV. **Data base**
  A. **History and physical examination.** Evaluate the infant for symptoms of hypoglycemia (see p 217). Are there signs of sepsis, shock, or Beckwith-Wiedemann syndrome?
  B. **Laboratory studies**
     1. **Initial studies for transient hypoglycemia**
        a. **A serum glucose level** should be obtained to confirm paper strip determination.
        b. **Complete blood count and differential** should be obtained to evaluate for sepsis and to rule out polycythemia.
     2. **Studies for persistent hypoglycemia.**
        a. **Initial studies.** A recent study recommends obtaining only serum glucose, insulin, and ketones. The ratio of insulin to glucose (I/G) is obtained. A level greater than 0.37 indicates a nonhyperinsulinemic cause of hypoglycemia. Serum ketones are absent in the presence of hyperinsulinemia.
        b. **Follow-up studies.** If further evaluation is needed, the following tests can be done to help differentiate a metabolic defect, hypopituitarism, and hyperinsulinism.
           (1) Insulin.
           (2) Growth hormone.
           (3) Cortisol.
           (4) Free fatty acids.
           (5) Thyroxine (T4) and thyroid-stimulating hormone (TSH).
           (6) Glucagon.
           (7) Uric acid.
           (8) Lactate.
           (9) Alanine.
           (10) Ketones.
  C. **Radiologic and other studies.** None are usually necessary.

V. **Plan**
  A. **Overall plan.** Attempt to maintain normoglycemia. Infants at risk for hypoglycemia and those with established hypoglycemia should have glucose screening every 1–2 hours until glucose levels are stable, then every 4 hours. Once the glucose level is stable, the next step is to determine why the patient is hypoglycemic. Sometimes the cause is obvious, as in the case of an infant of a diabetic mother or one with intrauterine growth retardation. If the cause is not obvious, further workup is necessary.
     1. **Asymptomatic hypoglycemia**
        a. **Draw a blood sample** and send it to the laboratory for a stat baseline serum glucose level.
        b. **For infants with Dextrostix values of less than 25 mg/dL or Chemstrip-bG values of less than 20 mg/dL** (confirmed by stat central serum level), **insert an intravenous line and start a glucose infusion** of 6 mg/kg/min (see calculation on p 74), even if the infant is asymptomatic. Initially, glucose levels should be checked every 30 minutes until stable. The infusion should be increased until normoglycemia is achieved. A bolus of glucose in the asymptomatic infant is contraindicated, because it is thought to result in hyperglycemia with rebound hypoglycemia (*controversial*).
        c. **For infants with Dextrostix values of 25–45 mg/dL or Chemstrip bG values of 20–40 mg/dL,** if there are no risk factors for hypoglycemia and

the infant is clinically stable, an **early feeding of D5W** or formula can be given. The glucose levels are followed every 30 minutes until stable, then every 4 hours. If the glucose remains low, an intravenous line will have to be started with a glucose infusion of 6 mg/kg/min.

2. **Symptomatic hypoglycemia (transient)**
   a. **Draw a sample for a baseline serum glucose level.**
   b. **Insert an intravenous line and start a glucose infusion.** Infuse a mini-bolus (usually not associated with rebound hypoglycemia) of 2 mL/kg of a 10% glucose solution over 2–3 minutes. Then give a continuous infusion of glucose at a rate of 6–8 mg/kg/min and increase the rate as needed to maintain a normal blood glucose (at least 40 mg/dL). The level should be followed every 30 minutes until stable. Remember, **the highest concentration of glucose that can be infused through a peripheral line is 12.5%. If a more concentrated solution is required, a central line will have to be placed.** Higher concentrations are hypertonic and may damage the veins.
   c. **If an intravenous line cannot be started, glucagon** (p 486) **can be given to infants with adequate glycogen stores.** This measure may be particularly effective in infants of diabetic mothers. It is not effective in infants who have growth retardation or are small for gestational age, because of poor glycogen stores.

3. **Persistent hypoglycemia.** Endocrinologic consultation should be obtained.
   a. **Continue administration of intravenous glucose.** Continue to increase the rate of intravenous glucose administration to 16–20 mg/kg/min. Rates higher than 20 mg/kg/min are not usually helpful. If it is evident at this point that the infant still has problems with hypoglycemia, further workup should be initiated as outlined below.
   b. **Perform a definitive workup.** First obtain blood samples to get the I/G level and serum ketones. If the diagnosis is still unclear, the definitive workup of an infant with persistent hypoglycemia consists in obtaining a set of laboratory determinations prior to and 15 minutes after the parenteral administration of glucagon (0.3 mg/kg/dose). Laboratory studies include serum glucose, ketones, free fatty acids, lactate, alanine, uric acid, insulin, growth hormone, cortisol, glucagon, T4, and TSH. The results are interpreted as shown in Table 39–1. The following methods of treatment can be initiated while waiting for results of the glucagon test.
      (1) **Consider a trial of corticosteroids.** The recommended drug is ei-

TABLE 39–1. DIAGNOSIS OF PERSISTENT HYPOGLYCEMIA BEFORE AND AFTER PARENTERAL GLUCAGON ADMINISTRATION[a]

	Hyperinsulinism		Hypopituitarism		Metabolic Defect	
	Before	After	Before	After	Before	After
Glucose	↓	↑↑↑	↓	↑/N	↓	↓/N
Ketones	↓	↓	N/↓	N	↑	↑
Free fatty acids	↓	↑	N/↓	N	↑	↑
Lactate	N	N	N	N	↑	↑↑
Alanine	N	?	N	N	↑	↑↑
Uric acid	N	N	N	N	↑	↑↑
Insulin	↑↑	↑↑↑	N/↑	↑	N	↑
Growth hormone	↑	↓	↓	↓	↑	↑
Cortisol	↑	↓	↓[b]	↓[b]	↑	↑
TSH and T₄	N	N	↓[b]	↓[b]	N	N

[a] N, normal or no change; ↑, elevated; ↓, lowered; ?, unknown.
[b] Response may vary, depending on the degree of hypopituitarism.
Courtesy of Marvin Cornblath, MD, Baltimore, Maryland.

ther hydrocortisone sodium succinate (Solu-Cortef), 5 mg/kg/d given intravenously in 4 divided doses, or prednisone, 2 mg/kg/d orally.

    (2) If hypoglycemia persists, the following can be tried for 3 days each (it is not necessary to stop corticosteroids).

        (a) Diazoxide, 8–15 mg/kg/d orally in 3–4 divided doses.

        (b) Human growth hormone (Somatrem, Protropin) 0.1 unit/d intramuscularly.

        (c) Surgery to remove most of the pancreas is the treatment of choice in patients with B-cell hyperplasia or nesidioblastosis.

B. Specific treatment plans

  1. Neonatal hyperinsulinism. Pancreatectomy, removing at least 95% of the organ, is usually necessary. Recent studies have shown that partial pancreatomy can be done in cases where hypersecretion can be shown to be confined to a small area of the pancreas.

  2. Congenital hypopituitarism usually responds to administration of cortisone and intravenous glucose. Administration of human growth hormone may be necessary. (See Chap 73 for dosages and other pharmacologic information.)

  3. Metabolic defects

    a. Type I glycogen storage disease. Frequent small feedings with fructose or galactose may be beneficial.

    b. Hereditary fructose intolerance. The infant should begin a fructose-free diet.

    c. Galactosemia. The infant should be placed on a galactose-free diet.

40 Hypokalemia

I. **Problem.** A serum potassium value is less than 3.5 meq/L. Normal serum potassium is 3.5–5.5 meq/L.

II. **Immediate questions**

    A. **What is the central serum potassium?** If a low value is obtained by heelstick, central values should be obtained because they may actually be lower than values obtained by heelstick due to the release of potassium from red cells during the heelstick.

    B. **Are potassium-wasting medications or digitalis being given?** Diuretics may cause hypokalemia. Hypokalemia may cause arrhythmias if digitalis is being given.

    C. **How much potassium is the infant receiving?** Normal maintenance dosages are 1–2 meq/kg/d.

    D. **Is diarrhea occurring or is a nasogastric tube in place?** Loss of large amounts of gastrointestinal fluids can cause hypokalemia.

III. **Differential diagnosis**

    A. **Inadequate maintenance infusion of potassium.** See Chapter 7 for a further discussion.

    B. **Abnormal potassium losses**

        1. **Medications.** Amphotericin B can cause direct renal tubular damage with resulting hypokalemia. Any thiazide diuretic may cause hypokalemia. High and continuous doses of spironolactone with hydrochlorothiazide (Aldactazide) have also resulted in hypokalemia. Gentamicin and carbenicillin are also associated with potassium losses.

        2. **GI tract losses.** Diarrhea and loss of fluid via nasogastric tube may cause hypokalemia.

        3. **Bartter's syndrome,** a rare form of potassium wasting, is characterized by hypokalemia, normal blood pressure, and increased levels of aldosterone and renin.

        4. **Hypercalcemia**

        5. **Hypomagnesemia**

        6. **Adrenogenital syndrome.** In certain forms of the disease, hypokalemia may occur.

        7. **Renal tubular defects.**

    C. **Redistribution of potassium by an increase in intracellular uptake.**

        1. **Alkalosis (metabolic or respiratory).** An increase in pH by 0.1 unit causes a decrease in the potassium level by 0.3–1.3 meq/L. The decrease is less in respiratory than in metabolic alkalosis.

        2. **Insulin.** An increase in insulin causes intracellular uptake in potassium with hypokalemia.

        3. **Medications.** Certain medications cause an increase in intracellular uptake of potassium. These include: Terbutaline, Albuterol, Isoproterenol, and catecholamines.

IV. **Data base**

    A. **Physical examination.** Hypokalemia may cause ileus. Symptoms of hypokalemia include muscle weakness and decreased tendon reflexes, but these are difficult to evaluate in an infant.

    B. **Laboratory studies**

        1. **Repeat measurement of serum potassium level.**

    2. Spot checks of urinary electrolytes. Perform periodic spot checks of urinary potassium levels to determine if urinary losses are high.

    3. Serum electrolytes and Creatinine. This will help to evaluate renal status.

    4. Blood gas levels. An alkalosis may cause or aggravate hypokalemia (ie, as hydrogen ions leave the cells, potassium ions enter the cells, causing decreased serum potassium levels).

C. Radiologic and other studies

    1. Abdominal x-ray study. If ileus is suspected, an abdominal x-ray film should be obtained.

    2. Electrocardiography. If hypokalemia is present and the infant is unstable, an ECG may show a prolonged QT interval, flat T wave, u waves, and depressed ST segment.

V. Plan

A. General measures. The problem of hypokalemia is increasing in NICUs because of the widespread use of diuretics. The goal of treatment is to increase the potassium intake so that normal blood levels are achieved and maintained. Short-term potassium administration may cause damage to the veins and, sometimes, hyperkalemia, because the potassium does not rapidly equilibrate. Therefore, corrections are given slowly, often over 24 hours. If too large a bolus is given, cardiac arrest may result. Serum potassium levels should be followed every 4–6 hours until correction is achieved. Once levels reach high normal, decrease the amount of potassium given.

B. Specific measures. Any specific defects, ie, renal defects, adrenal disorders, and certain metabolic problems, need specific evaluation and therapy.

    1. Inadequate maintenance infusion of potassium. Calculate the normal maintenance infusion of potassium that should be given and increase the amount accordingly (normal maintenance infusion is 1–2 meq/kg/d usually only necessary after the first day of life).

    2. Abnormal potassium losses

        a. Medications. If the infant is receiving potassium-wasting medications, increase the maintenance dose of potassium. Abnormal potassium loss often occurs in patients with bronchopulmonary dysplasia who are receiving long-term furosemide therapy. Oral supplementation in the form of potassium chloride may be given, 1–2 meq/kg/d in 3–4 divided doses (with feedings). This amount may be increased or decreased, depending on serum potassium levels. Often, a potassium-sparing diuretic (eg, spironolactone) may decrease the amount of potassium supplementation needed.

        b. Gastrointestinal losses.

            (1) Severe diarrhea leading to potassium losses in the stool can be corrected by treating the cause of the diarrhea, withholding oral feedings to allow the gut to rest, and giving intravenous fluids. Potassium supplementation may be given intravenously. The initial intravenous dosage of potassium chloride is 1–2 meq/kg/d. Serum potassium levels are followed, and the intravenous dosage is increased accordingly.

            (2) Nasogastric drainage. This amount should be measured each shift and replaced cc for cc with 1/2 normal saline with 20 meq potassium chloride.

            (3) Bartter's syndrome. Potassium supplementation is given orally, usually at a starting dosage of 2–3 meq/kg/d, which is increased as necessary to maintain a normal serum potassium level.

            (4) Hypercalcemia. See Chap 70.

C. Redistribution.

    1. Alkalosis. Determine the cause of metabolic or respiratory alkalosis and treat the underlying disorder.

    2. Medications. The medications should be discontinued if possible.

41 Hyponatremia

I. **Problem.** The serum sodium level is 127 meq/L, below the normal accepted value of 135 meq/L.

II. **Immediate questions**

A. **Is there any seizure activity?** Seizure activity is often seen in patients with extremely low serum sodium levels (usually < 120 meq/L). *This event is a medical emergency, and urgent sodium correction is needed.*

B. **How much sodium and free water is the patient receiving? Is weight gain or loss occurring?** Be certain that an adequate amount of sodium is being given and that free water intake is not excessive. The normal amount of sodium intake is 2–3 meq/kg/d. Weight gain with low serum sodium levels is most likely due to volume overload, especially in the first day or two of life, when weight loss is expected.

C. **What is the urine output?** With syndrome of inappropriate secretion of antidiuretic hormone (SIADH), urine output is decreased. If the urine output is increased (> 4 mL/kg/h), perform a spot check of urine sodium to determine if sodium losses are high.

D. **Are renal salt-wasting medications being given?** Diuretics such as furosemide may cause hyponatremia.

III. **Differential diagnosis**

A. **Volume overload (dilutional hyponatremia).** This can be seen in CHF, renal and liver failure, paralysis with fluid retention, use of diluted formulas, and nephrotic syndrome.

B. **Inadequate sodium intake.**

C. **Increased sodium loss.** In very low birth weight infants, renal tubular sodium losses are high and an increased amount of sodium is needed (see Chap 10). Sodium losses can also occur secondary to salt-losing nephropathies, gastrointestinal losses, skin losses with the use of a radiant warmer, third spacing, and adrenal insufficiency.

D. **Drug-induced hyponatremia.** Diuretics lead to sodium losses. Indomethacin causes water retention, which causes dilutional hyponatremia. Certain medications, such as opiates and barbiturates, can cause SIADH. Infusion of mannitol or hypertonic glucose can cause hyperosmolality with salt wasting.

E. **Syndrome of inappropriate secretion of antidiuretic hormone (SIADH).** SIADH is more commonly seen with central nervous system disorders such as intraventricular hemorrhage, hydrocephalus, birth asphyxia, and meningitis but may also be seen with lung disease. SIADH is often considered in the differential diagnosis of ill patients, but it is not frequently encountered in neonatal nurseries.

IV. **Data base**

A. **Evaluation of bedside chart.** Evaluate the pertinent information on the bedside chart. First, check for **weight loss or gain.** Weight gain is more likely to be associated with dilutional hyponatremia. Next, assess the **urine output and specific gravity.** A low urine output with a high specific gravity is more commonly seen with SIADH. Check the **fluid intake and output** over a 24-hour period. Normally, infants retain two-thirds of the fluid administered, and the rest is lost in the urine or by insensible water loss. If the input is much greater than the output, the patient may be retaining fluid, and dilutional hyponatremia should be considered.

B. **Physical examination.** Perform a complete physical examination. Note signs of seizure activity (abnormal eye movements, jerking of the extremities, tongue thrusting). Check for edema which would be found in volume overload. Look for decreased skin turgor and dry mucous membranes which would be seen in dehydration.

- **C. Laboratory studies**
    1. **Specific tests to order**
        a. **Serum sodium and osmolality.**
        b. **Urine spot sodium, osmolality, and specific gravity.**
        c. **Serum electrolytes, creatinine, and total protein** to assess renal function.
    2. **Laboratory results of specific diagnoses**
        a. **Volume overload (dilutional hyponatremia):** Decreased urine output and urine sodium and increased urine osmolality and specific gravity.
        b. **Increased sodium losses**
            (1) In renal losses, with diuretics and adrenal insufficiency: urine output is increased, urine Na^+ is increased, urine osmolality and specific gravity is decreased.
            (2) In skin and GI losses, and with third spacing: urine output and sodium are decreased, and urine osmolality and specific gravity are increased.
        c. **The diagnosis of SIADH** is made by documenting the following on simultaneous laboratory studies: low urine output, urine osmolality greater than serum osmolality, low serum sodium level and low serum osmolality, high urinary sodium level and high specific gravity.
- **D. Radiologic and other studies.** Usually, none are needed. Occasionally, an ultrasound of the head may reveal intraventricular hemorrhage as a cause of hyponatremia due to SIADH.

V. Plan
- **A. Emergency measures.** If the infant is having **seizures due to hyponatremia** (usually sodium < 120 meq/dL), hypertonic saline solution (3% sodium chloride) should be given. The total body deficit of sodium (see **C.3,** below) is calculated, and half of that is given over 12–24 hours. Rapid corrections may result in brain damage.
- **B. Volume overload (dilutional hyponatremia)** is treated with fluid restriction. The total maintenance fluids can be decreased by 20 mL/kg/d, and serum sodium levels should be followed every 6–8 hours. The underlying cause must be investigated and treated.
- **C. Inadequate sodium intake**
    1. **The maintenance sodium requirement for term infants is 2–4 meq/kg/d; it is higher in premature infants** (see p 73). Calculate the amount of sodium the patient is receiving, using the equations on p 74. Readjust the intravenous sodium intake if it is the cause of hyponatremia.
    2. **If the infant is receiving oral formula only, check the formula being used.** Low-sodium formulas include SMA 20 and PM 60/40. Use of supplemental sodium chloride or a formula with a higher sodium content may be necessary.
    3. **Calculate total sodium deficit** using the following equation:

Sodium value desired (130–135) – Infant's sodium value × Weight (kg) × 0.6

The result will be the amount of sodium needed to correct the hyponatremia. Usually only half of this amount is given over 12 to 24 hours.
- **D. Increased sodium losses.** Try to treat the underlying cause and increase sodium administered to replace the losses.
- **E. Drug-induced hyponatremia.** If a renal salt-wasting medication such as furosemide (Lasix) is being given, serum sodium levels will be low even though an adequate amount of sodium is being given in the diet. An increase in sodium intake may be required, often the case in infants with bronchopulmonary dys-

plasia who are receiving furosemide. Most are also receiving oral feedings, so an oral sodium chloride supplement can be used. Start with 1 meq 3 times per day with feedings and adjust as needed. Some infants may require as much as 12–15 meq/d. Indomethacin therapy needs to be treated with fluid restriction.

F. Syndrome of inappropriate secretion of antidiuretic hormone (SIADH). Restrict fluids, usually to 40–60 mL/kg/d. (This regimen does not allow for fluid loss that accompanies the use of a radiant warmer or phototherapy.) Follow the serum sodium level and osmolality and the urine output to determine if the patient is responding. The cause of SIADH is usually obvious, but if it is not, further investigation is needed—for example, ultrasonography of the head to diagnose or rule out intraventricular hemorrhage or hydrocephalus; chest x-ray studies to diagnose or rule out lung pathology. Use of furosemide can also be tried.

42 Hypotension and Shock

I. **Problem.** The blood pressure is more than 2 standard deviations below normal for age. (For normal blood pressure values, see Appendix C.)

II. **Immediate questions**

A. **What method of measurement was used?** If a cuff was used, be certain that it was the correct width (ie, covering two-thirds of the upper arm). A cuff that is too large will give falsely low readings. If measurements were obtained from an indwelling arterial line, a "dampened" waveform suggests there is air in the transducer or tubing or a clot in the system, and the readings may be inaccurate.

B. **Are symptoms of shock present?** Symptoms of shock include tachycardia, poor perfusion, cold extremities with a normal core temperature, lethargy, narrow pulse pressure, apnea and bradycardia, tachypnea, metabolic acidosis, and weak pulse.

C. **Is the urine output acceptable?** Normal urine output is approximately 1–2 mL/kg/h. Urine output is decreased in shock because of decreased renal perfusion. If the blood pressure is low but the urine output is adequate, aggressive treatment may not be necessary, because the renal perfusion is adequate. (***Note:*** An exception to this would be an infant with septic shock and hyperglycemia who has osmotic diuresis.)

D. **Is there a history of birth asphyxia?** Birth asphyxia may be associated with hypotension.

E. **At the time of delivery, was there maternal bleeding (eg, abruptio placentae or placenta previa) or was clamping of the cord delayed?** These factors may be associated with loss of blood volume in the infant.

III. **Differential diagnosis.** Hypotension, (diminished blood pressure) is distinct from shock, which is a clinical syndrome of inadequate tissue perfusion with the clinical signs noted above.

A. **Hypovolemic shock** may be secondary to antepartum or postpartum blood loss.
   1. **Antepartum blood loss**
      a. **Abruptio placentae.**
      b. **Placenta previa.**
      c. **Twin-twin transfusion.**
      d. **Feto-maternal hemorrhage.**
   2. **Postpartum blood loss**
      a. **Coagulation disorders.**
      b. **Vitamin K deficiency.**
      c. **Iatrogenic causes** (eg, loss of arterial line).
      d. **Birth trauma** (eg, liver injury, adrenal hemorrhage).

B. **Septic shock.** Endotoxemia occurs, with release of vasodilator substances and resulting hypotension. It usually involves gram-negative organisms such as *E coli* and *Klebsiella* but can also occur with gram-positive organisms such as in group B streptococcal and staphylococcal infections.

C. **Cardiogenic shock**
   1. **Birth asphyxia.**
   2. **Metabolic problems** (eg, hypoglycemia, hyponatremia, hypocalcemia) can cause decreased cardiac output with a decrease in blood pressure.
   3. **Congenital heart disease** (eg, hypoplastic left heart, aortic stenosis).
   4. **Arrhythmias** can cause a decrease in cardiac output.
   5. **Any obstruction of venous return** (eg, tension pneumothorax).

D. **Neurogenic shock.** Birth asphyxia and intracranial hemorrhage can both cause hypotension.

E. **Drug-induced hypotension.** Certain drugs (eg, tolazoline, tubocurarine, nitroprusside, sedatives, magnesium sulfate, digitalis, barbiturates) will cause vasodilation and a drop in blood pressure.

F. **Endocrine disorders.** Complete 21-hydroxylase deficiency and adrenal hemorrhage are the most notable endocrine disorders that can cause hypotension and shock. If there is a low serum sodium, high serum potassium, and hypotension, it is important to rule out adrenogenital syndrome.

IV. **Data base**

A. **Physical examination.** Particular attention is given to signs of blood loss (eg, intracranial or intra-abdominal bleeding), sepsis, or clinical signs of shock.

B. **Laboratory studies**

1. **Complete blood count with differential.** Decreased hematocrit will identify blood loss; however, the hematocrit can be normal in patients with acute blood loss. Elevated white blood count and differential may help identify sepsis as the cause.

2. **Coagulation studies (prothrombin time [PT] and partial thromboplastin time [PTT]) and platelet count** if disseminated intravascular coagulation is suspected.

3. **Serum glucose, electrolytes, and calcium levels** may reveal a metabolic disorder.

4. **Cultures.** Obtain blood and urine for culture and antibiotic sensitivity testing.

5. **Kleihauer-Betke test** should be performed if fetomaternal transfusion is suspected. The test detects the presence of fetal erythrocytes in the mother's blood by a slide elution technique. A smear of maternal blood is fixed and incubated in an acidic buffer. It causes adult hemoglobin to be eluted from erythrocytes; fetal hemoglobin resists elution. After the slide is stained, fetal hemoglobin cells, if present, appear dark, whereas maternal erythrocytes appear clear.

6. **Arterial blood gases** to assess for hypoxia and/or acidosis.

C. **Radiologic and other studies**

1. **Chest x-ray study.** An anteroposterior chest x-ray study should be done to assess the heart and lungs and rule out any mechanical cause of shock (eg, pneumothorax).

2. **Ultrasonography of the head is done** in infants in whom intracranial hemorrhage is suspected.

3. **Electrocardiography** should be performed if an arrhythmia is suspected.

4. **Echocardiography** is performed in birth-asphyxiated infants to assess myocardial function. If there is myocardial failure, drug therapy is needed to improve cardiac output. Echocardiography is also useful to rule out a congenital heart lesion.

5. **Central venous pressure measurement.** A venous umbilical catheter can be placed above the diaphragm to obtain central venous pressure readings. Normal values are 4–6 mm Hg. If these readings are low, hypovolemia is present and transfusion is usually necessary.

V. **Plan**

A. **General measures**

1. **Rapidly assess the infant and determine what is causing the hypotension** in order to direct treatment accordingly. The basic decision is whether the infant needs volume replacement or administration of inotropic agents. The decision is not difficult in the majority of patients. Four parameters are useful in making this decision.

a. **History.** A history should be obtained to rule out birth asphyxia, blood loss (antepartum or postpartum), drug infusion, and birth trauma (adrenal hemorrhage or liver injury).

b. **Physical examination.** A careful physical examination will often reveal which organ systems are involved.

     c. Chest x-ray. A small heart is seen in volume depletion; a large heart is seen in cardiac disease.

     d. Central venous pressure. If it is low (< 4 mm Hg), the infant is volume depleted. If it is high (eg, > 6 mm Hg), the infant probably has cardiogenic shock.

2. If you are still unsure of the cause, start empirical volume expansion with either intravenous colloid or crystalloid (10 mL/kg intravenously over 30 min).

     a. If there is a response, continue volume expansion.

     b. If there is no response, an inotropic agent (eg, dopamine) should be started (see p 229, **B.3**).

3. Provide respiratory support as needed. Blood gas determinations and clinical examinations will dictate whether supplemental oxygen will suffice or whether intubation and mechanical ventilation are necessary.

4. Correct any metabolic acidosis with sodium bicarbonate.

B. Specific measures

  1. Hypovolemic shock

     a. Volume expansion using either intravenous crystalloid or colloid (should be given (see **2,** above for dosage). Colloids such as albumin or plasma protein fraction (Plasmanate) are preferred, but agents such as normal saline or Ringer's lactate may be used in an emergency. The goal is to give a volume expander until adequate tissue perfusion is attained, as evidenced by good urine output and central nervous function. If blood loss has occurred and the patient is severely hypovolemic, immediate volume expansion with colloid or crystalloid is essential. Meanwhile a blood sample should be sent to the laboratory for a hematocrit value, which is used to determine the specific blood products that should be used in blood replacement therapy.

     b. Blood replacement therapy

       (1) Hematocrit less than 40%. Packed red blood cells should be given, 5–10 mL/kg over 30–40 minutes. The following formula may also be used to calculate the volume of packed red blood cells needed. This formula assumes that the total blood volume is 80 mL/kg and the hematocrit (Hct) of the packed red blood cells is 70%.

$$\text{Volume required} = \frac{(\text{Weight [kg]} \times \text{Total blood volume}) \times (\text{Desired Hct} - \text{Patient's Hct})}{\text{Hct of transfusion product}}$$

       (2) Hematocrit over 50%. Plasmanate, albumin, or fresh-frozen plasma (FFP) should be used. FFP is used only if clotting studies are also abnormal.

       (3) Hematocrit of 40–50%. Alternating transfusions of packed red blood cells and Plasmanate or albumin should be given.

  2. Septic shock

     a. Obtain cultures (blood and urine [unless in the first 24 hours of life, obtain only blood]; lumbar puncture for CSF culture and other culture studies as clinically indicated).

     b. Initiate empiric antibiotic therapy after culture specimens have been obtained. **Intravenous ampicillin and gentamicin** are recommended. **Vancomycin** may be substituted for ampicillin if staphylococcal infection is suspected (usually seen in infants more than 3 days old who have invasive monitoring lines or chest tubes in place). Some institutions are advocating the use of **cefotaxime** with vancomycin instead of gentamicin to avoid the nephrotoxicity. (See Chap 73 for dosages.)

     c. Use volume expansion and inotropic agents as needed to maintain adequate tissue and renal perfusion (see p 228, **B.1.a, and 3,** below).

     d. Use of corticosteroids. Intravenous corticosteroid therapy for sepsis is *controversial.* Agents such as dexamethasone have been used, however (see p 479).

    e. Use of naloxone. Naloxone has been used in patients with septic shock and persistent hypotension, but its use is *controversial* (see p 497 for dosage).

3. Cardiogenic shock. First treat any obvious cause.

    a. Air leak. If a tension pneumothorax is causing hypotension by obstructing venous return, immediate evacuation of the air is necessary.

    b. Arrhythmia. Recognize the arrhythmia and treat it.

    c. Metabolic etiology. Metabolic problems need to be corrected.

    d. Asphyxia. The hypotension usually responds to inotropic agents. See below.

    e. Then, in cardiogenic shock, the goal is to improve cardiac output. Inotropic agents should be used intravenously (see Chap 73 for dosages and other pharmacologic information).

        (1) Dopamine. Dopamine is the drug of first choice. Previous studies have suggested that higher than traditionally used dosages may be used without causing alpha-adrenergic side effects such as decreased renal perfusion and decreased urine output.

        (2) Dobutamine. If dopamine fails to improve blood pressure, dobutamine is recommended as a second-line drug. In neonates, it is usually given together with dopamine infusion.

        (3) Other agents. Epinephrine and isoproterenol are sometimes used.

4. Neurogenic shock. Neurogenic shock is treated with volume expansion (see p 228) and inotropic agents (see **3,** above).

5. Drug induced hypotension. Volume expansion (see p 228,) will usually maintain the blood pressure in cases of drug-induced vasodilatation. If the blood pressure cannot be maintained, the drug causing hypotension may need to be discontinued.

6. Endocrine disorders.

    a. Adrenal hemorrhage is treated with volume expansion and blood replacement (see p 000) and corticosteroids (see Chap 73).

    b. Congenital adrenal hyperplasia is treated with corticosteroids (see Chap 73).

43 No Stool in 48 Hours

I. **Problem.** No stool has been passed in 48 hours.

II. **Immediate questions**

A. **Has a stool been passed since birth?** If a stool has been passed since birth but not in the last 48 hours, constipation may be the cause. If a stool has never been passed, imperforate anus or some degree of intestinal obstruction may be present. Table 43–1 shows the time after birth at which the first stool is typically passed. In the first 48 hours of life, 94% of infants will pass a stool.

B. **What is the gestational age?** Prematurity may be associated with delayed passage of stool because of immaturity of the colon.

C. **Were maternal drugs used that could cause a paralytic ileus with delayed passage of stool?** Magnesium sulfate, which is used to slow the premature onset of labor, may cause paralytic ileus. Use of heroin by the mother may also cause delayed passage of stool in the infant.

III. **Differential diagnosis**

A. **Constipation.**

B. **Anorectal abnormalities such as imperforate anus.**

C. **Bowel obstruction**

1. **Meconium plug.** A meconium plug is an obstruction in the lower colon and rectum caused by meconium. It is more common in infants of diabetic mothers (as seen in neonatal small left colon syndrome where the plug extends to the splenic flexure) and in premature infants. (**Note:** A rectal biopsy should be done in all these patients, as they have an increased incidence of Hirschsprung's disease [10–15%].)

2. **Meconium ileus occurs** when meconium becomes obstructed in the terminal ileum. It is the most common presentation of cystic fibrosis in the neonatal period.

3. **Hirschsprung's disease** accounts for approximately 15% of infants who have delayed passage of stool. A functional obstruction is caused by aganglionosis of cells in Meissner's and Auerbach's plexus of the colon. The affected segment of colon is aperistaltic.

4. **Ileal atresia** can occur secondary to meconium ileus, Hirschsprung's disease, incarcerated hernia, or intussusception. Signs include abdominal distention, bilious vomiting, and failure to pass meconium.

5. **Inspissated milk syndrome.** In this syndrome, milk curds form and ob-

---

TABLE 43–1. PASSAGE OF FIRST STOOL

	Premature Infant		Term Infant	
	Percentage	Cumulative Percentage	Percentage	Cumulative Percentage
Delivery room	13	13	27.2	27.2
0–24 hours	31.5	44.5	41.8	69
12–24 hours	35.5	80	25	94
24–48 hours	14	94	5.8	99.8
Over 48 hours	6	100	1	100

Based on data from Sherry SN, Kramer I: *J Pediatr* 1955;**46**:158; and Kramer I, Sherry SN: *J Pediatr* 1957;**51**:373.

struct the gut. The infant initially has a normal stooling pattern and is being fed and then has abdominal distention, vomiting, and no stooling.

6. **Adhesions.** Postoperatively, such as after surgery for necrotizing enterocolitis, there is a 30% chance of having adhesions.

7. **Incarcerated hernia.** A hernia is obstructed when its contents cannot be reduced and the bowel is obstructed. Signs include irritability, cramps, bilious vomiting, and abdominal distention. The risk of incarceration for an inguinal hernia in infancy is 20–30%, the risk for bowel obstruction secondary to an inguinal hernia is 9%.

8. **Malrotation.** Malrotation is the failure of the GI tract to properly rotate and adhere. Volvulus is a specific malrotation of the gut and is a **surgical emergency** because it can cause ischemia of the gut, with resulting shock and possibly death. Malrotation without volvulus formation may present with intermittent episodes of vomiting and abdominal distention. The stooling pattern can be normal.

D. **Other causes**
1. **Ileus** can be secondary to:
    a. **Sepsis.**
    b. **Necrotizing enterocolitis.**
    c. **Hypokalemia.**
    d. **Pneumonia.**
    e. **Maternal use of magnesium sulfate.**
    f. **Hypothyroidism.**
2. **Prematurity** (see **II.B**, p 230).

IV. **Data base**
A. **Physical examination.** First, document the patency of the anus. Check for abdominal distention or rigidity, bowel sounds, and evidence of a mass. A rectal examination will determine whether muscle tone is adequate, and it may reveal hardened stool in the colon.

B. **Laboratory findings**
1. **A complete blood count and differential and blood culture** should be done to rule out sepsis. A sterile urine culture should also be done.
2. **Urinary drug screening** should be performed for mother and infant to detect maternal use of narcotics.
3. **The serum magnesium level** should be determined to detect hypermagnesemia.
4. **The serum thyroxine (T4) level and thyroid-stimulating hormone (TSH) level** should be determined to detect hypothyroidism.
5. **Serum electrolytes** should be measured, especially to rule out hypokalemia.

C. **Radiologic and other studies**
1. **Plain film abdominal x-rays.** A flat plate and upright film of the abdomen should be obtained to look for ileus or bowel obstruction in any infant who has not passed stool within 48 hours of birth. With Hirschsprung's disease or meconium plug, distention of the colon with multiple air-fluid levels is seen.
2. **Abdominal x-rays with barium enema** should be obtained in all cases of delayed passage of stool if the patient is symptomatic. It will help to define the disease process and may be therapeutic. Specific findings for each disease are described below under Plan.

V. **Plan**
A. **Constipation**
1. **Digital rectal stimulation** can be tried first.
2. **Glycerin suppositories** can be used if digital rectal stimulation is unsuccessful.

B. **Anorectal abnormality: imperforate anus**
1. **Obtain pediatric surgical consultation** immediately.
2. **Insert a nasogastric tube** for decompression.

3. Look for other congenital anomalies. Genitourinary tract abnormalities are frequently seen with imperforate anus.

C. Bowel obstruction

1. Meconium plug

a. Barium enema is performed to verify meconium plug. In infants with this problem, the study usually reveals a normal-sized colon with filling defects.

b. If meconium plug is verified by barium enema, repeated water soluble enemas are usually given every 4–6 hours.

c. Acetylcysteine (Mucomyst) enema. If water-soluble enemas are ineffective, a dilute 4% solution of acetylcysteine and water can be used as an enema to break down the meconium so that it can be passed.

d. If normal stooling occurs, no further workup is needed. However, some clinicians recommend rectal biopsy in these infants because up to 15% have Hirschsprung's disease.

e. If an abnormal pattern of stooling occurs, further workup (eg, rectal biopsy) is necessary to rule out Hirschsprung's disease.

2. Meconium ileus

a. Barium enema may reveal microcolon. Evidence of perforation, volvulus, or atresia may also be seen.

b. Mild obstruction can be treated with Mucomyst enemas (see above).

c. Complete obstruction may be relieved by Gastrografin enema. Adequate fluid and electrolyte replacement must be given.

d. Operative management may be necessary in cases not relieved by enemas.

3. Hirschsprung's disease

a. Barium enema examination usually shows a narrowed, aganglionic segment leading to a dilated proximal segment.

b. Rectal biopsy, the definitive diagnosis, is performed to confirm aganglionosis.

c. Colostomy is usually indicated once the diagnosis is confirmed.

4. Inspissated milk syndrome

a. Barium enema reveals a narrow colon with filling defects.

b. Gastrografin enema often relieves the obstruction.

c. Surgery may be necessary in rare cases.

5. Adhesions. Surgery is usually necessary to lyse the adhesions if a trial of nasogastric decompression fails.

6. Incarcerated hernia is a surgical emergency.

7. Malrotation

a. Barium enema reveals an abnormally placed cecum.

b. Surgical correction is necessary.

8. Volvulus

a. Barium enema reveals obstruction at the midtransverse colon.

b. Surgery should be an immediate intervention.

D. Ileus

1. Ileus caused by sepsis

a. Broad-spectrum antibiotics are initiated after a septic workup (see p 000,) is performed. Intravenous ampicillin and gentamicin are recommended. Vancomycin may be substituted for ampicillin if staphylococcal infection is suspected (see Chap 73 for dosages).

b. A nasogastric tube should be placed to decompress the bowel. The infant should not be fed enterally.

2. Ileus caused by necrotizing enterocolitis (see Chap 64).

3. Ileus caused by hypokalemia

a. Treat underlying metabolic abnormalities.

b. Place a nasogastric tube to rest the bowel.

E. Prematurity. Conservative treatment is usually recommended in infants who are not vomiting but have progressive abdominal distention, even if microcolon is seen. Treatment consists of a hyperosmolar contrast enema for passage of the stool. (***Note:*** Some institutions are advocating the use of low-osmolality contrast enemas because of fewer side effects. Low-osmolality contrast media include metrizamide, iohexol, iopamidol, and ioxaglate.)

F. Hypothyroidism. If the serum T4 and TSH levels confirm the presence of hypothyroidism, thyroid replacement therapy is indicated. However, consultation with an endocrinologist should be obtained before starting this therapy.

44 Decreased or No Urine Output

I. **Problem.** Urine output has been scant or absent for 48 hours. Oliguria is defined as urine output less than 20 mL/kg in a 24-hour period.

II. **Immediate questions**

    A. **Is the bladder palpable?** If a distended bladder is present, it is usually palpable and there is urine in the bladder. The **Crede maneuver** (manual compression of the bladder) may initiate voiding, especially in infants receiving medications causing muscle paralysis.

    B. **Has bladder catheterization been performed?** It will determine whether urine is present in the bladder.

    C. **What is the blood pressure?** Hypotension can cause decreased renal perfusion and urine output.

    D. **Has the infant ever voided?** If the infant has never voided, consider bilateral renal agenesis, renovascular accident, or obstruction. Table 44–1 shows the time after birth at which the first voiding occurs. 90.5% of infants will void within the first 24 hours of life.

III. **Differential diagnosis.** See Chap 68 for a complete discussion of acute renal failure.

    A. **Prerenal causes (inadequate blood supply to the kidneys)**

        1. **Sepsis.**

        2. **Hemorrhage.**

        3. **Hypotension.**

        4. **Asphyxia.**

        5. **Hypokalemia.**

        6. **Heart failure.**

        7. **Dehydration.**

        8. **Medications.** Certain medications (captopril and beta agonists), if given to the mother prior to delivery, can result in renal insufficiency.

    B. **Intrinsic renal failure (kidney failure because of intrinsic renal disease)**

        1. **Renal agenesis.**

        2. **Hypoplastic, dysplastic, or cystic kidneys.**

        3. **Pyelonephritis.**

        4. **Vascular accident (renal artery and vein thrombosis).**

        5. **Nephritis.**

        6. **Infections** such as congenital syphilis, CMV, Toxoplasmosis, and gram-negative infections.

TABLE 44–1. TIME TO FIRST VOIDING

	Premature Infant		Term Infant	
	Percentage	Cumulative Percentage	Percentage	Cumulative Percentage
Delivery room	21.5	21.5	17	17
0–12 hours	43	64.5	50.6	67.6
12–24 hours	26	90.5	24.8	92.4
24–48 hours	9.5	100	7	99.4
Over 48 hours			0.6	100

Based on data from Sherry SN, Kramer I: *J Pediatr* 1955;**46:**189; and Kramer I, Sherry SN: *J Pediatr* 1957;**51:**374.

      7. Acute tubular necrosis secondary to shock, dehydration, and asphyxia.

      8. Medications. Certain medications are nephrotoxic: Tolazoline, aminoglycosides, and indomethacin.

  C. Postrenal causes (urine is formed but not voided)

      1. Neurogenic bladder (from meningomyelocele, or medications such as Pancuronium or heavy sedation).

      2. Urethral stricture.

      3. Posterior urethral valves (males only).

IV. Data base

  A. Physical examination. Physical examination may reveal bladder distention, abdominal masses, or ascites. Signs of renal disorders (eg, Potter's facies [low-set ears, inner canthal crease, etc]) should be noted. Urinary ascites may be seen with posterior urethral valves. Oligohydramnios in the mother suggests possible renal problems.

  B. Laboratory studies. The following laboratory tests can be obtained to help establish the diagnosis. Interpret the results as outlined in Table 68–1, p 433.

      1. Urine osmolality.

      2. Urine sodium (meq/L).

      3. Urine/plasma creatinine ratio.

      4. Fractional excretion of sodium (see p 433, **B.2**).

      5. Renal failure index (see p 433, **B.2**).

      6. Serum creatinine

      7. Serum electrolytes and BUN will also help to evaluate renal function.

      8. CBC and platelet count. An abnormal CBC can be seen in sepsis. Thrombocytopenia can be seen in renal vein thrombosis.

      9. Urinalysis may reveal WBCs which suggest a urinary tract infection.

     10. Arterial blood ph. A metabolic acidosis can be seen in sepsis.

  C. Radiologic and other studies

      1. Ultrasonography of the abdomen and kidneys will rule out urinary tract obstruction and evaluate for other renal abnormalities.

      2. Abdominal x-ray studies may reveal spina bifida or absent sacrum, suggesting neurogenic bladder.

V. Plan. See also Chapter 68 for management of renal failure.

  A. Prerenal.

      1. Treat specific cause such as sepsis.

      2. A fluid challenge can be given (10–15 mL/kg of plasma expander).

      3. Treatment may involve volume therapy or inotropic agents.

  B. Renal

      1. Supportive measures.

      2. Treat specific cause.

      3. Fluid restriction and replace insensible losses.

  c. Postrenal

      1. If obstruction is distal to the bladder, perform initial catheterization.

      2. If obstruction is proximal to the bladder, surgical intervention should be considered.

      3. Neurogenic bladder is initially managed with catheterization.

      4. Medications may be stopped and bladder function is usually restored.

45 Pneumoperitoneum

I. **Problem.** A pneumoperitoneum (abnormal collection of air in the peritoneal cavity) is seen on an abdominal x-ray film.

II. **Immediate questions**

A. **Is mechanical ventilation being given?** High peak inspiratory pressures (PIP) (> mean of 34 cm water) can be associated with pneumoperitoneum.

B. **Are signs or symptoms of pneumoperitoneum present?** These findings can include abdominal distention, respiratory distress, deteriorating blood gas levels, and a decrease in blood pressure.

C. **Are signs or symptoms of necrotizing enterocolitis (NEC) present?** If so, the pneumoperitoneum is likely to be associated with gastrointestinal tract perforation.

D. **Is a pneumomediastinum present?** If a pneumomediastinum is present, the peritoneal air collection is more likely to be of respiratory tract origin. Also, the presence of PIE and/or pneumothorax suggests alveolar origin.

E. **Did the infant recently undergo abdominal surgery?** Intra-abdominal air is normal in the immediate postoperative period and usually resolves without treatment.

III. **Differential diagnosis.** Pneumoperitoneum develops secondary to air leak from the chest, from a perforated viscus or iatrogenic.

A. **Pneumoperitoneum associated with respiratory disorder (eg, pneumomediastinum, pneumothorax)**

B. **Pneumoperitoneum associated with gastrointestinal perforation**

1. **Spontaneous perforation** occurs most commonly in the stomach of a neonate. It may be due to a misplaced nasogastric tube. Perforation of the appendix and Meckel's diverticulum have also been reported.

2. **Necrotizing enterocolitis** may also be associated with perforation.

C. **Iatrogenic pneumoperitoneum** may be caused by improperly performed suprapubic bladder aspiration, paracentesis, or as a normal transient finding postexploratory laparotomy.

IV. **Data base**

A. **Physical examination.** Perform a complete physical examination. Clinical evaluation may not help in differentiating whether the pneumoperitoneum is of respiratory or gastrointestinal tract origin.

B. **Laboratory studies**

1. **Preoperative laboratory testing** should be performed, including **serum electrolyte levels and a complete blood count.** Elevation of the white blood cell count or a left shift may signify a gastrointestinal tract perforation.

2. **Arterial blood gas levels** should be obtained. They may reveal hypoxemia and increasing Pco_2 levels.

C. **Radiologic and other studies**

1. **Anteroposterior x-ray study of the abdomen** may show signs of necrotizing enterocolitis or ileus. Air-fluid levels in the peritoneal cavity usually indicate bowel perforation.

2. **Lateral decubitus x-ray study of the abdomen** with the right side up is the best examination for the detection of free abdominal air. Air rises anteriorly, so that a lucency will be seen over the liver if a perforation has occurred.

3. **Paracentesis.** Air obtained by paracentesis (see Chap 23) may be tested for its oxygen level. If the oxygen level is high, the air is probably from a respiratory tract leak. Fluid may be obtained by paracentesis if the diagnosis

is still undetermined. If more than 0.5 mL of green or brown fluid is obtained, the air is probably of gastrointestinal tract origin.

V. Plan
A. General measures. A nasogastric tube should be placed.
B. Specific measures
1. **Pneumoperitoneum of respiratory tract origin**
   a. **For asymptomatic patients,** observation is the treatment of choice, with follow-up x-ray studies usually performed every 8–12 hours but more frequently if the patient's clinical course changes.
   b. **For symptomatic patients,** paracentesis can be performed (see Chap 23).
2. **Pneumoperitoneum of gastrointestinal tract origin.** Unless the pneumoperitoneum is of a known iatrogenic etiology, **immediate surgical evaluation** is necessary. Exploratory laparotomy is usually the treatment of choice.
   a. **Preoperative laboratory values** should be available.
   b. **The infant should be stabilized** as much as possible before being taken to the operating room.
   c. **The surgical team may request a study with a water-soluble contrast medium given through the nasogastric tube** to try to localize the perforation (see below).
3. **Iatrogenic pneumoperitoneum**
   a. **Pneumoperitoneum caused by suprapubic bladder aspiration or paracentesis may require surgical exploration.**
   b. **Postexploratory laparotomy** pneumoperitoneum associated with an uncomplicated surgical procedure will resolve spontaneously.
4. **If the cause of the pneumoperitoneum is in doubt, a low osmolality water soluble contrast medium (such as metrizamide) can be given through a nasogastric tube.** If there is a pneumoperitoneum due to a gastrointestinal perforation, contrast material will pass into the peritoneal cavity.

46 Pneumothorax

I. **Problem.** An infant may have a pneumothorax (an accumulation of air in the pleural space).

II. **Immediate questions**

A. **Are symptoms of tension pneumothorax present?** Tension pneumothorax presents as a **medical emergency,** and the patient's status will deteriorate acutely. The following signs and symptoms may be seen with tension pneumothorax: cyanosis, hypoxia, tachypnea, sudden decrease in heart rate with bradycardia, sudden increase in systolic blood pressure followed by narrowing pulse pressure and hypotension, asymmetric chest (bulging on the affected side), distention of the abdomen (secondary to downward displacement of the diaphragm), decreased breath sounds on the affected side, and shift of the cardiac apical impulse away from the affected side.

B. **Is the patient asymptomatic?** Asymptomatic pneumothorax is present in 1–2% of neonates. Most of these cases are discovered on chest x-ray at admission. Up to 15% of these infants were meconium-stained at birth.

C. **Is mechanical ventilation being used?** The incidence of pneumothorax in patients receiving positive-pressure ventilation is 15%–30%. A life-threatening tension pneumothorax may result from mechanical ventilation.

III. **Differential diagnosis.** A pneumothorax may be spontaneous or it may develop secondary to mechanical ventilation causing barotrauma.

A. **Pneumothorax**
1. **Symptomatic** pneumothorax (includes tension pneumothorax).
2. **Asymptomatic** pneumothorax.

B. **Pneumomediastinum.** Air in the mediastinal space that may be confused with a true pneumothorax.

C. **Congenital lobar emphysema.** Overdistension of one lobe secondary to air trapping occurs most commonly in the left upper lobe (47%). Other lobe involvement is 20% right upper lobe, 28% right middle lobe, and rare in the lower lobes. The causes of congenital lobar emphysema are probably multifactorial.

D. **Atelectasis with compensatory hyperinflation.** Compensatory hyperinflation may appear as a pneumothorax on a chest x-ray film.

E. **Pneumopericardium.** In neonates, pneumopericardium and tension pneumothorax can both present as sudden and rapid clinical deterioration. In pneumopericardium, the blood pressure drops and heart sounds are distant or absent. In tension pneumothorax, the blood pressure may initially increase. The chest x-ray film easily differentiates between the two. A pneumopericardium has a halo of air around the heart.

IV. **Clinical findings**

A. **Physical examination.** Perform a thorough examination of the chest. Specific findings are discussed in **II.A,** above. Transillumination is a useful rapid technique in neonates. (see **C.** below).

B. **Laboratory studies.** Blood gas levels may show decreased Pao_2 and increased Pco_2, with resultant respiratory acidosis.

C. **Radiologic and other studies**
1. **Transillumination.** Transillumination of the chest will define the pneumothorax. The room lights are lowered, and a fiberoptic transilluminator is placed along the posterior axillary line on the side on which pneumothorax is suspected. If pneumothorax is present, the chest will "light up" on that side. The transilluminator may be moved up and down along the posterior

axillary line and may also be placed above the nipple. Transilluminate both sides of the chest and then compare the results. If severe subcutaneous edema is present, transillumination may be falsely positive. Premature infants with PIE may also have a false positive transillumination. Large infants with thick chest walls do not transilluminate well. **Always verify the diagnosis of pneumothorax by chest x-ray studies if time permits.**

2. **Chest x-ray studies** are the best method of choice for diagnosing pneumothorax. The following films will help in making the diagnosis.

   a. **Anteroposterior view** of the chest will show the following:

      (1) A shift of the mediastinum away from the side of pneumothorax (with tension pneumothorax).

      (2) Depression of the diaphragm on the side of the pneumothorax (with tension pneumothorax).

      (3) The lung on the affected side will be displaced away from the chest wall by a radiolucent band of air.

   b. **Cross table lateral view** will show a rim of air around the lung ("pancaking"). It will *not* help to identify the affected side. This film must be considered together with the anteroposterior view to identify the involved side.

   c. **Lateral decubitus view.** The infant should be positioned so that the side of the suspected pneumothorax is up (eg, if pneumothorax is suspected on the left side, the film is taken with the left side up). This view will detect even a small pneumothorax not seen on a routine chest x-ray film.

V. Plan

A. **Symptomatic (tension) pneumothorax is an emergency! A 1- to 2-minute delay could be fatal. If a tension pneumothorax is suspected, act immediately. It is better to treat in this setting, even if it turns out there is no pneumothorax. There is no time for X-ray confirmation.** If the patient's status is deteriorating rapidly, a needle or Angiocath can be placed for aspiration, followed by formal chest tube placement.

   1. The site of puncture should be at the second or third intercostal space along the midclavicular line. Cleanse this area with antibacterial solution (Betadine).

   2. Connect a 21- or 23-gauge scalp vein needle or a 22- or 24- gauge Angiocath to a 20-mL syringe with a stopcock attached. Have an assistant hold the syringe and withdraw the air.

   3. Palpate the third rib at the midclavicular line. Insert the needle above the rib and advance it until air is withdrawn from the syringe. The needle may be removed before the chest tube is placed if the infant is relatively stable, or it may be left in place for continuous aspiration while the chest tube is being placed. If an Angiocath is used, the needle may be removed and the catheter left in place.

   4. Chest tube placement is discussed in Chapter 17.

B. **Asymptomatic pneumothorax**

   1. **If positive-pressure mechanical ventilation is the cause of asymptomatic pneumothorax,** a chest tube *must* be inserted because the pressure being given by the ventilator will prevent resolution of the pneumothorax, and tension pneumothorax may develop. If a pneumothorax develops in a patient who is ready to be extubated, clinical judgment must be used in deciding whether a chest tube should be placed.

   2. **If positive-pressure mechanical ventilation is not being administered,** one of 2 treatments may be used:

      a. Close observation with follow-up chest x-ray studies every 8–12 hours, or sooner if the infant becomes symptomatic. The pneumothorax will probably resolve within 48 hours.

      b. For more rapid resolution of the pneumothorax in the asymptomatic patient, give the infant 100% oxygen for 8–12 hours, a procedure known as *nitrogen washout therapy.* Less nitrogen is able to enter the lungs, and, at the same time, absorption of nitrogen from the extrapleural space is increased and then exhaled. The total gas tension is decreased, which also facilitates absorption of nitrogen by the blood. *It should be used only in full-term infants in whom retinopathy or prematurity will not be a problem.*

C. Pneumomediastinum may progress to a pneumothorax or pneumopericardium. Close observation is required.

D. Congenital lobar emphysema
   1. **Asymptomatic.** Conservative management with observation is advocated.
   2. **Symptomatic.** If respiratory failure is occurring, the treatment is usually surgical excision of the affected lobe.

E. Atelectasis with compensatory hyperinflation
   1. Chest physiotherapy and postural drainage should be initiated.
   2. Treatment with bronchodilators is indicated (see p 57).
   3. Positioning the infant with the affected side (hyperinflated side) down may speed resolution.

F. Pneumopericardium should be treated emergently by pericardiocentesis (see Chap 24).

47 Polycythemia

I. **Problem.** The hematocrit is 68% in a newborn. (The upper limit of normal for a peripheral venous stick is 65%.)

II. **Immediate questions**

A. **What is the central hematocrit?** In blood obtained by heelstick, the hematocrit may be falsely elevated by 5–15%. Therefore, treatment should not be initiated based on heelstick hematocrit values alone; a central (peripheral venous stick) hematocrit is needed. If the sample is from the umbilical vein or radial artery, the upper limit of normal is 63%.

B. **Is the infant dehydrated?** Dehydration may cause hemoconcentration, resulting in a high hematocrit. It usually occurs in infants more than 48 hours old.

C. **Does the infant have symptoms of polycythemia?** Symptoms and signs of polycythemia include respiratory distress, tachypnea, hypoglycemia, lethargy, irritability, apnea, seizures, jitteriness, weak sucking reflex, poor feeding, and cyanosis.

D. **Is the mother diabetic?** Poor control of diabetes during pregnancy leads to chronic fetal hypoxia, which may result in increased neonatal erythropoiesis.

E. **What is the infant's age?** The hematocrit reaches a peak at 2–4 hours of age. After 48 hours of age, hemoconcentration due to dehydration may be present.

III. **Differential diagnosis.** (See also Chap 54)

A. **Falsely elevated hematocrit.** This finding occurs most often when blood is obtained by heelstick.

B. **Dehydration.** Weight loss and decreased urine output are sensitive indicators of dehydration. Hemoconcentration secondary to dehydration is suspected if more than than 8–10% of the birth weight has been lost. It usually occurs in the second or third day of life.

C. **True polycythemia**

1. **Placental transfusion** occurs with delayed cord clamping, twin-twin transfusion, or fetomaternal transfusion.

2. **Iatrogenic.** Too much blood was transfused.

3. **Intrauterine hypoxia** may be caused by placental insufficiency. It may be seen in postmature or small-for-gestational-age (SGA) infants, preeclampsia-eclampsia, and with maternal use of the drug propranolol. Maternal smoking and severe maternal heart disease may also cause intrauterine hypoxia.

4. **Other causes**

a. Infant of diabetic mother.

b. Chromosomal abnormalities such as Down's syndrome and trisomies 13 and 18.

c. Beckwith-Wiedemann syndrome.

d. Neonatal thyrotoxicosis.

e. Congenital adrenal hyperplasia.

IV. **Data base**

A. **Physical examination.** Evaluate for possible dehydration. The mucous membranes will be dry. Increased skin turgor is usually not seen. True polycythemia is often, but not always, associated with visible skin changes, Ruddiness, plethora, or "pink on blue" or "blue on pink" coloration may be present. In males, priapism may be seen secondary to sludging of red blood cells. Clinical signs are listed on page 241, **II.C.**

B. **Laboratory studies**

1. **A central hematocrit value** must be obtained.

2. **The serum glucose level** should be checked because hypoglycemia is commonly seen with polycythemia.

3. **Serum bilirubin level.** Infants with polycythemia have problems with hyperbilirubinemia because of the increased turnover of red blood cells.

4. **Serum sodium and blood urea nitrogen levels.** These levels should be obtained if dehydration is being considered. They are usually high, or higher than baseline values, if dehydration is present.

5. **Urine specific gravity.** A high specific gravity (> 1.015) is usually seen with dehydration.

6. **Blood gas levels.** Blood gas levels should be obtained to rule out inadequate oxygenation.

7. **Serum platelet count.** Thrombocytopenia can be seen.

8. **Serum calcium level.** Hypocalcemia can also be seen.

C. **Radiologic and other studies.** These studies are usually not indicated.

V. **Plan**

A. **Falsely elevated hematocrit (> 65%).** If the confirmatory central hematocrit is normal, no further evaluation is needed. If the central hematocrit is high, either dehydration or true polycythemia is present (see **B** and **C** below for treatment).

B. **Hemoconcentration secondary to dehydration.** If the infant is dehydrated and does not have symptoms or signs of polycythemia, a trial of rehydration over 6–8 hours can be attempted. The type of fluid used depends on the infant's age and serum electrolyte status and is discussed in Chapter 7. Usually 130–150 mL/kg/d is given. The hematocrit is checked every 6 hours and usually decreases with adequate rehydration.

C. **True polycythemia**

1. **Central hematocrit of 65–70% in asymptomatic infant.** If the central hematocrit is 65–70% and the infant is asymptomatic, only observation may be needed. Many of these patients respond to increased fluid therapy; increases of 20–40 mL/kg/d can be attempted. The central hematocrit must be checked every 6 hours. The hematocrit normally reaches a peak at 2–4 hours of age. If the hematocrit is 70% at birth, it may be 5–10% higher at 2–4 hours of age.

2. **Central hematocrit greater than 65% in symptomatic infant.** Partial exchange transfusion should be given. To calculate the volume of Plasmanate that must be exchanged, use the following formula (blood volume = 80 mL/kg).

$$\text{Volume exchanged} = \frac{(\text{Weight [kg]} \times \text{Blood volume}) \times (\text{Hct of patient} - \text{Desired Hct})}{\text{Hct of patient}}$$

Partial exchange transfusion may be administered via a low or high umbilical venous catheter (*care must be taken not to place it in the liver,* see page 165 for the technique). A low umbilical artery catheter may also be used. The fluid that can be used for a partial exchange transfusion in Plasmanate, 5% albumin, normal saline, or fresh-frozen plasma (FFP). FFP is usually not recommended because of the risk of HIV transmission. The decision about which fluid to use depends on a particular institution's preference. The exchange transfusion procedure is discussed in detail in Chapter 19. Serial hematocrits should be obtained following transfusion.

3. **Central hematocrit greater than 70% in aymptomatic infant.** Most neonatologists agree that partial exchange transfusion should be given, although some controversy still exists. Institutional guidelines should be followed.

D. **Infants who have a central hematocrit between 60–65% but symptoms of polycythemia.** If all other disease entities are ruled out, these infants may indeed by polycythemic and hyperviscous. In these cases, management is *controversial.* Use clinical judgment and institutional guidelines to decide whether or not this infant should have a partial exchange tranfusion.

48 Poor Perfusion

I. **Problem.** You receive a report an infant "doesn't look good," looks "mottled" or "washed out," or "perfusion is poor."

II. **Immediate questions**

  A. **What is the age of the infant?** Hypoplastic left heart syndrome may cause poor perfusion and a mottled appearance. It may be seen at days 1–21 of life (more commonly, day 2 or 3). In an infant less than 3 days old, sepsis may be a cause. Associated risk factors are premature rupture of the membranes or maternal infection and fever.

  B. **Are congenital anomalies present?** Persistent cutis marmorata may be seen in de Lange syndrome and trisomies 18 and 21.

  C. **What are the vital signs?** If the temperature is lower than normal, cold stress or hypothermia associated with sepsis may be present. Hypotension may cause poor perfusion (see normal blood pressure values in Appendix C). Decreased urine output (< 2 mL/kg/h) may indicate depleted intravascular volume or shock.

  D. **Is the liver enlarged and are metabolic acidosis, a poor peripheral pulse rate, and gallop present?** These problems are signs of failure of the left side of the heart **(such as hypoplastic left heart syndrome).** Poor perfusion occurs because of reduced blood flow to the skin.

  E. **If mechanical ventilation is being used, are chest movements adequate and are blood gas levels improving?** Inadequate ventilation can result in poor perfusion. Pneumothorax may also be a cause.

III. **Differential diagnosis**

  A. **Sepsis.**

  B. **Cold Stress** (in general, a skin temperature < 36.5 °C).

  C. **Hypotension, usually with shock.**

  D. **Hypoventilation.**

  E. **Pneumothorax.**

  F. **Necrotizing enterocolitis.**

  G. **Left-sided heart lesions** such as hypoplastic left heart syndrome, coarctation of the aorta, and aortic stenosis.

  H. **Cutis marmorata,** a marbling pattern of the skin (infant appears poorly perfused), may occur in a normal infant, especially when it is exposed to cold stress. Persistent cutis marmorata may be seen in de Lange syndrome and trisomies 18 (Edwards' syndrome) and 21 (Down's syndrome).

IV. **Data base**

  A. **Physical examination.** Note temperature and vital signs. Look for signs of sepsis. The cardiovascular and pulmonary examinations are important because they may suggest cardiac problems or pneumothorax. Signs of trisomy 18 include micrognathia and overlapping digits; signs of trisomy 21 include single palmar transverse crease and epicanthal folds.

  B. **Laboratory studies**

   1. **CBC and differential.** These studies suggest the presence of sepsis or decreased hematocrit.

   2. **Blood gas levels.** These studies reveal inadequate ventilation or the presence of acidosis, which may be seen in sepsis or necrotizing enterocolitis.

   3. **Cultures.** If sepsis is suspected, a complete workup should be considered, especially if antibiotics are to be started. This workup includes cultures of blood, urine, and spinal fluid (if indicated).

C. **Radiologic and other studies**

1. **Transillumination of the chest.** This study can be performed quickly to help determine whether or not pneumothorax is present (see p 238).

2. **Chest x-ray study.** A chest x-ray study should be obtained if pneumonia, pneumothorax, congenital heart lesion, or hypoventilation is suspected. In left-sided heart lesions, the x-ray film shows cardiomegaly with pulmonary venous congestion (except in hypoplastic left heart syndrome, when the size of the heart may be normal). If a view taken during lung expansion shows that the lungs are down only to the sixth rib or less, hypoventilation should be considered. With hyperventilation, lung expansion will be down to the ninth or tenth rib.

3. **Abdominal x-ray study.** A flat-plate x-ray film of the abdomen should be obtained if necrotizing enterocolitis is suspected.

4. **Echocardiography** should be performed if a congenital heart lesion is suspected. In hypoplastic left heart syndrome, a large right ventricle and a small left ventricle is seen on the echocardiogram, and there is failure to visualize the mitral or aortic valve. In aortic stenosis, the echocardiogram reveals a deformed aortic valve. In coarctation of the aorta, it reveals decreased aortic diameter.

5. **Karyotyping** is performed if trisomy 18 or 21 is suspected.

V. **Plan**

A. **General plan.** A quick workup should be performed initially. While checking vital signs and quickly examining the patient, order stat blood gas levels and a chest x-ray study. Initiate oxygen supplementation. Transillumination of the chest may need to be done if a pneumothorax is suspected.

B. **Specific plans**

1. **Sepsis.** If sepsis is suspected, a sepsis workup is indicated. Empiric antibiotic therapy may be started at the discretion of the physician.

2. **Cold stress.** Gradual rewarming is necessary, usually at a rate of no more than 1 °C per hour. It can be accomplished by means of a radiant warmer or incubator, or heating pad. (See also Chap 5.)

3. **Hypotension/shock.** If the blood pressure is low because of depleted intravascular volume, give colloid, 10 mL/kg IV 5–10 rnin. See Chap 42.

4. **Hypoventilation.** If hypoventilation is suspected, it may be necessary to increase the pressure being given by the ventilator. The amount of pressure must be decided on an individual basis. One method is to increase the pressure by 2–4 cm water and then obtain blood gas levels in 20 minutes. Another method is to use bag-and-mask ventilation, observing the manometer to determine the amount of pressure needed to move the chest.

5. **Pneumothorax.** (See Chap 46.)

6. **Necrotizing enterocolitis.** (See Chap 64.)

7. **Left-sided heart lesions.** Treat with oxygen, possibly diuretics and digoxin if congestive heart failure is present, and infusion of prostaglandin E_1. Surgery is usually indicated in all these patients except those with hypoplastic left heart syndrome, for whom it is *controversial*. A full discussion of cardiac abnormalities in located in Chapter 55.

8. **Cutis marmorata.** If this condition has occurred secondary to cold stress, treat the patient as described in 2, above. If the condition persists, consider formal karyotyping to rule out trisomies 18 and 21.

49 Premature Rupture of Membranes

I. **Problem.** A newborn whose mother had premature rupture of the membranes is admitted to the nursery. Should a sepsis workup be done and should antibiotics be started?

II. **Immediate questions**

A. **How long before delivery did the membranes rupture?** Rupture of the membranes occurring 24–48 hours before delivery is associated with an increased incidence of neonatal sepsis. If the rupture occurs 24 hours or less before delivery, there is no increased risk.

B. **Did the mother show signs of infection?** Fever, urinary tract infection, chorioamnionitis, pneumonia, or sepsis in the mother increase the risk of sepsis in the infant.

C. **Are signs of sepsis present in the infant?** Signs of sepsis include apnea and bradycardia, temperature instability (hypothermia or hyperthermia), feeding intolerance, tachypnea, jaundice, cyanosis, poor peripheral perfusion, hypoglycemia, lethargy, poor sucking reflex, increased gastric aspirates and irritability. Other signs include: tachycardia, shock, vomiting, seizures, abnormal rash, abdominal distention, and hepatomegaly.

D. **Was the infant monitored during labor?** Fetal tachycardia (greater than 160 beats/min), especially sustained, and decelerations (usually late) can be associated with neonatal infection. A biophysical profile score of less than 6 (see Table 1–1, p 1) can be associated with an increased incidence of infection.

E. **Are there any neonatal risks for infection?** Prematurity, male sex, twin birth, and low apgar scores (less than 5 at 5 minutes) are all associated with an increased incidence of infection in the infant. Low birth weight is the most hazardous risk for infection.

F. **Did the mother have a cerclage for cervical incompetence?** Presence of a cerclage increases the risk of infection in the infant.

III. **Differential diagnosis**

A. **Sepsis.** The patient is manifesting clinical signs of sepsis as noted above.

B. **Infant at increased risk for sepsis.** There are definitive signs of maternal infection, but the newborn is not clinically infected.

C. **Infant at low risk for sepsis.** PROM may have ocurred without any sign of maternal or newborn infection.

IV. **Data base**

A. **Physical examination.** Perform a complete physical examination, looking for signs of sepsis (see **II.C,** above). Maternal clinical exam should be reviewed with the OB/GYN service.

B. **Laboratory studies**

1. **Complete blood count and platelet count.** *An abnormally low or high white blood cell count is worrisome. Values less than 6000/* μL *or greater* than 30,000/μL in the first 24 hours of life are abnormal. A band neutrophil count greater than 20% is abnormal. A normal white blood cell count does not rule out sepsis. The total neutrophil count can be calculated and plotted on the White Cell Count Graph in Appendix L.

2. **Peripheral blood cultures.** Resin bottles should be used for antibiotic removal if the mother has been receiving antibiotics.

3. **Suprapubic aspiration of urine for urinalysis and culture** (*controversial*). Many institutions do not insist on this procedure in newborn infants with pos-

sible sepsis on day 1 of life, because newborns rarely present with urinary tract infection in the first day.

4. **Maternal endocervical culture.** Requested from obstetric service, this may help guide therapy. Standard cultures include gonococcal, chlamydia, and group-B strep.
5. **Arterial blood gas levels.**
6. **Baseline bilirubin and serum glucose levels.**
7. **Specialized "scoring" tests** as noted in **V.A.1.** below.

C. **Radiologic and other studies**
   1. **Chest x-ray study.** If there are signs of respiratory infection, obtain a chest x-ray film to rule out pneumonia.
   2. **Lumbar puncture** for cerebrospinal fluid examination is indicated if a decision is made to give antibiotics. This measure is *controversial*—some institutions perform a lumbar puncture only if the infant has signs of CNS infection.

V. **Plan**
   A. **General measures.** For the majority of cases, a decision about whether an infant requires a sepsis workup and antibiotics is usually straightforward. These infants are either clinically sick or have such a positive history of an increased risk for sepsis and some clinical signs of sepsis that the decision is easily made. However, if an infant does not have a clear-cut history and clinical presentation, the decision is difficult. Once the decision is made to treat the infant, treatment usually involves 3 days of antibiotics after obtaining cultures. The following guidelines can be used to help make the decision to treat.
      1. **Use of scoring systems.** Some institutions have devised their own septic scoring systems to help decide which infants should be treated. Listed below are 2 representative scoring systems.
         a. **Five tests whose results are available in less than 1 hour are used.** If 2 or more of these 5 tests are positive, the score is positive and the infant should receive a septic workup and antibiotics.
            (1) Total white blood count less than 5000/mm^3.
            (2) Immature neutrophils (bands) divided by total neutrophils $\geq$ 0.2.
            (3) Latex C-reactive protein positive.
            (4) Latex haptoglobin positive.
            (5) Mini-erythroctye sedimentation rate > 15 mm/h.
         b. The second scoring system includes 7 findings with a score of 1 for each; a total score of greater than or equal to 3 identifies a high-risk infant. In such cases, a workup should be done and antibiotics started.
            (1) Abnormal white blood count (< 5000/μL or > 25,000/μL at birth, > 30,000/μL at 12–24 hours of age, > 21,000/μL at 2 days of age or more).
            (2) Abnormal total neutrophil count (see Appendix L).
            (3) Elevated immature PMN (band) count (see Appendix L).
            (4) Elevated immature to total PMN ratio (see Appendix L).
            (5) Immature to mature PMN ratio > 0.3.
            (6) Platelet count < 150,000 mm^3
            (7) Degenerative changes in PMNs (> +3 for vacuolization, toxic granulation, or Dohle's bodies when quantified on 0 to 4+ scale).
      2. **If no septic scoring system is used,** a few general guidelines can be followed when deciding whether or not to treat the infant.
         a. **Send culture specimens to the laboratory and initiate empiric antibiotic therapy:**
            (1) If symptoms of infection are present, regardless of the history or laboratory value results.
            (2) If the white blood count is obtained and shows neutropenia.
            (3) If there is documented sepsis in the mother and she is receiving antibiotics.

    (4) If the membranes ruptured more than 48 hours before delivery and there is evidence of infection in the mother.

    (5) If the membranes ruptured 24–48 hours before delivery and the mother is asymptomatic, obtain a white blood count on the infant. If the count is abnormal, if the infant is symptomatic, or if there are perinatal risk factors for infection, obtain cultures and begin antibiotics.

  b. Observe the infant:

    (1) If the white blood cell count is elevated and the infant has no clinical signs of sepsis. However, a repeat white blood count must be obtained in 4–6 hours. The infant must be *closely* observed for any changes in clinical status.

    (2) If the membranes ruptured less than 24 hours before delivery and the mother is afebrile or is not receiving antibiotics and is doing well.

    (3) If the membranes ruptured more than 24 hours before delivery and the mother is asymptomatic, obtain a white blood count on the infant. If the count is normal, observe the infant.

B. Specific therapy

  1. If the decision is to treat

    a. Obtain cultures of the blood, urine, and spinal fluid (cultures of urine and spinal fluid are *controversial*).

    b. Ampicillin and gentamicin are the antibiotics most commonly used for empiric initial therapy in a newborn. (See Chap 73 for specific dosages and other pharmacologic information.)

  2. Discontinuing antibiotics is another *controversial* topic. The following guidelines may be used.

    a. If the cultures are negative and the patient is doing well, antibiotics are usually stopped after 3 days.

    b. If the cultures are negative but the infant had signs of sepsis, some clinicians treat the infant for 5–10 days.

    c. If the cultures are positive, treat accordingly (see Chap 73 for specific antibiotic agents, dosages, and other pharmacologic information).

50 Pulmonary Hemorrhage

I. **Problem.** Gross bleeding is seen in the endotracheal tube.

II. **Immediate questions**

   A. **Are any other signs or symptoms abnormal?** Typically, an infant with pulmonary hemorrhage is a low birth weight infant, 2–4 days old, who suddenly develops pallor, shock, apnea, bradycardia, and cyanosis. The infant is usually on the ventilator and has a sudden deterioration in respiratory status.

   B. **Is the infant hypoxic? Has a blood transfusion recently been given?** Hypoxia or hypervolemia (usually caused by overtransfusion) may cause an acute rise in the pulmonary capillary pressure and lead to pulmonary hemorrhage.

   C. **Is bleeding occurring from other sites?** If there is bleeding from multiple sites, coagulopathy may be present, and coagulation studies should be obtained. Volume replacement with colloid or blood may be needed.

   D. **What is the hematocrit of the blood?** If the hematocrit is the same as the venous hematocrit, it represents a true hemorrhage and the blood is usually from trauma, aspiration of maternal blood, or bleeding diathesis. If the Hct is between 5–10%, the bleeding probably represents hemorrhagic edema fluid. This is seen with the majority of cases of pulmonary hemorrhage (such as secondary to PDA, surfactant therapy, left heart failure, seen with the rest below).

III. **Differential diagnosis**

   A. **Direct trauma. Trauma to the airway** is usually due to nasogastric or endotracheal intubation. Vigorous suctioning can also cause trauma to tissues and bleeding. Trauma during chest tube insertion can cause hemorrhage.

   B. **Aspiration of gastric or maternal blood** is often seen following cesarean section. The majority of blood is usually obtained from the nasogastric tube, but blood may be seen in the endotracheal tube.

   C. **Coagulopathy.** May be related to sepsis or congenital.

   D. **Other disorders associated with pulmonary hemorrhage**

   1. **Hypoxia.**
   2. **Hypervolemia** is often the result of overtransfusion.
   3. **Congestive heart failure** (especially in pulmonary edema caused by patent ductus arteriosus).
   4. **Respiratory distress syndrome.**
   5. **Severe Rh incompatibility.**
   6. **Pneumonia.**
   7. **Hemorrhagic disease of the newborn** resulting from failure to administer vitamin K.
   8. **IUGR.**
   9. **Severe hypothermia.**
   10. **Surfactant administration.** Pulmonary hemorrhage has occurred within hours of surfactant therapy. The etiology is not definite but may be that the improved oxygenation of blood causes hemorrhagic pulmonary edema.
   11. **Mechanical ventilation.**

IV. **Data base**

   A. **Physical examination.** Note the presence of other bleeding sites, signs of pneumonia or other infection, or congestive heart failure.

   B. **Laboratory studies**

   1. **Complete blood count with differential and platelet count.** With pneumonia or other infection, results of these studies may be abnormal.

Thrombocytopenia may be seen. The hematocrit should be checked to determine whether excessive blood loss has occurred.

2. **Coagulation profile (prothrombin time [PT], partial thromboplastin time [PTT], thrombin time [TT], and fibrinogen level)** may reveal coagulation disorders.

3. **Arterial blood gas levels** will detect hypoxia.

4. **Apt test** if aspiration of maternal blood is suspected.

C. **Radiologic and other studies.** A chest x-ray study will rule out pneumonia, respiratory distress syndrome, and congestive heart failure. With massive pulmonary hemorrhage, the chest x-ray film shows a complete white-out.

V. Plan

A. **General measures**

1. **Support blood pressure** with volume expansion and colloids (see p 228, **B.1.a**).

2. **Treat the underlying cause.** The following measures may help to stop the bleeding.

   a. If mechanical ventilation is being used when the bleeding begins:

      (1) Increase the positive end-expiratory pressure (PEEP) to 4–8 cm water; it may cause tamponade of the capillaries.

      (2) Consider giving epinephrine through an endotracheal tube (*controversial*). This may cause constriction of the pulmonary capillaries.

   b. If mechanical ventilation is not being used, consider initiating its use in providing the treatments outlined in **a,** above.

B. **Specific therapy**

1. **Direct nasogastric or endotracheal trauma.** If there is significant bleeding immediately after an endotracheal or nasogastric intubation, trauma is the most likely cause; surgical consultation is indicated.

2. **Aspiration of maternal blood.** If the infant is stable, no treatment is needed, since the condition is typically self-limited.

3. **Coagulopathy**

   a. **Hemorrhagic disease of the newborn.** Vitamin K, 1 mg intravenously, should be given.

   b. **Other coagulopathies.** Fresh frozen plasma, 10 mL/kg every 12–24 hours, may be given. If the platelet count is low, give 1 unit/5 kg. Monitor the thrombin time (TT), partial thromboplastin time (PTT), platelet count, and fibrinogen level.

51 Seizure Activity

I. **Problem.** The nurse reports that an infant is having abnormal movements of the extremities consistent with seizure activity.

II. **Immediate questions**

A. **Is the infant really seizing?** This question is very important and is often initially difficult to answer. **Jitteriness** is sometimes confused with seizures. In a jittery infant, eye movements are normal. The hands will stop moving if they are grasped, and movements are of a fine nature. In an infant who is seizing, eye movements can be abnormal (staring, blinking, nystagmoid jerks, or tonic horizontal eye deviation). The hands continue to move if grasped, and movements are of a coarser nature. The EEG is normal with jitteriness and abnormal with seizure activity.

B. **Is there a history of birth asphyxia or risk factors for sepsis?** Asphyxia and sepsis with meningitis may cause neonatal seizures.

C. **What is the blood glucose level?** Hypoglycemia is an easily treatable cause of seizures in the neonatal period.

D. **How old is the infant?** The age of the infant is often the best clue to the cause of the seizures. Common causes for specific ages are given below.

1. **At birth.** Maternal anesthetic agents.

2. **Day 1.** Metabolic abnormalities such as hypoglycemia, hypocalcemia, hypoxic-ischemic encephalopathy (presenting at 6–18 hours after birth and getting more severe in the next 24–48 hours).

3. **Days 2–3.** Drug withdrawal, meningitis.

4. **Day 5 or greater.** Hypocalcemia, TORCH infections, developmental defects.

5. **More than 1–2 weeks.** Methadone withdrawal.

III. **Differential diagnosis.** (See also Chap 65.)

A. **Seizure activity** may be secondary to the following conditions.

1. **Hypoxic ischemic injury.**

2. **Intracranial hemorrhage** including subarachnoid, periventricular-intraventricular, or subdural.

3. **Metabolic abnormality**

a. **Hypoglycemia.**

b. **Hypocalcemia or hypercalcemia.**

c. **Hypomagnesemia.**

d. **Hyponatremia or hypernatremia.**

e. **Pyridoxine dependence.**

4. **Infection**

a. **Meningitis.**

b. **Sepsis.**

c. **TORCH infections.**

5. **Neonatal drug withdrawal** discussed in Chapter 57.

6. **Inborn errors of metabolism** (see also Chap 59).

a. Maple syrup urine disease.

b. Methylmalonic acidemia.

c. Nonketotic hyperglycinemia.

7. **Maternal anesthetic agents.** If mepivacaine is accidentally injected into the infant, seizures can occur at birth.

8. **Drug toxicity.** Agents such as theophylline.

9. **Developmental abnormalities.** Cerebral malformations can cause sei-

zures. Often, the infant will have obvious anomalies of the face or head if developmental abnormalities are present.

10. CNS trauma. Usually there is a history of a difficult delivery.

11. Hydrocephalus. 20% of infants with periventricular or intraventricular hemorrhage will develop posthemorrhagic hydrocephalus.

12. Polycythemia with hyperviscosity.

B. Jitteriness. This benign condition is differentiated from seizures as described in **II.A,** p 250.

C. Benign myoclonic activity. These isolated jerky, nonrepetitive movements of an extremity or other part of the body occur mainly during sleep and are benign.

IV. Data base

A. History. A detailed history will help in diagnosing seizure activity. The nurse or physician observing the activity should record a complete description of the event on the chart.

B. Physical examination. Perform a complete physical examination, with close attention to the neurologic status.

C. Laboratory studies

1. Metabolic workup

a. Serum glucose level. If the glucose level on paper-strip testing is less than 25 mg/dL, obtain a serum glucose value from the laboratory.

b. Serum sodium level.

c. Serum ionized and total calcium levels. Only an ionized calcium level is usually necessary, but if that test cannot be done, a total calcium study should be ordered. Ionized calcium is the most accurate measurement of calcium.

d. Serum magnesium level.

2. Infection workup

a. Complete blood count and differential. A hematocrit will also rule out polycythemia.

b. Blood, urine, and CSF cultures.

c. Serum IgM- and IgM-specific TORCH titers. The serum IgM titer may be elevated in TORCH infections.

3. Urine drug screening if drug withdrawal is suspected.

4. Theophylline level if the infant is on this medication and toxicity is suspected.

5. Blood gas levels to rule out hypoxia or acidosis.

D. Radiologic and other studies

1. Ultrasound examination of the head will confirm periventricular-intraventricular hemorrhage (PV-IVH). (**Note:** the coexistence of IVH and seizures does not necessarily mean they are related.)

2. CT scan of the head. A CT scan can be done to diagnose subarachnoid or subdural hemorrhage. It may also reveal a congenital malformation.

3. Lumbar puncture. The presence of blood in the cerebrospinal fluid suggests intraventricular hemorrhage. Cultures of the fluid should be done to diagnose infection. (See Chap 22.)

4. Electroencephalography. It is usually not possible to perform electroencephalography during the episode of seizure activity. This study should be done at some time after seizure activity has been documented. It may confirm seizure activity and may also be used as a baseline study.

V. Plan

A. General measures. Once it is determined that the infant is having seizures, because the other two diagnoses (jitteriness and benign myoclonic activity) are benign conditions, the following measures should be taken. Immediate management is necessary.

1. Rule out hypoxia. Send a blood sample to the laboratory for measurement of blood gases and start oxygen therapy. Assess the infant's airway and breathing. Intubation and mechanical ventilation may be necessary to maintain ventilation and oxygenation. Correct any metabolic acidosis.

2. **Check glucose level.** A **Dextrostix or Chemstrip-bG paper strip test** should be done to rule out hypoglycemia. Also, send a blood sample to the laboratory for a stat serum glucose level for confirmation of the paper-strip test result. If the paper-strip test shows low blood glucose, it is acceptable to give 10% glucose, 2–4 mL/kg intravenous push before obtaining results from the laboratory.

3. **Obtain stat serum calcium and sodium levels.** If these levels were low on earlier values and a metabolic disorder is strongly suspected to be the cause of the seizures, it is acceptable to go ahead and treat the infant before new laboratory values are available.

4. **Anticonvulsant therapy.** If hypoxia and all metabolic abnormalities have been treated or if blood gas and metabolic workup values are normal, start anticonvulsant therapy. See Chapter 73 for detailed pharmacologic information.

   a. **Give phenobarbital as the first-line drug.** Initially 20/mg/kg is given as the loading dose, but up to 40/mg/kg can be given if the seizures have not stopped.

   b. **If seizures persist,** give phenytoin (Dilantin) at 20 mg/kg/dose.

   c. **If seizures still persist,** the following drugs may be used: paraldehyde, lorazepam, or diazepam, depending on institutional preference. If a benodiazepam is used, respiratory depression is more likely to occur, but this is usually not a problem because most infants are already on mechanical ventilation.

B. **Specific measures**

1. **Hypoxic ischemic injury.** Seizures secondary to birth asphyxia usually present anywhere from 6 to 18 hours of age.

   a. Careful observation by the physician and nursing staff are required to detect seizure activity.

   b. Prophylactic phenobarbital is used at some institutions (*controversial*).

   c. Restrict fluids to approximately 60 mL/kg/d.

   d. If seizures begin, follow guidelines given in **A.4,** above.

2. **Hypoglycemia.** Treat and determine the cause, as outlined in Chapter 39.

3. **Hypocalcemia.** Slowly give 100–200 mg/kg calcium gluconate intravenously. Make certain the infant is receiving maintenance calcium therapy (usually 50 mg/kg every 6 hours). Monitor the heart rate continuously and make certain that the intravenous line is correctly positioned.

4. **Hypomagnesemia.** Give 0.2 meq/kg magnesium sulfate intravenously every 6 hours until magnesium levels are normal or symptoms resolve.

5. **Hyponatremia.** See Chapter 41.

6. **Hypernatremia.** Treat the seizure activity as described in **A.4,** above. If hypernatremia is secondary to decreased fluid intake, increase the rate of free water. The amount of sodium needs to be decreased; it should be reduced over 48 hours to decrease the possibility of cerebral edema.

7. **Hypercalcemia.** Usual treatment plans include:

   a. Increase intravenous fluids by 20 mL/kg/d.

   b. Administer a diuretic, eg, furosemide (Lasix), 1–2 mg/kg/dose every 12 hours.

   c. Administer phosphate, 30–40 mg/kg/d orally or intravenously.

8. **Pyridoxine dependence.** Pyridoxine, 50–100 mg, is given intravenously. If the seizures stop immediately, it is diagnostic.

9. **Infection.** If sepsis is suspected, a complete workup should be performed and empiric broad-spectrum antibiotic therapy started. A complete septic workup includes white blood count and differential, blood culture, urine and serum antigen test (Wellcogen), lumbar puncture (if indicated), and urinalysis and urine culture (if indicated).

10. **Drug withdrawal syndrome.** Supportive therapy and anticonvulsants are used. See Chapter 57.

11. **Subarachnoid hemorrhage.** Only supportive therapy is necessary.

12. **Subdural hemorrhage.** Only supportive therapy is necessary unless the infant has lacerations of the falx and tentorium or hemorrhage over cerebral convexities. Rapid surgical correction is necessary for lacerations of the falx and tentorium. Hemorrhage over cerebral convexities is treated by repeated subdural taps.
13. **CNS trauma.** If depressed skull fracture, elevation of the bone may be necessary.
14. **Hydrocephalus.** Repeated lumbar taps may be necessary or a shunt placed.
15. **Polycythemia.** Partial plasma exchange is necessary. See Chap 19.

52 Vasospasm of Leg

I. **Problem.** An infant with an indwelling umbilical artery catheter develops vasospasm in one leg.

II. **Immediate questions**

A. **Can the umbilical artery catheter be removed?** Evaluate the need for the catheter. If the catheter can be removed, this is the treatment of choice. **Vasospasm is most commonly related to the use of umbilical artery catheters.**

B. **Was a medication given recently through the catheter?** The majority of medications, if given too rapidly, can cause vasospasm.

III. **Differential diagnosis**

A. **Vasospasm.** Vasospasm is a muscular contraction of a vessel, manifested by acute color change (white or blue) in the lower extremity, sometimes only on the toes, sometimes over the entire extremity. Occasionally the color change extends to the buttocks and abdomen. The change in color may be transient or persistent. It may be caused by prior injection of medication or a thromboembolic phenomenon.

B. **Thromboembolic phenomenon.** A **thrombus** is a clot formation at a specific site in a vessel. It can cause complete obstruction, resulting in loss of pulses and an extremity that is white. An **embolus** is a clot that lodges in a blood vessel and may cause obstruction or vasospasm.

IV. **Data base**

A. **Physical examination.** The severity of the vasospasm must be assessed, as it dictates treatment. The areas on involvement, appearance of the skin over the involved areas, and pulses of the affected extremity are measures of severity.

1. **Severe vasospasm** involves a large area of one or both legs, the abdomen, or the buttocks. The skin may be completely white. Pulses of the affected extremity are present.

2. **Less severe vasospasm** involves a small area of one or both legs (usually some of the toes and part of the foot). The skin has a mottled appearance. Pulses of the affected extremity are present.

3. **Thrombosis.** If pulses are absent, thrombosis (a **medical emergency**) is likely.

B. **Laboratory studies.** Laboratory tests are not usually needed. However, the following laboratory tests should be obtained if thrombosis is suspected and streptokinase is to be used.

1. **Thrombin time (TT).**
2. **Activated partial thromboplastin time (PTT).**
3. **Prothrombin time (PT).**
4. **Hematocrit.**
5. **Platelet count.**

C. **Radiologic and other studies**

1. **Real-time ultrasonography** with or without color doppler flow imaging can be used to diagnose thrombosis.

2. **Angiography** performed through the umbilical artery catheter can be used to diagnose aorto-iliac thrombosis. (In one study, this procedure was found to be the most effective diagnostic technique).

3. **An x-ray study of the abdomen** should be done to determine catheter placement.

V. Plan

A. Vasospasm. (***Note:*** Treatment is highly *controversial* and guidelines vary extensively. Check with your institution's guidelines prior to initiating treatment.)

1. Severe vasospasm

   a. If possible, remove the catheter. The vasospasm should then resolve spontaneously.

   b. Tolazoline (Priscoline), 0.1 mg/mL by continuous infusion at a rate of 0.25 mg/kg/h, until the catheter is removed. This dosage was used in one series of 3 cases with success.

   c. Tolazoline, 0.1 mg/h through the catheter as a continuous infusion for 3–4 hours. If the vasospasm resolves, the infusion may be stopped. If the vasospasm does not resolve, remove the catheter. *This treatment is highly controversial!*

2. Less severe vasospasm

   a. Conservative. Wrap the entire *unaffected* leg in a warm—not hot— washcloth. This measure will cause reflex vasodilation of the vessels in the affected leg, and the vasospasm may resolve. Alternatively, immerse the affected leg in a sterilized container filled with warm water (*controversial*). A possible side effect of this method is increased oxygen consumption in the extremity. With either method, treatment should continue for 15–30 minutes before a beneficial effect will be seen.

   b. Papaverine. If the above treatment does not work, give papaverine hydrochloride, 1 mg intramuscularly, in the unaffected leg (*controversial*). Papaverine is a mild vasodilator; if it is going to work, the effect is usually apparent within 30 minutes.

   c. Tolazoline. If both of the above treatments fail, tolazoline may be given as described above in **1.b,c** for severe vasospasm.

   d. Catheter removal. If all of the above treatments fail, it is best to remove the catheter.

B. Thromboembolic phenomenon. If thrombosis is suspected and there is loss of pulses in the affected extremity, it is a **medical emergency.** *Management is highly controversial.*

1. Don't remove the catheter. Leave the catheter in place to facilitate arteriography and streptokinase infusion, if needed.

2. Emergency consultation with a vascular surgeon is recommended.

3. Infusion of intra-arterial streptokinase has been successful in some infants. See p 508 for dosage and other pharmacologic information.

4. Immediate surgery may be indicated.

53 Ambiguous Genitalia

I. **Definition.** Ambiguous genitalia are present (1) when the sex of an infant is not readily apparent after examination of the external genitalia or (2) when a gender role cannot be assigned on the basis of the appearance of the external genitalia alone (eg, microphallus in an apparent male, labial gonads in an apparent female, or bifid penis and scrotum as part of exstrophy of the bladder).

II. **Embryology.** Sexual differentiation of the external genitalia begins at 6–8 weeks' gestation and is virtually complete by 16 weeks. Differentiation of the external genitalia depends solely on the presence or absence of **androgen.** Adequate androgen will cause the external genitalia to differentiate along male lines. Absence of androgen causes a division of the urogenital sinus into the urethra and vagina with no further differentiation.

   A. In the normal male, androgen production is determined by differentiation of the gonad as testes or ovary. Gonadal differentiation is determined primarily by the absence or presence of a single gene, now thought to be the **SRY** gene, on the **Y chromosome.** If the Y or SRY gene is present, the gonad will differentiate as a testis, and chorionic gonadotropin will drive it to produce and release **testosterone.** Testosterone is taken into the target-organ cells and converted there to **dihydrotestosterone,** the most potent of the androgens involved with sexual differentiation. At each step of this process, developmental or metabolic disorders may cause inadequate androgen production and incomplete male differentiation or pseudohermaphroditism.

   B. In the female fetus, where the Y chromosome and the SRY gene are absent, the gonad forms an ovary (even in 45,X Turner syndrome, a histologically normal ovary is present at birth). The ovary does not produce testosterone and female differentiation proceeds. Excessive androgen can mimic the effect of testosterone and dihydrotestosterone in the male, but the effect is usually partial, leading to phallic (clitoral) enlargement, incomplete fusion of the labioscrotal folds, and incomplete separation of the urethra and vagina.

III. **Pathophysiology**

   A. **Virilization of female infants**

      1. The **most common cause** of excess fetal androgen is an **enzymatic deficiency in the cortisol pathway** leading to excessive ACTH stimulation, adrenal hyperplasia, and excessive production of adrenal androgens (dihydroepiandrosterone and androstenedione) and testosterone (see Fig 53–1). Virilization is most commonly caused by **absence of the 21-hydroxylase enzyme.** Relative or absolute **aldosterone deficiency** is usually present, producing salt loss and subsequent shock. **11-Hydroxylase enzyme deficiency** is less common and is not associated with salt loss.

      2. **Other less common causes** are virilizing maternal or fetal tumors or inadvertent maternal androgen ingestion.

   B. **Inadequate virilization of male infants.** This problem is caused by inadequate androgen production or incomplete end-organ response to androgen. All of these abnormalities are uncommon, and most require extensive laboratory investigation before a final diagnosis can be confirmed.

      1. **Decreased androgen production** can be caused by one of 5 rare enzyme defects. Three of these defects also cause cortisol deficiency and **non-virilizing adrenal hyperplasia,** and 2 are specific to the testosterone pathway. The association of **micropenis** and **hypoglycemia** suggests **pituitary**

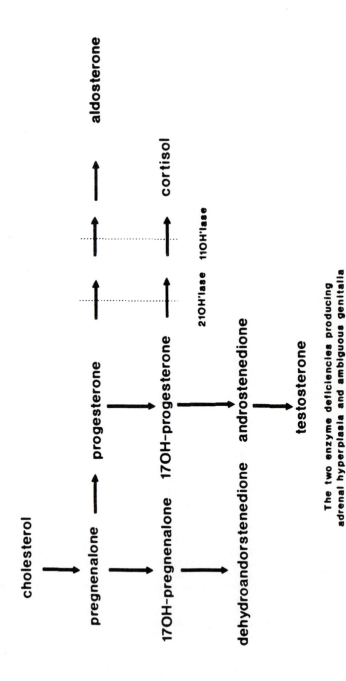

FIGURE 53–1. Adrenal metabolic pathways involved in virilization and ambiguous genitalia.

    deficiency with absence of gonadotropins, adrenocorticotropic hormone (ACTH), and/or growth hormone.

    2. Decreased end-organ response to androgen is often called **testicular feminization** and can be caused by a defect in the androgen receptor or an unknown defect with normal receptors. It can be total (labial testes with otherwise normal-appearing female genitalia) or partial (incomplete virilization of a male).

  C. True hermaphroditism. The presence of both testis and ovary (or ovotestes) in the same individual is a rare cause of ambiguous genitalia. Most individuals with true hermaphroditism have a 46,XX karyotype, but mosaics of 46,XX, 45,X, 46,XY, and multiple X/multiple Y have all been reported. The appearance of the genitalia is variable, but about three-fourths of these babies have adequate phallus size to be raised as males.

  D. Chromosome abnormalities do not usually lead to ambiguous genitalia.

    1. Turner syndrome (45,X chromosomes) and its variants do not cause an increase in androgen production, so differentiation of the genitalia is unambiguously female.

    2. Klinefelter syndrome (47,XXY) and its variants cause differentiation of the gonad as a testes followed by male differentiation of the external genitalia.

    3. Mixed gonadal dysgenesis, the presence of a normal or partially differentiated testis and an undifferentiated or streak gonad, is usually associated with 45,X/46,XY mosaicism and ambiguity of the external genitalia. Mixed gonadal dysgenesis is associated with a high incidence of gonadal malignancy in mid to late childhood, and it should be recognized and treated (with removal of the dysfunctional gonads) as early as possible to reduce the risk of future malignancy.

IV. Risk factors. Maternal ingestion or topical application of androgens and some progestational agents can cause sexual ambiguity in the fetus. Others causes are chromosomal, hormonal, or structural and can be sporadic or familial.

V. Clinical presentation. Ambiguous genitalia usually are noted immediately at birth, when the first person to see the infant cannot readily assign a sex to the child. Occasionally the abnormality of genital development is noted later when a careful examination discloses the presence of labial gonads (suggesting testes and testicular feminization) or a micropenis (usually defined as less than 2.0 cm in length, pubis to tip) or perineoscrotal hypospadius.

VI. Diagnosis

  A. Laboratory studies

    1. Chromosome analysis. Most laboratories can now determine sex chromosome status from a blood sample in 24–48 hours, and this is the most appropriate first test. Buccal smears provide a fast answer but are notoriously unreliable. The remainder of the diagnostic evaluation depends on the sex chromosome status; accuracy is paramount.

      a. Normal 46,XX karyotype. This finding implies virilization of a genetic female and is caused by excessive maternal or fetal androgen. If the mother is not virilized, the infant almost always has **virilizing adrenal hyperplasia.** To confirm the diagnosis, measure:

        (1) 17-hydroxyprogesterone (17-OHP). This is the immediate precursor to the enzyme defect in 21-hydroxylase enzyme deficiency and one step prior to that in 11-hydroxylase enzyme deficiency. In infants with either defect, the serum or plasma level of 17-OHP will be 100 to 1000 times the normal infant level.

        (2) Daily serum measurements of sodium and potassium. Infants with 21-hydroxylase enzyme deficiency will usually have relative or absolute aldosterone deficiency and will begin to demonstrate hyperkalemia at days 3–5 and hyponatremia a day or two later. If hyperkalemia becomes clinically significant before the 17-OHP result is available, begin treatment empirically with intravenous saline, cortisol, and Florinef, since the diagnosis is virtually certain (see p 261).

(3) **Serum testosterone.** About 3% of infants with ambiguous genitalia will be true hermaphrodites and most will have 46,XX chromosomes. If the 17-OHP is not elevated and there is no maternal virilization, elevated testosterone suggests hermaphroditism or fetal testosterone-producing tumor.

b. **Normal 46,XY karyotype.** The differential diagnosis of an **incompletely virilized genetic male** is extremely complex and includes in utero testicular damage, defects of testosterone synthesis, end-organ resistance, or an enzymatic defect in conversion of testosterone to dihydrotestosterone. The laboratory evaluation is correspondingly complex and usually proceeds through a number of steps before the results of the preceding step become available.

(1) **Testosterone (T) and dihydrotestosterone (DHT).** These hormone levels should be measurable and higher in newborns than later in childhood. The T:DHT ratio should be between 5:1 and 20:1 when expressed in similar units. High T:DHT ratio suggests 5_α-reductase deficiency.

(2) **Luteinizing hormone (LH) and follicle-stimulating hormone (FSH).** These hormones are also higher in infancy than they are in childhood. A diagnosis of gonadotropin deficiency is suspected if these values are low in a reliable assay but can be confirmed in infancy only if there are other pituitary hormone deficits. Remember, growth hormone and ACTH deficiency are manifested in the newborn period as hypoglycemia.

(3) **Human chorionic gonadotropin.** Human chorionic gonadotropin should be administered to stimulate further gonadal steroid production when testosterone values are low (as in gonadotropin deficiency or a defect in testosterone synthesis). HCG is often given empirically, before the basal steroid measurements have returned. Recommendations vary, but a dose of 500–1000 units every day or every other day for 3 doses is most common. Then measure T and DHT again to demonstrate adequate gonadal response. Particularly after HCG, it is wise to obtain enough blood to measure other steroid intermediates if the testosterone is low. In national reference laboratories, multiple steroid hormone measurements can be made on as little as four mL of blood. Be sure to ask the laboratory to freeze any remaining serum or plasma.

(4) **Testosterone.** Depo-Testosterone should be administered. The usual dose is 25 mg intramuscularly at 3–4 week intervals for 3 doses. This regimen is followed to demonstrate adequate growth of the phallus and is essential before a final decision is made to raise an ambiguous child as a male.

c. **Abnormal karyotype.** Mixed gonadal dysgenesis with a dysplastic gonad is the great risk for infants with abnormal karyotype and ambiguous genitalia. Hormone studies are likely to be unrevealing in this circumstance. Sex of rearing should be determined by the appearance of the external genitalia after consultation with a pediatric or urologic surgeon and detailed discussion with the family. Surgical exploration should be done before age 2 to look for dysplastic gonads and remove gonadal tissue incompatible with the sex of rearing.

B. **Radiographic studies.** Ultrasonography of the pelvis sometimes demonstrates the presence of a uterus. Contrast studies to outline the internal anatomy (sinography, urethrography, intravenous urography) should be done prior to any reconstructive surgery.

VII. **Management**

A. **General considerations.** The most important aspect of the treatment of ambiguous genitalia in an infant is to protect the privacy of the parents and child while diagnostic studies are in progress. Once a diagnosis has been established, gender identity can be unambiguously assigned and steroid replacement, gonadal removal, and reconstructive surgery can be started to make the appearance and function of the child fit the gender assignment.

B. Initial measures

   1. Early instructions for the parents. As soon as the abnormality is noted, a physician responsible for the infant should be identified and the parents should be informed. The family should be told their infant is generally healthy (if it is true) but that the genitalia are "incompletely developed" and that it is not possible, at present, to identify the sex of their child. It is best to use gender-nonspecific nouns such as baby, infant, or child rather than gender-specific pronouns such as he or she, him or her at this point to avoid showing your biases to the parents. All attempts to identify the sex of the child on the basis of appearance should be resisted, although there is likely to be great pressure to do so from parents, relatives, and professional personnel. It is important not to complete the birth certificate or make any reference to gender in any of the permanent medical records of mother or child.

   2. Isolation of the infant. The next objective should be to isolate the child from the inquiries of the community. *Tell the parents not to send out birth announcements and not to tell anyone outside the immediate family that the baby has been born until a gender assignment has been made.* Whatever the final gender assignment, the child will probably live the majority of its life in the community of birth, and confusion about gender assignment because of premature release of information will never be completely forgotten.

   3. Early referral. It is advisable to seek consultation from a specialist in the evaluation of children with ambiguous genitalia (usually an endocrinologist or geneticist) as soon as feasible. It is never acceptable to discharge a child from the nursery prior to detailed evaluation of the causes of ambiguous genitalia. In most cases, complete diagnosis, assignment of sex of rearing, and a plan for surgical reconstruction should be initiated before discharge to home.

C. Medical management. Most causes of ambiguous genitalia are not acute medical or surgical emergencies, and therapy is variable.

   1. Congenital adrenal hyperplasia. All forms of adrenal hyperplasia have absolute or relative cortisol deficiency and require early diagnosis and replacement therapy to prevent vascular collapse.

   a. Glucocorticoid therapy. Standard replacement therapy is **cortisone acetate,** 10–25 mg intramuscularly daily for 2–3 days followed by 37.5 mg/M^2 intramuscularly every 3 days. Oral hydrocortisone is erratically absorbed in infants but is the common agent for children after 6 months of age.

   b. Mineralocorticoid therapy. Deoxycorticosterone actetate (DOCA) is no longer being manufactured. **9$_\alpha$-Fluorocortisol (Florinef)** is the drug of choice. The usual dose is 0.05–0.1 mg orally daily. Most endocrinologists also give 15–20 meq oral sodium daily as 25% sodium chloride or 1 g table salt (about 1/4 tsp) added to the formula.

   2. Incompletely virilized genetic male. See p 259.

D. Gender assignment. Gender assignment is beyond the scope of this brief discussion, but in general, the sex of rearing should be determined only when the final diagnosis is secure. The decision is generally made primarily on the basis of external anatomy. If the phallic length is less than 2.0 cm, it is best to raise the child as a female, whatever the chromosomal and gonadal sex. In the very rare circumstances of 5$_\alpha$-reductase deficiency, or pituitary deficiency with concomitant growth hormone deficiency, the child may be raised as a male even with a very small phallus in infancy. In androgen resistance syndromes, the phallus may not enlarge with the increasing androgen levels of adolescence, and a final decision on the sex of rearing may have to await the results of a 2–3 month trial of testosterone therapy (see p 260). In any case, the decision must be made in conjunction with surgical colleagues and with the goal of appropriate sexual function, if not fertility, as an adult. The parents must have a complete understanding of the options, and achieving this understanding can be a very time-consuming process.

VIII. Prognosis. Morbidity and mortality are largely dependent on associated anomalies. Although most children with ambiguous genitalia are fertile as adults, in some cases the gonads are dysplastic or must be removed to prevent malignant degeneration or to allow normal functional development compatible with assigned sex of rearing. Despite gonadal dysfunction or absence, anyone with a normal uterus is now a candidate for pregnancy using the steadily advancing techniques of in vitro fertilization.

REFERENCES

Berkovitz GD: Abnormalities of gonadal determination and differentiation. *Semin Perinatol* **1992(5)**;289–98.

Charest NJ (ed): *Semin Perinatol* **1992(5)**;265–339. (entire issue on sexual differentiation and evaluation of ambiguous genitalia).

Griffin JE: Androgen resistance—the clinical and molecular spectrum. *N Engl J Med* **1992;326(9)**:611–18.

Grumbach MM, Conte FA: Disorders of sexual differentiation. Pages 853–951 in: *Williams Textbook of Endocrinology,* 8th ed. Wilson JD, Foster DW (eds). Saunders, 1992.

Josso N: Hormonal regulation of sexual differentiation *Semin Perinatol* **1992(5)**;279–88.

Kupfer SR, Quigley CA, French FA: Male Pseudohermaphroditism. *Semin Perinatol* **1992(5)**;319–31.

McGillivray BC: Genetic aspects of ambiguous genitalia. *Pediatr Clin North Am* **1992; 39(2)**:307–17.

Meyers-Seifer CH, Charest NJ: Diagnosis and management of patients with ambiguous genitalia. *Semin Perinatol* **1992(5)**;332–39.

Moore CCD, Grumbach MM: Sex determination and gonadogenesis: A transcription cascade of sex chromosome and autosome genes. *Semin Perinatol* **1992(5)**;266–78.

New MI: Female pseudohermaphroditism. *Semin Perinatol* **1992(5)**;299–318.

Stradtman EW Jr: Female gender reconstruction surgery for ambiguous genitalia in children and adolescents. *Curr Opin Obstet Gynecol* **1991;3(6)**:805–12.

54 Blood Abnormalities

ABO INCOMPATIBILITY

I. **Definition.** Isoimmune hemolytic anemia may result when ABO incompatibility occurs between the mother and the newborn infant. This disorder is most common with blood type A or B infants born to type O mothers. The hemolytic process begins in utero and is the result of active placental transport of maternal isoantibody. In type O mothers, isoantibody is predominantly 7S-IgG and is capable of crossing the placental membranes. Because of its larger size, the 19S-IgM isoantibody found in type A or type B mothers cannot cross. Symptomatic clinical disease, which usually does not present until after birth, is a compensated mild hemolytic anemia with reticulocytosis, microspherocytosis, and early-onset unconjugated hyperbilirubinemia.

II. **Incidence.** Risk factors for ABO incompatibility are present in 12–15% of pregnancies, but evidence of fetal sensitization (positive direct Coombs' test) occurs in only 3–4%. Symptomatic ABO hemolytic disease occurs in less than 1% of all newborn infants but accounts for approximately two-thirds of observed cases of hemolytic disease in the newborn.

III. **Pathophysiology.** Transplacental transport of maternal isoantibody results in an immune reaction with the A or B antigen on fetal erythrocytes, which produces characteristic **microspherocytes.** This process eventually results in complete extravascular hemolysis of the end-stage spherocyte. The ongoing hemolysis is balanced by compensatory reticulocytosis and shortening of the cell-cycle time, so that there is overall maintenance of the erythrocyte indices within physiologic limits. A paucity of A or B antigenic sites on the fetal (in contrast to the adult) erythrocytes and competitive binding of isoantibody by soft tissues may explain the often mild hemolytic process that occurs and the usual absence of progressive disease with subsequent pregnancies.

IV. **Risk factors**
  A. **A$_1$ antigen in infant.** Of the major blood group antigens, the A$_1$ antigen has the greatest antigenicity and is associated with a greater risk of symptomatic disease.
  B. **Elevated isohemagglutinins.** Antepartum intestinal parasitism or third-trimester immunization with tetanus toxoid or pneumococcal vaccine may stimulate isoantibody titer to A or B antigens.
  C. **Birth order.** Birth order is not considered a risk factor. Maternal isoantibody exists naturally and is independent of prior exposure to incompatible fetal blood group antigens. First-born infants have a 40–50% risk for symptomatic disease. Progressive severity of the hemolytic process in succeeding pregnancies is a rare phenomenon.

V. **Clinical presentation**
  A. **Symptoms and signs**
    1. **Jaundice.** Icterus is often the sole physical manifestation of ABO incompatibility with a clinically significant level of hemolysis. The onset is usually within the first 24 hours of life. The jaundice evolves at a faster rate over the early neonatal period than nonhemolytic physiologic pattern jaundice.
    2. **Anemia.** Because of the effectiveness of compensation by reticulocytosis in response to the ongoing mild hemolytic process, erythrocyte indices are maintained within a physiologic range that is normal for asymptomatic in-

fants of the same gestational age. Additional signs of clinical disease (hepatosplenomegaly, hydrops fetalis) are extremely unusual but may be seen with a more progressive hemolytic process (see Rh Incompatibility, p 274).

Exaggerated physiologic anemia may occur at 8–12 weeks of age, particularly when treatment during the neonatal period required phototherapy or exchange transfusion.

VI. Diagnosis. Obligatory screening for infants with unconjugated hyperbilirubinemia include the following studies.

A. Blood type and Rh factor in mother and infant. These studies establish risk factors for ABO incompatibility.

B. Reticulocyte count. Elevated values following adjustment for gestational age and degree of anemia, if any, will support the diagnosis of hemolytic anemia. For term infants, normal values are 4–5%; for preterm infants of 30–36 weeks' gestational age, 6–10%. In ABO hemolytic disease of the newborn, values range from 10% to 30%.

C. Direct Coombs' test. The direct Coombs test (see definition under Rh incompatibility, p 275) is usually weakly positive. If negative, it may raise doubt about ABO incompatibility as the cause of clinical disease or may indicate a lack of analytic sensitivity of the test. A strongly positive test is distinctly unusual and would direct attention to other isoimmune or autoimmune hemolytic processes.

D. Blood smear. The blood smear typically demonstrates **microspherocytes, polychromasia** proportionate to the reticulocyte response, and **normoblastosis** above the normal values for gestational age.

E. Bilirubin levels (fractionated or total and direct). Indirect hyperbilirubinemia is mainly present and provides an index of the severity of disease. The rate at which unconjugated bilirubin levels are increasing suggests the required frequency of testing, usually every 4–8 hours until values plateau.

F. Additional laboratory studies. Supportive diagnostic studies may be indicated on an individual basis if the nature of the hemolytic process remains unclear.

1. Antibody identification (indirect Coombs' test). The indirect Coombs test is more sensitive than the direct Coombs test in detecting the presence of maternal isoantibody and will identify antibody specificity. The test is performed on an eluate of neonatal erythrocytes, which is then tested against a panel of type-specific adult cells.

2. Maternal IgG titer. The absence in the mother of elevated IgG titers against the infant's blood group will tend to exclude a diagnosis of ABO incompatibility.

VII. Management

A. Antepartum treatment. Because of the low incidence of moderate to severe ABO hemolytic disease, invasive maneuvers before term is reached (eg, amniocentesis, early delivery) are usually not indicated.

B. Postpartum treatment

1. General measures. The maintenance of adequate hydration (see Chap 7) and evaluation for potentially aggravating factors (eg, sepsis, drug exposure, or metabolic disturbance) should be considered.

2. Phototherapy. Once a diagnosis of ABO incompatibility is established, phototherapy may be initiated before exchange transfusion is given. Because of the usual mild to moderate hemolysis, phototherapy may entirely obviate the need for exchange transfusion or may reduce the number of transfusions required. See Appendix I for guidelines on phototherapy.

3. Exchange transfusion. See Chapter 19 and Chapter 35.

VIII. Prognosis. For infants with ABO incompatibility, the overall prognosis is excellent. Timely recognition and appropriate management of the rare infant with aggressive ABO hemolytic disease may avoid any potential morbidity or severe hemolytic anemia and secondary hyperbilirubinemia and the inherent risks associated with exchange transfusion and with the use of blood products.

ANEMIA

I. **Definition.** Anemia developing during the neonatal period (0–28 days of life) in infants older than 34 weeks' gestational age is indicated by a central venous hemoglobin less than 13 g/dL or a capillary venous hemoglobin less than 14.5 g/dL.

II. **Normal physiology.** At birth, normal values for the central venous hemoglobin in infants older than 34 weeks' gestational age are 14–20 g/dL, with an average value of 17 g/dL. In term infants, these values remain unchanged until 3 weeks of age, when hemoglobin begins to decline. In preterm infants of 30–36 weeks' gestational age, a similar process begins slightly earlier, at the end of the second week. Fetal **stress erythropoiesis** present at birth is reflected by reticulocytosis and macrocytic red cell indices. In anemia of prematurity, there is a similar physiologic adaptation in hemoglobin, but the lowest levels (7–9 g/dL) are reached earlier in the postnatal period (4–8 weeks). In the absence of clinical complications associated with prematurity, infants will remain asymptomatic during this process.

III. **Pathophysiology.** Anemia in the newborn infant results from one of 3 processes: (1) loss of red blood cells, or hemorrhagic anemia, the most common cause; (2) increased destruction of red blood cells, or hemolytic anemia; or (3) underproduction of red blood cells, or hypoplastic anemia.

 A. **Hemorrhagic anemia**

  1. **Antepartum period** (1:1000 live births).

   a. **Loss of placental integrity.** Abruptio placentae, placenta previa, or traumatic amniocentesis (acute or chronic) may result in loss of placental integrity.

   b. **Anomalies of umbilical cord or placental vessels.** Velamentous insertion of the umbilical cord occurs in 10% of twin gestations and almost all gestations with 3 or more fetuses. Communicating vessels (vasa previa), umbilical cord hematoma (1:5500 deliveries), or entanglement of the cord by the fetus may also cause hemorrhagic anemia.

   c. **Twin-twin transfusion.**

  2. **Intrapartum period**

   a. **Fetomaternal hemorrhage.** Fetomaternal hemorrhage occurs in 30–50% of pregnancies. The risk is increased with preeclampsia-eclampsia, with the need for instrumentation, and with cesarean section. In approximately 8% of pregnancies, the volume of the hemorrhage is more than 10 mL.

   b. **Cesarean section.** In elective cesarean deliveries, there is a 3% incidence of anemia. The incidence is increased in emergency cesarean deliveries. Delay in cord clamping beyond 30 seconds is associated with an increased risk of fetomaternal hemorrhage.

   c. **Traumatic rupture of the umbilical cord.** Rupture may occur if delivery is uncontrolled or unattended.

   d. **Failure of placental transfusion.** Failure is usually caused by umbilical cord occlusion (nuchal cord, entangled or prolapsed cord) during vaginal delivery. Blood loss may be 25–30 mL in the newborn.

   e. **Obstetric trauma.** During a difficult vaginal delivery, occult visceral or intracranial hemorrhage may occur. It may not be apparent at birth. Difficult deliveries are more common with large-for-gestational-age (LGA) infants, breech presentation, or difficult extraction.

  3. **Neonatal period**

   a. **Enclosed hemorrhage.** Hemorrhage severe enough to cause neonatal anemia suggests obstetric trauma, perinatal distress, or a defect in hemostasis.

    (1) **Caput succedaneum** is relatively common and may result in benign hemorrhage.

    (2) **Cephalohematoma** is found in up to 2.5% of births. It is associated with vacuum extraction and primiparity (5% risk of associated linear nondepressed skull fracture).

        (3) Intracranial hemorrhage may occur in the subdural, subarachnoid, or subependymal space.

        (4) Visceral parenchymal hemorrhage is uncommon. It is usually the result of obstetric trauma to an internal organ, most commonly the liver but also the spleen, kidneys, or adrenal glands.

    b. Defects in hemostasis. Defects in hemostasis may be congenital, but more commonly hemorrhage occurs secondary to consumption coagulopathy, which may be caused by:

        (1) Congenital coagulation factor deficiency.

        (2) Consumption coagulopathy

           (a) Disseminated congenital or viral infection.

           (b) Bacterial sepsis or hypotension.

           (c) Intravascular embolism of thromboplastin (due to dead twin, maternal toxemia, necrotizing enterocolitis (NEC), others).

        (3) Deficiency of vitamin K–dependent coagulation factors (factors II, VII, IX, and X).

           (a) Failure to administer vitamin K at birth usually results in a bleeding diathesis at 3–4 days of age.

           (b) Use of antibiotics may interfere with the production of vitamin K by normal gastrointestinal flora.

        (4) Thrombocytopenia

           (a) Immune thrombocytopenia may be isoimmune or autoimmune.

           (b) Congenital thrombocytopenia with absent radii is a syndrome frequently associated with hemorrhagic anemia in the newborn.

    c. Iatrogenic blood loss. Anemia may occur if blood loss due to repeated venipuncture is not replaced routinely. Symptoms may develop if a loss of 20% or more occurs within a 48-hour period.

B. Hemolytic anemia

    1. Immune hemolysis

        a. Isoimmune hemolytic anemia is due to ABO, Rh, or minor blood group incompatibility.

        b. Autoimmune hemolytic anemia.

    2. Nonimmune hemolysis

        a. Bacterial sepsis may cause primary microangiopathic hemolysis.

        b. Congenital TORCH infections (see p 345).

    3. Congenital erythrocyte defect

        a. Metabolic enzyme deficiency.

           (1) Glucose-6-phosphate dehydrogenase (G6PD) deficiency.

           (2) Pyruvate kinase deficiency.

        b. Thalassemia.

        c. Hemoglobinopathy may be characterized as unstable hemoglobins or congenital Heinz-body anemias.

        d. Membrane defects are usually autosomal dominant.

           (1) Hereditary spherocytosis (1:5000 neonates) commonly presents with jaundice and less often with anemia.

           (2) Hereditary elliptocytosis (1:2500 neonates) rarely presents in the newborn infant.

    4. Systemic diseases

        a. Galactosemia.

        b. Osteopetrosis.

    5. Nutritional deficiency. Vitamin E deficiency occurs in association with prematurity or chronic malabsorption but usually does not present until after the neonatal period.

C. Hypoplastic anemia

    1. Congenital disease

        a. Diamond-Blackfan syndrome (congenital hypoplastic anemia).

        b. Atransferrinemia.

      c. Congenital leukemia.

      d. Sideroblastic anemia.

  2. Acquired disease

      a. Infection. Rubella and syphilis are the most common causes.

      b. Aplastic crisis.

      c. Aplastic anemia.

IV. Clinical presentation

  A. Symptoms and signs. The 3 major forms of neonatal anemia may be demonstrated by determination of the following factors: (1) age at presentation of anemia, (2) associated clinical features at presentation, (3) hemodynamic status of infant, and (4) presence or absence of compensatory reticulocytosis.

    1. Hemorrhagic anemia. Hemorrhagic anemia is often dramatic in clinical presentation when acute but may be more subtle when chronic. Both forms have significant rates of perinatal morbidity and mortality if they remain unrecognized. Neither form has significant elevation of bilirubin levels or hepatosplenomegaly.

      a. Acute hemorrhagic anemia presents at birth or with internal hemorrhage after 24 hours. There is pallor unassociated with jaundice and often without cyanosis (< 5 g deoxyhemoglobin) and unrelieved by supplemental oxygen. Tachypnea or gasping respirations are present. Vascular instability ranges from decreased peripheral perfusion ($\leq$ 10% loss of blood volume) to hypovolemic shock (20–25% loss of blood volume). There is also decreased central venous pressure and poor capillary refill. Normocytic or normochromic red blood cell indices are present, with reticulocytosis developing within 2–3 days of the hemorrhagic event.

      b. Chronic hemorrhagic anemia presents at birth with unexplained pallor, often without cyanosis (< 5 g deoxyhemoglobin) and unrelieved by supplemental oxygen. Minimal signs of respiratory distress are present. The central venous pressure is normal or increased. Microcytic or hypochromic red blood cell indices are present, with compensatory reticulocytosis. Hydrops fetalis or stillbirth may occur with failure of compensatory reticulocytosis or intravascular volume maintenance.

      c. Asphyxia pallida (severe neonatal asphyxia) is not associated with hemorrhagic anemia at presentation. This disorder must be distinguished clinically from acute hemorrhage because specific immediate therapy is needed for each disorder. Asphyxia pallida presents at birth with pallor and cyanosis that improves with supplemental oxygen delivery, respiratory failure, bradycardia, and normal central venous pressure.

    2. Hemolytic anemia. Jaundice is often seen before diagnostic levels of hemoglobin are obtained, in part because of the compensatory reticulocytosis that is invariably present. The infant usually presents with pallor after 48 hours of age. However, severe Rh isoimmune disease or homozygous alpha thalassemia will present at birth with severe anemia and, in many cases, hydrops fetalis. Unconjugated hyperbilirubinemia exceeding 10–12 mg/dL, tachypnea, and hepatosplenomegaly may be seen with hemolytic anemia.

    3. Hypoplastic anemia. Hypoplastic anemia is uncommon. It is characterized by presentation after 48 hours of age, absence of jaundice, and reticulocytopenia.

    4. Other forms of anemia

      a. Anemia associated with twin-twin transfusion. If chronic hemorrhage is occurring, there is often more than a 20% difference in the birth weights of the 2 infants, with the donor being the smaller twin.

      b. Occult (internal) hemorrhage

         (1) Intracranial hemorrhage. Signs include a bulging anterior fontanelle and neurologic signs (eg, change in consciousness, apnea, or seizures).

       (2) **Visceral hemorrhage.** Most commonly, the liver has been injured. An abdominal mass or distention is seen.

       (3) **Pulmonary hemorrhage.** Partial or total radiographic opacification of a hemithorax and bloody tracheal secretions are seen.

B. History

  1. Anemia at birth

    a. Hemorrhagic anemia. There may be a history of third-trimester vaginal bleeding or amniocentesis. Hemorrhagic anemia may be associated with multiple gestation, maternal chills or fever postpartum, and nonelective cesarean section.

    b. Hemolytic anemia may be associated with intrauterine growth retardation (IUGR) and Rh-negative mothers.

  2. Anemia presenting after 24 hours of age is often associated with obstetric trauma, unattended delivery, precipitous delivery, perinatal fetal distress, or a low Apgar score.

  3. Anemia presenting with jaundice suggests hemolytic anemia. There may be evidence of drug ingestion late in the third trimester; IUGR; a family member with splenectomy, anemia, jaundice, or cholelithiasis; maternal autoimmune disease; or Mediterranean or Oriental ethnic background.

V. Diagnosis

A. Obligatory initial studies

  1. Hemoglobin

  2. Red blood cell indices

    a. Microcytic or hypochromic red blood cell indices suggest fetomaternal or twin-twin hemorrhage or alpha thalessemia (MCV < 90 fl).

    b. Normocytic or normochromic red blood cell indices are suggestive of acute hemorrhage, systemic disease, intrinsic red cell defect, or hypoplastic anemia.

  3. Reticulocyte count (corrected). The following formula is used.

Corrected reticulocyte count =

$$\frac{\text{Observed reticulocyte count} \times \text{Observed hematocrit}}{\text{Normal hematocrit for age}}$$

An elevated reticulocyte count is associated with antecedent hemorrhage or hemolytic anemia. A low count is seen with hypoplastic anemia.

  4. Blood smear

    a. Spherocytes are associated with ABO isoimmune hemolysis or hereditary spherocytosis.

    b. Elliptocytes are seen in hereditary elliptocytosis.

    c. Pyknocytes may be seen in G6PD deficiency.

    d. Schistocytes or helmet cells are most often seen with consumption coagulopathy.

  5. Direct antiglobin test (direct Coombs' test). This test is positive in isoimmune or autoimmune hemolysis.

B. Other selected laboratory studies

  1. Isoimmune hemolysis. The blood type and Rh type should be determined, and an eluate of neonatal cells should be prepared

  2. Fetomaternal hemorrhage. The **Kleihauer-Betke test** should be performed. Using an acid elution technique, a maternal blood smear is stained with eosin. Fetal red blood cells stain darkly. Adult red blood cells do not stain and appear as "ghost cells." ABO incompatibility between mother and infant will result in increased clearance rate of fetal cells from the maternal circulation, giving a falsely low result.

$2400 \times$ Ratio of fetal to maternal cells =

           mL of fetal blood lost into maternal circulation

  3. Pulmonary hemorrhage. Perform the Apt test (see p 182).

4. **Congenital hypoplastic or aplastic anemia.** Bone marrow aspiration is usually indicated.
5. **TORCH infection**
   a. Skull and long bone films.
   b. IgM levels.
   c. Acute or convalescent serologic.
   d. Urine culture for cytomegalovirus.
6. **Consumption coagulopathy**
   a. Prothrombin time (PT) and partial thromboplastin time (PTT).
   b. Platelet count.
   c. Thrombin time (TT) or fibrinogen assay.
   d. Factor V and factor VIII levels.
   e. Fibrin split products.
7. **Occult hemorrhage**
   a. Pathologic examination of placenta.
   b. Cranial or abdominal ultrasonography will help identify the site of bleeding.
8. **Intrinsic red blood cell defect**
   a. Red blood cell enzyme studies.
   b. Analysis of globin chain ratio.
   c. Studies of red blood cell membrane.

VI. **Management.** Treatment of neonatal anemia may involve, individually or in combination, simple replacement transfusion, exchange transfusion, nutritional supplementation, or treatment of the underlying primary disorder.
   A. **Simple replacement transfusion**
      1. **Indications**
         a. Acute hemorrhagic anemia.
         b. Ongoing deficit replacement.
         c. Maintenance of effective oxygen-carrying capacity (hemoglobin, 15 g/dL) in high-risk infants with apnea, or compromised tissue oxygenation (eg, NEC, cardiopulmonary instability).
      2. **Emergency transfusion at birth only**
         a. Use type O, Rh-negative packed red blood cells.
            (1) Adjust the hematocrit to 50%.
            (2) *If a medical emergency exists, blood that has not been cross-matched may be given.*
            (3) Blood drawn from the placental vein and heparinized (1 unit/mL) can be utilized if given through a blood filter. If time permits, blood may be cross-matched to the mother's blood.
         b. Alternative replacement fluids include fresh-frozen plasma, 5% albumin in saline, and dextran. Timely infusion of packed red blood cells or partial exchange transfusion should follow.
         c. Perform umbilical vein catheterization to a depth of 2–3 cm or until free blood flow is established (see p 000).
         d. Measure the central venous pressure, if time and technical capabilities allow, after advancing the catheter to the level of T6–T9.
         e. Draw initial blood samples for diagnostic studies. Obtain a hemogram and differential, blood type and Rh type, direct Coombs' test, and, if indicated, total bilirubin levels. In a medical emergency, transfusion may be started before the results of laboratory testing are known.
         f. Infuse 10–15 mL/kg of replacement fluid over 10–15 minutes if emergency measures are needed. Once the infant's status has stabilized, reassess the diagnostic studies, physical examination, and obstetric history.
         g. Calculate the red blood cell volume. Under controlled circumstances or if simple transfusion is indicated, calculate the volume of packed red blood cells needed to achieve the desired increase in red blood cell mass (see p 227).

h. The volume of a single transfusion should not exceed 10 mL/kg unless the central venous pressure is monitored.

B. Exchange transfusion

1. Indications

a. Chronic hemolytic anemia or hemorrhagic anemia with increased central venous pressure.

b. Severe isoimmune hemolytic anemia with circulating sensitized red blood cells and isoantibody.

c. Consumption coagulopathy.

2. Technique. See Chapter 19.

C. Nutritional replacement

1. Iron. Iron replacement is useful in the following situations.

a. Fetomaternal hemorrhage of significant volume.

b. Chronic twin-twin transfusion (in the donor twin).

c. Incremental external blood loss (if unreplaced).

d. Preterm infant (< 36 weeks gestational age).

2. Folate (especially with serum levels < 0.5 ng/mL).

a. Premature infants weighing less than 1500 g or younger than 34 weeks' gestational age.

b. Chronic hemolytic anemias or conditions involving "stress erythropoiesis."

c. Infants receiving phenytoin (Dilantin).

3. Vitamin E. Preterm infants younger than 34 weeks' gestational age, unless they are being breast-fed.

D. Prophylactic nutritional supplementation

1. Elemental iron, 1–2 mg/kg/d, beginning at 2 months of age and continuing through 1 year of age.

2. Folic acid, 1–2 mg/wk for preterm infants; 50 μg/d for term infants.

3. Vitamin E, 25 IU/d, until a corrected age of 4 months is reached.

E. Treatment of selected disorders

1. Consumption coagulopathy

a. Treat the underlying cause, eg, sepsis.

b. Give blood replacement therapy. Perform exchange transfusion or give fresh-frozen plasma, 10 mL/kg every 12–14 hours. Platelet concentrate, 1 unit, may be used as a substitute for plasma transfusion.

c. Perform coagulation studies. Monitor the PTT, TT, and fibrinogen levels and the platelet count.

2. Immune thrombocytopenia

a. Isoimmune thrombocytopenia

(1) Consider performing cesarean section if the diagnosis has been confirmed and there is an older sibling with immune thrombocytopenia (75% risk of recurrence).

(2) Give maternal washed platelets when indicated for bleeding diathesis in an infant with a platelet count less than 20,000–30,000/μL. Exchange transfusion may be used as an alternative.

(3) Corticosteroid therapy is *controversial.*

b. Autoimmune thrombocytopenia

(1) Consider performing cesarean section if the maternal platelet count is less than 100,000/μL or the fetal platelet count is less than 50,000/μL.

(2) Use of corticosteroids is *controversial.* Under the above conditions, consider giving corticosteroids to the mother several weeks before delivery.

(3) Transfusion of random donor platelets may be given when indicated.

POLYCYTHEMIA AND HYPERVISCOSITY

I. Definitions. Polycythemia is increased total red blood cell mass. Polycythemic hyperviscosity is increased viscosity of the blood resulting from increased numbers of red blood cells.

A. **Polycythemia.** Polycythemia of the newborn is defined as a central venous hematocrit of 65% or more. The clinical significance of this value results from the curvilinear relationship between the circulating red cell volume (hematocrit) and whole blood viscosity. Above a hematocrit of 65%, blood viscosity rises exponentially.

B. **Hyperviscosity.** Hyperviscosity is a more direct cause of clinical symptoms in most polycythemic infants. Factors other than hematocrit may sometimes exacerbate or occur independently of increased red cell volume, causing hyperviscosity. The terms *polycythemia* and *hyperviscosity* are thus not interchangeable. Although most polycythemic infants are also hyperviscous, it is not invariably the case.

II. Incidence

A. **Polycythemia.** Polycythemia occurs in 2–4% of the general newborn population; half of these patients are symptomatic. Determining the hematocrit only in symptomatic newborn infants tends to underestimate the incidence of polycythemia.

B. **Hyperviscosity.** Hyperviscosity without polycythemia occurs in an additional 1% of normal newborns. In infants with a hematocrit of 60–64%, one-fourth have hyperviscosity.

III. Pathophysiology.

Symptomatic clinical disease in a polycythemic infant results from the regional effects of hyperviscosity, including tissue hypoxia, acidosis, and hypoglycemia, and from the formation of microthrombi within the microcirculation. More commonly involved structures include the central nervous system, the kidneys and adrenal glands, the cardiopulmonary system, and the gastrointestinal tract. The degree to which clinical disease is expressed depends on the interaction of frictional forces in the whole blood. These forces are defined as **shear stress** and **shear rate,** a measure of blood flow velocity. The frictional forces identified within whole blood and their relative contributions to hyperviscosity in the newborn include the following.

A. **Hematocrit.** Increase in the hematocrit is the most important single factor contributing to hyperviscosity in the neonate. An increased hematocrit results from either an absolute increase in circulating red blood cell volume or a decrease in plasma volume.

B. **Plasma viscosity.** A direct linear relationship exists between plasma viscosity and the concentration of plasma proteins, particularly those of high molecular weight, such as fibrinogen. Term infants and, to a greater degree, preterm infants have low plasma fibrinogen levels compared to those of adults. Consequently, except for the rare case of primary hyperfibrinogenemia, plasma viscosity does not contribute to increased whole blood viscosity in the neonate. Under normal conditions, low plasma fibrinogen levels and correspondingly low plasma viscosity actually may protect the microcirculation of the neonate by facilitating perfusion and contributing to low whole-blood viscosity.

C. **Red blood cell aggregation.** Aggregation of erythrocytes occurs only in areas of low blood flow and is usually limited to the venous microcirculation. Because fibrinogen levels are typically low in term and preterm infants, red cell aggregation does not contribute significantly to whole blood viscosity in newborn infants. There is some recent concern that the use of adult fresh-frozen plasma for partial exchange transfusion in neonates might critically alter the concentration of fibrinogen and limit the expected fall of whole blood viscosity within the microcirculation.

D. **Deformability of red blood cell membrane.** There are apparently no differences between term infants, preterm infants, and adults in terms of the membrane deformability of erythrocytes.

IV. Risk factors

A. **Conditions that alter incidence**

1. **Altitude.** There is an absolute increase in red blood cell mass as part of physiologic adaptation to high altitude.

2. **Neonatal age.** The normal pattern of fluid shifts during the first 6 hours of life

is away from the intravascular compartment. The period of maximum physiologic increase in the hematocrit occurs at 2–4 hours of age.

3. Obstetric factors. A delay in cord clamping beyond 30 seconds or stripping of the umbilical cord, if that is the prevailing practice, will result in a higher incidence of polycythemia.

4. High-risk delivery. High-risk delivery is associated with an increased incidence of polycythemia, particularly if precipitous or uncontrolled.

B. Perinatal processes

1. Enhanced fetal erythropoiesis. Elevated erythropoietin levels result from a direct stimulus, usually related to fetal hypoxia, or from altered regulation of erythropoietin production.

  a. Placental insufficiency

    (1) Maternal hypertensive disease (preeclampsia-eclampsia) or primary renovascular disease.

    (2) Abruptio placentae (chronic recurrent).

    (3) Postmaturity.

    (4) Cyanotic congenital heart disease.

    (5) Intrauterine growth retardation.

    (6) Maternal cigarette smoking.

  b. Endocrine disorders. Increased oxygen consumption is the suggested mechanism by which hyperinsulinism or hyperthyroxinemia creates fetal hypoxemia and stimulates erythropoietin production.

    (1) Infant of a diabetic mother (> 40% incidence of polycythemia).

    (2) Infant of a mother with gestational diabetes (> 30% incidence of polycythemia).

    (3) Congenital thyrotoxicosis.

    (4) Congenital adrenal hyperplasia.

    (5) Beckwith-Wiedemann syndrome (secondary hyperinsulinism).

  c. Genetic trisomies (trisomies 13,18, and 21).

2. Hypertransfusion. Conditions that enhance placental transfusion at birth may create hypervolemic normocythemia, which evolves into hypervolemic polycythemia as the normal pattern of fluid shift occurs. A larger transfusion may create hypervolemic polycythemia at birth, with acute symptoms present in the infant. Conditions associated with hypertransfusion include the following.

  a. Delay in cord clamping. Placental vessels contain up to one-third of the fetal blood volume, half of which will be returned to the infant within 1 minute after birth. Representative blood volumes for term infants with a variable delay in cord clamping are:

    (1) 15-second delay, 75–78 mL/kg.

    (2) 60-second delay, 80–87 mL/kg.

    (3) 120-second delay, 83–93 mL/kg.

  b. Gravity. Positioning the infant below the placental bed (> 10 cm below the placenta) enhances placental transfusion via the umbilical vein. Elevation of the infant more than 50 cm above the placenta will prevent placental transfusion.

  c. Maternal use of medications. Drugs that enhance uterine contractility—specifically oxytocin—do not significantly alter the gravitational effects on placental transfusion during the first 15 seconds after birth. With further delay in clamping of the cord, however, blood flow toward the infant will accelerate to a maximum at 1 minute of age.

  d. Cesarean section. In cesarean delivery, there is usually a lower risk of placental transfusion if the cord is clamped early because of the absence of active uterine contractions in most cases and because of gravitational effects.

  e. Twin-twin transfusion. Interfetal transfusion (**parabiosis syndrome**) is observed in monochorionic twin pregnancy with an incidence of 15%.

The recipient twin, on the venous side of the anastomosis, becomes poly-cythemic and the donor, on the arterial side, becomes anemic. Simultaneous venous hematocrits obtained following delivery differ by more than 12–15%, and both twins will have a high risk of intrauterine or neonatal death.

    f. Maternal-fetal transfusion. Approximately 10–80% of normal newborn infants receive a small volume of maternal blood at the time of delivery. The "reverse" Kleihauer-Betke acid elution technique (see p 268) will document maternal red blood cell "ghosts" on a neonatal blood smear. With large transfusions, the test will be positive for several days.

    g. Intrapartum asphyxia. Prolonged fetal distress enhances the net umbilical blood flow toward the infant until cord clamping occurs.

V. Clinical presentation. *Clinical signs observed in polycythemia are nonspecific and reflect the regional effects of hyperviscosity within a given microcirculation. The conditions listed below may occur independently of polycythemia or hyperviscosity and must be considered in the differential diagnosis.*

    A. Central nervous system. There is an altered state of consciousness, including lethargy and decreased activity or hyperirritability. Proximal muscle hypotonia, vasomotor instability, vomiting, seizures, thrombosis, and cerebral infarction may also be seen.

    B. Cardiopulmonary system. Respiratory distress syndrome may be present. Tachycardia and low-output congestive heart failure with cardiomegaly may be seen. There may be primary pulmonary hypertension.

    C. Gastrointestinal tract. Feeding intolerance, abdominal distention, or necrotizing enterocolitis may be present.

    D. Genitourinary tract. Oliguria, acute renal failure, renal vein thrombosis, or priapism may occur.

    E. Metabolic disorders. Hypoglycemia, hypocalcemia, or hypomagnesemia may be seen.

    F. Hematologic disorders. There may be hyperbilirubinemia, thrombocytopenia, or reticulocytosis (with enchanced erythropoiesis only).

VI. Diagnosis

    A. Venous (not capillary) hematocrit. Polycythemia is present when the central venous hematocrit is 65% or more.

    B. The following screening studies may be used.

        1. A cord blood hematocrit greater than 56% indicates polycythemia.

        2. A warmed capillary hematocrit greater than 65% indicates polycythemia.

VII. Management. Clinical management of the polycythemic infant is based on the presence of symptoms, the age of the infant, central venous hematocrit, and associated conditions.

    A. Asymptomatic infants. Only expectant observation is required for most asymptomatic infants. The exceptions are infants with a central venous hematocrit over 70%, in which case partial exchange transfusion is recommended. Meticulous clinical examination is necessary to detect subtle clinical signs of polycythemia or hyperviscosity. The absence of even subtle signs does not preclude some risk of neurologic sequelae, however.

    B. Symptomatic infants. When the central venous hematocrit is 65% or more, partial exchange transfusion is indicated at any age. When the central venous hematocrit is 60–64% and the infant is less than 2 hours of age, monitor the hematocrit closely and consider partial exchange transfusion in anticipation of physiologic fluid shifts and further decrease in plasma volume. See p 152, for the procedure for partial exchange transfusion. The efficacy of partial exchange transfusion in polycythemic infants remains controversial.

VIII. Prognosis. The long-term outcome of infants with polycythemia or hyperviscosity and response to partial exchange transfusion is as follows.

    A. A causal relationship exists between partial exchange transfusion and an increase in gastrointestinal tract disorders and necrotizing enterocolitis.

   B. Randomized controlled prospective studies of polycythemic and hyperviscous infants indicate that partial exchange transfusion may reduce but not eliminate the risk of neurologic sequelae.
   C. Infants with "asymptomatic" polycythemia have an increased risk for neurologic sequelae.
   D. The natural spectrum of neurologic sequelae observed in polycythemic infants not undergoing partial exchange transfusion includes abnormalities in speech, delay in acquiring both fine and gross motor control, and general neurologic deficits.

Rh INCOMPATIBILITY

I. Definition. Isoimmune hemolytic anemia of variable severity may result when Rh incompatibility develops between an Rh-negative mother previously sensitized to the Rh antigen and her Rh-positive fetus. The onset of clinical disease begins in utero as the result of active placental transfer of maternal IgG-Rh antibody. It is manifested as a partially compensated, moderate to severe hemolytic anemia at birth, with unconjugated hyperbilirubinemia developing in the early neonatal period.

II. Incidence. Historically, Rh hemolytic disease of the newborn accounted for up to one-third of symptomatic cases seen and was associated with detectable antibody in approximately 15% of Rh-incompatible mothers. The use of Rh immunoglobulin (RhoGAM) prophylaxis has reduced the incidence of Rh sensitization to less than 1% of Rh-incompatible pregnancies. Isoimmunization may still occur when incompatibility for Rh antigens other than the D antigen exists, notably C and E, which occur in low frequency in the population and cannot be prevented by the use of D-antigen-specific Rh immunoglobulin.

III. Pathophysiology. Initial exposure of the mother to the Rh antigen occurs most often during parturition, miscarriage, or abortion or following traumatic amniocentesis. If recognition of the antigen by the immune system ensues following initial exposure, reexposure to the Rh antigen will induce a maternal anamnestic response and elevation of specific IgG-Rh antibody. Active placental transport of this antibody and immune attachment to the Rh antigenic sites on the fetal erythrocyte are followed by extravascular hemolysis of erythrocytes within the fetal liver and spleen. The rate of the hemolytic process is proportionate to the levels of the maternal antibody titer but is more accurately reflected in the antepartum period by elevation of the amniotic fluid bilirubin concentration, and in the postpartum period by the rate of rise of unconjugated bilirubin. In contrast to ABO incompatibility, the greater antigenicity and density of the Rh antigen loci on the fetal erythrocyte will facilitate progressive, rapid clearance of fetal erythrocytes from the circulation. A demonstrable phase of spherocytosis will be absent. Compensatory reticulocytosis and shortening of the erythrocyte generation time, if unable to match the often high rate of hemolysis in utero, will result in anemia in the newborn infant and a risk of multiple systemic complications.

IV. Risk factors
   A. Birth order. The first-born infant is at minimum risk (< 1%) unless sensitization has occurred previously. Once sensitization has occurred, subsequent pregnancies are at a progressive risk for fetal disease.
   B. Fetomaternal hemorrhage. The volume of fetal erythrocytes entering the maternal circulation correlates directly with the risk of sensitization. The risk is approximately 8% with each pregnancy but ranges from 3% to 65%, depending on the volume of fetal blood (0.1 mL to > 5 mL) that passes into the maternal circulation.
   C. ABO incompatibility. Coexistent incompatibility for either the A or B blood group antigen will reduce the risk of maternal Rh sensitization to 1.5–3.0%. Rapid immune clearance of these fetal erythrocytes following their entry into the maternal circulation exerts a protective effect that decreases with increasing parity.

D. **Obstetric factors.** Cesarean section or trauma to the placental bed during the third stage of labor increases the risk of significant fetomaternal transfusion and subsequent maternal sensitization.

E. **Gender.** Male infants are reported to have an increased risk of more severe disease than females, although the basis for this observation is unclear.

F. **Ethnicity.** Approximately 15% of Caucasians are Rh-negative compared to 5.5% of blacks. The risk to the fetus varies accordingly. Rh-negativity is not seen in Asians.

G. **Maternal immune response.** A significant proportion of Rh-negative mothers (10–50%) fails to develop specific IgG-Rh negative antibody despite repeated exposure to Rh antigen.

V. **Clinical presentation**

A. **Symptoms and signs**

1. **Jaundice.** Unconjugated hyperbilirubinemia is the most common presenting neonatal sign of Rh disease, usually appearing within the first 24 hours of life.

2. **Anemia.** A low cord blood hemoglobin at birth reflects the relative severity of the hemolytic process in utero and is present in approximately 50% of cases.

3. **Hepatosplenomegaly.** Enlargement of the liver and spleen are seen in severe hemolysis, sometimes occurring in association with ascites, with an increased risk for splenic rupture.

4. **Hydrops fetalis.** Severe Rh disease has an historical association with hydrops fetalis and at one time was its most common cause. Clinical features in the fetus include progressive hypoproteinemia with ascites or pleural effusion, or both; severe chronic anemia with secondary hypoxemia; and cardiac failure. There is an increased risk of late fetal death, stillbirth, and intolerance of active labor. The neonate frequently has generalized edema, notably of the scalp, which can be detected by antepartum ultrasound; cardiopulmonary distress often involving pulmonary edema; congestive heart failure; hypotension and peripheral perfusion defects; cardiac rhythm disturbances; and severe anemia with secondary hypoxemia and metabolic acidosis. Currently, nonimmune conditions are more commonly associated with hydrops fetalis. Severe anemia per se is not the controlling factor in the clinical development of fetal hydrops. It may be that several systemic disturbances must be present in combination to produce the clinical expression of disease. Secondary involvement of other organ systems may result in hypoglycemia or thrombocytopenic purpura.

VI. **Diagnosis.** Obligatory screening in an infant with unconjugated hyperbilirubinemia includes the following studies.

A. **Blood type and Rh type (mother and infant).** These studies establish the likelihood of Rh incompatibility and will exclude the diagnosis if the infant is Rh-negative, with one exception (see direct Coombs' test, below).

B. **Reticulocyte count.** Elevated reticulocyte levels, adjusted for the degree of anemia and gestational age in preterm infants, reflect the degree of compensation and support a diagnosis of an ongoing hemolytic process. Normal values are 4–5% for term infants, and 6–10% for preterm infants (30–36 weeks' gestational age). In symptomatic Rh disease, expected values are 10–40%.

C. **Direct Coombs' test.** A strongly positive direct Coombs test on fetal red blood cells, indicative of an active immune reaction occurring against fetal erythrocytes, is diagnostic of Rh incompatibility in the presence of the appropriate setup and an elevated reticulocyte count. If Rh immunoglobulin was given at 28 weeks' gestation, subsequent passive transfer of antibody will result in a false-positive direct Coombs test, without associated reticulocytosis. Rarely, a falsely Rh-negative infant will present with a strongly positive direct Coombs test, resulting from blockage of the Rh antigenic sites by high-titer maternal antibody.

D. **Blood smear.** Polychromasia and normoblastosis proportionate to the reticulocyte count are typically present. Hypochromia in proportion to the severity of the hemolytic process and anemia are seen. Spherocytes are not usually present.

E. Bilirubin levels. Progressive elevation of unconjugated bilirubin on serial testing provides an index of the severity of the hemolytic process. In severe disease, an elevated direct fraction may be secondary to a laboratory artifact or coexisting hepatobiliary damage.

F. Bilirubin-binding capacity is currently investigational.

G. Glucose and blood gas levels should be followed closely.

H. Supplementary laboratory studies. Supportive diagnostic studies may be required when the basis of the hemolytic process remains unclear.

1. **Direct Coombs' test in mother.** This study will be negative in Rh disease but often is positive if maternal autoimmune hemolytic disease is present, particularly collagen vascular disease.

2. **Antibody identification (indirect Coombs' test in infant).** An eluate of antibody attached to neonatal erythrocytes is tested against a type-specific panel of adult erythrocytes to determine the antibody specificity.

VII. Management

A. Antepartum treatment. Verification of the Rh-negative status at the first prenatal visit may be obtained by the following measures.

1. **Maternal antibody titer (indirect Coombs' test).** Detection of specific IgG-Rh antibody will document prior sensitization. Serial antibody titer determinations are required every 1–4 weeks (depending on gestational age) during pregnancy. A negative indirect Coombs test signifies absence of sensitization. This test should be repeated at 28–34 weeks' gestation.

2. **Rh immunoglobulin (RhoGAM).** Current obstetric guidelines suggest giving immunoprophylaxis at 28 weeks' gestation in the absence of sensitization.

3. **Amniocentesis.** If maternal antibody titers indicate a risk of fetal death (usual range, 1:16–1:32), amniocentesis should be performed. To reasonably predict the risk of moderate to severe fetal disease, serial determinations of amniotic fluid bilirubin levels present photometrically at 450 nm are plotted on standard graphs according to gestational age.

4. **Ultrasonography.** As a screening study in pregnancies at risk, serial fetal ultrasound examinations allow detection of scalp edema, ascites, or other signs of developing hydrops fetalis.

5. **Intrauterine transfusion.** Based on the above studies, intrauterine transfusion may be indicated because of possible fetal demise or the presence of fetal hydrops. This procedure must be performed by an experienced team. The goal is maintenance of effective erythrocyte mass within the fetal circulation and maintenance of the pregnancy until there is a reasonable chance for successful extrauterine survival of the infant.

B. Postpartum treatment

1. **Resuscitation.** Moderately to severely anemic infants with or without hydropic features are at risk for high-output cardiac failure, hypoxemia secondary to decreased oxygen-carrying capacity, and hypoglycemia. These infants may require immediate single-volume exchange blood transfusion at delivery to improve oxygen-carrying capacity, mechanical support of ventilation, and an extended period of monitoring for hypoglycemia.

2. **Cord blood studies.** A cord blood bilirubin level greater than 4 mg/dL or a cord hemoglobin less than 12 g/dL, or both, usually suggests moderate to severe disease. The cord blood is used for these and initial screening studies, including blood typing, Rh typing, and Coombs' test.

3. **Serial unconjugated bilirubin studies.** Determination of the rate of increase in unconjugated bilirubin levels will provide an index of the severity of the hemolytic process and the need for exchange transfusion. Commonly used guidelines include a rise of more than 0.5 mg/dL/h or more than 5 mg/dL over 24 hours within the first 2 days of life, or projection of a serum level that will exceed a predetermined "exchange level" for a given infant (usually 20 mg/dL in term infants).

4. **Phototherapy.** In Rh hemolytic disease, because of its frequently severe

course, phototherapy is used only as an adjunct to exchange transfusion and should not be instituted until a decision has been made regarding exchange transfusion. Phototherapy may reduce the number of total exchange transfusions required.

5. **Exchange transfusion.** (See Chap 19 for procedure.) Exchange transfusion is indicated if the unconjugated bilirubin level is likely to reach a predetermined "exchange level" for that patient. Optimally, exchange transfusion is done well before this "exchange level" is reached, to minimize the entry of unconjugated bilirubin into soft tissues. Consideration should be given to irradiation of blood before the transfusion is given, particularly in preterm infants or infants expected to require multiple transfusions, to reduce the risk of graft vs host disease.

C. **Rh immunoglobin (RhoGAM) prophylaxis.** Most cases of incompatibility involve the D antigen. RhoGAM given at 28 weeks' gestation or within 72 hours of suspected Rh antigen exposure, or both, will reduce the risk of sensitization to less than 1%; the recommended dosage should be well in excess of the amount of Rh antigen transfused. In massive fetomaternal hemorrhage, however, conventional doses may be insufficient. The amount of fetal blood entering the maternal circulation may be estimated using the Kleihauer-Betke acid elution technique (p 268) during the immediate postpartum period.

No treatment equivalent to RhoGAM is available for maternal Rh sensitization to non-D antigens, notably C and E antigens. These antigens, however, are significantly less antigenic than the D antigen, and clinical manifestations of incompatibility are frequently milder and the risk of severe disease considerably less.

D. **Hydrops fetalis.** Skilled resuscitation and anticipation of selective systemic complications may prevent early neonatal death.

1. **Isovolumetric partial exchange transfusion** with type O Rh-negative packed erythrocytes will raise the hematocrit and improve the oxygen-carrying capacity .

2. **Central arterial and venous catheterization** may be performed to provide the following measures.
   a. Isovolumetric exchange transfusion.
   b. Monitoring of arterial blood gas levels and central venous and systemic blood pressures.
   c. Monitoring of fluid and electrolyte balance, particularly renal and hepatic function, the calcium:phosphorus ratio, and serum albumin levels as well as appropriate hematologic studies and serum bilirubin levels.

3. **Positive-pressure mechanical ventilation.** This measure may include increased levels of positive-end expiratory pressure, if pulmonary edema is present, as a means of stabilizing alveolar ventilation.

4. **Therapeutic paracentesis or thoracentesis** may be performed to remove fluid that may further compromise respiratory effort. Attention to the volume removed and progressive systemic hypotension is important.

5. **Volume expanders** may be necessary in addition to erythrocytes to improve peripheral perfusion defects. Only **fresh-frozen plasma containing high-molecular-weight proteins** should be used. *Albumin is contraindicated* and may aggravate existing ascites or pleural effusion. Transfused volumes should be small to avoid further cardiac embarrassment.

6. **Drug treatment** may include diuretics such as furosemide for pulmonary edema and pressor agents including dopamine, which may also benefit renal perfusion (for dosages, see Chap 73). In the case of cardiac rhythm disturbances, appropriate drugs may be used if indicated.

7. **Electrocardiography or echocardiography** may be needed to determine whether cardiac abnormalities are present.

VIII. **Prognosis.** Prenatal mortality for infants at risk of anti-DRH isoimmunization is currently approximately 1.5% and has decreased significantly over the past 2 decades. Antenatal immune prophylaxis and improved management techniques including amniotic fluid spectrophotometry, intrauterine transfusion, and advances in neonatal intensive care have been largely responsible for this reduction. Isolated cases of severe isoimmunization still occur due to isoimmunization by other than anti-D antibody or failure to receive immune prophylaxis and may exhibit the full spectrum of disease, including an increased risk of stillbirths and early neonatal morbidity and mortality.

THROMBOCYTOPENIA AND PLATELET DYSFUNCTION

I. **Definition.** Thrombocytopenia is defined as a platelet count less than 150,000/μL, although a few normal neonates may have counts as low as 100,000/μL in the absence of clinical disease. The best measure of platelet function is the standardized (Ivy) bleeding time. Normal values for the Ivy bleeding time are the same as for older children (1.5–5.5 minutes).

II. **Normal platelet physiology.** The rate of platelet production and turnover in neonates is similar to that of older children and adults. The platelet life span is approximately 8 days, and the mean platelet count is greater than 200,000/μL. Platelet counts are slightly lower in low birth weight infants, in whom platelet counts less than 100,000/μL have occasionally been observed in the absence of a clinical disorder. Low platelet counts should nonetheless be investigated in low birth weight infants. Platelet counts vary according to the method of determination. Phase microscopy determinations are generally 25,000–50,000/μL lower than those obtained by direct microscopy.

III. **Etiology**
  A. **Thrombocytopenia**
    1. **Maternal disorders causing thrombocytopenia in infant**
      a. Drug use (eg, digoxin, chlorothiazide, sulfonamide derivatives).
      b. Infections (eg, TORCH infections, bacterial or viral infections).
      c. Disseminated intravascular coagulation (DIC).
      d. Severe hypertension.
      e. Antiplatelet antibodies.
        (1) Antibodies against maternal platelets (autoimmune thrombocytopenia).
          (a) Idiopathic thrombocytopenic purpura (ITP).
          (b) Drug-induced thrombocytopenia.
          (c) Systemic lupus erythematosus.
        (2) Antibodies against fetal platelets (isoimmune thrombocytopenia).
          (a) Isolated isoimmune thrombocytopenia.
          (b) Isoimmune thrombocytopenia associated with erythrohblastosis fetalis.
    2. **Placental disorders causing thrombocytopenia in infant (rare)**
      a. Chorioangioma.
      b. Vascular thrombi.
      c. Placental abruption.
    3. **Neonatal disorders causing thrombocytopenia**
      a. Decreased platelet production or congenital absence of megakaryocytes.
        (1) Isolated.
        (2) Thrombocytopenia–absent radius syndrome.
        (3) Fanconi's anemia.
        (4) Rubella syndrome.
        (5) Congenital leukemia.
        (6) Trisomies 13, 18, or 21.
      b. **Increased platelet destruction**
        (1) Bacterial sepsis.
        (2) TORCH infections.
        (3) DIC.
        (4) Necrotizing enterocolitis.

(5) Platelet destruction associated with giant hemangiomas (**Kasabach-Merritt syndrome**).

B. Platelet dysfunction

1. Drug-induced platelet dysfunction.
   a. Maternal use of aspirin.
   b. Indomethacin.
   c. Perhaps penicillins, furosemide, theophylline.
2. Metabolic disorders.
   a. Hyperbilirubinemia.
   b. Phototherapy-induced metabolic abnormalities.
   c. Acidosis.
   d. Fatty acid deficiency.
   e. Maternal diabetes.
3. Inherited thrombasthenia (Glanzmann's disease).

IV. Clinical presentation

A. Symptoms and signs

1. Generalized superficial petechiae are often present, particularly in response to minor trauma or pressure or increased venous pressure. Platelet counts are usually less than 60,000/μL.
2. Mucosal bleeding and spontaneous hemorrhage may be occurring from other sites with platelet counts less than 20,000/μL.
3. Intracranial hemorrhage may occur with severe thrombocytopenia.
4. Large ecchymoses and muscle hemorrhages are more likely to be due to coagulation disturbances than to platelet disturbances.
5. Petechiae in normal infants tend to be clustered on the head and upper chest, do not recur, and are associated with normal platelet counts. They are a result of a transient increase in venous pressure during birth.

B. History

1. There may be a family history of thrombocytopenia.
2. Maternal drug ingestion may be a factor.
3. A history of infection should be noted.
4. Previous episodes of bleeding may have occurred.

C. The placenta should be carefully examined for evidence of choriangioma, thrombi, or abruptio placentae.

D. Physical examination

1. Petechiae and bleeding should be noted.
2. Physical malformations may be present in thrombocytopenia—absent radius syndrome, rubella syndrome, giant hemangioma, or trisomy syndromes.
3. Hepatosplenomegaly may be caused by viral or bacterial infection or congenital leukemia.

V. Diagnosis

A. Laboratory studies

1. Test for maternal thrombocytopenia. A low maternal count suggests autoimmune thrombocytopenia or inherited thrombocytopenia (X-linked recessive thrombocytopenia or autosomal dominant thrombocytopenia).
2. Neonatal platelet count.
3. Complete blood count.
4. Blood typing.
5. Coombs' test.
6. Coagulation studies.
7. Other studies (if indicated).
   a. TORCH titers.
   b. Bacterial cultures.
   c. Bone marrow studies if decreased platelet production is present.

B. Decreased platelet production vs increased platelet destruction

1. **Decreased platelet production**

      a. Platelet size is normal.
      b. Platelet survival time is normal.
      c. Megakaryocytes are decreased in a bone marrow sample.
      d. A sustained increase in the platelet count over a period of 4–7 days is seen following platelet transfusion.
   2. Increased platelet destruction
      a. Platelet size is increased.
      b. Platelet survival time is decreased.
      c. Megakaryocytes in the bone marrow are normal or increased.
      d. There is little or no sustained increase in platelet count following platelet transfusion.
 C. Evaluation of platelet function as indicated by prolonged Ivy bleeding time caused by:
   1. Platelet dysfunction.
   2. Thrombocytopenia with platelet counts less than 80,000/μL.

VI. Management

 A. Obstetric management of maternal autoimmune thrombocytopenia
   1. Treatment is aimed at prevention of intracranial hemorrhage during vaginal delivery.
   2. There is an increased risk of severe neonatal thrombocytopenia and intracranial hemorrhage if antibody is present in the maternal plasma or if fetal scalp platelet counts are less than 75,000–100,000/μL.
   3. Cesarean delivery may be indicated.
   4. Administering corticosteroids to the mother has been beneficial in preliminary studies.

 B. Management of isoimmune thrombocytopenia
   1. Transfuse platelets lacking the incompatible antigen. Although these platelets are usually obtained from the mother, transfusion of unmatched platelets from a random donor may be helpful if matched platelets cannot be obtained.
   2. Intravenous gamma globulin is useful (see Chap 73 for dosage and other pharmacologic information).
   3. The risk of recurrence in siblings is greater than 75%. In subsequent pregnancies, the administration of intravenous gamma globulin weekly during the third trimester may be effective (see Chap 73 for dosage and other pharmacologic information). These infants are usually delivered by cesarean section.

 C. Treatment of infants with thrombocytopenia
   1. Treat the underlying cause (eg, sepsis). If drugs are the cause, stop administration.
   2. Platelet transfusions are indicated (1) if active bleeding is occurring with any degree of thrombocytopenia or (2) if there is no active bleeding but platelet counts are less than 20,000/μL. It may be desirable to transfuse "sick" premature infants if the platelet count is less than 50,000/μL. Random donor platelets are given in a dosage of 10 mL/kg of standard platelet concentrates. The platelet count should increase to over 100,000/μL. Failure to achieve or sustain such a rise suggests a destructive process.
   3. Exchange transfusion is given for immune thrombocytopenia. The platelet count may rise only transiently. There is considerable risk involved.
   4. Prednisone, 2 mg/kg/d, may also be beneficial in immune thrombocytopenia.

REFERENCES

Black VD, Lubchenco LO: Neonatal polycythemia and hyperviscosity. *Pediatr Clin North Am* 1982;**29:**1137.

Black VD, Lubchenco LO et al: Neonatal hyperviscosity: Randomized study of effect of partial plasma exchange transfusion on long-term outcome. *Pediatrics* 1985;**75:**1048.

Bowman, JM: Rh erythroblastosis fetalis 1975. *Semin Hematol* 1975;**12:**189.

Bussel JB et al: Antenatal treatment of neonatal alloimmune thrombocytopenia *N Engl J Med* 1988;**319:**1374.

Castle V et al: Frequency and mechanism of neonatal thrombocytopenia. *J Pediatr* 1986;**108:**749.

Dickerman JF: Anemia in the newborn infant. *Pediatr Rev* 1984;**6:**131.

Glader BE: Erythrocyte disorders in infancy. In: *Schaffer's Diseases of the Newborn,* 5th ed. Avery ME, Taeusch HW (editors). Saunders, 1984.

Gross S, Shurin SB, Gordon EM: The blood and hematopoietic system. Pages 708–752 in: *Behrman's Neonatal Perinatal Medicine,* 3rd ed. Fanaroff AA, Martin RJ (editors). Mosby, 1983.

Klemperer MR: Hemolytic anemias: Immune defects. In *Blood Diseases of Infancy and Childhood,* 5th ed. Miller DR, Baehner RL, McMillan CW (editors). Mosby, 1984.

Linderkamp O: Placental transfusion: Determinants and effects. *Clin Perinatol* 1982;**9:**559.

Linderkamp O et al: Contributions of red cells and plasma to blood viscosity in preterm and full-term infants and adults. *Pediatrics* 1984;**74:**45.

Martin JN, Morrison JC, Files FC: Autoimmune thrombocytopenic purpura: Current concepts and recommended practices. *Am J Obstet Gynecol* 1984;**150:**86.

Mentzer WC: Polycythemia and hyperviscosity syndrome in newborn infants. *Clin Haematol* 1978;**7:**63.

Miller DR (editor): Normal values and examination of the blood: Perinatal period, infancy, childhood, and adolescence. Pages 22–47 in: *Blood Diseases of Infancy and Childhood,* 5th ed. Miller DR, Baehner RL, McMillan CW (editors). Mosby, 1984.

Naiman JL: Disorders of the platelets. In: *Hematologic Problems in the Newborn,* 3rd ed. Oski FA, Naiman JL (editors). Saunders, 1982.

Naiman JL: Erythroblastosis fetalis. In: *Hematologic Problems in the Newborn,* 3rd ed. Oski FA, Naiman JL (editors). Saunders, 1982.

Oh W: Neonatal polycythemia and hyperviscosity. *Pediatr Clin North Am* 1986;**33:**523.

Oski FA: Hematologic problems. In: *Neonatology Pathophysiology and Management of the Newborn,* 2nd ed. Avery GB (editor). Lippincott, 1981.

Oski FA: Hydrops fetalis. In: *Schaffer's Diseases of the Newborn,* 5th ed. Avery ME, Taeusch HW (editors). Saunders, 1984.

Oski FA, Naiman JL: Polycythemia and hyperviscosity in the neonatal period. In: *Hematologic Problems in the Newborn,* 3rd ed. Saunders, 1982.

Pearson HA: Posthemorrhagic anemia in the newborn. *Pediatr Rev* 1982;**4:**40.

Pearson HA, McIntosh S: Neonatal thrombocytopenia. *Clin Haematol* 1978;**7:**111.

Peddle LJ: The antenatal management of the Rh sensitized woman. *Clin Perinatol* 1984;**11:**251.

Polesky HF: Diagnosis, prevention and therapy in hemolytic diseases of the newborn. *Clin Lab Med* 1982;**2:**107.

Shohat M, Merlob P, Reisner S: Neonatal polycythemia: I. Early diagnosis and incidence related to time of sampling. *Pediatrics* 1984;**73:**7.

Stuart MJ: Platelet function in the neonate. *Am J Pediatr Hematol Oncol* 1979;**1:**227.

55 Cardiac Abnormalities

CONGENITAL HEART DISEASE

The diagnostic dilemma of the newborn with congenital heart disease must be resolved quickly since therapy may prove lifesaving for some of these infants. Congenital heart disease occurs in approximately 1% of live-born infants. Nearly half of all cases of congenital heart disease are diagnosed during the first week of life. The most frequently occurring anomalies seen during this first week are patent ductus arteriosus, D-transposition of the great arteries, hypoplastic left heart syndrome, tetralogy of Fallot, and pulmonary atresia.

I. **Classification.** Symptoms and signs in newborns with heart disease permit grouping according to levels of arterial oxygen saturation. Further classification (based on other physical findings and laboratory tests) facilitates delineation of the exact cardiac lesion present.

   A. **Cyanotic heart disease.** Infants with cyanotic heart disease are usually unable to achieve a PaO_2 above 100 mm Hg after breathing 100% inspired oxygen for 10–20 minutes.

   B. **Acyanotic heart disease.** Infants with acyanotic heart disease will achieve PaO_2 levels of over 100 mm Hg under the same conditions as noted in **A,** above.

II. **Cyanotic heart disease** (Table 55–1)

   A. **100% oxygen test.** Because of intracardiac right-to-left shunting, the newborn with cyanotic congenital heart disease (in contrast to the infant with pulmonary disease) is unable to raise the arterial saturation, even in the presence of increased ambient oxygen.

   1. Determine PaO_2 while infant is on room air.

   2. Give 100% oxygen for 10–20 minutes by mask, hood, or endotracheal tube.

   3. Obtain an arterial blood gas level while the infant is breathing 100% oxygen.

   B. **Cyanosis.** Care must be taken in evaluating cyanosis by skin color, since polycythemia, jaundice, racial pigmentation, or anemia may make clinical recognition of cyanosis difficult.

   C. **Murmur.** The infant with cyanotic congenital heart disease often does not have a distinctive murmur. In fact, the most serious of these anomalies may not be associated with a murmur at all.

   D. **Other studies.** Cyanotic infants may be further classified on the basis of pulmonary circulation on chest x-ray and electrocardiographic findings.

   E. **Diagnosis and treatment.** Table 55–1 outlines the diagnosis and treatment of cyanotic heart disease.

   F. **Specific cyanotic heart disease abnormalities**

   1. **D-Transposition of the great arteries** is the most common cardiac cause of cyanosis in the first year of life, with a male:female ratio of 2:1. The aorta comes from the right ventricle and the pulmonary artery from the left ventricle. With modern newborn care, 1-year survival approaches 80%.

      a. **Physical examination.** Typical presentation is a large, vigorous infant with cyanosis but little or no respiratory distress. There may be no murmur or a soft, systolic ejection murmur.

      b. **Chest x-ray study.** This study may be normal, but typically it reveals a very narrow upper mediastinal shadow ("egg on a stick" appearance).

      c. **Electrocardiography.** There are no characteristic ECG findings.

      d. **Echocardiography is diagnostic.** Typical findings are branching of the

TABLE 55-1. CYANOTIC CONGENITAL HEART DISEASE (Pao$_2$ < 100 mm Hg in 100% F$_I$o$_2$)*

	Decreased blood flow with small heart (or normal heart)		Decreased pulmonary blood flow with large heart		Increased pulmonary blood flow with small heart	Increased pulmonary blood flow with large heart		Normal pulmonary blood flow, with normal-sized heart. No thymus
Chest x-ray								
ECG	RVH	LVH, LAD	LVH, normal axis	RBBB	RVH	RVH or normal	LVH or normal	Normal
Differential diagnosis	Pulmonary atresia with VSD, TOF	Tricuspid atresia	Pulmonary atresia with intact septum	Ebstein's anomaly	TAPVR	HLHS	TGA with VSD. Truncus arteriosus	TGA
Physical examination	Short, soft ejection murmur may only be heard in back	Faint PDA murmur or systolic murmur of sm VSD	Systolic and diastolic murmurs at xiphoid TS/TI	Widely split S$_2$, scratchy diastolic murmur at xiphoid	No murmur. Quadruple rhythm often due to pulmonary ejection sound, split S$_2$, diastolic filling sound	Poor peripheral pulses	Systolic murmur	No murmur
Treatment	If PaO$_2$ low, start PGE$_1$ infusion. Then perform further cardiac evaluation. Operation may or may not be needed					Consider PGE$_1$ infusion. Then perform further cardiac evaluation. Operation may or may not be needed		Immediate balloon septostomy

*AS, aortic stenosis; EFE, endocardial fibroelastosis; HLHS, hypoplastic left heart syndrome; LAD, left axis deviation; LVH, left ventricular hypertrophy; PDA, patent ductus arteriosus; PS, pulmonary stenosis; RBBB, right bundle branch block; RVH, right ventricular hypertrophy; SEM, systolic ejection murmur; TAPVR, total anomalous pulmonary venous return; TGA, transposition of great arteries; TI, tricuspid incompetence; TOF, tetralogy of Fallot; TS, tricuspid stenosis; VSD, ventricular septal defect.

anterior great vessel into the inominate, subclavian, and carotid vessels and branching of the posterior great vessel into the right and left pulmonary arteries.

   e. Cardiac catherization. Like echocardiography, this study is diagnostic and often therapeutic as outlined in **f,** below.

   f. Treatment. Urgent cardiac catherization with balloon septostomy and later Mustard or Senning procedures (transposing venous return via an intra-arterial baffle) or early arterial switch operation are the methods of treatment.

2. **Tetralogy of Fallot (TOF).** TOF is characterized by 4 anomalies: pulmonary stenosis, ventricular septal defect, overriding aorta, and right ventricular hypertrophy (RVH). There is a slight male predominance. Cyanosis usually signifies complete or partial atresia of the right ventricular overflow tract or extremely severe pulmonary stenosis with hypoplastic pulmonary arteries. The degree of right ventricular outflow obstruction is inversely proportional to pulmonary blood flow and directly proportional to the degree of cyanosis. TOF with absent pulmonary valve may present later in infancy due to poor feeding (due to very large pulmonary arteries causing esophageal compression).

   a. Physical examination. The patient is cyanotic with a systolic ejection murmur along the left sternal border. Loud murmurs are associated with more flow across the right ventricular outflow tract, and softer murmurs, with less flow.

   b. Chest x-ray study. A small, often "boot-shaped" heart, with decreased pulmonary vascular markings. A right aortic arch is seen in about 20% of these infants.

   c. Echocardiography. The echocardiogram may be normal or demonstrate right ventricular hypertrophy (RVH). The only sign of RVH may be an upright T wave in V4R or V1 after 72 hours of age.

   d. Echocardiography is usually diagnostic, with the demonstration of an overriding aorta, ventricular septal defect (VSD), and small right ventricular outflow tract.

   e. Treatment. Pulmonary blood flow may be ductal-dependent with severe cyanosis and may respond to ductal dilation using prostaglandin E_1 (see Chap 73). This measure allows more flexibility for planning cardiac catherization and surgical correction. Surgery (shunting or total correction) may be palliative.

III. Acyanotic heart disease. (Table 55–2.)

   A. 100% oxygen test. (See **II.A,** above.)

   B. Murmur. The infant who is not cyanotic will present with either a heart murmur or symptoms of congestive heart failure.

   C. Diagnosis and treatment. (Table 55–2.)

   D. Specific acyanotic heart disease abnormalities

   1. **Ventricular septal defect (VSD)** is the most common congenital heart abnormality, with equal sex distribution. Murmurs are not heard at birth but typically appear between 3 days and 3 weeks of age. Congestive heart failure is unusual before 4 weeks of age but may develop earlier in premature infants. Symptoms and physical findings vary with the age of the patient and the size of the defect. Spontaneous closure occurs in half. Surgical correction is reserved for large, symptomatic VSD only.

   2. **Atrial septal defect (ASD)** is not an important cause of morbidity or mortality in infancy. Occasionally, congestive heart failure can occur in infancy but not usually in the neonatal period.

   3. **Endocardial cushion defects** include ostium primum–type ASD with or without cleft mitral valve and atrioventricular (AV) canal. These defects are commonly associated with multiple congenital anomalies, especially Down's syndrome. If marked AV-valve insufficiency is present, the patient may present with congestive heart failure at birth or in the neonatal period.

TABLE 55–2. ACYANOTIC CONGENITAL HEART DISEASE (Pao$_2$ > 100 mm Hg in 100% F$_I$o$_2$)*

	Normal pulmonary blood flow with normal-sized heart		Normal pulmonary blood flow with large heart				Increased pulmonary blood flow with large heart
Chest x-ray							
ECG	RVH or normal	LVH or normal	Normal arrhythmia or complete heart block	LVH	RVH or LVH	RVH	LAD
Differential diagnosis	Valvar PS	Noncritical valvar AS; VSD; PDA	Intrauterine arrhythmia	AV malformation; Common sites are head, liver, placenta; AS, critical	AV valve insufficiency; Primary myocardial disease (including EFE)	HLHS, coarctation of aorta	AV canal
Physical examination	SEM	SEM-AS; VSD, no murmur; PDA, continuous murmur	May be hydropic or normal	AVM, usually continuous murmur over site; Increased pulses; Critical AS, decreased pulses; Not much murmur	TI; MI; Pansystolic murmur with rumble; EFE, gallop	HLHS; poor pulses, perfusion, and color; gallop; Coarctation of aorta, decreased femoral pulses	SEM, diastolic rumble
Treatment	Observe	Observe	Treat arrhythmia with drugs or cardioversion; May need furosemide; Congenital complete heart block may need pacemaker	AVM, ultrasound, CT scanning, angiography; AS; PGE, infusion; Digoxin, furosemide	Digoxin, furosemide	Anticongestives if in heart failure; HLHS, consider PGE; infusion	Observe; Anticongestives if in heart failure

→ Further cardiac evaluation

*Abbreviations are explained in Table 55–1 footnote.

  a. **Physical examination.** A systolic murmur due to AV-valve insuffi-
     ciency. Cyanosis may be present but is often not severe.
  b. **Chest x-ray study.** Variable findings may include a dilated pulmonary
     artery or a large heart due to atrial dilatation.
  c. **Electrocardiography.** Left axis deviation (left superior vector) is *always*
     found; the PR interval may be long or there may be a R-S-R' pattern in
     V4R and V1.
  d. **Echocardiography** is usually diagnostic; the echocardiogram usually
     demonstrates a common AV valve with inlet ventricular septal defect or
     a defect in the septum primum with an abnormal mitral valve.
  e. **Treatment.** Congestive heart failure is treated with diuretics and digoxin
     (see Chap 73); early cardiac catheterization with corrective surgery may
     be needed to prevent the development of pulmonary vascular obstruc-
     tive disease.

IV. **Hypoplastic left heart syndrome (HLHS)** occurs in both cyanotic and acyanotic
    forms. In 15% of cases, the foramen ovale is intact and thus prevents mixing at
    the atrial level, causing cyanosis. The infants with free mixing at the atria are
    acyanotic. Hypoplastic left heart syndrome accounts for 25% of all cardiac deaths
    during the first week of life.
    A. **Physical examination.** The baby is typically pale, tachypneic with poor per-
       fusion, and poor to absent peripheral pulses. A loud single S2 is present,
       usually with a gallop and no murmur. There is hepatomegaly, and metabolic
       acidosis is usually present by 48 hours of age.
    B. **Electrocardiography** demonstrates a small or absent left ventricular vector.
    C. **Chest x-ray study.** Moderate cardiomegaly is present, often with large main
       pulmonary artery shadow.
    D. **Echocardiography.** A diagnostic study demonstrates a small or slitlike left
       ventricle with a hypoplastic ascending aorta.
    E. **Treatment.** Systemic blood flow is ductal dependent; therefore prostaglandin
       E_1 may be of value. Surgical correction is done in 2 stages. The first is pallia-
       tion (Norwood procedure), redirecting the blood flow so that the right ventricle
       serves as the "systemic ventricle," and is high-risk intervention. The second
       stage (Fontan procedure) directs systemic venous return directly to the pul-
       monary circulation and the ASD is closed. The second stage has variable
       results; survival is only fair after both procedures. Infant transplantation is
       available, with good results at some centers, but shortage of donors is a prob-
       lem.

V. **Associated anomalies and syndromes** (Table 55–3). No discussion of heart
   disease in neonates would be complete without the inclusion of common multiple
   congenital anomaly (MCA) syndromes associated with heart defects. Many
   times, recognition of MCA syndrome will facilitate identification of the heart defect. Syndromes that tend to present after the newborn period have not been
   included.

VI. **Teratogens and heart disease.** Several teratogens associated with congenital
    heart disease have been identified (Table 55–4), although there is not a 100%
    relationship between exposure and heart defects. A history of teratogen expo-
    sure may help in the diagnosis.

VII. **Abnormal situs syndromes.** Syndromes of abnormal situs relationships are as-
     sociated with congenital heart disease. For example, an infant with situs inversus
     totalis and dextrocardia has the same incidence of congenital heart disease as
     the general population. If, however, there is disparity between thoracic and ab-
     dominal situs, the incidence of congenital heart disease is more than 90%.
     (Check the chest x-ray film to see if the cardiac apex and the stomach bubble are
     on the same side.) Some of these syndromes involve bilateral left-sidedness (2
     bilobed lungs, multiple spleens) and complex cyanotic congenital heart disease,
     while others have bilateral right-sidedness (2 trilobed lungs, absent spleen) and
     complex cyanotic congenital heart disease.

VIII. **General principles of management**

TABLE 55–3. CONGENITAL ANOMALIES ASSOCIATED WITH HEART DEFECTS

Congenital Anomaly	Heart Defect
CHROMOSOMAL ANOMALY	
Trisomy 21 (Down's syndrome)	Atrioventricular canal, ventricular septal defect
Trisomy 13, 15, 18	Ventricular septal defect, patent ductus arteriosus
Syndrome associated with 4p—	Atrial septal defect, ventricular septal defect
Syndrome associated with 5p— (cri du chat syndrome)	Variable
XO (Turner's syndrome)	Coarctation of aorta, aortic stenosis
SYNDROMES WITH PREDOMINANTLY SKELETAL DEFECTS*	
Ellis-van Creveld syndrome	Atrial septal defect, single atrium
Laurence-Moon-Biedl syndrome	Tetralogy of Fallot, ventricular septal defect
Carpenter's syndrome	Patent ductus arteriosus, ventricular septal defect
Holt-Oram syndrome	Atrial septal defect, ventricular septal defect
Fanconi's syndrome	Patent ductus arteriosus, ventricular septal defect
Thrombocytopenia-absent radius syndrome	Atrial septal defect, tetralogy of Fallot
SYNDROMES WITH CHARACTERISTIC FACIES*	
Noonan's syndrome	Pulmonary stenosis
DiGeorge's syndrome	Tetralogy of Fallot, aortic arch anomalies
Smith-Lemli-Opitz syndrome	Ventricular septal defect, patent ductus arteriosus
de Lange's syndrome	Tetralogy of Fallot, ventricular septal defect
Goldenhar's syndrome	Tetralogy of Fallot, variable
William's syndrome	Supravalvular aortic stenosis, peripheral pulmonary artery stenosis
Asymmetric crying facies	Variable

*Not all infants with these syndromes have heart defects.

A. Fetal echocardiography

1. **General considerations.** Fetal echocardiography is now possible in many centers. The optimal gestational age to perform echocardiography is between 18 and 24 weeks, when structural abnormalities and arrhythmias can be detected. With early detection of cardiac abnormalities, arrangements can be made for delivery at a center with pediatric cardiac and surgical facilities. If the anomaly is not consistent with life, some families may elect termination of pregnancy.

2. **Indications**
   a. **Maternal factors.** Oligo- or polyhydramnios, diabetes, collagen vascular disease or teratogen exposure (Table 55–4).
   b. **Fetal factors.** Suspected cardiac abnormality on obstetric ultrasound examination, pleural fluid, pericardial fluid, heart rate abnormalities, intrauterine growth retardation, or other abnormality on obstetric ultrasound examination.

TABLE 55–4. TERATOGENS ASSOCIATED WITH HEART DEFECTS

Teratogen	Heart Defect
DRUGS	
Alcohol	Ventricular septal defect, tetralogy of Fallot, atrial septal defect
Phenytoin	Variable
Thalidomide	Tetralogy of Fallot, truncus arteriosus
Trimethadione	Ventricular septal defect, tetralogy of Fallot
OTHER TERATOGENS	
Maternal diabetes	Variable
Maternal systemic lupus erythematosus	Congenital heart block
Rubella syndrome	Patent ductus arteriosus, peripheral pulmonary stenosis

     c. **Genetic factors.** Familial history of chromosomal disorders or congenital heart disease.
  B. Emergency therapy. Once the specific lesion has been identified as emergent, a decision about therapy must be made. If, for example, one is confronted with a very cyanotic infant with no murmur, a normal chest x-ray film, and a normal ECG and believes the diagnosis of D-transposition of the great arteries is likely, it is necessary to prepare the catheterization laboratory for a **balloon septostomy.**
  C. Prostaglandins. As a general principle, if an infant is cyanotic and has decreased pulmonary blood flow, the Pao_2 will be improved by promoting flow through the ductus arteriosus via a drip of **prostaglandin E$_1$** (Alprostadil, Prostin VR Pediatric). Maintaining patency of the ductus will enable stabilization of the infant and allow cardiac catheterization and subsequent surgery to be planned on an urgent rather than emergent basis. Similarly, if poor peripheral pulses and acidosis from poor perfusion are present, infusion of prostaglandin, utilizing the same dose, will open the ductus arteriosus and allow right ventricular blood flow to augment the systemic circulation. This measure is beneficial in critical aortic stenosis, coarctation of the aorta, and hypoplastic left heart syndrome. (See Chap 73 for dosage and other pharmacologic information.)
  D. Antiarrhythmic drugs. Arrhythmias may occur during intrauterine life or after delivery. They are a cause of fetal hydrops and intrauterine death; most often the rhythm disturbance is a rapid supraventricular tachycardia with a 1:1 ventricular response. Occasionally, atrial flutter with 2:1 block presents before or just after birth. **Digitalis** (see Chap 73) has been a successful antiarrhythmic agent in this situation, but electrical cardioversion is also sometimes necessary.
  E. Pacemaker. In congenital complete heart block with imminent cardiovascular demise, **temporary transvenous ventricular pacing may be lifesaving.** It should be followed by urgent surgical placement of a permanent pacemaker.

PATENT DUCTUS ARTERIOSUS

  I. Definition. Patent ductus arteriosus (PDA) results from failure of the ductus arteriosus to close or from its reopening after functional closure. The ductus arteriosus is an artery that normally closes functionally at birth. In the fetus, the majority of the blood supply bypasses the pulmonary circulation, going from the pulmonary artery to the aorta via the ductus. After birth, if the ductus remains patent, a left-to-right shunt may develop, sometimes creating pulmonary overload and left ventricular failure.
 II. Incidence
  A. Prematurity. There is an increased incidence of PDA in premature infants weighing less than 1500 g (40–60%), and especially in those weighing less than 1000 g.
  B. Congenital rubella. PDA is present in 60–70% of infants with congenital rubella syndrome.
  C. Other forms of congenital heart disease. PDA in the term infant is a distinct lesion accounting for 5–10% of congenital heart disease. It occurs in approximately 1 in 2000 live births. PDA is common in other forms of congenital heart disease such as coarctation of the aorta, total anomalous pulmonary venous return, transposition of the great vessels, and pulmonic stenosis with intact septum.
 III. Pathophysiology
  A. Increased oxygen concentration. The most important factor stimulating functional closure of the ductus arteriosus at birth is the increased oxygen concentration, which has a direct action on smooth muscle in the wall of the ductus. This response increases with increasing gestational age.
  B. Other factors affecting closure of the ductus are **levels of circulating prostaglandins** and the **available muscle mass.** The fetus has high levels of

circulating prostaglandins (eg, PGE_2, PGI_2) as compared to the adult. These are products of arachidonic acid metabolism and have been shown to cause opening of an oxygen-constricted ductus arteriosus. Ductal wall tone is therefore mainly determined by the interaction between oxygen, which produces constricting effects, and endogenous prostaglandins, which produce dilating effects.

   C. Physiology of PDA. At birth, there is a decrease in pulmonary vascular resistance and an increase in systemic resistance. If there is a PDA, the shunt thus becomes left-to-right. A small PDA may be of minimal significance, but a moderate size ductus may produce a significant shunt. This may lead to decreased effective systemic blood flow due to aorta to pulmonary artery shunting. The result is increased left ventricular end-diastolic volume and pressure, increased left atrial pressure and, eventually, if untreated, congestive heart failure.

IV. Risk factors. The major risk factor for PDA is prematurity. There is a slightly higher incidence in females and in infants born at higher altitudes. Congenital rubella and other forms of congenital heart disease are also risk factors (see **II,** above).

V. Clinical presentation. The initial presentation may be at birth or after the first few days of life, depending on the hemodynamics. In neonates, the cardiopulmonary signs and symptoms are as follows.

   A. Heart murmur. The murmur is usually systolic and is heard best in the second or third intercostal space at the left sternal border. There may be a mid-diastolic flow rumble as well because of increased flow across the mitral valve in diastole. The presentation may vary with the degree of shunting (from a soft high frequency continuous murmur to a loud noisy machinery-type murmur) and in a collaborative PDA study, a murmur was found in only 20% of the cases.

   B. Hyperactive precordium. The increased left ventricular stroke volume may result in a hyperactive precordium.

   C. Bounding peripheral pulses. A PDA results in a widened pulse pressure that may produce bounding peripheral pulsations.

   D. Other signs. The disease, if untreated, may progress to left ventricular failure with tachycardia, tachypnea, rales, and congestive hepatomegaly.

VI. Diagnosis

   A. Laboratory studies. In the presence of an increasing left-to-right shunt, **arterial blood gas determinations** will demonstrate progressive hypercarbia and metabolic acidosis.

   B. Radiologic studies. The chest x-ray in an infant with a moderate to large shunt will often show cardiomegaly with prominence of the left ventricle and left atrium. Increased pulmonary vascular markings may be seen and may eventually lead to gross pulmonary edema.

   C. Echocardiography. Two-dimensional and pulsed Doppler echocardiography are highly sensitive and specific in making the diagnosis of PDA. Hemodynamic significance may be estimated by documenting the left atrial and ventricular enlargement along with clinical evidence of respiratory insufficiency. However, the most sensitive method of detecting a shunt is with the use of real-time Doppler color flow mapping.

VII. Management

   A. Ventilatory support. If the infant has deteriorating blood gases and is in respiratory distress, ventilatory support may be needed or increased if the infant has been on mechanical ventilation. If the infant is on mechanical ventilation, increasing the positive end-expiratory pressure may also help to decrease the shunt.

   B. Medical therapy. Medical therapy may be tried initially.

      1. Fluid restriction and diuretics. This measure attempts to minimize the effects of the cardiovascular volume overload by restricting fluid intake, sometimes in association with diuretics. Furosemide (Lasix) is often considered the drug of choice for short-term management (see Chap 73).

      2. Indomethacin (Indocin). Indomethacin is a prostaglandin synthetase inhibitor that blocks the effect of arachidonic acid metabolites on the ductus. In multiple clinical trials, it has proved to be safe and effective. Closure rates as high as 79% have been reported. (See Chap 73 for full dosage information.) Indomethacin should be given if fluid management and ventilator changes fail to significantly lessen the degree of left-to-right ductal shunting. Some clinicians advocate prophylactic indomethacin therapy after initial echocardiographic demonstration of a PDA in the absence of an associated ductal-dependent cyanotic heart lesion.

- **a. Contraindications.** Relative contraindications to the use of indomethacin are as follows.
    - **(1)** Serum creatinine > 1.7 mg/dL or urine output < 1 mL/kg/h.
    - **(2)** Frank renal or gastrointestinal bleeding.
    - **(3)** Signs of necrotizing enterocolitis.
    - **(4)** Suspected or proven sepsis.
- **b. Complications.** There is some short-term toxicity associated with indomethacin treatment.
    - **(1) Transient renal effects.** A transient decrease in glomerular filtration rate and urine output may occur.
    - **(2) Gastrointestinal tract effects.** The few reports of gastrointestinal tract bleeding with indomethacin are not statistically significant. Bleeding has usually been transient, without an increased incidence of necrotizing enterocolitis.
    - **(3) Intracranial hemorrhage.** Despite early reports to the contrary, there is no increased incidence of intracranial hemorrhage after indomethacin therapy. Indomethacin prolongs bleeding time and disturbs platelet function for 7–9 days, irrespective of the platelet number.

C. Surgical therapy. Surgical ligation should be performed for a hemodynamically significant PDA if medical treatment fails. Depending on the condition of the patient, a second course of indomethacin may be considered prior to surgery. Ligation is done through a thoracotomy incision and requires a general anesthetic and paralysis. There is a higher incidence of pneumothorax and grades III and IV cicatricial retinopathy of prematurity in surgically treated infants.

VIII. Prognosis. The outcome is related to many factors, including the degree of prematurity, the underlying lung disease, the ease with which the ductus responds to medical therapy, and other events such as intraventricular hemorrhage. Because there often are associated problems, the mortality rate for the effects of PDA alone cannot be determined. Perioperative mortality for PDA ligation is less than 2%.

PERSISTENT PULMONARY HYPERTENSION (PERSISTENT FETAL CIRCULATION)

I. Definition. Persistent pulmonary hypertension (PPH) evolves when pulmonary vascular resistance increases, resulting in pulmonary hypertension. This, in turn, causes a right-to-left shunt through the ductus arteriosus and/or foramen ovale. This condition usually lasts 3–5 days. If the patient can be managed through this acute period, persistent fetal circulation will usually resolve spontaneously.

II. Incidence. Because of the many underlying causes of pulmonary artery hypertension and the clinical settings from which it may evolve, the incidence varies from center to center and is broad.

III. Pathophysiology. At birth, a sequence of events occurs, allowing the normal transition from fetal to adult circulation. Normally, there is expansion and oxygenation of the lungs, a decrease in pulmonary vascular resistance, and an increase in Pao_2, which aids in constriction of the ductus arteriosus. The systemic vascular resistance increases, and the foramen ovale closes functionally. However, if pulmonary hypertension occurs during this normal process, the foramen ovale and ductus arteriosus will remain open because the pulmonary vascular resistance remains higher than systemic. A right-to-left shunt develops, hypoxia and acidosis result, which further increase pulmonary artery pressure. The following factors are involved in the pathogenesis of pulmonary artery hypertension.

  A. Pulmonary vasoconstriction. Pulmonary vasoconstriction may be caused by hypoxia, acidosis, or premature closure of the ductus arteriosus, which may be due to intrauterine exposure to prostaglandin synthetase inhibitors such as aspirin or indomethacin.

  B. Pathologic changes in the pulmonary arterial smooth muscle. Abnormal muscularization and proliferation may occur secondary to abnormal development or intrauterine hypoxia or stress.

  C. Humoral agents. Thromboxane A_2, a powerful pulmonary vasoconstrictor and a product of the lipoxygenase pathway of arachidonic acid metabolism, may play a role in the development of pulmonary artery hypertension. Other local vasoactive mediators such as prostaglandins, thromboxanes, and endothelium-derived relaxation factor (EDRF) may be involved in the balance between pulmonary vasoconstriction and relaxation.

IV. Risk factors. The following factors or conditions may be associated with an increased risk of persistent fetal circulation.

  A. Lung disease or meconium aspiration syndrome. Hypoxia, hypercarbia, and acidosis may result from lung disease or from meconium aspiration.

  B. Decreased pulmonary vascular bed may occur as primary congenital pulmonary hypoplasia as a result of chronic oligohydramnios (Potter syndrome), or it may be secondary to a diaphragmatic hernia, for example.

  C. Hyperviscosity (polycythemia) may cause functional obstruction of the pulmonary vascular bed with resultant increased arterial pressures.

  D. Congenital heart disease. Any cardiac disease that produces increased pulmonary blood flow (eg, D-transposition of the great arteries), pulmonary venous obstruction (eg, left ventricular failure), or decreased pulmonary blood flow (eg, pulmonic stenosis) may be a cause.

  E. Sepsis. Septic infants frequently develop severe metabolic acidosis with secondary pulmonary vasoconstriction.

  F. Hypocalcemia or hypoglycemia. These metabolic abnormalities may cause decrease in cardiac output, leading to hypoxia and acidosis.

  G. Perinatal factors

    1. Gestational age. The muscular layers of the small pulmonary arterioles develop near term. This developmental change causes a decrease in the cross-sectional area of the pulmonary vascular bed and subsequent increase in resistance to blood flow to the lung.

    2. Fetal distress. Intrauterine fetal distress may be a result of acute or chronic hypoxia.

    3. Repeat elective cesarean section. Labor acts as a stimulus for reduction of pulmonary vascular resistance, resorption of lung fluid, lung maturation, and release of surfactant. If labor is bypassed by cesarean section, these mechanisms fail to occur, which may result in pulmonary hypertension.

V. Clinical presentation

  A. Signs and symptoms. The following signs and symptoms are found in infants with pulmonary artery hypertension.

    1. Increasing alveolar-arterial gradient (A-aDO_2). Normal values are < 20 mm Hg. Values in the range of 250–650 mm Hg may be seen, depending on the degree of the shunt.

    2. Marked lability of oxygenation. Readings on transcutaneous oxygen monitoring or pulse oximeter fall during routine nursing care, drawing of blood, or during periods of stress, loud noise, movement, and crying.

    3. Progressive hypoxia leading to fixed hypoxemia with Pa_{O_2} < 40 mm Hg.

      a. Intermittent cyanosis gives way to persistent cyanosis.

      b. Fixed acidemia (pH < 7.25) may develop secondary to worsening lactic acidosis.

4. Difficulty in maintaining adequate intravascular volume. Central venous and systemic blood pressure are low even with continuous infusion of colloid. Urine output decreases.

5. Single, loud S2 upon auscultation of the heart.

VI. Diagnosis

A. Laboratory studies. The following tests should be closely monitored in a patient with persistent fetal circulation.

   1. Arterial blood gas levels. Without adequate ventilation, blood gas levels will demonstrate fixed hypoxemia, progressive hypercarbia, and metabolic acidosis. Close monitoring of blood gas values is necessary to calculate the alveolar-arterial gradient and the degree of metabolic acidosis, and carbon dioxide retention.

   2. Total and ionized calcium levels. Hypocalcemia, if present, may cause decreased cardiac output, hypoxia, and systemic hypotension.

   3. Serum glucose levels. Hypoglycemia also potentiates hypoxia from decreased cardiac output.

B. Radiologic studies. A chest x-ray study will help detect lung disease. It is often said that oxygen requirements in persistent fetal circulation are out of proportion to the degree of disease seen on a chest x-ray film. Findings may include pneumonia, air leak syndrome (pneumothorax, pulmonary interstitial emphysema, pneumomediastinum, pneumopericardium), aspiration, or retained lung fluid. The lungs may also appear normal but underperfused.

C. Echocardiography. Echocardiography is necessary to rule out congenital cyanotic heart disease. Once congenital heart disease has been excluded, the test is not diagnostic in persistent fetal circulation as the echocardiogram can be normal. Abnormalities may included right ventricular dilatation, hypertrophy, and poor contractility with bowing of the interventricular septum. With pulsed color Doppler echocardiography, however, the shunt may be seen and determined to be at the ductal and/or foraminal level. In addition, the pulmonary artery pressure may be estimated from the flow velocity across a regurgitant tricuspid or pulmonic valve.

D. Differential oximeter readings. Oximetry helps to diagnose the presence of a right-to-left shunt, which is suggestive of persistent fetal circulation. Two transcutaneous oximeters are used, with one sensor placed on the right upper chest wall (preductal) and the other on the left lower abdomen (postductal). Alternately, a pulse oximeter can be used with one sensor on the right thumb (preductal) and a sensor on the left great toe (postductal). If there is a difference of 20 mm Hg in the two readings (correlated to simultaneous blood gases via the right radial and umbilical arteries), a right-to-left ductal shunt should be expected.

E. Response to hyperventilation. The right-to-left shunt may be reversed by hyperventilation or infusion of alkali (bicarbonate) to increase the pH > 7.50. A significant increase in PaO_2 (generally to > 100 torr) with hyperventilation and alkalinization favors the diagnosis of pulmonary artery hypertension rather than cyanotic heart disease, in which the PaO_2 usually does not increase significantly.

VII. Management

A. Drug therapy. For dosages, see Chapter 73.

   1. Fluids and electrolytes. Normal glucose and calcium levels are essential for maintaining cardiac output. Alkali is frequently needed to maintain a normal blood pH, since acidosis is a major cause of pulmonary vasoconstriction. The decision to use sodium bicarbonate or tromethamine (THAM) will depend on serum electrolyte levels, respiratory status, and urinary output. THAM may be preferred if the serum sodium is high and the serum PCO_2 is high. To use THAM, the urine output must be satisfactory.

   2. Sedatives. Sedation is often used in infants exhibiting marked lability and resistance to ventilation. Phenobarbital or lorazepam is useful in stabilizing the infant and reducing the incidence of air leak problems.

3. **Paralyzing agents.** The use of these agents is *controversial*. They may be tried in infants who have not responded to sedation and are still labile and resisting the ventilator. Pancuronium (Pavulon) has been used, since it does not have the hypotensive effects seen with curare. Some infants, however, may worsen with paralysis due to increased ventilation-perfusion mismatch.

4. **Volume expanders.** Blood pressure should be maintained by colloid transfusions (5% albumin or whole blood, depending on the hematocrit). Use whole blood if the hematocrit is low. Maintenance of blood pressure increases the systemic vascular resistance, which helps to decrease the right-to-left shunt.

5. **Pressor agents.** Dopamine is used when the blood pressure is difficult to maintain and there is decreased renal perfusion. Dopamine in higher doses may increase the pulmonary vascular resistance (shown in animal studies), resulting in increased right-to-left shunt. Dobutamine may also be added for its inotropic effect if cardiac contractility is decreased significantly.

6. **Pulmonary vasodilators.** Tolazoline (Priscoline) is an alpha-adrenergic blocking agent and should be used only when oxygenation is difficult to maintain. It is thought to cause dilation of the pulmonary vascular bed. A test dose is usually given, and if there is an increase in oxygenation (usually > 10–25 torr), a drip infusion is started. It is, however, a systemic vasodilator and may cause severe systemic hypotension. Colloid and pressor agents should be readily available if hypotension occurs. Other vasodilator drugs that have been used with occasional success include PGE_1, prostacyclin, PGD_2, sodium nitorprusside, nitroglycerine, isoproteronol, hydralazine, magnesium sulfate, and calcium channel blockers. There is, however, no selective pulmonary vasodilator that is clinically available for use. Nitric oxide, which is synthesized from L-arginine, has been found to be the EDRF and acts on vascular smooth muscle. There are currently ongoing clinical trials using inhaled nitric oxide as a selective pulmonary vasodilator.

B. **Mechanical ventilation**

1. **Ventilatory support** is instituted when the alveolar-arterial gradient is high (usually > 250 mm Hg) and adequate ventilation can no longer be maintained. The goal is to provide ventilation using the **lowest mean airway pressure possible.** Ideally, blood gas levels should be maintained within the following ranges: pH, 7.40–7.50; $Paco_2$, 25–35 mm Hg; PaO_2, over 50 mm Hg. Initially, 100% inspired oxygen should be used, since most of these infants are term, and retinopathy of prematurity is not of major concern. With clinical improvement, the oxygen may then be slowly decreased to maintain acceptable PaO_2 with oxygen saturation > 90%.

2. **Rapid-rate ventilation** may be used in an attempt to hyperventilate the patient and achieve the critical $Paco_2$ (ie, pulmonary artery vasodilatation and a secondary rise in Pao_2). It must be remembered, however, that overventilation may reduce venous return and pulmonary blood flow. Pulmonary vasodilatation may be attained with ventilation in the normal range in conjunction with alkali infusions. Recent work has shown that high-frequency jet ventilation and high-frequency oscillatory ventilation may be used successfully if maximal conventional therapy fails. In approximately 40–60% of patients treated with high-frequency ventilation, the need for extracorporeal membrane oxygenation (ECMO) therapy can be averted. High-frequency ventilation should be attempted when conventional ventilation fails (ie, PaO_2 cannot be maintained at a level $\geq$ 50 mm Hg). (See Chap 10.)

3. **Air leaks** occur frequently when high mean airway pressures are used. Close monitoring for pneumothorax and other forms of barotrauma is essential.

4. **Bag-and-mask ventilation,** using different rates and pressures to determine which combination gives the best oxygenation, is often helpful.
5. **Continuous negative pressure ventilation (CNP).** CNP using a body-enclosing chamber has also been shown to be effective in improving oxygenation and diminishing the need for extracorporeal membrane oxygenation (ECMO) in infants with pulmonary artery hypertension.

C. **Extracorporeal membrane oxygenation (ECMO).** (See Chap 11.) It is recommended for infants less than 7 days old, greater than 34 weeks' gestation, and greater than 2 kg in weight. It involves cannulation of the internal jugular vein and common carotid artery and placing the infant on cardiopulmonary bypass. There is currently an 82% rate of successful outcome. The decision to send an infant to an ECMO center depends on many factors; ECMO should be considered when:

1. The infant is unable to maintain adequate oxygenation (PaO_2 50 mm Hg).
2. The A-aDO_2 gradient is increasing.
3. Increasing support is required to maintain blood pressure.
4. The infant meets the ECMO criteria specified on page 122.

VIII. **Prognosis.** Prognosis depends on the underlying condition; for example, an infant with RDS usually does better than one with pulmonary hypoplasia. For all causes, survival is now in the range of 50–70%. Outcome also depends on other factors such as the presence of asphyxia, duration of hyperventilation, and central nervous system dysfunction. The condition of infants seen at follow-up can range from normal to severe neurodevelopmental delay, and sensorineural hearing loss.

REFERENCES

Abu-Osba YK: Treatment of persistent pulmonary hypertension of the newborn: update. *Arch Dis Child* 1991;**66**:74.

Clarke WR: The transitional circulation: physiology and anesthetic implications. *J Clin Anesth* 1990;**2**:192.

Cotton RB, Haywood JL, FitzGerald GA: Symptomatic patent ductus arteriosus following prophylactic indomethacin. A clinical and biochemical appraisal. *Biol Neonate* 1991;**60**:273.

Cvetnic WG, Shoptaugh M, Sills JH: Intermittent mandatory ventilation with continuous negative pressure compared with positive end-expiratory pressure for neonatal hypoxemia. *J Perinatol* 1992;**XII**:316.

Cvetnic WG, Sills JH: Neonatal lung disease. *Clin Anesth* 1992;**6**:395.

Edwards AD et al: Effects of indomethacin on cerebral hemodynamics in very preterm infants. *Lancet* 1990;**335**:1491.

Evans N: Diagnosis of patent ductus arteriosus in the preterm newborn. *Arch Dis Child* 1993;**68**:58.

Geggel RL: Inhalational nitric oxide: A selective pulmonary vasodilatory for treatment of persistent pulmonary hypertension of the newborn. *J Pediatr* 1993;**123**:76.

Keszler M et al: Severe respiratory failure after elective repeat cesarean delivery: a potentially preventable condition leading to extracorporeal membrane oxygenation. *Pediatrics* 1992;**89**:670.

Kinsella JP, Abman SH: Inhalational nitric oxide therapy for persistent pulmonary hypertension of the newborn. *Pediatrics* 1993;**91**:997.

Knight DB: Patent ductus arteriosus: How important to which babies? *Early Hum Dev* 1992;**29**:287.

Marron MJ et al: Hearing and neurodevelopmental outcome in survivors of persistent pulmonary hypertension of the newborn. *Pediatrics* 1992;**90**:392.

Meinert CL: Extracorporeal membrane oxygenation trials. *Pediatrics* 1990;**85**:365.

Reller MD et al: The timing of spontaneous closure of the ductus arteriosus in infants with respiratory distress syndrome. *Am J Cardiol* 1990;**66**:75.

Renfro WH, Burr JM, Rawlings J: Criteria for use of indomethacin injection in neonates. *Clin Pharm* 1993;**12**:232.

Satur CR, Walker DR, Dickinson DF: Day case ligation of patent ductus arteriosus in preterm infants: a 10 year review. *Arch Dis Child* 1991;**66**:477.

Stefano JL et al: Closure of the ductus arteriosus with indomethacin in ventilated neonates with respiratory distress syndrome. Effects of pulmonary compliance and ventilation. *Am Rev Respir Dis* 1991;**143**:236.

Van Bel F, Van Zwieten PH, Den Ouden LL: Contribution of color Doppler flow imaging to the evaluation of the effect of indomethacin on neonatal cerebral hemodynamics. *J Ultrasound Med* 1990;**9**:107.

Varnholt V et al: High frequency oscillatory ventilation and extracorporeal membrane oxygenation in severe persistent pulmonary hypertension of the newborn. *Eur J Pediatr* 1992;**151**:769.

Walsh-Sukys MC: Persistent pulmonary hypertension of the newborn. The black box revisited. *Clin Perinatol* 1993;**20**:127.

Weigel TJ, Hageman JR: National survey of diagnosis and management of persistent pulmonary hypertension of the newborn. *J Perinatol* 1990;**X**:369.

Zanardo V et al: Early screening and treatment of "silent" patent ductus arteriosus in prematures with RDS. *J Perinat Med* 1991;**19**:291.

56 Common Multiple Congenital Anomaly Syndromes

The intensive care newborn nursery is a busy place where quick decisions must often be made. For many disorders, treatment is the same regardless of the underlying problem. However, in the management of multiple congenital anomaly (MCA) syndromes, the neonatologist must deal with complex clinical issues calling for a wide range of diagnostic skills. Without a correct diagnosis of MCA syndrome, many available forms of therapy go underutilized and others may be tried when they will be relatively ineffective. Furthermore, unrealistic counseling may be given about prognosis and recurrence risk.

Only a few MCA syndromes are life-threatening in the neonatal period. It is important to note, however, that malformations are second only to prematurity as a cause of death at this critical point in the life span.

I. **Clinical presentation.** Table 56–1 lists symptoms and signs that should alert the clinician to the possibility of cryptogenic malformations or disorders. Obviously, if overt malformations are present, an MCA syndrome will be immediately recognized and diagnostic efforts will shortly follow. However, if external features of the disorder are subtle or nonspecific and the usual procedures associated with intensive newborn support have been started, findings may go unrecognized early. Each manifestation listed in Table 56–1 is more common in infants with MCA syndromes.

Tables 56–2 through 56–5 list the more common neonatal MCA syndromes, many of which share some of the features set forth in Table 56–1.

II. **General approach to diagnosis.** The diagnostic approach to malformations in neonates is no different from that in older children except that the effects of delivery and excess baby fat must be considered. Because so many of these children are intubated and have protective eye patches, the face may be obscured. Early and accurate documentation of physical characteristics, including photographs, is essential. If the infant is critically ill, confirmatory tests (chromosome studies, renal ultrasonography, echocardiography) become a priority equal in importance to on-

---

TABLE 56–1. SYMPTOMS AND SIGNS IN NEONATES THAT MIGHT INDICATE CRYPTIC MULTIPLE CONGENITAL ANOMALY SYNDROME

Prenatal
Oligohydramnios
Polyhydramnios
Decreased or unusual fetal activity
Abnormal fetal problem

Postnatal
Abnormalities of size: SGA or LGA, microcephaly or macrocephaly, large or irregular abdomen, small chest, limb-trunk disproportion, asymmetry
Abnormalities of tone: Hypotonia, hypertonia
Abnormalities of position: Joint contractures, fixation of joints in extension, hyperextension of joints
Midline aberrations: Hemangiomas, hair tufts, dimples or pits
Problems of secretion, excretion, or edema: No urination, no passage of meconium, chronic nasal or oral secretions, edema (nuchal, pedal, generalized, ascites)
Symptoms: Unexplained seizures, resistant or unexplained respiratory distress
Metabolic disorders: Resistant hypoglycemia, unexplained hypo- or hypercalcemia, polycythemia

---

TABLE 56–2. MOST COMMON CHROMOSOME DISORDERS DIAGNOSED IN THE NEONATAL PERIOD

Trisomy 21 (Down's syndrome)
Trisomy 18
Trisomy 13
45,X (Turner's) syndrome

going therapy. **The basis of diagnosis of MCA syndromes in the neonate is knowing which disorders are most common plus documentation of the physical manifestations and appropriate exclusion tests such as chromosomal analysis.** This somewhat "overkill" approach is necessary because a significant percentage of infants with MCA syndromes die in the neonatal period, often before a diagnosis is made, and because the parents in such cases often refuse to permit autopsy. Diagnostic problems also occur because immediate efforts tend to emphasize therapy. Nevertheless, diagnosis will often facilitate or guide therapy in a more efficient manner. If clinical geneticists or dysmorphologists are locally available, they should be asked to examine the infant as soon after delivery as possible. If specialists in these fields are not available, a phone call to a university medical center asking for expert advice is often useful.

III. **Chromosomal syndromes** (Table 56–2). Chromosomal syndromes are by far the most common MCA syndromes diagnosed in the neonatal period.
  A. **Trisomy 21 (Down's syndrome)**
    1. **Incidence.** Trisomy 21 is by far the most common MCA syndrome, occurring in about 1:600 live births. Only about 80% of cases are diagnosed accurately in the newborn nursery, which means that there is a 20% rate of diagnostic error for this most common cause of MCA and mental retardation. The reason for missing the diagnosis is probably that most of the features of trisomy 21 may occur as isolated features in otherwise normal infants.
    2. **Physical findings.** Findings include epicanthus, hypotelorism, a tendency to protrude the tongue, Brushfield's spots, single transverse palmar crease, and mongoloid slant of the palpebral fissures. Although each of these features may occur in normal individuals, it is the combination of features forming a recognizable pattern that usually permits early diagnosis.
    3. **Associated anomalies** include congenital heart defects and increased frequency of duodenal atresia, esophageal atresia, and imperforate anus. Patients may have many immediate medical problems because of these anomalies.
    4. **Hyptonia** may be associated with breathing difficulties, poor swallowing, and aspiration.
  B. **Trisomy 18 (Edwards' syndrome)**
    1. **Incidence.** About 1:5000 live births.
    2. **Morbidity.** Highly lethal within the first 3 months of life.
    3. **Physical findings.** Manifested by micrognathia, overlapping digits, rockerbottom feet, congenital heart disease (usually VSD or PDA), abnormal ears, short sternum, ptosis, and generalized hypertonicity.
  C. **Trisomy 13 (Patau's syndrome)**
    1. **Incidence.** About 1:7000 live births.
    2. **Morbidity.** Highly lethal within the first 3 months of life.

TABLE 56–3. MOST COMMON NONCHROMOSOMAL DEFORMATION/DISRUPTION SEQUENCES DIAGNOSED IN THE NEONATAL PERIOD

Potter's oligohydramnios sequence
Amniotic band syndrome
Arthrogryposis
Pierre Robin sequence

TABLE 56–4. OTHER MCA SYNDROMES OF SPECIAL INTEREST IN THE NEONATE

VATER association
CHARGE association
Lethal short-limb, short-rib dwarfism
DiGeorge association
Beckwith syndrome

    3. Physical findings. Manifested by cleft lip and palate, polydactyly, microphthalmia, and congenital heart disease (usually VSD or PDA).

  D. 45,X (Turner's) syndrome

    1. Incidence. About 1:10,000 live-born females.

    2. Morbidity. The 45,X syndrome is usually compatible with survival if the child reaches term.

    3. Physical findings. Neck webbing, pedal and nuchal edema, and short stature are the hallmarks of this disorder.

IV. Nonchromosomal syndromes (Table 56–3)

  A. Oligohydramnios sequence (Potter's oligohydramnios sequence)

    1. Incidence. This syndrome is the second most common MCA (1:3000 live births). Most cases are nonsyndromic and have a 2–7% recurrence risk, depending on the specific urinary tract defect. Some may be associated with the prune belly syndrome (absent abdominal musculature, urinary tract abnormalities, cryptorchidism) if the kidneys were hydronephrotic early in gestation and later decompress, leaving a wrinkled abdomen and the effects of oligohydramnios (pulmonary hypoplasia and Potter' sequence). About 5% of cases are part of an MCA syndrome with primary defects outside the urinary system.

    2. Morbidity. Almost all of these infants die.

    3. Pathophysiology. Renal agenesis leads to decreased production of amniotic fluid (oligohydramnios). Deficient amniotic fluid is believed to be responsible for associated pulmonary hypoplasia.

    4. Clinical presentation

      a. History. The history of oligohydramnios must be solicited from the obstetrician. Anuria is typically present in the newborn.

      b. Placental examination. The placenta must be examined for yellowish plaques ("**amnion nodosum**").

      c. Physical findings. Unexplained and highly refractory respiratory distress coupled with pneumothoraces, club feet, hyperextensible fingers, large cartilage-deficient ears, lower inner eye folds, and a beak nose are classic manifestations associated with prolonged and severe oligohydramnios.

    5. Diagnosis is usually confirmed by renal ultrasonography and autopsy disclosure of the urinary tract abnormality. It is advisable to do chromosome studies on the propositus to exclude a chromosomal basis for the disorder. The recurrence risk depends on the specific syndrome diagnosis. In either case, future pregnancies should be monitored by ultrasonography unless the risk of recurrence is definitely ruled out.

  B. Amniotic band syndrome

    1. Incidence. About 1:4000 live births. Because in some newborns many body

TABLE 56–5. TERATOGENIC SYNDROMES COMMONLY SEEN IN NOENATES

Fetal alcohol syndrome
Fetal hydantoin syndrome
Fetal valproate syndrome
Fetal cocaine syndrome
Infant of diabetic mother

areas are involved and because the bands dissipate before delivery in 90% of cases, the diagnosis is often missed or a misdiagnosis is made.

2. Pathophysiology. This syndrome is poorly understood, but the effects of early amnion rupture with entanglement of body parts in bands or strands of amnion are well appreciated. The resulting biomechanical forces can cause deformities of the limbs, digits, and craniofacies. Viscera that are normally outside the fetus in early embryologic development may be hindered in their return, giving rise to omphalocele and other anomalies.

3. Physical findings

a. Extremities. Limb and digit amputations, constrictions, distal swellings.

b. Craniofacies. Facial clefts, encephaloceles.

c. Viscera. Omphalocele, gastroschisis, ectopia cordis.

4. Placental examination. It is always important to examine the placenta, but especially in these cases. The amnion is often small, absent, or rolled into strands. Not all amniotic bands cause intrauterine problems. Recent ultrasound studies of routine pregnancies have identified amniotic bands that were not attached to the fetus. Follow-up of these pregnancies has revealed normal newborns.

5. Management. Surgical removal of the constricting band and plastic surgical reconstruction should be done if possible.

C. Arthrogryposis (multiple joint fixations)

1. Incidence. About 1:3000 live births.

2. Pathophysiology. Ninety percent of children with arthrogryposis have a neurologic (brain, spinal cord) basis for the disorder. Many syndromes associated with fetal inactivity (akinesia) may be characterized by arthrogryposis also, because normal fetal joint development depends on adequate fetal movement.

3. Clinical presentation. The newborn infant is afflicted by a combination of joint contractures, joint extensions, and joint dislocations. Those with arthrogryposis of central nervous system origin are at increased risk for aspiration and inadequate respiratory movement.

4. Management. Early treatment and rehabilitation can result in remarkable improvement.

D. Pierre Robin sequence

1. Incidence. About 1:8000 live births.

2. Pathophysiology. The basis of this sequence is severe hypoplasia of the mandible, which does not support the tongue. The accompanying glossoptosis results in severe upper airway obstruction and early intrauterine cleft palate.

3. Clinical presentation. These infants present with a short jaw or receding chin associated with cleft palate. Respiratory distress due to upper airway obstruction may occur.

4. Differential diagnosis. Many syndromes (eg, **Stickler, Catel-Manzke**) have the craniofacial features of Pierre Robin sequence. If noncraniofacial primary defects (malformations) are present, an MCA syndrome other than Pierre Robin sequence is present. Some syndromes (eg, Stickler syndrome) may be manifested only by craniofacial features in infancy. Examinations for myopia and malar flattening should be done to support a diagnosis of Stickler syndrome rather than Pierre Robin sequence.

5. Management. Intubation, obturators, tracheostomy, and suturing of the tongue tip to the lower gingiva are effective temporary measures for glossoptosis. As the mandible grows out, the glossoptosis eventually will resolve. Oral feedings may result in choking or respiratory distress, and gavage feedings or gastrostomy tube feedings may be needed. Most cases of Pierre Robin sequence are nonsyndromic and have little or no recurrence risk.

V. Miscellaneous syndromes (Table 56–4)

A. VATER association

1. Incidence. About 1:5000 live births.

2. **Clinical presentation.** Major features include Vertebral anomalies, Anal atresia, Tracheoesophageal fistula, Esophageal atresia, and Radial defects. The **V** in VATER can also represent vascular (cardiac) defects and the **R** renal defects, since these 2 areas are also commonly involved. The presence of additional features, except for atresia of the small intestine, rules out a diagnosis of VATER association. This nonrandom association is usually not of genetic origin and requires exclusion of other similar disorders, including chromosomal syndromes.

B. **CHARGE association**
   1. **Incidence.** While not as common as the VATER association, CHARGE often presents as a medical emergency because about half the patients have choanal atresia.
   2. **Clinical presentation**
      a. **CHARGE** stands for **C** coloboma, **H** heart disease, **A** choanal atresia, **R** retarded growth and development with or without CNS anomalies, **G** genital anomalies with or without hypogonadism, and **E** ear abnormalities and/or deafness.
      b. **Choanal atresia.** The infant may present with unexplained respiratory distress.
      c. **Associated anomalies.** Patients with CHARGE association also have heart defects, small ears, and retinal colobomas; males have micropenis. A smaller percentage have unilateral facial palsies and swallowing difficulties, the latter potentially as lethal as choanal atresia. Postnatal growth deficiency and psychomotor delay round out the major features of this nonrandom and nongenetic association.
   3. **Diagnosis.** Any newborn with unexplained breathing difficulties should have nasogastric tubes passed through its nasal passages, particularly if there are multiple congenital anomalies. Exclusion of other similar entities and chromosomal disorders is essential before the diagnosis of CHARGE association can be accepted.

C. **Lethal short-limb, short-rib dwarfism**
   1. **Incidence.** About 1:5000 live births.
   2. **Pathophysiology.** The 3 most common lethal dwarfing conditions are **achondrogenesis, thanatophoric dysplasia,** and **type II osteogenesis imperfecta.** However, at least 7 other disorders can be lethal in neonates. All of these disorders are of genetic origin.
   3. **Clinical presentation.** These conditions commonly present clinical and diagnostic difficulties in neonates. Recognition of disproportionate parameters in a newborn with respiratory distress should immediately suggest the possibility of a lethal dwarfing condition. Because many newborns have a lot of fat, chest size may be difficult to assess.
   4. **Diagnosis.** If the babygram (chest and abdominal x-ray film) shows a small chest and long bone metaphyseal or epiphyseal abnormalities, a potentially lethal dwarfing condition is present and accurate diagnosis is essential for prognosis estimation of recurrence risk. A full skeletal x-ray study is mandatory in all cases.

D. **DiGeorge association**
   1. **Clinical presentation**
      a. **Physical findings** include heart defects; small, abnormally shaped ears; and mild nonspecific facial dysmorphology.
      b. **Laboratory findings** usually consist of hypocalcemia secondary to absence or hypoplasia of the parathyroid glands. Hypocalcemia is often diagnosed before other features are recognized, and this finding should immediately stimulate a search for abnormalities of the heart and craniofacial area. A decreased lymphocyte count may also be seen.
   2. **Associated anomalies.** Total or partial **thymic absence** is a hidden feature of the DiGeorge association that should be investigated because it may be the most serious of all the abnormalities.

E. Beckwith's syndrome
   1. Clinical presentation
      a. Physical findings typically include macroglossia and omphalocele, but about 20% of patients have only one or neither of these 2 features. Unilateral limb hypertrophy may also be seen.
      b. Laboratory findings. Refractory hypoglycemia is frequently present regardless of the presence of external features and should immediately raise the possibility of Beckwith's syndrome.
   2. Management. Making the diagnosis early in the postnatal period and immediate institution of aggressive hypoglycemic therapy may prevent mental retardation.
VI. Teratogenic malformations (Table 56–5)
   A. Fetal alcohol syndrome may be suspected on the basis of the phenotype alone or may present only as an SGA infant. It may also present with microcephaly, microphthalmia, and a flattened maxillary area. A thorough history of maternal drug intake is important to rule out a teratogenic cause of malformations.
   B. Fetal hydantoin syndrome is characterized by a typical facies (broad, low nasal bridge, hypertelorism, epicanthal folds, ptosis, and prominent malformed ears), and these infants also have a high incidence of absence or hypoplasia of the fifth fingernail and toenail.
   C. Fetal valproate syndrome was recently recognized after the association of neural tube defects (ie, spina bifida) in offspring of mothers taking valproic acid was established in 1982. Other anomalies comprising the fetal valproate syndrome include prominent or fused metopic suture, trigonencephaly, epicanthal folds, midface hypoplasia, anteverted nostrils, oral cleft, heart defect, hypospadius, club feet, and psychomotor retardation.
   D. Fetal cocaine syndrome is characteristically seen in small-for-gestational-age (SGA) infants, who may show hyperirritability or withdrawal symptomatology. There is an increased incidence of genitourinary tract anomalies such as hydronephrosis, hypospadias, and prune belly sequence and central nervous system abnormalities such as microcephaly, porencephaly, and infarction. There have been reports of gastrointestinal and cardiac anomalies. No well-established facial phenotype is known at this time.
   E. Infants of diabetic mothers
      1. Incidence. These infants are at 3 times the risk for malformations compared with the offspring of nondiabetic mothers. Infants of diabetic mothers present with anomalies in approximately 1:2000 consecutive deliveries.
      2. Clinical presentation. The well-known malformations are sacral agenesis, femoral hypoplasia, heart defects, and cleft palate. Others include preaxial radial defects, microtia, cleft lip, microphthalmia, holoprosencephaly, microcephaly, anencephaly, spina bifida, hemivertebra, urinary tract defects, and hallical polydactyly. Some infants of diabetic mothers have many anomalies, which may not be recognized as related to maternal diabetes.
VII. Genetic counseling for multiple congenital anomaly syndromes is complex and requires a great deal of bona fide sensitivity. It is first important to have a secure diagnosis, if one is possible. The next step is to establish where the parents are with the entire situation and what they have been told by other professionals. Be sure you know what questions the parents want answers to before the factual counseling begins. Do not give excessive details relative to the facts and try to avoid specific predictions, particularly timing and the presence or absence of certain problems relative to the future. Leave some degree of hope, but be honestly realistic; particularly if the parents clearly demand it. Assume frequent follow-up counseling sessions and outline a long-term program for the child's care and evaluations. Recurrence risk figures and the availability of prenatal diagnosis for subsequent pregnancies are mandatory areas to cover. Remember, you may well view the child's problems much differently than the parents. Consequently, work with the family from their perspective.

REFERENCES

Aase JM: *Diagnostic Dysmorphology.* Plenium Medical Publishers, 1990.

Hall BD: The twenty-five most common multiple congenital anomaly syndromes. Pages 141–150 in: *Genetic Issues in Pediatric, Obstetric, and Gynecologic Practice.* Kaback MM (editor). Year Book, 1981

Myrianthopoulos NC, Chung CS: Congenital malformations in singletons: Epidemiologic survey. *Birth Defects* 1974;**10:**1.

Smith DW: *Recognizable Patterns of Human Malformations,* 3rd ed. Saunders, 1982.

Van Regemorter N et al: Congenital malformations in 10,000 consecutive births in a university hospital: Need for genetic counseling and prenatal diagnosis. *J Pediatr* 1984;**104:**386.

57 Infant of Drug-Abusing Mother

I. **Definition.** An infant of a drug-abusing mother (IDAM) is an infant whose mother has taken drugs that may potentially cause neonatal withdrawal symptoms. The constellation of signs and symptoms associated with withdrawal is called the neonatal abstinence syndrome (NAS). Table 57–1 lists drugs that have been associated with NAS.

II. **Incidence.** Maternal drug abuse has increased over the past decade. It is estimated that about 10% of deliveries nationwide are to women who have abused drugs during pregnancy. The incidence is considerably higher in inner-city hospitals.

III. **Pathophysiology.** Drugs of abuse are of low molecular weight and are usually water-soluble and lipophilic. These features facilitate their transfer across the placenta and accumulation in the fetus and amniotic fluid. Half-life of drugs is usually prolonged in the fetus compared to an adult. Most drugs of abuse either bind to various CNS receptors or effect the release and reuptake of various neurotransmitters. This may have a long-lasting trophic effect on developing dendritic structures. In addition, some drugs are directly toxic to fetal cells. The developing fetus may also be effected by the direct physiologic effects of a drug. Many of the fetal effects of cocaine, including its putative teratogenic effects, are thought to be due to its potent vasoconstrictive property.

Some drugs appear to have a partially beneficial effect. The incidence of RDS is decreased following maternal use of heroin and possibly cocaine also. These effects are probably a reflection of fetal stress rather than a direct maturational effect of these drugs. Particularly in the case of cocaine, the decreased incidence of RDS is more than offset by the considerable increase in preterm deliveries following its use. The major concern in IDAMs is the long-term outcome. The importance of direct and indirect effects of drugs on the developing CNS predominate and the risks of drug abuse far outweigh the benefits.

IV. **Limitations of studies on drug abuse.** Existing studies on neonatal effects of drug exposure in utero are subject to many confounding factors. Many studies have relied on history obtained from the mother and this is notoriously inaccurate.

TABLE 57–1. DRUGS CAUSING NEONATAL WITHDRAWAL SYNDROME

Opiates	Barbiturates	Miscellaneous
Codeine	Butalbital	Alcohol
Heroin	Phenobarbital	Amphetamine
Meperidine	Secobarbital	Cocaine
Methadone		Chlordiazepoxide
Morphine		Clomipramine
Pentazocine		Desmethylimipramine
Propoxyphene		Diazepam
		Diphenhydramine
		Ethchlorvynol
		Fluphenazine
		Glutethimide
		Hydroxyzine
		Imipramine
		Meprobamate
		Phencyclidine

In addition to recall bias there is a considerable incentive to withhold information. Testing of urine for drugs of abuse does not reflect drug exposure throughout pregnancy and does not provide quantitative information. Many women who abuse drugs are poly-drug abusers and also drink alcohol and smoke cigarettes. It is thus difficult to isolate the effects of any one drug. Social and economic deprivation is common among drug abusers and this factor compounds not only perinatal data but has a major effect on long-term studies of infant outcome.

V. **Risk factors.** Associated with an increased incidence of drug abuse:
   A. **Poor social and economic circumstances.**
   B. **Poor antenatal care.**
   C. **Teenage or unwed mothers.**
   D. **Poor education.**

VI. **Associated conditions**
   A. **Infectious diseases** (hepatitis B, syphilis, and other STD).
   B. **HIV positive serology.**
   C. **Multiple drug abuse.**
   D. **Poor nutritional status.**
   E. **Anemia.**

VII. **Obstetric complications**
   A. **Premature delivery.**
   B. **Premature rupture of membranes.**
   C. **Chorioamnionitis.**
   D. **Fetal distress.**
   E. **IUGR.**
   F. **With cocaine use** (in addition to above):
      1. **Hypertension.**
      2. **Abruptio placentae.**
      3. **Cardiac:** arrhythmias, myocardial ischemia and infarction.
      4. **Cerebrovascular accident.**
      5. **Respiratory arrest.**
      6. **Fetal demise.**

VIII. **Diagnosis.**
   A. **History.** Many, if not most, drug abusers withhold this information. Details of extent and quantity and duration of abuse is unreliable. It is, however, the simplest and most convenient means of diagnosis.
   B. **Laboratory tests.** The most commonly used tests to detect drugs of abuse are immunoassays (enzymatic or radio-). They are, however, subject to a low rate of false-negative and, due to cross-reactivity, false-positive testing. They are thus viewed as screening tests. In cases where it is either medically or legally important these tests should be supplemented by the more sensitive and specific chromatographic and/or mass spectrometric tests.
      1. **Urine.** This is easily obtained and is the most common substance used at present for drug-testing. Reflects intake only in the last few days prior to delivery. Urine may be obtained from both mother and baby (where it may persist for a longer time).
         a. **False-negative immunoassays.** May be due to dilution (low specific gravity) or high NaCl content (detected by high specific gravity). Various adulterants may also effect detection; this is unlikely in the neonate but may occur in maternal urine.
         b. **False-positive immunoassays.** While these depend on the specific assay used, the following have been reported:
            (1) **Detected as morphine:** Codeine (found in many cold and cough medications and in analgesics). About 10% of codeine is metabolized to morphine in the liver. Consumption of baked goods containing poppy seeds (eg, bagels) can result in detectable amounts of morphine in the urine. These are 'physiologic' false positives but chromatography/mass spectrometry may determine the source by quantitative assays of other metabolites.

(2) **Detected as amphetamines:** ranitidine, chlorpromazine, ritodrine, phenylpropanolamine, ephedrine, pseudoephedrine, phenylephrine, phentermine, phenmetrazine. Some of these (eg, phenylpropanolamine, pseudoephedrine, phenylephrine) are found in many "over-the-counter" preparations.

(3) **Very high concentrations of nicotine** (probably higher than those obtained in smokers) have shown false-positive in-vitro testing for morphine and benzoylecgonine.

2. **Meconium.** This is easily obtained and drugs may be found up to 3 days following delivery. Is a more sensitive test than urine for detecting drug abuse and reflects usage over a longer period than is detectable by urine testing. Its main disadvantage is that the specimen requires processing prior to testing and hence places an additional burden on the laboratory.

3. **Hair.** This is by far the most sensitive test available for detection of drug abuse. Hair grows at 1–2 cm/month; hence maternal hair can be segmented and each segment analyzed for drugs. Thus details of drug abuse throughout pregnancy may be obtained. There is a quantitative relation between amounts of drug used and amounts incorporated in growing hair. Hair may be obtained from the mother or infant (where it will reflect usage only during the last trimester). Hair may also be obtained from the infant a long time after delivery should symptoms occur that suggest in-utero drug exposure which was previously unsuspected. The test requires processing prior to assay, is more expensive and is, at present, not as widely available.

IX. **Signs and symptoms of drug withdrawal.** These are listed in Table 57–2. These signs essentially reflect CNS "irritability," altered neurobehavioral organization, and abnormal sympathetic activation. While each drug may have its own effects, these signs and symptoms must be noted for every infant of a drug-abusing mother (because of poly-drug abuse) and, conversely, drug abuse should be suspected in infants exhibiting these signs and symptoms.

A scoring system has been devised for assessment of withdrawal signs; this is commonly called the **"Finnegan score"** after its originator. However the score had been devised for neonates exposed to opiates in utero. Its utility for assessing signs following exposure to other drugs or to guide management in these cases has not been established, but can be used as a guide. The scoring system is in Table 57–3.

No laboratory tests are routinely required in IDAM (other than tests to confirm

---

TABLE 57–2. SIGNS AND SYMPTOMS OF NEONATAL ABSTINENCE

Hyperirritability
   Increased deep-tendon and primitive reflexes
   Hypertonus; hyperacusis
   Tremors
   High-pitched cry
Seizures
Wakefulness
Increased rooting reflex
Uncoordinated/ineffectual sucking and swallowing
Regurgitation and vomiting
Loose stools and diarrhea
Tachypnea; apnea
Yawning; hiccups
Sneezing; stuffy nose
Mottling
Fever
Failure to gain weight
Lacrimation

TABLE 57–3. MODIFIED FINNEGAN'S SCORING SYSTEM FOR NEONATAL WITHDRAWAL[a,b]

Signs and symptoms are scored between feedings.

Cry:	High-pitch (2)															
	Continuous (3)															
Sleep hours after feed:	1 hour (3)															
	2 hours (2)															
	3 hours (1)															
Moro reflex:	Hyperactive (2)															
	Marked (3)															
Tremors when disturbed:	Mild (2)															
	Marked (3)															
Tremors when un-disturbed:	Mild (3)															
	Marked (4)															
Muscle tone increased:	Mild (3)															
	Marked (6)															
Convulsions:	(8)															
Feedings:																
Frantic sucking of fists	(1)															
Poor feeding ability	(1)															
Regurgitation	(1)															
Projectile vom-iting	(1)															
Stools:	Loose (2)															
	Watery (3)															
Fever:	100–101 °F (2)															
	Over 101 °F (2)															
Respiratory rate:	> 60/minute (1)															
	Retractions (2)															
Excoriations:	Nose (1)															
	Knees (1)															
	Toes (1)															
Frequent yawning:	(1)															
Sneezing:	(1)															
Nasal stuffiness:	(1)															
Sweating:	(1)															
Total scores per day																

[a]Initiated by Loretta Finnegan, MD, and modified by J. Yoon, MD
[b]Once an objective score has been attained a dose for treatment can be decided upon.
Reproduced with permission.

the diagnosis). Laboratory tests are required to rule out other etiologies of particular signs and symptoms (eg, calcium and glucose for cases of jerky movements) or to follow-up and manage some particular complication of drug abuse appropriately.

X. **Specific drugs**

    A. **Opiates.** Opiates bind to opiate receptors in the CNS while part of the clinical manifestations of narcotic withdrawal result from alpha-2-adrenergic supersensitivity (particularly in the locus ceruleus). Infants born to opiate-addicted mothers show an increased incidence of IUGR and perinatal distress. Even when not SGA they have lower weight and head circumference compared to drug-free babies.

Signs and symptoms of withdrawal occur in 60–90% of exposed babies. Onset of symptoms may be minutes following delivery up to 1–2 weeks of age but most infants will exhibit signs by 2–3 days of life. Onset of withdrawal may be delayed beyond 2 weeks in infants exposed to methadone.

Clinical course is variable ranging from mild symptoms of brief duration to severe symptoms. Clinical course may be protracted with exacerbations or recurrence of symptoms after discharge. Restlessness, agitation, tremors, wakefulness, and feeding problems may persist for 3–6 months. A blunted ventilatory response to carbon dioxide has been shown. There is reduced incidence of RDS and of hyperbilirubinemia.

Prognosis: There is increased risk of SIDS and of strabismus. A substantial proportion of children will demonstrate good catch-up growth by 1–2 years of age although they may still be below the mean. There is no firm evidence for long-term cognitive impairment but a higher proportion of these children will have some psychomotor retardation and require special education classes. Behavioral dysfunction and poor attention span have been reported.

B. **Cocaine.** Cocaine prevents the reuptake of neurotransmitters (epinephrine, norepinephrine, dopamine, serotonin) at nerve endings and causes a supersensitivity or exaggerated response to neurotransmitters at the effector organs. It also effects the permeability of nerves to sodium ions. Cocaine is a CNS stimulant and a sympathetic activator with potent vasoconstrictive properties. It causes a decrease in uterine and placental blood flow with consequent fetal hypoxemia. It causes hypertension in mother and fetus with a reduction in fetal cerebral blood flow.

Symptoms seen in neonates exposed to cocaine in utero are: irritability, tremors, hypertonia, high-pitched cry, hyperreflexia, frantic fist sucking, feeding problems, sneezing, tachypnea, and abnormal sleep patterns. A specific cocaine-withdrawal syndrome has not been described. The symptoms mentioned above may be a reflection of cocaine intoxication rather than withdrawal, and following an initial period of irritability and over-activity, a period of lethargy and decreased tone has been described.

In the neonate the following have been described: NEC, transient hypertension and reduced cardiac output (1st day of life), intracranial hemorrhages and infarcts, seizures, apneic spells, periodic breathing, abnormal EEG, abnormal brainstem auditory evoked potentials, abnormal response to hypoxia and carbon dioxide, and ileal perforation.

Cocaine has been suggested as a teratogen. A list of malformations attributed to cocaine is presented in Table 57–4. Most of these reports are based on insufficiently controlled observations. A recent meta-analysis on this subject concluded that the only (statistically) significant effects were an increased incidence of genitourinary malformations and of in utero death.

Prognosis: By 1 year of age most infants will have achieved catch-up growth. At 3–4 years there are problems with expressive and receptive speech and children are reported to be hyperactive, distractable, irritable, and to have problems socializing. There is, however, very limited data and many of these problems appear to be related to a deprived environment.

C. **Alcohol.** This is probably the foremost drug of abuse today. Ethanol is an anxiolytic-analgesic with a depressant effect on the CNS. Both ethanol and its metabolite, acetaldehyde, are toxic. Alcohol crosses the placenta and also impairs its function. The risk of effecting the fetus is related to alcohol dose but there is a continuum of effects and there is no known safe limit. The risk that an alcoholic woman will have a child with the fetal-alcohol syndrome (FAS) is about 35–40%. But even in the absence of FAS, and also with lower alcohol intakes, there is an increased risk of congenital anomalies and impaired intellect. It is estimated that alcohol is the major cause of congenital mental retardation today.

FAS consists of (1) pre- or postnatal growth retardation; (2) CNS involvement such as irritability in infancy or hyperactivity in childhood, developmental

TABLE 57–4. MALFORMATIONS ASSOCIATED WITH COCAINE ABUSE

CNS
Microcephaly
Agenesis of corpus callosum
Absence of septum pellucidum
Septo-optic dysplasia
Schizencephaly
Neuronal heterotopias
Encephalocele
Optic nerve hypoplasia
Exencephaly
Porencephaly

Cardiovascular
Pulmonary atresia/stenosis
Septal defects (ASD, VSD)
Hypoplastic heart
Biventricular hypertrophy
PDA
Conduction defects
Transposition of great arteries
Aortic valve leaflet prolapse

Gastrointestinal
Ileal atresia
Jejunal atresia
Colonic atresia
Imperforate anus

Ophthalmic
Ptosis
Abnormal vascularization of the iris

Genitourinary
Prune belly
Hydronephrosis
Cryptorchidism
Hypospadias
Hydroureter
Horseshoe kidney
Renal agenesis
Pseudohermaphroditism
Bifid scrotum
Rectovesical fistula

Others
Limb reduction defects
Parietal bone defects
Polydactyly
Syndactyly
Cleft lip/palate
Ankyloglossia
Cutis aplasia
Skin tags

delay, hypotonia, or intellectual impairment; and (3) facial dysmorphology: microcephaly, microphthalmia, and/or short palpebral fissures, poorly developed philtrum, thin upper lip (vermillion border), and hypoplastic maxilla. Numerous congenital anomalies have been described following exposure to alcohol in utero both with and without a full-blown FAS. CNS symptoms may appear within 24 hours after delivery and include: tremors, irritability, hypertonicity, twitching, hyperventilation, hyperacusia, opisthotonus, and seizures. Symptoms may be severe but are usually of short duration. Abdominal distention and vomiting are less frequent than with most other drugs of abuse.

D. **Barbiturates.** Symptoms and signs of withdrawal are similar to those observed in narcotic-exposed babies but symptoms usually appear later. Most infants become symptomatic toward the end of the 1st week of life although onset may be delayed up to 2 weeks. Duration of symptoms is usually 2–6 weeks.

E. **Benzodiazepines.** Symptoms are indistinguishable from those of narcotic withdrawal, including seizures. Onset of symptoms may be shortly after birth.

F. **Phencyclidine (PCP).** Symptoms usually begin within 24 hours of birth and the infant may show signs of CNS "hyperirritability" as in narcotic withdrawal. Gastrointestinal symptoms of withdrawal are less common. Very few studies have been done, but at 2 years of age these infants appear to have lower scores in fine motor, adaptive, and language areas of development. Although weight, length, and head circumference are somewhat reduced at birth, most children demonstrate adequate catch-up growth.

G. **Marijuana.** Studies have suggested a slightly shorter duration of gestation and somewhat reduced birthweight but the extent of these differences was of no clinical importance. Although the drug may have some mild effect on a variety of newborn neurobehavioral traits there is no evidence of long-term dysfunction.

XI. **Treatment.** Manifestations of drug withdrawal in many infants will resolve within a few days and drug therapy is not required. Supportive care will suffice in many, if not most, babies. It is not appropriate to treat prophylactically babies of drug-dependent mothers. The infant's withdrawal score should be assessed to monitor progression of symptoms and adequacy of treatment.

A. **Supportive care**

1. **Minimal stimulation.** Attempt to keep the baby in a darkened and quiet environment.

2. **Swaddling.**

3. **Prevent excessive crying** with pacifier, cuddling etc.

B. **Drug treatment.** The general aim of treatment is to allow sleep and feeding patterns to be as close to normal as possible. When supportive care is insufficient to do this, or if symptoms are particularly severe, drugs are used. Indications for drug treatment are progressive irritability, continued feeding difficulty, and significant weight loss. A score above 6 on the "Finnegan score" may also be regarded as an indication for treatment. Drugs used for withdrawal are discussed below. Additional treatment may be required for some symptoms (eg, dehydration or convulsions). With the exception of a few small trials comparing paregoric to phenobarbital for narcotic withdrawal, drug therapy is largely based on anecdotal evidence and hence is variable.

1. **Paregoric (camphorated opium tincture).** This has 0.4 mg/mL anhydrous "physiological" than nonnarcotic agents. Treated infants have a more physiologic sucking pattern, higher calorie intake, and better weight gain than infants treated with phenobarbital. Will control seizures related to narcotic withdrawal better than phenobarbital. Paregoric will control symptoms in over 90% of babies with withdrawal following narcotic exposure. Potential disadvantages are due to other constituents present in the preparation: camphor is a CNS stimulant and paregoric also contains alcohol, anise oil, and benzoic acid, a metabolite of benzyl alcohol. **Dosage** in full-term babies: Start with 0.2 mL q 3–4 hrs; if no improvement is seen within 4 hours increase dose by 0.05 mL steps up to a maximum of 0.5 mL q 3–4 hrs. In premature babies: Start 0.05 mL/kg q 4 hrs and increase with increments of 0.02 mL/kg q 4 hrs until symptoms are controlled, up to a maximum of 0.15 mL/kg q 4 hrs. Once withdrawal score is stable for 48 hours, dosage may be tapered by 10% each day.

2. **Tincture of opium.** Similar to paregoric and has the advantage of fewer additives than paregoric. It has 10 mg/mL morphine equivalent and should be diluted to provide the same (morphine) dosage as paregoric.

3. **Phenobarbital.** An adequate drug for controlling withdrawal from narcotics

especially those of irritability, fussiness, and hyperexcitability. Not as effective as paregoric for control of gastrointestinal symptoms or seizures following narcotic exposure. It is not suitable for dose titration because of a long half-life. Is mainly useful for treatment of withdrawal from nonnarcotic agents. **Dosage:** 20 mg/kg loading dose followed by 4 mg/kg/d maintenance. Once symptoms have been controlled for 1 week, decrease daily dose by 25% every week.

4. **Chlorpromazine.** Is quite effective in controlling symptoms of withdrawal from both narcotics and nonnarcotics. It has multiple untoward side effects (reduces seizure threshold, cerebellar dysfunction, hematologic problems) that make it potentially undesirable for use in neonates when alternatives can be used. **Dosage:** 3 mg/kg/d divided into 3–6 doses/d.

5. **Clonidine.** Has been used for withdrawal from both narcotic and nonnarcotic agents. **Dosage:** 3–4 microgram/kg/d divided in 4 doses/d.

6. **Diazepam.** Has been used to treat withdrawal from narcotics. In one study there was a greater incidence of seizures following methadone withdrawal when babies were treated with diazepam rather than paregoric. When used to treat methadone withdrawal it also impairs nutritive sucking more than does methadone alone. It may produce apnea when used with phenobarbital. It may be used for treatment of withdrawal from benzodiazepines and possibly also for the hyperexcitable phase following cocaine exposure. **Dosage:** 0.5–2 mg q 6–8 hrs.

C. **Long-term management.** During the first few years of life infants exposed to drugs in utero may have various neurobehavioral problems. Minor signs and symptoms of drug withdrawal may continue for a few months following discharge. This places a difficult infant in a difficult home situation. There are a few reports of an increased incidence of child abuse in these circumstances. Thus, frequent follow-up visits and close involvement of social services may be required.

XII. **Breast-feeding.** The various drugs of abuse may be presumed to enter breast milk and there have been reports of intoxication in breast-fed babies whose mothers had continued to abuse drugs. Mothers on low-dose methadone have been allowed to breast feed but this required closed supervision and there was a constant concern that unsupervised weaning would precipitate withdrawal. The cautious course would be to dissuade these mothers from breast feeding unless there is reasonable certainty that they will discontinue their habits.

XIII. **WARNING. Naloxone (Narcan) may precipitate acute drug withdrawal in babies exposed to narcotics. It should thus not be used in mothers suspected of abusing opiates.**

REFERENCES

Azuma SD, Chasnoff IJ: Outcome of children prenatally exposed to cocaine and other drugs: A path analysis of three-year data. *Pediatrics* 1993;**92**:396–402.

Callahan CM, Grant TM, Phipps P, Clark G, Novack AH, Streissguth AP, Raisys VA: Measurement of gestational cocaine exposure: Sensitivity of infants' hair, meconium, and urine. *J Pediatr* 1992;**120**:763–68.

Fried PA: Prenatal exposure to tobacco and marijuana: Effects during pregnancy, infancy, and early childhood. *Clin Obstet Gynecol* 1993;**36**:319–37.

Kain ZN, Kain TS, Scarpelli E: Cocaine exposure in utero: Perinatal development and neonatal manifestations—review. *Clin Toxicol* 1992;**30**:607–36.

Lutiger B, Graham K, Einarson T, Koren G: Relationship between gestational cocaine use and pregnancy outcome: A meta-analysis. *Teratology* 1991;**44**:405–14.

Pierog S, Chandavasu O, Wexler I: Withdrawal symptoms in infants with the fetal alcohol syndrome. *J Pediatr* 1977;**90**:630–33.

Pietrantoni M, Knuppel RA: Alcohol use in pregnancy. *Clin Perinatol* 1991;**18**:93–111.

Vega WA, Kolody B, Hwang J, Noble A: Prevalence and magnitude of perinatal substance exposure in California. *N Engl J Med* 1993;**329**:850–54.

Volpe JJ: Effect of cocaine use on the fetus. *N Engl J Med* 1992;**327**:399–407.

58 Hyperbilirubinemia

Hyperbilirubinemia is a common finding in the majority of newborn premature and full-term infants. An elevation of serum bilirubin concentration > 2 mg/dL is found in most newborns in the first several days of life.

Bilirubin is the end product of the catabolism of heme and is produced chiefly by the breakdown of red cell hemoglobin. Other sources of heme include myoglobin and certain liver enzymes. Bilirubin exists in several forms in the blood but is predominantly bound to serum albumin. In this form, unconjugated bilirubin cannot cross the blood-brain barrier. Free unconjugated bilirubin, and possible other forms, may enter the central nervous system and become toxic to cells. The precise mechanism is unknown.

Inside liver cells, unconjugated bilirubin is bound to ligandin, Z-protein, and other proteins; it is conjugated by uridine diphosphate glucuronyl transferase. In the fetus, most unconjugated bilirubin crosses the placenta and is metabolized by the maternal liver. The capacity of the fetal liver to conjugate bilirubin is limited.

Conjugated bilirubin is water soluble and can be excreted in the urine, but most of it is rapidly excreted as bile into the intestine. In children and adults, conjugated bilirubin is further metabolized by bacteria in the intestine and excreted in the feces. Newborns have increased β-glucuronidase in the intestine and lack bacterial flora. β-glucuronidase hydrolyzes conjugated bilirubin back to unconjugated bilirubin. Therefore, the newborn intestine contains excessive amounts of unconjugated bilirubin and, through enterohepatic uptake, contributes to the serum unconjugated bilirubin load.

Hyperbilirubinemia presents in one of 2 forms in the neonate: unconjugated hyperbilirubinemia or conjugated hyperbilirubinemia. The 2 forms have different causes and potential complications; their treatment will be discussed separately.

UNCONJUGATED (INDIRECT) HYPERBILIRUBINEMIA

I. **Definition.** Unconjugated hyperbilirubinemia is the most common form in the newborn. Elevations of indirect serum bilirubin are related to bilirubin load less bilirubin excretion and are therefore dependent on the gestational age and chronologic age of the infant.

II. **Classification and pathophysiology.** The causes of unconjugated hyperbilirubinemia are listed in Table 58–1.

A. **Physiologic jaundice.** In almost every newborn infant, elevation of serum unconjugated bilirubin develops during the first week of life and resolves spontaneously. This form is referred to as physiologic jaundice. However, jaundice that develops in the first 24 hours of life is pathologic until proven otherwise.

1. **Bilirubin levels**

a. **In normal term infants beyond 24 hours of age,** levels of unconjugated bilirubin rise slowly and peak at 6–8 mg/dL by about the third to fourth day of life. In premature infants, liver function is less mature and jaundice is more frequent and more pronounced than in term infants. For most jaundiced newborns, the bilirubin level may peak at 10–12 mg/dL, usually by the fifth day of life.

b. **Physiologic jaundice** is defined as serum bilirubin not exceeding 12 mg/dL in full-term infants or 15 mg/dL in premature infants during the first week of life. Criteria that would rule out physiologic jaundice include clinical jaundice in the first 24 hours of life, conjugated bilirubin levels exceeding 2 mg/dL, total serum bilirubin concentrations increasing by more

TABLE 58–1. CAUSES OF UNCONJUGATED HYPERBILIRUBINEMIA

PHYSIOLOGIC JAUNDICE

HEMOLYTIC ANEMIA
Congenital: hereditary spherocytosis, infantile pynknocytosis, pyruvate kinase deficiency, G6PD deficiency, sickle cell disease (rarely seen in newborn period)
Acquired: ABO or Rh incompatibility, infection, drugs

POLYCYTHEMIA
Placental hypertransfusion: twin-twin transfusion, maternal-fetal transfusion, delayed cord clamping
Placental insufficiency: postmaturity, pregnancy-induced hypertension, SGA infant
Endocrine disorders: maternal diabetes, congenital adrenal hyperplasia, neonatal thyrotoxicosis
Other disorders: Down's syndrome, Beckwith-Wiedemann syndrome

BLOOD EXTRAVASATION

GLUCURONYL TRANSFERASE DEFECT
Congenital: Crigler-Najjar syndrome (type I deficiency), type II deficiency, Gilbert's syndrome
Acquired: Lucey-Driscoll syndrome

BREAST MILK AND BREAST-FEEDING JAUNDICE

METABOLIC DISORDERS: galactosemia, hypothyroidism, maternal diabetes

INCREASED ENTEROHEPATIC CIRCULATION: ileus, intestinal obstruction, swallowed blood at delivery

DRUGS: aspirin, sulfonamides, furosemide, and chloral hydrate

than 5 mg/dL/d, and clinical jaundice persisting for longer than 1 week in full-term or 2 weeks in preterm infants.

2. **Mechanisms.** A number of mechanisms have been suggested.
   a. **An increased bilirubin load** owing to the larger red blood cell volume, the shorter life span of red blood cells, and increased enterohepatic circulation in newborn infants.
   b. **Defective uptake** of bilirubin by the liver.
   c. **Defective conjugation.**
   d. **Impaired excretion into bile.**
   e. **Overall impairment of liver function.**

B. **Hemolytic anemia**
   1. **Red blood cell defects.** Hemolytic anemia may result from a congenital red blood cell defect such as hereditary spherocytosis, infantile pyknocytosis, pyruvate kinase deficiency, glucose-6-phosphate dehydrogenase (G6PD) deficiency, thalassemia, or vitamin K–induced hemolysis.
   2. **Acquired hemolytic anemia** may be seen in ABO or Rh incompatibility (eg, erythroblastosis fetalis) between infant and mother. It may also be associated with the use of certain drugs (eg, sulfonamides) or with infection.

C. **Polycythemia.** Polycythemia in the newborn infant may cause hyperbilirubinemia because the liver may not have the capacity to metabolize the increased bilirubin load (see p 271).

D. **Blood extravasation.** A large hematoma in the newborn period **may overload the bilirubin degradation pathway.** It may be seen with cephalohematoma, intraventricular and pulmonary hemorrhage, subcapsular hematoma of the liver, excessive ecchymoses or petechiae, or occult gastrointestinal hemorrhage.

E. **Defects of conjugation.**
   1. **Congenital deficiency of glucuronyl transferase**
      a. **Type 1 deficiency (Crigler-Najjar syndrome)** is an autosomal recessive disorder with a poor prognosis.
      b. **Type II glucuronyl transferase** is an autosomal dominant benign deficiency.
      c. **Gilbert's syndrome** is autosomal dominant, benign, and relatively common.

    2. Glucuronyl transferase inhibition
      a. Drugs such as novobiocin.
      b. Lucey-Driscoll syndrome. In this syndrome, a maternal gestational hormone found in the infant's serum interferes with the conjugation of bilirubin. This problem appears to resolve spontaneously.

F. Breast milk jaundice (late onset) is characterized by a higher peak and slower decline in the serum bilirubin concentration and rarely appears before the end of the first week of life for term or preterm infants. Factors associated with an abnormality of the milk itself may include pregnanediol in the milk, increased concentration of fatty acids, or increased enteric absorption of unconjugated bilirubin. Levels of unconjugated bilirubin may be elevated for weeks to several months. Interruption of breast feeding for 24–48 hours at unacceptable bilirubin levels results in a rapid decline. Resumption of breast feeding increases bilirubin levels slightly but usually below previous levels. Breast milk jaundice may recur in 70% of future pregnancies.

G. Metabolic disorders. Galactosemia, hypothyroidism, and maternal diabetes may be associated with unconjugated hyperbilirubinemia.

H. Increased enterohepatic circulation of unconjugated bilirubin may result in jaundice. It may be seen with **pyloric stenosis, duodenal atresia, annular pancreas, cystic fibrosis, and any form of gastrointestinal obstruction or ileus.** Blood swallowed during delivery and decreased caloric intake may also be contributing factors.

I. Substances and disorders affecting binding of bilirubin to albumin. Certain drugs occupy bilirubin-binding sites on albumin and increase the amount of free unconjugated bilirubin that can cross the blood-brain barrier. Drugs in which this effect may be significant include aspirin and sulfonamides. Fatty acids in nutritional products (eg, Intralipid) may also influence bilirubin binding to albumin, as may asphyxia, acidosis, sepsis, hypothermia, hyperosmolality, and hypoglycemia. Chloral hydrate is shown to compete for hepatic glucuronidation with bilirubin and thus increase serum unconjugated bilirubin.

J. Kernicterus. Kernicterus, a postmortem diagnosis, is characterized by yellow pigmentation of the brain, which occasionally occurs when the amount of free unconjugated (indirect) bilirubin (from various causes) increases to the extent that it crosses the blood-brain barrier and is deposited in the central nervous system. The basal ganglia, hypothalamus, hippocampus, and cranial nuclei are usually stained with the greatest intensity. Cerebral, cerebellar, and spinal nuclei may also become stained in severe cases of hyperbilirubinemia (usually when levels are in excess of 25 mg/dL). Bilirubin toxicity to the brain may be reversible if bilirubin levels fall before saturation of the CNS nuclei occur. Bilirubin, not bound to albumin and not conjugated, is left in a "free" state. It is believed that CNS uptake of "free bilirubin" accounts for clinical and pathological findings of bilirubin toxicity.

K. Bilirubin encephalopathy. The effect of bilirubin upon neurons begins with an aggregation of bilirubin at nerve terminals. This lowers membrane potentials, and is best exhibited by decreased auditory brainstem conduction. This process is usually reversible if serum bilirubin reduction is prompt. If not, bilirubin subsequently binds to neuronal cell components impairing substrate transport, synthesis of neurotransmitters, and profoundly decreasing mitochondrial functions. This phase may be reversible depending upon availability of equimolar albumin. Irreversible stages of bilirubin encephalopathy include retrograde bilirubin uptake by neuronal bodies, pyknosis and gliosis of neurons, and eventual neuron death.

L. Clinical manifestations of bilirubin encephalopathy. Early (acute) and late (chronic) stages occur. Acute bilirubin encephalopathy occurs generally at levels above 20 mg/dL in sick full-term infants and at levels between 10–20 mg/dL in preterm infants. It is usually associated with some form of hemolytic disease. It presents as apathy, lethargy, and ultimately stupor. A poor suck and feeding intolerance are notable. Episodic fever and alternating hypotonia and hypertonia are found. Subsequently, chronic postkernicteric bilirubin encephalopathy develops in untreated hyperbilirubinemic situations. It is marked by extrapyramidal signs of athetosis, dysarthria, grimacing, drooling, and dysphagia. Hearing loss is pronounced due to cochlear nuclei death and loss of brainstem auditory conduction. Finally, oculomotor nuclei are affected and loss of upward gaze is peculiar to kernicteric infants with bilirubin encephalopathy.

A third form of bilirubin encephalopathy, occurring at levels below 20 mg/dL in near-term and term infants is known as non-hyperbilirubinemic chronic postkernicteric encephalopathy. It is usually associated with sepsis and vasculitis, anoxia, hypercarbia, acidosis, hyperosmolar states, and certain drugs.

Controversy exists over what level of unconjugated bilirubin is associated with a significant risk of kernicterus. Historically, most authors agree that clinical manifestations of kernicterus are unlikely to occur if the serum bilirubin level is kept lower than 20 mg/dL in full-term infants with hemolytic disease. The "magic number" in full-term infants without hemolysis or for preterm infants is less clear. Most clinicians try to keep serum bilirubin levels below 15 mg/dL in preterm infants.

M. Prolonged indirect hyperbilirubinemia may be due to Crigler-Najjar syndrome, intestinal obstruction, ongoing hemolytic disease, breast milk jaundice, or hypothyroidism.

III. Clinical presentation

A. History

1. **Family history.** A family history of jaundice, anemia, splenectomy, or metabolic disorders is significant. A history of a previous sibling with jaundice may suggest blood group incompatibility, breast milk jaundice, or G6PD deficiency. A familial nature of neonatal hyperbilirubinemia is present regardless of breast feeding and other risk factors, and the excess risk of neonatal hyperbilirubinemia in siblings is most notable for severe neonatal jaundice.

2. **Maternal history.** Neonatal jaundice is increased with a history of maternal diabetes or infection. Use of oxytocin, sulfonamides, antimalarials, and nitrofurantoins by the mother may initiate hemolysis in G6PD deficient infants. Delivery trauma, asphyxia, delayed cord clamping, and prematurity are associated with an increased risk of hyperbilirubinemia in the infant.

3. **Infant's history.** Factors associated with the gastrointestinal tract may affect the bilirubin level. Factors include the history and frequency of breast feeding. Poor breast feeding may be associated with lethargy or abnormalities of the face and mouth, leading to a weak or absent suck. Poor caloric intake by the infant may increase the enterohepatic uptake of bilirubin. Vomiting may be an early presentation in sepsis, intestinal obstruction, or metabolic disorders, all of which may increase the risk of bilirubin load and toxicity. Delayed passage of meconium and infrequent stooling are seen with intestinal obstruction.

B. Symptoms and signs.

Clinical jaundice is visible when the serum bilirubin level approaches 5–7 mg/dL. Jaundice is often apparent first in the face, especially the nose, then descending to the torso and lower extremities as the degree of jaundice increases. Some infants appear "orange" in color because of the combination of "red" from a high neonatal hemoglobin concentration and "yellow" from the bilirubin. Jaundice can be demonstrated in some infants by pressing lightly on the skin with a finger. The yellow color is seen more easily in the "fingerprint" area than in the surrounding skin. Pressing upon the buccal mucosa or gums are also good sites for noting jaundice. These signs should not appear within the first 24 hours of birth in otherwise healthy infants.

Besides confirming the presence of jaundice, physical examination may also be helpful in determining the cause of hyperbilirubinemia. Areas of bleeding such as cephalohematoma, petechiae, or ecchymoses indicate blood extravasation. Hepatosplenomegaly may signify hemolytic disease, liver disease, or infection. Physical signs of prematurity, intrauterine growth retardation (IUGR), and postmaturity may be helpful in elucidating a cause for hyperbilirubinemia.

Plethora is seen with polycythemia, pallor with hemolytic disease, and large infants with maternal diabetes—all associated with hyperbilirubinemia. Omphalitis, chorioretinitis, microcephaly, and petechial and purpuric lesions all suggest infectious causes of increased serum bilirubin.

C. **Neurologic examination.** The appearance of abnormal neurologic signs heralds the onset of early bilirubin encephalopathy. Beginning with lethargy, poor feeding, vomiting, and hypotonia the hyperbilirubinemic infant goes on to experience seizures. Left untreated a high-pitched cry and irritability lead to spasticity, opisthotonus, hyperpyrexia, and respiratory irregularity. Finally, spasticity lessens, intermittent fevers diminish, and the untreated kernicteric infant is left with permanent neurologic deficits. They include nerve deafness, loss of upward gaze, and mental retardation. The progression of neurologic changes parallel the stages of bilirubin encephalopathy from acute to chronic and irreversible changes.

IV. Diagnosis

A. **Laboratory studies.** Hyperbilirubinemia should be investigated whenever pathologic causes are suspected. The presence of a serum bilirubin level of 13 mg/dL or higher in any infant requires initial evaluation.

1. **Total and direct bilirubin**
   a. **Direct bilirubin** = conjugated.
   b. **Indirect bilirubin** = unconjugated.
   c. **Total minus direct** = indirect fraction.
2. **Hemoglobin or hematocrit.** Hemolytic anemia can be detected by a low hemoglobin or hematocrit associated with a high reticulocyte count and the presence of nucleated red blood cells. Polycythemia is defined as venous blood hematocrit greater than 65%. **Use of capillary blood samples may cause underestimation of venous bilirubin values when the latter exceeds 10 mg/dL.** This may be explained by the increased **light penetration and photoisomerization** of capillary unconjugated bilirubin and less penetration in the deeper venous vascular beds.
3. **Peripheral blood smear.** The peripheral blood smear aids in the diagnosis of hereditary spherocytosis and other red blood cell defects.
4. **Reticulocyte count.**
5. **Blood type and Rh status in mother and infant.** ABO and Rh incompatibility can be easily diagnosed by comparing infant and maternal blood types.
6. **Direct Coombs' test in the infant.** The direct Coombs test is usually positive in isoimmunization disorders.
7. **Measurement of serum albumin** may help to assess total bilirubin binding sites available and whether there is a need for an albumin infusion.
8. **Other laboratory tests.** The white blood cell count or platelet count can be helpful in suggesting infection. The urine should be tested for reducing substances to rule out galactosemia if the infant is receiving a galactose-containing formula. If hemolysis is present in the absence of ABO or Rh incompatibility, hemoglobin electrophoresis, G6PD screening, or osmotic fragility testing may be required to diagnose red blood cell defects. Persistent jaundice (> 2 weeks of life) may call for further investigation into possible causes. Thyroid and liver function tests, blood and urine cultures, direct Coombs' test and a blood smear, and serum and urine amino acids and organic acid measurements may help in this search.

B. **Radiologic studies.** Radiologic studies for suspected intestinal obstruction or blood extravasation into internal organs and ultrasonography of the head to document intraventricular or subdural hemorrhage may be indicated.

C. **Transcutaneous bilirubinometry.** The transcutaneous bilirubinometer measures the degree of yellow color in the skin and subcutaneous tissues by selective wavelength reflection. Standardization has not been achieved, which makes correlation with serum bilirubin levels difficult to interpret.

V. Management. Three methods of treatment are commonly used to decrease the level of unconjugated bilirubin: exchange transfusion, phototherapy, and pheno-

barbital therapy. As noted above, however, controversy persists as to what levels of serum bilirubin warrant therapy, especially in otherwise healthy full-term infants.

A. Phototherapy

1. **Indications.** Most infants with pathologic jaundice are treated initially with phototherapy. Phototherapy is usually started when it is felt that bilirubin levels could enter the toxic range. No firm recommendations are universally accepted regarding serum bilirubin levels and the initiation of phototherapy. The following guidelines are related to the first week of life and large birth weight groups. The authors do attempt to maintain bilirubin levels below 15 mg/dL in low birth weight (< 2500 g) infants. Phototherapy would be considered for bilirubin greater than 5 mg/dL in infants weighing less than 1500 g. Infants weighing 1500 to 2500 g may be considered for phototherapy when serum levels exceed physiologic range, that is above 12 mg/dL. Consistent with the authors' concern to maintain levels of bilirubin below 20 mg/dL, we would use phototherapy in term, formula-fed well newborns with levels above 15 mg/dL in the first week of life. If the infant is being breast-fed, and is well (not dehydrated) and peak bilirubin is below 18 mg/dL through the first week of life, we would withold phototherapy under conditions of continuing observation. See Appendix H to determine when to begin phototherapy.

2. **Technique**
   a. **Light source and dosage.** The infant is exposed to light in the blue part of the spectrum (410–460 nm). The light causes a photochemical reaction in the skin (**photoisomerization**) that changes unconjugated bilirubin into photobilirubin, which is excreted by the liver into the bile. In addition, photooxidation produces bilirubin products that are excreted in the urine; however, this is not the mechanism by which phototherapy exerts its major effect. The effectiveness of phototherapy is related to the amount of **irradiation** to which the skin is exposed. Blue lamps are most efficient, but a combination of blue and cool white lamps is also effective; furthermore, this combination does not cause overheating and does not cause the infant to appear cyanotic. Bulbs must be changed regularly to ensure adequate irradiance. A radio meter may be used to measure the exact amount of irradiance delivered. The desired amount is 5–9 $\mu W/cm^2/nm$ at 425–475 nm. The infant's eyes must be covered with opaque patches, because animal experiments have shown that retinal damage can occur from phototherapy. Phototherapy is usually given continuously. To maximize the surface area, exposed infants should be naked, except for eye patches. Fiber optic phototherapy blankets (**"biliblankets"**) can be wrapped around infants or placed beneath them. They allow for more handling by parents and continuation of breast feeding.

   b. **Supportive management.** Small infants require use of a servocontrolled incubator to maintain body temperature. Fluid balance and temperature must be monitored closely. Tungsten bulbs have been shown to decrease insensible water loss. Phototherapy may be interrupted for feedings and parental visits. Once phototherapy is started, skin color cannot be used as a guide to the presence of hyperbilirubinemia. Because melanin and bilirubin both strongly absorb the blue end of the visible spectrum, increased pigmentation in the epidermis lowers the effectiveness of treatment. Moist skin is less translucent to light therapy and reduces its penetration.

   Other simple measures to aid in elimination of bilirubin during phototherapy include maintenance of hydration status to ensure adequate urine and stool output to decrease enterohepatic uptake of bilirubin.

3. **Fluid management during phototherapy.** Use of phototherapy increases insensible water loss, and increased fluids must therefore be given to maintain fluid balance. For infants weighing less than 1500 g, increase fluid by 0.5 mL/kg/h; for those weighing more than 1500 g, increase by 1 mL/kg/h.

4. **Termination of phototherapy.** Phototherapy is stopped when the following criteria are met:

   a. The bilirubin level is low enough to eliminate the risk of kernicterus.

   b. The risk factors for the infant have resolved.

   c. The infant is old enough to handle the bilirubin load.

5. **Side effects.** No major toxicity has been associated with phototherapy thus far. Minor side effects include loose stools, skin erythema, transient skin rashes, and tanning. The eye shields may obstruct the airway and must be closely observed. If conjugated hyperbilirubinemia is present and phototherapy is used, a dark gray to brown discoloration may appear on the skin and in the serum and urine (**"bronze baby syndrome"**). The presence of cholestasis causes elevated copper and porphyrin serum concentrations. Copper porphyrins are sensitized by bilirubin and, under phototherapy, undergo photodestruction to degradation products, which are responsible for the brown discoloration of the skin.

B. **Exchange transfusion.** Exchange transfusion is used when the risk of kernicterus for a particular infant is significant. A double-volume exchange replaces 85% of the circulating red blood cells and decreases the bilirubin level to about half of the preexchange value. Besides removing bilirubin, an exchange transfusion can be used to correct anemia.

   1. **General guidelines.** It appears that no specific level of bilirubin can be considered safe or dangerous for all infants, since variations in the permeability of the blood-brain barrier exist. The current recommendation (from *Guidelines for Perinatal Care,* 3rd ed, American Academy of Pediatrics and American College of Obstetrics and Gynecologists) is that both aggressive approaches (keeping bilirubin levels below 20 mg/dL with exchange transfusion) and conservative approaches (allowing bilirubin levels to approach 20 mg/dL before performing exchange transfusion) are acceptable for nonhemolytic, well infants above 2000 g. The guidelines further suggest that bilirubin levels as high as 25 mg/dL may be well tolerated without the need for exchange transfusion in well, nonhemolytic, full-term infants. The current debate for upper limits of serum bilirubin is directed to full-term infants with no evidence for associated disease. Levels as high as 25 to 29 mg/dL before considering exchange transfusion are under discussion currently for these infants.

   Low birth weight infants are excluded from those considerations. The authors urgently suggest that each institution and its practicing physicians must establish their criteria for phototherapy and exchange transfusion by weight groups, age, and conditions of infants consistent with standard current pediatric reference materials.

   2. **Indications**

      a. **Early exchange transfusions in term infants**

         (1) Cord bilirubin levels greater than 4.5 mg/dL and hemoglobin less than 11 g/dL.

         (2) Bilirubin levels rising over 0.5 mg/dL/h.

         (3) Bilirubin levels of 20 mg/dL or a likelihood that bilirubin levels will reach 20/mg/dL in term infants with hemolytic disease.

         (4) Intrauterine exchange transfusions may reduce bilirubin levels in severe blood incompatibilities. Percutaneous umbilical blood sampling (PUBS) and amniotic fluid bilirubin levels are used to monitor fetal bilirubin levels. Umbilical vessel catheterization for intrauterine exchange transfusions is now routinely used at some centers to reduce bilirubin levels in the fetus with severe blood incompatibility.

      b. **Indications for later exchange transfusion.** If there is no hemolytic process or if hemolysis is mild, exchange transfusion is used to reduce toxicity from hyperbilirubinemia that is not being adequately controlled by phototherapy. In these cases, indications for exchange transfusion are:

  (1) Unconjugated bilirubin levels exceeding 20 mg/dL in a full-term infant without evidence of hemolysis, acidosis, or respiratory distress.

  (2) Bilirubin levels of 10–15 mg/dL in a premature infant with hypoxia, acidosis, or respiratory distress.

  (3) Clinical signs of bilirubin encephalopathy at any bilirubin level.

3. Factors that may affect the decision to perform exchange transfusion include the infant's maturity, birth weight, age, the rate of rise in bilirubin levels, and the presence of hypoxia, acidosis, sepsis, or hypoproteinemia.

4. Albumin transfusions may be useful if bilirubin levels are above 20 mg/dL and serum albumin levels are below 3 g/dL. Infusion of 1 g of albumin 1 hour prior to exchange transfusion may improve the yield of bilirubin removal. Fluid volume and cardiovascular status must be carefully considered before giving albumin.

C. Phenobarbital therapy

  1. Action. Phenobarbital affects the metabolism of bilirubin by increasing the concentration of ligandin in liver cells, inducing production of glucuronyl transferase, and enhancing bilirubin excretion. Because it takes 3–7 days to become effective, phenobarbital is usually not helpful in treating unconjugated hyperbilirubinemia in the newborn infant.

  2. Indications

    a. Prenatal indications. It may be useful to give phenobarbital 1–2 weeks before delivery to a mother whose fetus has **documented hemolytic disease** to aid in reducing bilirubin levels in the affected neonate.

    b. Other indications. Phenobarbital is also used to treat type II glucuronyl transferase deficiency and Gilbert's syndrome in the infant.

  3. Dosage. See Chapter 73 for dosage and other pharmacologic information.

D. Interruption of breast feeding. Most breast-fed infants do not develop bilirubin levels of 20 mg/dL or higher in the first 8 days of life. For infants 6–8 days old, breast-fed and otherwise well, consider holding breast feeding for 48 hours and use phototherapy if bilirubin exceeds 18 mg/dL.

CONJUGATED (DIRECT) HYPERBILIRUBINEMIA

I. Definition. Conjugated hyperbilirubinemia is a sign of hepatobiliary dysfunction. It usually appears in the newborn infant after the first week of life, when the indirect hyperbilirubinemia of physiologic jaundice has receded. **When the direct bilirubin level exceeds 2.0 mg/dL and is greater than 10% of the total serum bilirubin, it is clinically significant.**

II. Classification and pathophysiology. Conjugated hyperbilirubinemia results from inability to remove bilirubin that has been conjugated from the body. This excretion process normally involves the liver, the biliary system, and the small intestine. **Cholestasis** refers to disorders of bile excretion that result in retention of conjugated bilirubin, bile acids, and other bile components. It is helpful diagnostically to separate extrahepatic biliary obstruction from intrahepatic biliary disease. Causes of conjugated hyperbilirubinemia are listed in Table 58–2.

A. Intrahepatic biliary obstruction. Most cases of conjugated hyperbilirubinemia in newborn infants are due to disorders involving the liver.

  1. Intrahepatic cholestasis with paucity of bile ducts

    a. Arteriohepatic dysplasia.

    b. Syndromatic paucity of interlobular bile ducts (eg, Alagille syndrome).

  2. Intrahepatic cholestasis with normal bile ducts

    a. Total parenteral nutrition (TPN) may cause cholestasis. The pathologic process is not clearly defined, although amino acids may influence bile flow. Most abnormalities resolve once TPN is stopped.

    b. Idiopathic neonatal hepatitis (giant cell hepatitis) may account for up to two-thirds of cases of cholestasis in newborn infants. It is a histologic diagnosis; there is no known explanation for the inflammatory process.

    c. Infection

TABLE 58–2. CAUSES OF CONJUGATED HYPERBILIRUBINEMIA

EXTRAHEPATIC BILIARY OBSTRUCTION
Biliary atresia: polysplenia syndrome, trisomies 13 and 18
Choledochal cyst
Spontaneous rupture of bile duct
External compression of bile duct: enlarged lymph nodes, tumors, annular pancreas, hepatic cyst, pancreatic cyst
Others: hemangioendothelioma of pancreas or liver, inspissation of bile from cystic fibrosis, severe erythroblastosis fetalis

INTRAHEPATIC CHOLESTASIS WITH PAUCITY OF BILE DUCTS
Alagille's syndrome, nonsyndromatic form, biliary atresia

INTRAHEPATIC CHOLESTASIS WITH NORMAL BILE DUCTS
Infection
Viral: hepatitis B virus, non-A, non-B hepatitis virus, cytomegalovirus, herpes simplex virus, coxsackievirus, Epstein-Barr
  virus, adenovirus
Bacterial: *Treponema pallidum, Escherichia coli*, group B streptococcus, *Staphylococcus aureus, Listeria*; urinary tract infec-
  tion caused by *E coli* or *Proteus* sp, pneumococcus
Other: *Toxoplasma gondii*
Genetic disorders and inborn errors of metabolism: Dubin-Johnson syndrome, Rotor's syndrome, galactosemia, heredi-
  tary fructose intolerance, tyrosinemia, alpha₁-antitrypsin deficiency, Byler disease, recurrent cholestasis with lymph-
  edema, cerebrohepatorenal syndrome, congenital erythropoietic porphyria, Niemann–Pick disease, Menkes' kinky hair
  syndrome
Idiopathic neonatal hepatitis (giant cell hepatitis)

TPN-INDUCED CHOLESTASIS

- (1) **Hepatitis.** Hepatitis B virus, rubella virus, non-A, non-B hepatitis, cytomegalovirus, herpes simplex virus, coxsackievirus, Epstein-Barr
virus, and adenovirus are known causes of neonatal hepatitis with elevated conjugated bilirubin fractions.
- (2) **Congenital syphilis or toxoplasmosis** may rarely present with cholestasis.
- (3) **Direct bacterial infection of the liver** may occur with overwhelming
sepsis. Toxic cholestasis with no direct invasion of the liver by microorganisms may be seen with urinary tract infection.
  - d. **Genetic disorders and inborn errors of metabolism**
    - (1) **Alpha₁-antitrypsin deficiency** is the most common genetic cause of
cholestasis.
    - (2) **Dubin-Johnson syndrome** is due to a genetic defect in the canalicu-
lar transport system. It is a relatively benign autosomal recessive disorder characterized by jaundice and dark gray pigmentation of the
liver.
    - (3) **Rotor's syndrome** is also inherited in an autosomal recessive man-
ner but is believed to involve a defect in hepatic uptake and storage of
organic anions, such as bilirubin. There is no abnormal pigmentation
of the liver.
    - (4) **Inborn errors of metabolism** include galactosemia, hereditary fruc-
tose intolerance, and tyrosinemia.
    - (5) **Byler disease, or recurrent familial cholestasis,** is a progressive
autosomal recessive disorder characterized by recurring episodes of
cholestasis, each of which increases scarring of the liver and leads to
cirrhosis and death. It has a high incidence in Amish populations.
    - (6) **Recurrent cholestasis with lymphedema** may be benign, or cirrho-
sis may develop.
    - (7) **Cerebrohepatorenal (Zellweger's) syndrome, Niemann-Pick dis-
ease, and Menkes' syndrome** may also be causes.
    - (8) **Congenital erythropoietic porphyria** presents with anemia and con-
jugated hyperbilirubinemia in the first month of life. Bullous skin lesions may form on areas exposed to light because of sensitization by
accumulated porphyrins.

     e. Extracorporeal membrane oxygenation (ECMO). Infants on ECMO may show an increase in prevalence and severity of cholestasis.

B. Extrahepatic biliary obstruction

1. **Biliary atresia.** Biliary atresia accounts for 90% of cases of extrahepatic obstruction in neonates. The lumen of all or a portion of the bile duct system, including the gallbladder, is absent. The exact cause of this disease is unknown. Recent evidence suggests a process of obliterative inflammation that begins in utero or shortly after birth and then progresses.

2. **Choledochal cyst.** Choledochal cyst is dilitation of a portion of the extrahepatic biliary tree in association with complete or nearly complete segmental biliary obstruction.

3. **Spontaneous rupture of bile duct** may occur with ascites. The clinical presentation is identical to that of biliary atresia.

4. **External compression of the bile duct.** Enlarged lymph nodes, tumors, annular pancreas, or hepatic or pancreatic cysts can also cause extrahepatic biliary obstruction.

5. **Hemangioendothelioma** of the pancreas or liver may be a cause.

6. **Cystic fibrosis** may produce true inspissation of bile.

7. **Severe erythroblastosis fetalis** may present with elevated direct bilirubin levels at birth or later in the first week of life.

III. Clinical presentation

A. General findings

1. **Age.** Infants with conjugated hyperbilirubinemia tend to become jaundiced after 5–7 days of life. Alternatively, physiologic jaundice may not disappear as usual, and the infant may become increasingly icteric.

2. **Urine.** The urine is dark because of the presence of bilirubin.

3. **Stools** tend to be pale because bilirubin is not excreted into the small intestine. However, even in total extrahepatic obstruction, there may be some stool pigmentation. Persistence of acholic stools in an otherwise healthy infant is characteristic of biliary atresia or choledochal cyst.

4. **Liver and spleen.** The liver is usually enlarged. The spleen may also be enlarged, depending on the cause of cholestasis.

B. Specific findings in selected diseases

1. **Biliary atresia.** Hepatomegaly may be present but is not prominent. Splenomegaly is often absent. These infants are usually of normal birth weight, with good initial weight gain. Approximately 75% will have acholic stools, which may not be seen until 1–2 weeks after the appearance of conjugated hyperbilirubinemia.

    Biliary atresia may be isolated or may occur with a choledochal cyst. Ten percent of cases of biliary atresia are associated with malformations such as **polysplenia syndrome.** In these cases, the infants have multiple right-sided spleens, a midline liver, absent inferior vena cava, a preduodenal portal vein, and cardiac malformations. About half of infants with polysplenia have extrahepatic biliary atresia. Trisomies 13 and 18 are also associated with biliary atresia.

2. **Spontaneous rupture of the bile duct** may present with early ascites. There may be greenish-yellow discoloration of the scrotum, hernia sac, or umbilicus. Other causes of extrahepatic biliary obstruction have no specific clinical characteristics.

3. **Hepatitis.** Hepatomegaly may or may not be present, and acholic stools may be absent. There may be splenomegaly if a congenital infection such as cytomegalovirus is involved. Such infants may also have petechiae because of thrombocytopenia. Congenital infections may also cause microcephaly and chorioretinitis.

4. **Alagille's syndrome.** Facial features consisting of a prominent forehead, deep-set eyes, mild hypertelorism, a straight nose, and a small pointed chin may be seen. The face has a triangular shape. Butterfly vertebrae and cardiac anomalies such as peripheral pulmonic stenosis, pulmonary valve ste-

nosis, and ventricular septal defect occur. An abnormality in the anterior chamber of the eye (posterior embryotoxon) may be seen.

    5. **Metabolic disorders**

        a. **Galactosemia and hereditary fructose intolerance** are associated with failure to thrive, vomiting, diarrhea, hypoglycemia, hemolysis, hepatosplenomegaly, ascites, and bacterial sepsis. These disorders present only after sugar that cannot be metabolized is introduced into the diet.

        b. **Tyrosinemia** is characterized by failure to thrive, vomiting, diarrhea, hepatosplenomegaly, and rickets. The urine has an odor of decaying cabbage.

        c. **Alpha$_1$-antitrypsin deficiency.** The presentation is variable. There may be acholic stools and hepatomegaly, as in biliary atresia, or the symptoms may be very mild.

IV. Diagnosis

  A. **Laboratory studies**

    1. **Bilirubin levels (total and direct)** must be obtained.

    2. **Liver function tests.** SGOT (AST), SGPT (ALT), and alkaline phosphatase may be helpful in following the course of the disease.

    3. **Prothrombin time (PT) and partial thromboplastin time (PTT)** may be reliable indicators of liver function.

    4. **Gamma-glutamyl transpeptidase, 5′-nucleotidase, and serum bile acids** are also usually elevated in cholesatsis. Once the diagnosis of cholestasis is made, measurement of these markers of cholestasis may not add any further information.

    5. **A complete blood count and reticulocyte count** may be helpful if hepatitis is a possibility, since hemolysis may be found.

    6. **Serum cholesterol, triglycerides, and albumin levels.** Triglyceride and cholesterol levels may aid in nutritional management. Albumin is a long-term indicator of hepatic function.

    7. **Ammonia levels** should be checked if liver failure is suspected.

    8. **Serum glucose levels** should be checked if the infant appears ill.

    9. **Urine testing for reducing substances** is a simple screening test that should always be performed to detect for metabolic disease.

    10. **TORCH titers.** The use of TORCH titers (see p 345) should be guided by the clinical presentation, keeping in mind that cytomegalovirus infection may be asymptomatic and congenital syphilis is treatable.

    11. **Other tests.** More specific tests are indicated in the investigation of the specific causes of conjugated hyperbilirubinemia.

        a. **Hepatitis.** The maternal HBsAg status should be known, and the infant should also be tested. Cytomegalovirus IgM and IgG, Venereal Disease Research Laboratory (VDRL), and IgM-specific titers for herpes simplex, rubella, and toxoplasmosis may be useful in some cases.

        b. **Sepsis.** If bacterial sepsis or urinary tract infection is suspected, appropriate cultures should be obtained.

        c. **Metabolic disorders**

            (1) **Galactosemia and hereditary fructose intolerance.** The urine should be tested for nonglucose-reducing substances. Enzymes involved in these disorders can also be assayed in the blood.

            (2) **Tyrosinemia.** High concentrations of tyrosine and methionine, and their metabolic derivatives, will be seen in the urine.

            (3) **Alpha$_1$-antitrypsin deficiency.** The serum alpha$_1$-antitrypsin level can be measured.

            (4) **Cystic fibrosis.** A sweat test may diagnose cystic fibrosis.

  B. **Radiologic studies.** Diagnosis of biliary atresia and other forms of extrahepatic biliary obstruction by 8 weeks of age is required to prevent progression of the disease.

    1. **Ultrasonography** is the method of choice. It can be used to view the liver parenchyma and to diagnose dilatation of the biliary tree. In extrahepatic

obstruction, half of the infants will have dilated proximal ducts within the liver. Choledochal cysts are seen. Inability to identify the gallbladder on ultrasonography may be due to obliteration of its lumen in biliary atresia. However, the presence of a gallbladder does not rule out biliary atresia.

2. **Hepatobiliary imaging.** Contrast agents are taken up by the liver and excreted into the bile. HIDA (hepatobiliary iminodiacetic acid), EHIDA (ethyl hepatobiliary iminodiacetic acid), and PIPIDA (p-isopropylacetanilido iminodiacetic acid) are technetium-labeled and provide a clear image of the biliary tree after intravenous injection. Neonatal hepatitis, hyperalimentation, and septo-optic dysplasia are reported causes of absent gastrointestinal contrast excretion and must be considered in the diagnosis of biliary atresia. Administration of phenobarbital, 5 mg/kg/d for 5 days, in conjunction with hepatobiliary scanning, may be helpful in distinguishing infants who do not have biliary atresia, since excretion of the contrast medium may improve after this maneuver.

C. **Other studies**
   1. **Intubation of the duodenum** for collection of a 24-hour sample of fluid may be helpful. In this procedure an 8F radiopaque feeding tube is positioned between the second and third portions of the duodenum by fluoroscopy. Fluid is withdrawn from the tube every 2 hours and visually examined for the presence of bile pigment. If bile pigment is not observed in 24 hours, biliary atresia is a strong possibility. The presence of any amount of bile pigment rules out extrahepatic biliary atresia. This study may be repeated after a course of phenobarbital.
   2. **Percutaneous liver biopsy,** using a Menghini-type suction needle, is a safe procedure in experienced hands. Biopsy findings must be correlated with clinical and laboratory data.
   3. **Exploratory laparotomy** is sometimes indicated to correct biliary atresia as soon as possible if the above tests are not diagnostic.

V. **Management**
   A. **Medical management**
      1. **General plan.** In cholestatic jaundice, promotion of bile flow and prevention of malnutrition, vitamin deficiencies, and bleeding are goals of treatment.
      2. **Phenobarbital and cholestyramine** will promote bile flow and decrease serum bilirubin and bile salt levels. Cholestyramine is a nonabsorbable anion exchange resin that irreversibly binds salts in the intestine. This leads to increased fecal excretion of bile salts and increased hepatic synthesis of bile salts from cholesterol, which may lower serum cholesterol levels.
   B. **Dietary management**
      1. **Medium-chain triglycerides.** Long-chain triglycerides are poorly absorbed in the absence of sufficient bile salts. Therefore, infants with cholestasis often require a diet that includes medium-chain triglycerides, which can be absorbed without the action of bile salts. Formulas containing medium-chain triglycerides include Portagen and Pregestimil.
      2. **Vitamin supplementation.** Fat malabsorption will also interfere with maintenance of adequate levels of fat-soluble vitamins in these infants. Supplementation of vitamins A, D, E, and K is suggested. Extra vitamin K supplementation may be necessary if a bleeding tendency develops.
      3. **Dietary restrictions.** Removal of galactose plus lactose and fructose plus sucrose may prevent the development of cirrhosis and other manifestations of galactosemia and hereditary fructose intolerance, respectively. Dietary restrictions may also be used to treat tyrosinemia but usually are less successful. Most other metabolic causes of cholestatic jaundice have no specific therapy.
   C. **Surgical management**
      1. **Laparotomy with biopsy.** If extrahepatic biliary obstruction is strongly suspected after completion of an appropriate evaluation, exploratory laparotomy should be performed with operative cholangiography and liver biopsy.

Other causes of extrahepatic biliary obstruction that may be diagnosed and treated during exploratory laparotomy include choledochal cyst, spontaneous rupture of the bile duct, lymph node enlargement, tumors, annular pancreas, pancreatic and hepatic cysts, and hemangioendothelioma of the pancreas or liver. Inspissated bile syndrome caused by cystic fibrosis also requires surgical removal of tenacious bile from the bile ducts.

2. **Kasai procedure.** Attempts should be made to establish biliary drainage with the use of hepatic portoenterostomy (Kasai procedure). Optimal results are obtained before 8 weeks of age. Even if the Kasai procedure is successful, however, most infants will eventually progress to cirrhosis and death as a result of the ongoing intrahepatic inflammatory sclerosing process. The procedure is now used as a bridge to transplantation.

3. **Liver transplantation.** When end-stage liver disease is inevitable, liver transplantation may be performed. Currently, 50–70% of infants with liver transplants are alive 1 year after operation.

D. **Other treatments**

1. **Infectious diseases.** Some of the infectious causes of hepatitis such as hepatitis B virus, herpes simplex virus, congenital syphilis, and bacterial infections have specific therapeutic regimens. Most other forms of infectious hepatitis resolve with no specific therapy.

2. **Total parenteral nutrition (TPN)-induced conjugated hyperbilirubinemia** will usually resolve once TPN is stopped. The decision to continue TPN in an infant with cholestasis must be carefully considered.

REFERENCES

Auerbach KG, Gartner LM: Breast feeding and human milk: Their association with jaundice in the neonate. *Clin Perinatol* 1987;**14(1)**:89.

Cashore WJ: The neurotoxicity of bilirubin. *Clin Perinatol* 1990;**17(2)**:437.

Connolly AM, Volpe JJ: Clinical features of bilirubin encephalopathy. *Clin Perinatol* 1990;**17(2)**:371.

Ferry GD, et al: Guide to early diagnosis of biliary obstruction in infancy: Review of 143 cases. *Clin Pediatr* 1985;**24**:305.

Martinez JC, et al: Hyperbilirubinemia in the breast-fed newborn: A controlled trial of form interventions. *Pediatrics* 1993; **91(2)**:470.

Newman TB, Maisels MJ: Evaluation and treatment of jaundice in the term newborn: A kinder, gentler approach. *Pediatrics* 1992;**89(5)**:809.

Perlman M, Frank J: Bilirubin beyond the blood brain barrier. *Pediatrics* 1988;**81(2)**:304.

Salamy A, Eldredge L, Tooley WA: Neonatal status and hearing loss in high-risk infants. *J Pediatr* 1989;**114(5)**:847.

Schuman AJ, Karush G: Fiber optic vs. conventional home phototherapy for neonatal hyperbilirubinemia. *Clin Pediatr* 1992;**31(6)**:345.

Sirota L, et al: Breast milk jaundice in preterm infants. *Clin Pediatr* 1988;**27(4)**:195.

Vohr BR: New approaches to assessing the risks of hyperbilirubinemia. *Clin Perinatol* 1990;**17(2)**:293.

Watchko JF, Oski FA: Kernicterus in preterm newborns: Past, present, and future. *Pediatrics* 1992; **90(5)**:707.

59 Inborn Errors of Metabolism

It is well recognized that a number of inborn errors of metabolism can be treated, and their irreversible complications prevented, if diagnosed early in life. Additionally, potential damage to other organ systems may be prevented if inborn errors are discovered quickly.

I. **Classification**

It is helpful to divide the **inborn errors of metabolism (IEM)** into three distinct groups based on the time of presentation.

A. **Neonatal onset.** These diseases will be covered in this chapter (Table 59–1).

1. Although individually rare, inherited metabolic diseases collectively represent a frequent cause of disease in the newborn period.
2. Early recognition may be difficult but can lead to effective therapies, thus minimizing morbidity and mortality.
3. The possibility that a metabolic disease exists should be considered in every sick neonate.

B. **Insidious onset during infancy and childhood.** Newborn screening programs help to detect some diseases in this category. Although some disorders are ultimately fatal (Tay Sachs), immediate early intervention is available for others.

C. **Onset of symptoms in late childhood, adolescence, or adulthood** (hyperlipidemias).

II. **Incidence.** By some estimates, inborn errors of metabolism may account for as much as 20% of disease among full-term infants not known to have been born at risk. Cumulatively, IEM may represent more than 1 in 500 live births.

III. **Pathophysiology.** Metabolic processes are carried out by genetically controlled enzymes. When these enzymes are lacking, substrates accumulate and may be converted to products not usually present. In addition, end-products of the normal pathway will be deficient. Symptoms may result from an increased level of the normal substrate (eg, in urea cycle disorders, the substrate ammonia is toxic and leads to cerebral edema and death). Additionally, a lack of normal end-products of metabolism can lead to symptoms (eg, lack of cortisol in 21-hydroxylase deficiency). The alternative products may also interfere with normal metabolic processes (eg, accumulated propionyl-COA may participate in reactions normally utilizing acetyl-COA in propionic acidemia). Lastly, an inability to degrade end-products of a metabolic pathway may lead to symptoms (eg, myocardial dysfunction in glycogen storage disease type II, hydrops fetalis in Neiman-Pick and Gaucher's diseases).

IV. **Clinical Presentation**

A. **High-risk infant.** A high index of suspicion must be maintained under the following circumstances:

1. A history of unexplained neonatal deaths in the family (prior siblings or male infants on the mother's side of the family).
2. The onset of signs and symptoms as listed in Table 59–2 after a period of good health.
3. Failure of usual therapies to alleviate the symptoms.
4. The progression of signs and symptoms as listed in Table 59–2 despite the absence of evidence suggesting sepsis, CNS hemorrhage, or other congenital or acquired conditions.

B. **Signs and symptoms** (See Tables 59–2, 59–3.)

1. **Difficulty in diagnosis.** The infant offers a limited number of symptoms that may resemble commonly occurring disorders.
2. **Time of onset.** It is not uncommon for infants with IEM to have experienced an uneventful perinatal and newborn course prior to the manifestation of

TABLE 59–1. LABORATORY SELECTED METABOLIC DISEASES PRESENTING IN THE NEWBORN PERIOD

Disorders of Carbohydrate Metabolism
Galactosemia
Fructose-1,6-diphosphatase deficiency
Glycogen storage diseases (types IA, IB, II, III)
Hereditary fructose intolerance

Disorders of Amino Acid Metabolism
Maple syrup urine disease (MSUD)
Nonketotic hyperglycinemia
Hereditary tyrosinemia
Pyroglutamic acidemia (5-oxoprolinuria)
Periodic hyperlysinemia
Hyperornithinemia-hyperammonemia-homocitrullinemia syndrome
Lysinuric protein intolerance

Disorders of Organic Acid Metabolism
Isovaleric acidemia
Propionic acidemia (ketotic hyperglycinemia)
Methylmalonic acidemia
Multiple carboxylase deficiency
Glutaric acidemia, type II (multiple acyl-CoA dehydrogenase deficiencies)
3-Methyl crotonyl-CoA carboxylase deficiency

Disorders of Pyruvate Metabolism and the Electron Transport Chain
Pyruvate carboxylase deficiency
Pyruvate dehydrogenase deficiency
Electron transport chain deficiencies

Disorders of Urea Synthesis
Carbamyl phosphate synthetase (CPS) deficiency
Ornithine transcarbamylase (OTC) deficiency
Argininosuccinate synthetase (AS) deficiency (citrullinemia)
Argininosuccinate lyase (AL) deficiency
Arginase deficiency
N-Acetylglutamate synthetase (NAGS) deficiency
Transient hyperammonemia of the newborn (THAN)

Lysosomal Storage Disorders
GM₁ gangliosidosis, type I (beta-galactosidase deficiency)
Gaucher's disease (glucocerebrosidase deficiency)
Niemann-Pick disease, types A and B (sphingomyelinase deficiency)
Wolman disease (acid lipase deficiency)
Mucopolysaccharidosis, type VII (beta-glucuronidase deficiency)
I-cell disease (mucolipidosis, type II)
Sialidosis, type II (neuraminidase deficiency)

Peroxisomal Disorders
Zellweger syndrome
Neonatal adrenoleukodystrophy

Miscellaneous Disorders
Adrenogenital syndrome (21-hydroxylase deficiency)
Pyridoxine-responsive seizures
Alpha₁-antitrypsin deficiency
Disorders of bilirubin metabolism (eg, Crigler-Najjar syndrome)
Fatty acyl-CoA dehydrogenase deficiencies (short chain, medium chain, and long chain)

symptoms. Symptoms may also be related to the introduction and progression of enteral feedings.

    3. Term vs. preterm. These diseases are found principally in full-term infants with the exception of transient hyperammonemia of the newborn.

V. Diagnosis (if a known proband exists).

    A. Prenatal. The ability to diagnose enzyme defects prenatally has increased in recent years. In some cases, treatment while in utero can be accomplished (dietary control in PKU). Otherwise, appropriate therapies can begin quickly subsequent to delivery of the infant. When no effective therapy exists, parents

TABLE 59–2. SIGNS AND SYMPTOM COMPLEXES SUGGESTING CLASSES OF METABOLIC DISORDERS

1. Neurologic (hypotonia, lethargy, poor sucking, seizures, coma)
    Glycogen storage disease, galactosemia, organic acidemias, hereditary fructose intolerance, maple syrup urine disease, urea cycle disorders, hyperglycinemia, pyridoxine dependency, peroxisomal disorders.
2. Hepatomegaly
    Lysosomal Storage diseases, galactosemia, hereditary fructose intolerance, glycogen storage disease, tyrosinemia, Alpha-1-Antitrypsin deficiency, Gaucher's disease, Neiman-Pick disease, Wolman's disease, fatty acid oxidation defects.
3. Hyperbilirubinemia
    Galactosemia, hereditary fructose intolerance, tyrosinemia, Alpha-1-Antitrypsin deficiency.
4. Non-Immune Hydrops
    Gaucher's disease, Neiman-Pick disease.
5. Cardiomegaly
    Glycogen storage disease Type II, fatty acid oxidation defects.
6. Coarse Facial Features
    GM1 Gangliosidosis, Beta glucuronidase deficiency, I- Cell Disease, sialidosis.
7. Macroglossia
    GM1 Gangliosidosis, Glycogen storage disease Type II.
8. Abnormal Odor
    Maple Syrup Urine Disease (odor of maple syrup)
    Isovaleric Acidemia, Glutaric Acidemia (odor of sweaty feet)
    Hydroxymethylglutaryl COA Lyase Deficiency (odor of cat urine)
9. Abnormal Hair
    Arginosuccinic Acidemia, lysinuric protein intolerance, Menke's kinky hair syndrome
10. Hypoglycemia
    Galactosemia, hereditary fructose intolerance, tyrosinemia, Maple Syrup Urine Disease, Glycogen storage disease, methylmalonic acidemia, proprionic acidemia.
11. Ketosis
    Organic acidemias, tyrosinemia, methylmalonic acidemia.
12. Metabolic Acidosis
    Galactosemia, hereditary fructose intolerance, Maple Syrup Urine Disease, Glycogen storage disease, organic acidemias.

may use this information to help make an informed decision regarding continuation of the pregnancy.

1. **Chorionic villus sampling.** Over 50% of all prenatal diagnoses of enzyme defects can now be made using chorionic villus sampling. Adequate samples may be obtained prior to 8 weeks gestation.
2. **Amniocentesis.** Many metabolic disorders can be diagnosed through the detection of specific metabolites in the amniotic fluid.
3. **Fetal cells in the maternal circulation.** Attempts are now being made to analyze enzymatic defects using fetal cells obtained from the mother. If this proves successful, it will provide a noninvasive method of diagnosing metabolic disorders without risk to the fetus.
4. **Testing of preimplantation embryos.** This strategy has been used when X-linked disorders are known to exist in the family. Sexing embryos is facilitated by using Y-specific DNA amplification and transferring only female embryos for implantation.

B. **Postnatal** (See Tables 59–4, 59–5, 59–6.)

TABLE 59–3. MISDIAGNOSIS OF METABOLIC DISEASE IN THE NEWBORN INFANT

Sepsis (bacterial or viral)
Asphyxia
Gastrointestinal tract obstruction
Hepatic failure, hepatitis
Central nervous system catastrophe
Persistent pulmonary hypertension
Myocardiopathy

TABLE 59–4. LABORATORY FINDINGS SUGGESTIVE OF METABOLIC DISEASE

	Galactosemia	Fructose-1,6-diphosphatase Deficiency	Glycogen storage Disease[a]	Maple Syrup Urine Disease	Nonketotic Hyperglycinemia[b]	Glutaric Acidemia[c] Type II	Pyroglutamic Acidemia	Organic Acidemias	Disorders of Pyruvate[c] Metabolism	Disorders of Urea Synthesis	Transient Hyperammonemia of the Newborn
Hypoglycemia	−	+	+	±	−	±	−	±	±	−	−
Metabolic acidosis with or without elevated anion gap	−	+	+	+	−	±	+	+	+	−	±
Respiratory alkalosis	−	−	−	−	−	−	−	−	−	+	+
Hyperammonemia	−	−	−	N−1+	−	N−1+	−	N−3+	N−1+	1−3+	2−4+
Hyperlactatemia	−		±	−	−	±	−	N−1+	1+2+	−	±
Direct hyperbilirubinemia	1	−	−	−	−	−	−	−	−	−	−
Urine											
Clinitest +	+	+	+	−	−	−	−	−	−	−	−
Acetest + or Ketostix +	−	+	+	+	−	±	−	+	±	−	−
DNPH	−	±	±	+	−	−	−	+	±	−	−
Abnormal odor or color	−	−	−	+[d]	−	+[e]	−	±[e,f]	−	−	−
Neutropenia or thrombocytopenia	−	−	−	−	−	−	−	±	−	−	−

N = Normal

[a] Hypercholesterolemia. Hypertriglyceridemia. hyperuricemia.
[b] Elevated plasma glycine only metabolic abnormality.
[c] Dysmorphic features.
[d] Maple syrup or burnt sugar.
[e] Sweaty feet (isovaleric acidemia).
[f] Cat urine (3 methyl crotonyl CoA carboxylase deficiency).

327

TABLE 59–5. PROCEDURES FOR URINE TESTS HELPFUL IN THE DIAGNOSIS OF METABOLIC DISEASE

Clinitest (Ames)
1. Mix 5 drops of urine and 10 drops of water in a clean test tube. Add 1 tablet. Fifteen seconds after the end of the reaction, gently shake the test tube.
2. Compare the color after the reaction with the chart supplied. A negative test gives a blue color. Tests that produce green, brown, yellow, or red solutions may indicate the presence of carbohydrate reducing substances (eg, glucose, galactose), amino acids, or a variety of exogenous drugs.

Acetest (Ames)
1. Place 1 tablet on a clean white filter paper. Apply 1 drop of urine; wait 30 seconds.
2. Test is positive only if the tablet turns purple. Result is coded as small, moderate, or large amount of ketones by comparison to a color chart.

Ketostix (Ames)
1. Dip the reagent strip into urine.
2. Compare the color to the chart on the bottle.

Dinitrophenylhydrazine (DNPH)
1. Mix 10 drops of reagent (refrigerated solution of 100 mg 2,4-dinitrophenylhydrazine in 100 mL of 2-N HCl) with 1 mL of urine.
2. Yellow-white precipitates indicate the presence of ketoacids. This test is usually highly positive with maple syrup urine disease, though it may be positive with glycogen storage disease, fructose-1,6-diphosphatase deficiency, organic acidemias, phenylketonuria, or tyrosinemia.

   1. **Laboratory testing**
      a. **Blood:** CBC, glucose, blood gas, ammonium level, amino acids, lactate, pyruvate.
      b. **Urine:** ferric chloride, nonglucose-reducing substances, organic acids.
   C. **Postmortem**
      1. **Indications.** If death appears imminent, it is important to gather as much information as possible about the child's disorder.
      2. **Specific Diagnostic Steps**
         a. **Blood**
            (1) Collect 20–25 mL of whole blood. Separate the plasma from the cells and freeze in 1–2 mL aliquots at –20 °C (quantitative amino acids, carnitine, ketone bodies).
            (2) Refrigerate an erythrocyte fraction at 4 °C (enzyme and peroxisomal studies). In addition, refreeze an erythrocyte fraction at –20 °C (enzyme/DNA studies).
         b. **Urine.** Collect 20–30 mL and store in 5 mL aliquots at –20 °C (organic, orotic, and amino acid screening).

TABLE 59–6. ANALYSIS OF AMINO AND ORGANIC ACIDS IN PLASMA AND URINE

	Organic Acids	Amino Acids
Isovaleric acidemia	Isovalerylglycine 3-Hydroxyisovalerate	Normal
Propionic acidemia	3-Hydroxypropionate Methylcitrate	Elevated glycine
Methylmalonic acidemia	Methylmalonate	Elevated glycine
Multiple carboxylase deficiency	3-Methylcrotonyl 3-Hydroxyisovalerate 3-Hydroxypropionate	
Glutaric acidemia, type II	Glutaric acid 2-Hydroxyglutarate Ethylmalonate 2-Hydroxyisovalerate	Elevated lysine
5-Oxoprolinuria (pyroglutamic acidemia)	Pyroglutamate	Normal or elevated oxoproline
Nonketotic hyperglycinemia	Normal	Elevated glycine

  c. Vitreous humor (for chemistries).

  d. Skin. 3–4 mm should be taken as a full thickness sterile biopsy (cleansed with alcohol, not iodine). Store in a sterile culture medium (or sterile D5NS). Transport immediately to a tissue culture laboratory for fibroblast culture and enzyme/DNA analysis.

  e. CSF. Store a sample at –20 °C.

  f. Liver sample. May biopsy percutaneously as necessary and store at –20 °C.

  g. Tissue biopsies of liver, heart, muscle, and brain stored at –20 °C. Tissue should be evaluated by light and electron microscopy (peroxisomes, liposomes, mitochondria).

  h. Complete autopsy including x-ray films.

 D. Differential diagnosis (See Figs 59–1 and 59–2.)

VI. Management. There are currently no cures available for inborn errors of metabolism beyond experimental trials. However, certain defects are amenable to specific modes of therapy.

 A. While awaiting results

  1. Supportive care. General measures include correction of acid-base balance, electrolyte abnormalities, and hydration status. Assisted ventilation may be required in severely affected neonates and aggressive antibiotic therapy is occasionally indicated (galactosemia is associated with an increased risk of *E coli* (sepsis).

  2. Nutritional

   a. Protein and carbohydrate restriction. Accomplished by eliminating oral formula intake, thus removing the source of the offending metabolite.

   b. Provide adequate caloric intake. A high energy intake (80–120 Kcal/kg/d) using intravenous glucose, lipids, and insulin may help to initiate an anabolic state. (**Note:** Lipids may be contraindicated in certain fatty acid oxidation defects.)

   c. Megavitamin cocktail. Several inborn errors of metabolism have vitamin responsive forms. Often, a combination of vitamin cofactors (vitamin B12, biotin, riboflavin, thiamine, pyridoxine, and folate) are given to a sick infant while specific test results are still outstanding. (**Note:** Consider this approach only after appropriate specimens have been obtained for full metabolic investigation.)

   d. Carnitine. May be useful acutely in aiding the excretion of conjugates of accumulated metabolites in organic acidemias.

  3. Removal of toxic metabolites. Hemodialysis or peritoneal dialysis may be started in cases where acidosis is intractable. Exchange transfusions are less effective and their benefits are transient.

 B. Long-term therapy

  1. Provision of a deficient substance. This is effective when the deficient product is readily available and can reach the deficient tissue (ie, cortisol and mineralocorticoid in 21 hydroxylase deficiency).

  2. Vitamin therapies. Large doses of specific cofactors may increase the activity of deficient enzymes.

   a. Vitamin B6 (homocystinuria).

   b. Vitamin B12 (methylmalonic acidemia).

   c. Biotin (multiple carboxylase deficiency).

   d. Thiamine (maple syrup urine disease).

   e. Riboflavin (glutaric acidemia 11).

  3. Diet. Restrict the intake of a dietary substance leading to the accumulation of a toxic metabolite (ie, phenylalanine in PKU). Careful monitoring is necessary as some dietary intake of the substance may be needed for adequate growth.

  4. Supportive. May help to reduce the morbidity associated with specific inborn errors of metabolism.

   a. Splinting reduces deformities in mucopolysaccharidoses.

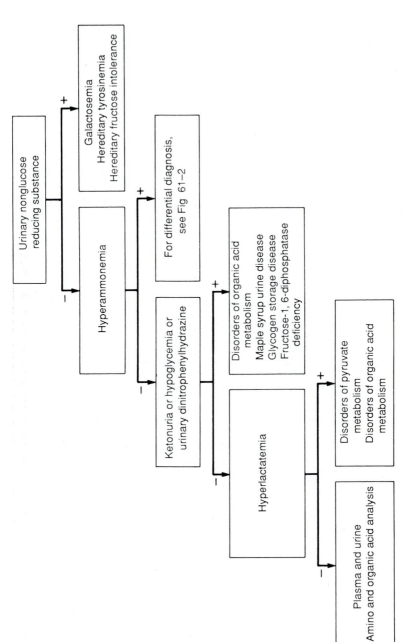

FIGURE 59-1. Algorithm for initial diagnosis of metabolic disease with acute neonatal onset.

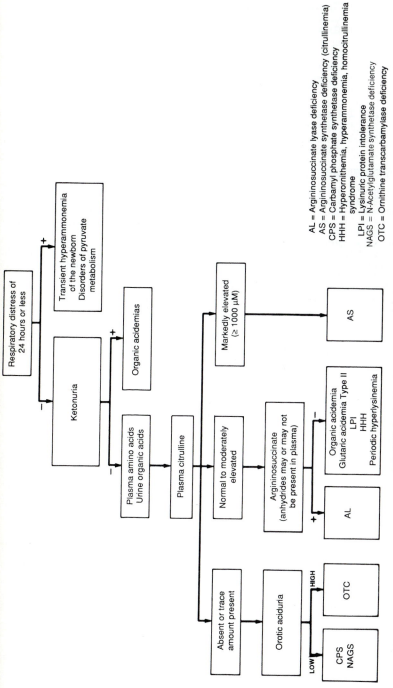

FIGURE 59–2. Algorithm for differential diagnosis of hyperammonemia.

AL = Argininosuccinate lyase deficiency
AS = Argininosuccinate synthetase deficiency (citrullinemia)
CPS = Carbamyl phosphate synthetase deficiency
HHH = Hyperornithemia, hyperammonemia, homocitrullinemia syndrome
LPI = Lysinuric protein intolerance
NAGS = N-Acetylglutamate synthetase deficiency
OTC = Ornithine transcarbamylase deficiency

      b. Splenectomy may be indicated for thrombocytopenia associated with Gaucher's disease.

      c. Early intervention and special education programs may be beneficial in those disorders characterized by intellectual impairment.

   5. **Alternative pathways.** Provide substances which can serve as alternative carriers for accumulated substrates and promote their excretion. For example, significant amounts of waste nitrogen excretion, independent of the urea cycle, may be achieved by providing arginine in citrullinemia and arginosuccinic acidemia.

   6. **Long-term.** These disorders require life-long nutritional, medical, and laboratory monitoring by a team of specialists in these disorders. Factors such as reintroduction of restricted substances into the diet, intercurrent illnesses, and stress may precipitate the recurrence of symptoms.

REFERENCES

Burton BK: Inborn errors of metabolism: The clinical diagnosis in early infancy. *Pediatr* 1987;**79:**359–69.

Goodman SL: Inherited metabolic disease in the newborn. *Adv Pediatr* 1986;**33:**197–224.

Goodman SL, Greene CL: Inborn errors as causes of acute disease in infancy. *Semin Perinatol* 1991;**15:**31–34.

Iafolla AK, McConkie-Rosell A: Prenatal diagnosis of metabolic disease. *Clin Perinatol* 1990;**17:**761–77.

Salle HM, Rosenbaum KN: Screening the newborn for anatomic and metabolic defects. *Pediatr Ann* 1988;**17:**467–76.

Waber L: Inborn errors of metabolism. *Pediatr Ann* 1990;**19:**105–18.

Ward JC: Inborn errors of metabolism of acute onset in infancy. *Pediatr Rev* 1990;**11:**205–16.

Wraith JE: Diagnosis and management of inborn errors of metabolism. *Arch Dis Child* 1989;**64:**1410.

60 Infant of Diabetic Mother

Good control of maternal diabetes is the key factor in determining fetal outcome. Recent data indicate that perinatal morbidity and mortality rates in the offspring of women with diabetes mellitus have improved with dietary management and insulin therapy. However, when adequate control of diabetes has not been accomplished, the physician must be aware of possible complications in the infant, including hypoglycemia, hypocalcemia, hypomagnesemia, perinatal asphyxia, respiratory distress syndrome, other respiratory illnesses, hyperbilirubinemia, polycythemia, renal vein thrombosis, macrosomia, birth injuries, and congenital malformations. Because of better current understanding of the pathophysiology of diabetic pregnancies, these complications can be recognized and treated.

I. **Classification**
   A. **White's classification.** In earlier descriptions of diabetic pregnancies, physicians relied on White's classification (Table 60–1). This nomenclature is based on the age at onset, the duration of the disorder, and the complications. It is used today chiefly to compare groups of infants delivered.
   B. **National Diabetes Data Group classification.** Table 60–2 presents the nomenclature of the National Diabetes Data Group. It replaces the older White classification and is a simpler method for characterizing diabetic pregnancies.

II. **Incidence.** Insulin-dependent diabetes occurs in 0.5% of all pregnancies. In addition, 1–3% of women exhibit biochemical abnormalities during pregnancy consistent with gestational diabetes.

III. **Pathophysiology**
   A. **Macrosomia.** Macrosomia is the classic presentation of the infant of a diabetic mother (IDM). It is the result of biochemical events along the maternal hyperglycemia–fetal hyperinsulinemia pathway as described by Pedersen (1971). Infants born to mothers described by White's classification as having class A (insulin-dependent), B, C, or D diabetes are often macrosomic. Complications are minimal in gestational diabetes and in class A diabetes controlled by diet.
   B. **Small for gestational age (SGA).** Mothers with renal, retinal, or cardiac diseases are more likely to have SGA or premature infants, poor fetal outcome, fetal distress, or fetal death.

TABLE 60–1. WHITE'S CLASSIFICATION OF DIABETES

Class	Description
A	Chemical diabetes with positive glucose tolerance test before or during pregnancy
B	Onset after age 20; less than 10 years' duration
C	Onset at age 10–19
D1	Onset before age 10
D2	Duration longer than 20 years
D3	Calcification of vessels of the leg
D4	Benign retinopathy
D5	Hypertension
E	Calcification of pelvic vessels (not used)
F	Nephropathy
G	Pregnancy failures
H	Vascular lesions developing in childbearing years; includes patients with cardiopathy
R	Malignant retinopathy

Adapted, with permission, from White P: Diabetes mellitus in pregnancy. *Clin Perinatol* 1974;**1**:331.

TABLE 60–2. NOMENCLATURE OF NATIONAL DIABETES DATA GROUP

Class	Description
Type I: Insulin-dependent diabetes mellitus (IDDM)	Ketosis-prone, insulin-deficient owing to islet cell loss. Often associated with specific HLA types, with predisposition to viral insulitis or diabetes autoimmune phenomena. Occurs at any age. Common in youth.
Type II: Non-insulin-dependent diabetes mellitus (NIDDM)	Ketosis-resistant. More common in adults but occurs at any age. Many patients are overweight. May be seen in family aggregates as an autosomal dominant genetic trait. May require insulin for hyperglycemia during stress. Invariably requires insulin during pregnancy.
Gestational diabetes mellitus (GDM)	Diabetes begins (or is recognized) during pregnancy. Above normal risk of perinatal complications. Glucose intolerance may be transitory but frequently recurs. Diagnosis requires at least 2 abnormal plasma glucose values on a 3-hour oral glucose tolerance test (100 g glucose). Fasting: 105 mg/dL or more 1 hour: 190 mg/dL or more 2 hours: 160 mg/dL or more 3 hours: 145 mg/dL or more

Adapted, with permission, from National Diabetes Data Group: Classification and diagnosis of diabetes mellitus and other categories of glucose intolerance. *Diabetes* 1979;**28**:1039.

C. Specific disorders frequently encountered in IDMs
1. Metabolic disorders
  a. Hypoglycemia is defined as a blood glucose level less than 45 mg/dL in a preterm or term infant. It is present in up to 40% of IDMs, most commonly in macrosomic infants. It usually presents within 1–2 hours after delivery. According to Pedersen, at birth, the transplacental glucose supply is terminated, and, because of high concentrations of plasma insulin, blood glucose levels fall. Mothers with well-controlled blood glucose levels have fewer infants with hypoglycemia. Hypoglycemia in the SGA infants born to mothers with diabetic vascular disease is due to decreased glycogen stores; it appears 6–12 hours after delivery.

  b. Hypocalcemia. Serum calcium levels less than 7 mg/dL associated with symptoms or less than 6 mg/dL without symptoms—or an ionized calcium level less than 3 mg/dL—is considered hypocalcemic. The incidence is up to 50% of IDMs (Tsang, 1979). The severity of hypocalcemia is related to the severity of maternal diabetes and involves decreased function of the parathyroid glands (Tsang, 1975). Serum calcium levels are lowest at 24–72 hours of age.

  c. Hypomagnesemia. A serum magnesium level less than 1.52 mg/dL in any infant is an indication of hypomagnesemia. It is related to maternal hypomagnesemia and the severity of maternal diabetes.

2. Cardiorespiratory disorders
  a. Perinatal asphyxia. Perinatal asphyxia occurs in up to 25% of IDMs. It may be due to prematurity, cesarean delivery, intrauterine hypoxia caused by maternal vascular disease, or macrosomia.

  b. Hyaline membrane disease or respiratory distress syndrome (RDS)
    (1) Incidence. The incidence has decreased to only 3% of IDM owing to better management of diabetes during pregnancy (Frantz, 1979). Most cases are due to premature delivery, delayed maturation of pulmonary surfactant production, or delivery by elective cesarean section.

    (2) Fetal lung maturity. Pulmonary surfactant production in the IDM is deficient or delayed principally in class A, B, and C diabetics. Fetal hyperinsulinism may adversely affect the lung maturation process in the IDM by antagonizing the action of cortisol (Smith, 1975).

    (3) Cesarean section. Infants delivered by elective cesarean section are at risk for RDS because of decreased prostaglandin production and increased pulmonary vascular resistance (Csaba, 1978).

  c. Other causes of respiratory distress

    (1) Transient tachypnea of the newborn (TTN) occurs especially after elective cesarean section. This disorder may or may not require oxygen therapy and usually responds by 72 hours of age.

    (2) Hypertrophic cardiomyopathy occurs in up to 50% of IDMs (Way, 1979). It occurs secondary to increased fat and glycogen deposition in the myocardium and may lead to congestive heart failure.

3. Hematologic disorders

  a. Hyperbilirubinemia. Bilirubin production is apparently increased in the IDM secondary to prematurity, macrosomia, hypoglycemia, and polycythemia.

  b. Polycythemia and hyperviscosity. The cause of polycythemia is unclear but may be related to increased levels of erythropoietin in the IDM, increased red blood cell production secondary to chronic intrauterine hypoxia in mothers with vascular disease, and intrauterine placental transfusion due to acute hypoxia during labor and delivery.

  c. Renal venous thrombosis is a rare complication most likely due to hyperviscosity, hypotension, or disseminated intravascular coagulation. It is usually diagnosed by ultrasonography and may present with hematuria and an abdominal mass.

4. Morphologic and functional problems

  a. Macrosomia and birth injury

    (1) Macrosomia is due to fetal hyperglycemia, resulting in increased glucose uptake in insulin-sensitive tissues. It is seen in the offspring of gestational and class A, B, and C diabetics. Macrosomia is rarely seen in the other classes because of maternal vascular disease.

    (2) Birth injury. Macrosomia may lead to shoulder dystocia, which may cause birth asphyxia. Birth injuries include fractures of the clavicle or humerus, Erb's palsy, phrenic nerve palsy, and, rarely, central nervous system injury.

  b. Congenital malformations. Congenital malformations occur in 6.4% of IDMs (Molsted-Pedersen, 1980)—a much higher incidence than in the general population. It is suspected that poor diabetic control in the first trimester is associated with a higher percentage of congenital malformations. Congenital malformations now account for up to 50% of perinatal deaths and include cardiac defects (transposition of the great vessels, ventricular septal defect, atrial septal defect), renal defects (agenesis), gastrointestinal tract defects (small left colon syndrome, situs inversus), neurologic defects (anencephaly, meningocele syndrome), skeletal defects (hemivertebrae, caudal regression syndrome), unusual facies and microophthalmia.

IV. Risk factors. The following factors or conditions may be associated with an increased risk for problems in IDMs.

  A. Maternal class of diabetes

    1. In gestational diabetes and class A diabetes controlled by diet alone, infants have few complications.

    2. Women with class A diabetes controlled with insulin and class B, C, and D diabetes are prone to deliver macrosomic infants if diabetes is inadequately controlled.

    3. Diabetic women with renal, retinal, cardiac, and vascular disease have the most severe fetal problems.

  B. Hemoglobin A$_{1c}$. To decrease perinatal morbidity and mortality rates, the diabetic woman should attempt to achieve good metabolic control before conception. Elevated hemoglobin A$_{1c}$ levels during the first trimester appear to be associated with a higher incidence of congenital malformations (Miller, 1979).

C. Diabetic ketoacidosis. Pregnant women with insulin-dependent diabetes are apt to develop diabetic ketoacidosis. The onset of this complication may be life-threatening for the mother and fetus or may lead to preterm delivery.

D. Preterm labor. Premature onset of labor in a diabetic woman is a serious problem because of the increased likelihood of respiratory distress syndrome in the fetus. Furthermore, beta-sympathomimetic agents used to prevent preterm delivery may be associated with maternal hyperglycemia, hyperinsulinemia, and acidosis.

E. Immature fetal lung profile. Diabetic women who present at 36 weeks' gestation or later should undergo amniocentesis to evaluate fetal lung maturity. A mature lecithin:sphingomyelin ratio may not ensure normal respiratory function in the IDM. However, the presence of phosphatidylglycerol in the amniotic fluid is more apt to be associated with normal neonatal respiratory function (see also Chap 1).

V. Clinical presentation

A. At birth, the infant may be large for gestational age, or if the mother has vascular disease, small for gestational age. The size of most infants is appropriate for gestational age; however, if macrosomia is present, birth trauma may occur.

B. After birth, hypoglycemia can present as lethargy, poor feeding, apnea, or jitteriness in the first 6–12 hours after birth. Jitteriness that occurs after 24 hours of age may be due to hypocalcemia or hypomagnesemia. Signs of respiratory distress due to immature lungs can be noted on examination. Cardiac disease may be present as an enlarged cardiothymic shadow on a chest x-ray film or by physical evidence of heart failure. Gross congenital anomalies may be noted on physical examination.

VI. Diagnosis

A. Laboratory studies. The following tests *must* be closely monitored in the IDM.

1. **Serum glucose levels** should be checked at delivery and at ½, 1, 1½, 2, 4, 8, 12, 24, 36, and 48 hours of age. Glucose levels should be checked with Chemstrip-bG or Dextrostix. Readings below 40 mg/dL on Chemstrip-bG or below 45 mg/dL on Dextrostix should be verified by serum glucose measurements.

2. **Serum calcium levels** should be obtained at 6, 24, and 48 hours of age. If serum calcium levels are low, **serum magnesium levels** should be obtained as they may also be low.

3. **The hematocrit** should be checked at birth and at 4 and 24 hours of age.

4. **Serum bilirubin levels** should be checked as indicated by physical examination.

5. **Other tests.** Arterial blood gas levels, complete blood counts, cultures, and Gram stains should be obtained as clinically indicated.

B. Radiologic studies are not necessary unless there is evidence of cardiac, respiratory, or skeletal problems.

C. Electrocardiography and echocardiography should be performed if hypertrophic cardiomyopathy or a cardiac malformation is suspected.

VII. Management

A. Initial evaluation. Upon delivery, the infant should be evaluated in the usual manner. In the transitional nursery, blood glucose levels and the hematocrit should be obtained. The infant should be observed for jitteriness, tremors, convulsions, apnea, weak cry, and poor sucking. A physical examination should be performed, paying particular attention to the heart, kidneys, lungs, and extremities.

B. Continuing evaluation. Over the first several hours after delivery, the infant should be assessed for signs of respiratory distress. During the first 48 hours, observe for signs of jaundice and for renal, cardiac, neurologic, and gastrointestinal tract abnormalities.

C. Metabolic management

1. **Hypoglycemia.** See Chapter 39.

2. **Hypocalcemia**
a. **Calcium therapy.** Symptomatic infants should receive 10% calcium gluconate intravenously. The infusion should be given slowly to prevent cardiac arrhythmias, and the infant should be monitored for signs of extravasation. Following the initial dose, a maintenance dose is given by continuous intravenous infusion. The hypocalcemia should respond in 3–4 days, but until then, serum calcium levels should be monitored every 12 hours.
b. **Magnesium maintenance therapy.** Magnesium is usually added to intravenous fluids or given orally as magnesium sulfate 50%, 0.2 mL/kg/d (4 meq/mL).

D. **Management of cardiorespiratory problems**
1. **Perinatal asphyxia.** Close observation for fetal distress should continue (see Chap 66).
2. **Hyaline membrane disease.** Obtaining amniotic fluid for a fetal lung maturity profile can decrease the incidence of hyaline membrane disease. However, some infants must be delivered even if the lung profile is immature.
3. **Cardiomyopathy.** The treatment of choice is with propranolol. See Chapter 73 for dosage information. Digoxin is contraindicated due to possible ventricular outflow obstruction.

E. **Hematologic therapy**
1. **Hyperbilirubinemia.** Frequent monitoring of serum bilirubin levels may be necessary. Phototherapy and exchange transfusion for infants with hyperbilirubinemia is discussed in Chapter 58.
2. **Polycythemia.** See Chapter 54.
3. **Renal venous thrombosis.** Treatment consists in fluid restriction and close monitoring of electrolytes and renal status. Supportive therapy is indicated to insure adequate blood circulation. Nephrectomy is usually only a last resort in unilateral disease.

F. **Management of morphologic and functional problems**
1. **Macrosomia and birth injury**
a. **Fractures of the extremities** should be treated with immobilization.
b. **Erb's palsy** can be treated with range-of-motion exercises.
2. **Congenital malformations.** If a gross malformation is discovered, a specialist should be consulted.

VIII. **Prognosis.** Less morbidity and mortality occur with adequate control during the diabetic pregnancy. Preconceptual counseling is used as an adjunct to preventive health care of the diabetic patient. The known pregnant diabetic is currently receiving better health care than before, but the challenge is early identification of women with biochemical abnormalities of gestational diabetes. The risk of subsequent diabetes in the infants of these women is at least 10 times greater than in the normal population.

REFERENCES

Csaba IF, Sulyok E, Ertl T: Relationship of maternal treatment with indomethacin to persistence of fetal circulation syndrome. *J Pediatr* 1978;**92**:484.

Cummins M, Norrish M: Follow-up of children of diabetic mothers. *Arch Dis Child* 1980;**55**:259.

Frantz IO III, Epstein MF: Fetal lung development in pregnancies complicated by diabetes. In: *The Diabetic Pregnancy: A Perinatal Perspective.* Merkatz IR, Adam PAJ (editors). Grune & Stratton, 1979.

Hollingsworth DR: Diabetes. In: *Medical Counseling Before Pregnancy.* Hollingsworth DR, Resnik R (editors). Churchill, 1988.

Kitzmiller JL, Cloherty JP, Graham CA: Management of diabetes and pregnancy. In: *Clinical Diabetes Mellitus.* Kozak GP (editor). Saunders, 1982.

Kulovich MV, Gluck L: The lung profile. 2. Complicated pregnancy. *Am J Obstet Gynecol* 1979;**135**:64.

Miller JM, Crenshaw MC Jr, Welt SI: Hemoglobin A$_{1c}$ in normal and diabetic pregnancy. *JAMA* 1979;**242**:2785.

Molsted-Pedersen L: Pregnancy and diabetes: A survey. *Acta Endocrinol [Suppl]* 1980;**238**:13.

Pedersen J: *The Pregnant Diabetic and Her Newborn,* 2nd ed. Williams & Wilkins, 1971.

Smith BT et al: Insulin antagonism of cortisol action on lecithin synthesis by cultured fetal lung cells. *J Pediatr* 1975;**87**:953.

Tsang RC, Brown DR, Steichen JJ: Diabetes and calcium: Calcium disturbances in infants of diabetic mothers. In: *The Diabetic Pregnancy: A Perinatal Perspective.* Merkatz IR, Adam PAJ (editors). Grune & Stratton, 1979.

Way GL et al: The natural history of hypertrophic cardiomyopathy in infants of diabetic mothers. *J Pediatr* 1979;**95**:1020.

White P: Diabetes mellitus in pregnancy. *Clin Perinatol* 1974;**1**:331.

61 Infectious Diseases

Isolation precautions for all infectious diseases, including maternal and neonatal precautions, breast-feeding and visiting issues, can be found in Appendix G, page 000.

NEONATAL SEPSIS

I. **Definition.** Neonatal sepsis is a clinical syndrome of systemic illness accompanied by bacteremia occurring in the first month of life.

II. **Incidence.** The incidence of primary sepsis is 1–10 per 1,000 live births. The mortality rate is high (13–50%), with the higher rates seen in premature infants and those with early fulminant disease.

III. **Pathophysiology.** In considering the pathogenesis of neonatal sepsis, 3 different clinical situations may be defined: early-onset, late-onset, and nosocomial disease.

A. **Early-onset disease** presents in the first 5–7 days of life and is usually a multisystem fulminant illness with prominent respiratory symptoms. In this situation, the infant is colonized with the pathogen in the perinatal period. Several infectious agents, notably treponemes, viruses, Listeria, and probably Candida, can be acquired transplacentally via hematogenous routes. Acquisition of other organisms is associated with the birth process. With rupture of the membranes, vaginal flora or various bacterial pathogens may ascend to reach the amniotic fluid and fetus. Chorioamnionitis develops, leading to fetal colonization and infection. Aspiration of infected amniotic fluid by the fetus or neonate may play a role in resultant respiratory symptoms. The presence of vernix or meconium impairs the natural bacteriostatic properties of amniotic fluid. Finally, the infant may be exposed to vaginal flora as it passes through the birth canal. The primary sites of colonization tend to be the skin, nasopharynx, oropharynx, conjunctiva, and umbilical cord. Trauma to these mucosal surfaces may lead to infection.

B. **Late-onset disease** may occur as early as five days of age; however, it is more common after the first week of life. Although these infants may have a history of obstetrical complications, these are associated less frequently than with early-onset disease. These babies usually have an identifiable focus, most often meningitis in addition to sepsis. Bacteria responsible for late-onset sepsis and meningitis include those acquired after birth from maternal genital tract, as well as organisms acquired after birth from human contact or from contaminated equipment. Therefore, horizontal transmission appears to play a significant role in late-onset disease. The reasons for delay in development in clinical illness, the predilection for central nervous system disease, and the less severe systemic and cardiorespiratory symptoms are unclear. Transfer of maternal antibodies to her own vaginal flora may play a role in determining which exposed infants become infected, especially in the case of group B streptococcal infections.

C. **Nosocomial sepsis.** This form of sepsis occurs in high-risk newborn infants. Its pathogenesis is related to the underlying illness and debilitation of the infant, the flora in the NICU environment, and invasive monitoring and other techniques used in neonatal intensive care. Infants, especially premature infants, have an increased susceptibility to infection due to immature immune defenses which are less efficient at localizing and clearing bacterial invasion.

D. **Causative organisms.** The principal pathogens involved in neonatal sepsis have tended to change with time. Primary sepsis must be contrasted with nosocomial sepsis. The agents associated with primary sepsis are usually the vaginal flora. Most centers report **group B streptococci** as the most common, followed by **gram-negative enteric** organisms, especially **Escherichia coli.** Other pathogens include *Listeria monocytogenes, Staphylococcus,* other streptococci (including the **enterococci**), **anaerobes,** and *Haemophilus influenzae.* In addition, many unusual organisms are documented in primary neonatal sepsis, especially in premature infants. The flora causing nosocomial sepsis varies in each nursery. *Staphylococci* (especially *Staphylococcus epidermidis*), gram-negative rods (including *Pseudomonas, Klebsiella, Serratia,* and *Proteus*) and fungal organisms predominate.

IV. Risk factors
   A. Prematurity and low birth weight. Prematurity is the single most significant factor correlated with sepsis. The risk increases in proportion to the decrease in birth weight.
   B. Rupture of membranes. Premature or prolonged (> 24 hours) rupture of membranes.
   C. Maternal peripartum fever/infection: chorioamnionitis, UTI, and other obstetric complications.
   D. Amniotic fluid problems. Meconium-stained or foul-smelling, cloudy amniotic fluid.
   E. Resuscitation at birth. Infants who had fetal distress, were born by traumatic delivery, or were severely depressed at birth and required intubation and resuscitation.
   F. Multiple gestation.
   G. Invasive procedures. Invasive monitoring and respiratory or metabolic support.
   H. Infants with galactosemia (predisposition to *E coli* sepsis), immune defects, or asplenia.
   I. Iron therapy (iron added to serum in vitro enhances the growth of many organisms).
   J. Other factors. Males are more commonly affected than females. Variations in immune function may play a role. Sepsis is more common in black than white infants, but this may be explained by a higher incidence or premature rupture of membranes, maternal fever, and low birth weight. Low socioeconomic status is often reported as an additional risk factor, but again this may be explained by low birth weight.

V. Clinical presentation. The initial diagnosis of sepsis is by necessity a clinical one, because it is imperative to begin treatment before results of culture are available. Clinical signs and symptoms of sepsis are nonspecific, and the differential diagnosis is broad, including respiratory distress syndrome (RDS), metabolic diseases, hematologic disease, central nervous system disease, cardiac disease, and other infectious processes (ie, TORCH infections). Clinical signs and symptoms most often mentioned include the following:
   A. Temperature irregularity. Hypo- or hyperthermia (greater heat output required by incubator or radiant warmer to maintain neutral thermal environment or frequent adjustments of infant servo-control probe).
   B. Change in behavior. Lethargy, irritability, or change in tone.
   C. Skin. Poor peripheral perfusion, cyanosis, mottling, pallor, petechiae, rashes, sclerema, jaundice.
   D. Feeding problems. Feeding intolerance, vomiting, diarrhea (water loss stool), abdominal distension with or without visible bowel loops.
   E. Cardiopulmonary. Tachypnea, respiratory distress (grunting, flaring, retractions), apnea especially within the first 24 hours or new onset, especially after one week of age, tachycardia, hypotension (tends to be a late sign).
   F. Metabolic. Hypo- or hyperglycemia, metabolic acidosis.

VI. Diagnosis
   A. Laboratory studies
      1. Cultures. Blood and other normally sterile body fluids should be obtained for culture. (In neonates less than 24 hours of age, sterile urine specimen is

not necessary given that the occurrence of UTIs is exceedingly rare in this age group). Positive bacterial cultures will confirm the diagnosis of sepsis. Results may vary because of a number of factors, including maternal antibiotics administered before birth, organisms that are difficult to grow and isolate (ie, anaerobes), and sampling error with small sample volumes. Therefore, in many clinical situations, infants are treated for "presumed" sepsis despite negative cultures, with apparent clinical benefit. Some controversy currently exists whether spinal tap need be performed on asymptomatic newborns that are being worked up for presumptive sepsis. Many institutions are only performing lumbar punctures on babies who are clinically ill or who have documented positive blood cultures.

2. **Antigen detection tests.** Tests are available for **group B streptococci, Neisseria menningitidis, H influenzae,** and **Streptococcal pneumoniae.** Urine and cerebrospinal fluid are generally the specimens that can be tested. These tests can be especially helpful, secondary to their rapid turnaround time as an adjunct to making the definitive diagnosis. They can also be valuable if mother or baby have received antibiotics prior to cultures being obtained. It is, however, important to become familiar with the techniques used in a particular laboratory, and their rate of false-positive or false-negative results. The N meningitidis B polysaccharide is a sialic acid polymer which is chemically and immunologically identical to the K1 capsular polysaccharide of E coli K1 and K92. Therefore, a positive N meningitidis latex agglutination may signify E coli infection as long as sample is not contaminated with stool. It has also been shown that contamination of bag specimens of urine with group B strep from perineal and rectal colonization may produce a positive **urine latex** agglutination test in an infant with no systemic signs of infection. Bladder aspiration or urinary catheterization may be more effective in improving the specificity of the test.

3. **Gram's stain of various fluids.** Gram's staining is especially helpful for study of cerebrospinal fluid. Gram-stained smears and cultures of amniotic fluid or of material obtained by gastric aspiration is often performed. White cells in the samples can be maternal in origin, and their presence along with bacteria indicates exposure and possible colonization but not necessarily actual infection.

4. **Adjunctive laboratory tests**
   a. **White cell count and differential.** These values alone are very nonspecific. There are references for total white count and absolute neutrophil count (probably a better measure) as a function of postnatal age in hours (see Appendix L). Neutropenia may be a significant finding with an ominous prognosis when associated with sepsis. The presence of immature forms is more specific but still rather insensitive. Ratios of bands to segmented forms > 0.3 and of bands to total PMNs > 0.1 have good predictive value if present. Serial white counts followed several hours apart may be helpful in establishing a trend.
   b. **Platelet count.** A decreased platelet count is usually a late sign and is very nonspecific.
   c. **Acute phase reactants**
      (1) **C-reactive protein (CRP)** is an acute phase reactant that increases in the presence of inflammation caused by infection or tissue injury. There is a variable lag time between clinical onset of disease and elevated serum concentrations. Therefore, an elevated CRP may be helpful in the assessment of neonatal sepsis. However, it appears that three serial measurements may be needed to optimize sensitivity.
      (2) **The standard erythrocyte sedimentation rate (ESR)** may be elevated but usually not until well into the illness, and therefore is used rather infrequently in the initial workup.
      (3) **Depression of plasma fibronectin** may become a useful marker for late-onset sepsis, especially in very low birth weight infants.

d. Miscellaneous tests. Abnormal values for bilirubin, glucose, and sodium may, in the proper clinical situation, provide supportive evidence for sepsis.

B. Radiologic studies

1. **A chest x-ray** should be obtained in cases with respiratory symptoms, although it is often impossible to distinguish group B streptococcal or *Listeria* pneumonia from uncomplicated RDS. (Group B streptococcal pneumonia will often have associated pleural effusions present.)

2. **Urinary tract imaging. Imaging with renal ultrasound examination, intravenous pyelography, renal scan, or voiding cystourethrography** should be part of the evaluation when urinary tract infection accompanies sepsis. Sterile urine for culture must be obtained either by a suprapubic (p 140) or catheterized specimen (p 142). Bag urine samples should not be used to diagnose urinary tract infection.

C. Other studies. Examination of the placenta and fetal membranes may disclose evidence of chorioamnionitis and thus an increased potential for neonatal infection.

VII. Management

A. Universal precautions have been mandated by OSHA, and apply to blood, semen, vaginal secretions, wound exudate, and cerebrospinal and amniotic fluids. Precautions include caution to prevent injuries when using or disposing of needles or other sharp instruments. Protective barriers appropriate for procedures should be used including gloves, goggles, gowns, face shields, and other types of protection. Hands and exposed skin surfaces should be immediately and thoroughly washed after contamination with blood or other body fluids.

B. Initial therapy. Treatment is most often begun before a definite etiologic agent is identified. It consits of a **penicillin,** usually **ampicillin,** plus an **aminoglycoside** such as gentamicin. In nosocomial sepsis, the flora of the NICU must be considered, however, generally staphylococcal coverage with **vancomycin plus either an aminoglycoside** or a third-generation cephalosporin is usually begun. Dosages are presented in Chapter 73.

C. Continuing therapy is of course based on culture and sensitivity results. Monitoring for antibiotic toxicity is important as well as following levels of aminoglycosides and vancomycin. When group B streptococci is documented as the causative agent, a penicillin is the drug of choice; however, an aminoglycoside is often given as well due to documented synergism in vitro.

D. Complications and supportive therapy

1. **Respiratory.** Assure adequate oxygenation with blood gas monitoring and initiate O_2 therapy or ventilator support if needed.

2. **Cardiovascular.** Support blood pressure and perfusion to prevent shock. Use volume expanders 10–20 mL/kg (normal saline, albumin, blood) and follow intake of fluids and output of urine. Pressor agents such as dopamine or dobutamine may be needed (see Chap 73).

3. **Hematologic**

   a. **DIC.** With disseminated intravascular coagulation, one may observe generalized bleeding at puncture sites, GI tract, or CNS sites. In the skin, large vessel thrombosis may cause gangrene. Laboratory parameters consistent with DIC include thrombocytopenia, increased prothrombin time (PT), and increased partial thromboplastin time (PTT). There is an increase in fibrin split products (FSP) or D-dimers. Measures include treating the underlying disease, fresh frozen plasma (FFP) 10 mL/kg, vitamin K (p 000), platelet infusion, and possible exchange transfusion (p 000).

   b. **Neutropenia.** Granulocyte transfusions have proven effective in treatment of some neutropenic septic newborns; however, it appears that documentation of bone marrow neutrophil storage pool depletion may be a criteria in addition to the absolute neutropenia. The ability to obtain and interpret such samples as well as the difficulties in obtaining leuka-pheresed white cell preparations prevents the widespread use of this treatment. Studies are ongoing with recombinant human granulocyte-macrophage and granulocyte colony-stimulating factors as possible adjunctive therapies to enhance the infant's endogenous white blood cell kinetics and function. Intravenous immune globulin does appear useful as an adjunct to antibiotic therapy in serious neonatal infection.

4. **CNS.** Seizure control (use phenobarbital 20mg/kg loading dose) and monitor for syndrome of inappropriate antidiuretic hormone (SIADH) (decreased urine output, hyponatremia, decreased serum osmolarity, increased urine specific gravity and osmolarity)

5. **Metabolic.** Monitor for and treat hypo/hyperglycemia. Metabolic acidosis may accompany sepsis and is treated with bicarbonate and fluid replacement.

E. **Future developments.** Immunotherapy progress continues in the development of various hyperimmune globulins monoclonal antibodies to the specific pathogens causing neonatal sepsis. They may prove to be significant adjuvants to the routine use of antibiotics for treatment of sepsis.

MENINGITIS

I. **Definition.** Neonatal meningitis is infection of the meninges and central nervous system in the first month of life. This is the most common time of life for meningitis to occur.

II. **Incidence.** The incidence is about 1:2500 live births.The **mortality rate** is 30–60%, and there is a high incidence (up to 50% or more) of neurodevelopmental sequelae in survivors.

III. **Pathophysiology.** In most cases, infection occurs because of hematogenous seeding of the meninges and central nervous system. In cases of central nervous system or skeletal anomalies (myelomeningocele, etc) there may be direct inoculation by flora on the skin or in the environment. Neonatal meningitis is often accompanied by **ventriculitis**, which makes resolution of infection more difficult. There is also a predilection for vasculitis, which may lead to hemorrhage, thrombosis, and infarction. Subdural effusions and brain abscess may also complicate the course.

Most organisms implicated in neonatal sepsis also cause neonatal meningitis. Some have a definite predilection for central nervous system infection. **Group B streptococcus** (especially type III) and the gram-negative rods (especially *Escherichia coli* with K1 antigen) are the **most common causative agents.** Other causative organisms include *Listeria monocytogenes,* other streptococci (*Enterococci*), other gram-negative enteric bacilli (*Klebsiella, Enterobacter, Serratia* species).

With central nervous system anomalies involving open defects or indwelling devices (such as ventriculoperitoneal shunts), staphylococcal disease (***Staphylococcus aureus*** and ***Staphylococcus epidermidis***) is more common, as is disease caused by other skin flora, including streptococci and diphtheroids. Many unusual organisms, including fungi and anaerobes are described in case reports of neonatal meningitis in debilitated and normal neonates.

IV. **Risk factors.** Premature infants with sepsis have a much higher incidence (up to threefold that of term infants) of central nervous system infection. Infants with central nervous system defects necessitating ventriculoperitoneal shunt procedures also are at increased risk.

V. **Clinical presentation.** The clinical presentation is usually nonspecific. Meningitis must be excluded in any infant being evaluated for sepsis or infection. Signs and symptoms of meningitis generally are similar to those reported for sepsis. A full or bulging fontanelle is often a late finding in meningitis. The syndrome of inappropriate antidiuretic hormone (SIADH) may accompany meningitis.

VI. **Diagnosis**

A. **Laboratory studies.** Cerebrospinal fluid examination is critical in the investigation of possible meningitis. The technique for obtaining fluid is discussed in Chapter 22. Normal values are found in Appendix D.

1. **Culture** may be positive in association with normal or minimally abnormal cerebrospinal fluid on inspection.

2. **A gram-stained** smear can be helpful in making a more rapid definitive diagnosis and identifying the initial classification of the causative agent.

3. **Cerebrospinal glucose levels must be compared with serum glucose levels.** Normal cerebrospinal fluid values are one-half to two-thirds of serum values.

4. **Cerebrospinal fluid protein** is usually elevated, although normal values for infants, especially prematures, may be much higher (up to 150 mg/dL) than in later life and the test may be confounded by the presence of blood in the specimen.

5. **Cerebrospinal fluid pleocytosis** is variable. There are usually more cells with gram-negative rod than with group B streptococcal disease. Normal values range from 8 to 32 white cells in various studies, some of which may be PMNs. Pleocytosis (with neutrophils early) may also be an irritant reaction to central nervous system hemorrhage.

6. **Rapid antigen tests** are available for several organisms and should be done on spinal fluid.

7. **Ventricular tap,** with culture and examination fluid, is indicated in cases not responding to treatment.

B. **Radiologic studies**

1. **Cranial ultrasound examination** has been useful in the diagnosis of ventriculitis. (Echogenic strands can be seen in the ventricles.)

2. **CT scan** of the head may be indicated to rule out abscess, subdural effusion, or an area of thrombosis, hemorrhage, or infarction.

VII. Management

A. **Drug therapy.** (See Chap 73 for drug dosages and other pharmacologic information). (*Note:* Dosages for Ampicillin, Nafcillin, and Penicillin G are doubled when treating meningitis.)

1. **Empiric therapy.** Optimal antibiotic selection depends on culture and sensitivity testing of etiologic organisms. **Ampicillin and gentamicin** are usually started as empirical therapy for suspected sepsis or meningitis. (See Chap 73 for dosages.)

2. **Gram-positive meningitis (group B streptococci and *Listeria*).** Penicillin or ampicillin is the drug of choice. These infections usually respond well to treatment. Administration for 14–21 days is indicated. (See Chap 73 for dosages.)

3. **Staphylococcal disease.** This is mainly seen in infants with neurosurgical disorders. **Nafcillin, methicillin, or vancomycin** should be substituted for penicillin or ampicillin as initial coverage. (See Chap 73 for dosages.)

4. **Gram-negative meningitis.** The optimal treatment is still under investigation. Many organisms may be ampicillin-resistant, and penetration of CSF (even in the inflamed neonatal meninges) may be inadequate with aminoglycosides. Studies have shown no advantage to using intrathecal or intraventricular aminoglycosides. A better choice may be third-generation cephalosporins (eg, cefotaxime, cefuroxime). Currently, most would use **ampicillin plus cefotaxime** as initial therapy. This infection may be difficult to eradicate and 5–7 days of drug therapy may be needed to sterilize the cerebrospinal fluid, even with adequate therapy. Follow-up cerebrospinal fluid examination is recommended until sterility is documented. External ventricular drainage may be indicated in certain cases complicated by ventriculitis. Treatment may be indicated in certain cases complicated by ventriculitis. Treatment would continue until 14 days after cultures are negative or for 21 days, whichever is longer. Screening for relapse of infection should continue for at least 48–72 hours of therapy.

B. **Supportive measures and monitoring for complications.** Head circumference should be measured daily, and transillumination off the head and neurologic examination should be performed frequently.

TORCH INFECTIONS

TORCH is an acronym (**T**oxoplasma, **O**thers such as syphilis, hepatitis B, coxsackie virus, Epstein-Barr, varicella-zoster, and human parvovirus, **R**ubella virus, **C**ytomegalovirus, **H**erpes simplex virus) that denotes chronic nonbacterial perinatal infection. Herpetic disease in the neonate does not fit the pattern of chronic intrauterine infection but is traditionally grouped with the others. This group of infections may present in the neonate with similar clinical and laboratory findings (ie, SGA, hepatosplenomegaly, rash, central nervous system manifestations, early jaundice, low platelets)—hence the usefulness of the TORCH concept.

TOXOPLASMOSIS

I. **Definition.** *Toxoplasma gondii* is a parasite capable of causing intrauterine infection.

II. **Incidence.** The incidence of congenital infection is 1:1000 live births.

III. **Pathophysiology.** *T gondii* is a coccidian parasite ubiquitous in nature. The primary natural host is the cat family. The organism exists in 3 forms: oocyst, tachyzoite, and tissue cyst. The **oocysts** are excreted in cat feces. Ingestion of oocyst is followed by penetration of gastrointestinal mucosa by sporazoites, and circulation of tachyzoites, the ovoid unicellular organism characteristic of acute infections. Most maternal organs, including the placenta are "seeded" by the protazoan. Actual transmission to the fetus is by the transplacental-fetal hematogenous route. In the chronic form of the disease, organisms invade certain body tissues, especially those of the brain, eye, and striated muscle forming **tissue cysts.**

Acute infection in the adult is often subclinical. If symptoms are present, they are generally nonspecific: mononucleosis-like illness with fever, lymphadenopathy, fatigue, malaise, myalgia, fever, skin rash, and splenomegaly. Fetal infection is believed to occur solely associated with nonimmune mothers experiencing their primary acute infection. Placental infection occurs and persists throughout gestation. The infection may or may not be transmitted to the fetus. The later in pregnancy infection is acquired, the more likely is transmission to the fetus, (first trimester, 14%; second trimester, 29%; and third trimester, 59% transmission). Infections transmitted earlier in gestation are likely to cause more severe fetal effects (abortion-stillbirth, severe disease with teratogenesis). Those transmitted later are more apt to be subclinical. Rarely, a parasite may be transmitted via an infected placenta during parturition. Infection in the fetus or neonate usually involves disease in one of 2 forms: infection of the central nervous system and/or eyes, or infection of the central nervous system with disseminated infection.

IV. **Risk factors.** *T gondii* may be ingested during contact with soil or litter boxes contaminated with cat feces. It may also be transmitted in unpasteurized milk, in raw or undercooked meats (especially pork), and via blood product transfusion (white blood cells). Premature infants have a higher incidence of congenital toxoplasmosis than term infants (25–50% of cases in some series).

V. **Clinical presentation.** Congenital toxoplasmosis may be manifested as clinical neonatal disease, disease in the first few months of life, late sequelae or relapsed infection, or subclinical disease.

A. **Clinical disease.** Those who present with evident clinical disease may have disseminated illness or isolated central nervous system (CNS) or ocular disease. Late sequelae are primarily related to ocular or central nervous system disease. Obstructive hydrocephalus, chorioretinitis, and intracranial calcifications form the **classic triad** of toxoplasmosis.

B. Prominent signs and symptoms in infants with congenital toxoplasmosis include chorioretinitis, abnormalities of cerebrospinal fluid (high protein value), anemia, seizures, intracranial calcifications, direct hyperbilirubinemia, fever, hepatosplenomegaly, lymphadenopathy, vomiting, microcephaly or hydrocephaly, diarrhea, cataracts, eosinophilia, bleeding diathesis, hypothermia, glaucoma, optic atrophy, microphthalmia, rash, and pneumonitis.

C. Associated findings. Toxoplasmosis has been associated with congenital nephrosis, various endocrinopathies (due to hypothalamic or pituitary effects), myocarditis, erythroblastosis with hydrops fetalis, and isolated mental retardation.

D. Subclinical disease. Subclinical infection is believed to be the most common. Studies of these infants (in whom infection is identified by serologic testing or documented maternal infection) indicate that a large percentage may have minor cerebrospinal fluid abnormalities at birth and later develop visual or neurologic sequelae or learning disabilities.

VI. Diagnosis

A. Laboratory studies. The diagnosis of congenital toxoplasmosis is most often based on clinical suspicion plus serologic tests that may be complex and difficult to interpret.

1. **Direct isolation of the organism from body fluids or tissues** requires inoculating blood, body fluids, or placental tissue into mice or tissue culture and is not readily available. Isolation of the organism from placental tissue correlates strongly with fetal infection.

2. **Cerebrospinal fluid examination** should be performed in suspected cases. The most characteristic abnormalities are xanthochromia, mononuclear pleocytosis, and a very high protein level. Tests for cerebrospinal fluid IgM to toxoplasmosis may also be performed.

3. **Serologic tests.** These include a maternal skin tests (a positive test indicates chronic or latent infection and little risk of transmission to the fetus). The **indirect fluorescent antibody (IFA)** test has largely replaced the **Sabin-Feldman dye tests** as it is relatively easy to perform. It measures antibodies to surface antigen. A mother with a high IFA (1 to 512 or greater) and a positive IGM-IFA is highly suspect for recently acquired infection. In the absence of a placenta leak and a positive (1 to 2 or more) IGM-IFA test in the newborn is firm evidence for congenital toxoplasmosis. A negative test does not rule out congenital toxoplasmosis, as most neonates with congenital disease do not have detectible IGM yet, and they must be followed by subsequent serologic testing.

B. Radiologic studies

1. **A skull film or CT scan of the head** may demonstrate characteristic intracranial calcifications (speckled throughout the central nervous system), including the meninges.

2. **Long-bone films** may show abnormalities, specifically, metaphyseal lucency and irregularity of the line of calcification at the epiphyseal plates without periosteal reaction.

C. Other studies. Ophthalmologic examination characteristically shows chorioretinitis. Other ocular features are often present at some stages.

VII. Management.
The efficacy of treatment of pregnant women and infants with congenital infection is unclear. Treatment of acute maternal toxoplasmosis appears to reduce the risk of fetal wastage, and decreases the likelihood of congenital infection. In most cases, maternal infection is not suspected.

A. Specific treatment. Treatment is with **pyrimethamine,** 1 mg/kg/d orally plus **sulfadiazine,** 50–100 mg/kg/d in 2 divided doses for a total of 21 days. For overt and subclinical infection, therapy should be continued for the first year as 3–4 courses of 21 days of each of these medications. These are potentially teratogenic and should only be used after the first trimester. Pyrimethamine is a folic acid antagonist and can cause marrow suppression that may be ameliorated by the concurrent administration of leucovorin. A third agent,

spiramycin, is a macrolide antibiotic related to erythromycin, and can be alternated with the pyrimethamine-sulfadiazine combination during the year of therapy. Steroids may alleviate some of the inflammatory processes (ie, chorioretinitis).

B. Prevention. Pregnant women should avoid eating raw meat or raw eggs and exposure to cat litter boxes or cat feces.

RUBELLA

I. **Definition.** Rubella is a viral infection capable of causing chronic intrauterine infection and damage to the developing fetus.

II. **Incidence.** The incidence varies from 0.1–2% of births, with the higher incidence after rubella epidemics.

III. **Pathophysiology.** Rubella virus is an RNA virus that typically has an epidemic seasonal pattern of increased frequency in the spring. Epidemics have occurred at 6- to 9-year intervals and major pandemics every 10 to 30 years. Humans are the only known hosts with an incubation period of approximately 18 days following contact. Virus is spread by respiratory secretions and is also spread from stool, urine, and cervical secretions. A live virus vaccine has been available since 1969. Five to 20% of women in childbearing age are susceptible to rubella. There is a high incidence of subclinical infections. Maternal viremia is a prerequisite for placental infection, which may or may not spread to the fetus. Most cases occur following primary disease. Maternal antibody to previous infection is protective for the fetus.

Fetal infection rate varies according to timing of maternal infection during pregnancy. If infection occurs at 1–12 weeks, there is an 81% risk of fetal infection, at 13–16 weeks, 54% risk; at 17–22 weeks, 36% risk; at 23–30 weeks, 30% risk; and there is a rise to 60% at 31–36 weeks; and 100% in the last month of pregnancy. No correlation exists between the severity of maternal rubella and teratogenicity. However, the incidence of fetal effects is greater the earlier in gestation infection occurs, especially at 1–8 weeks, when 85% of infected fetuses will be damaged. Rarely are rubella defects noted in those infected after the 16th week. The virus sets up chronic infection in the placenta and fetus. Placental or fetal infection may lead to resorption of the fetus, spontaneous abortion, stillbirth, fetal infection from multisystem disease, congenital anomalies, or inapparent infection.

The pathology involves angiopathy as well as cytolytic changes. Other viral effects include chromosome breakage, decreased cell multiplication time, and mitotic arrest in certain cell types. There is little inflammatory reaction.

IV. **Risk factors.** Women in childbearing age group who are rubella nonimmune.

V. **Clinical presentation.** Congenital rubella has a wide spectrum of presentations ranging from acute disseminated infection to deficits and defects not evident at birth.

A. **Teratogenic effects.** These include intrauterine growth retardation, congenital heart disease (PDA, pulmonary artery stenosis), sensorineural hearing loss, cataracts or glaucoma, neonatal purpura, dermatoglyphic abnormalities.

B. **Systemic involvement** can be manifested by adenitis, hepatitis, hepatosplenomegaly, jaundice, anemia, decreased platelets with or without petechiae, bony lesions, encephalitis, meningitis, myocarditis, eye lesions (iridocyclitis, retinopathy), or pneumonia.

C. **Later presenting defects.** Over one-half of all newborns with congenital rubella are normal at birth, however, the majority later develop one or more signs and symptoms of disease. These include immunologic dyscrasias, hearing deficit, psychomotor retardation, autism, brain syndromes such as subacute sclerosing panencephalitis, diabetes mellitus, and thyroid disease.

VI. **Diagnosis**

A. **Laboratory studies**

1. **Open cultures.** The virus can be cultured for up to a year despite measurable antibody titer. The best specimens for viral recovery are from nasal

pharyngeal swabs, conjunctival scrapings, urine, and cerebrospinal fluid, in decreasing order of usefulness.

   2. **Cerebrospinal fluid examination** may reveal encephalitis with an increased protein:cellular ratio in some cases.
   3. **Serologic studies** may be helpful, but the disease itself may cause immunologic aberrations and delay the infant's ability to mount IgM or IgG responses. An IgM hemagglutination inhibition antibody test is available, as well as an IgG hemagglutination inhibition titer.
   B. **Radiologic studies.** Long-bone films may show metaphyseal radiolucencies that correlate with metaphyseal osteoporosis. This is caused by virus-induced inhibition of mitosis of bone-forming cells.
VII. **Management.** There is no specific treatment for rubella. Long-term follow-up is needed secondary to late-onset symptoms. Prevention consists of vaccination of the susceptible population (especially young children). Vaccine should not be given to pregnant women. Passive immunization does not prevent fetal infection when maternal infection occurs.

CYTOMEGALOVIRUS

   I. **Definition.** Cytomegalovirus (CMV) is a DNA virus and a member of the herpesvirus group.
  II. **Incidence.** It is an important cause of intrauterine infection in infants with a 1–2% incidence of congenital CMV infection in the United States.
 III. **Pathophysiology.** CMV is a ubiquitous virus that may be transmitted in secretions, blood (white cells), and urine, and perhaps by sexual contact. More than 90% of primary CMV infections are asymptomatic. Those with symptoms usually have a mononucleosis-like illness. Seroconversion and initial infection often occur around the time of puberty, and shedding of the virus may continue for a long time. CMV can also become latent and reactivate periodically. Ten to 30% of pregnant women have cervical colonization with CMV. CMV is capable of penetrating the placental barrier as well as the blood-brain barrier. Both primary and recurrent maternal CMV can lead to transmission of virus to the fetus. Infants with symptomatic disease usually are born to women with primary CMV infection. One to 2% of all newborns in the United States are infected with CMV and of these, 10% are symptomatic, 90% have subclinical infection. **Symptomatic infants have a mortality rate of 20 to 30%.** Maternal virus infected leukocytes are the proposed vehicle of transplacental transmission to the fetus. Fetal viremia is spread by the hematogenous route. The primary target organs are CNS, eye, liver, lung, and kidney. Characteristics histopathologic feature of CMV include focal necrosis, inflammatory response, and the formation of enlarged cells with intranuclear inclusions (cytomegalic cells) and the production of multinucleated giant cells. CMV may also be transmitted to the infant at delivery (with cervical colonization), via breast milk, and via transfusion of seropositive blood to an infant whose mother is seronegative. There is no definite evidence of CMV transmission among hospital personnel.
 IV. **Risk factors.** CMV infection in neonates has been associated with lower socioeconomic status, drug abuse, and sexual promiscuity in the mother. Premature infants are more often affected than full-term infants. Transfusion with unscreened blood is an additional risk factor for neonatal disease.
  V. **Clinical presentation**
   A. **Subclinical infection** is 10 times more common than clinical illness.
   B. **Low birth weight.** Maternal CMV infection is associated with low birth weight and SGA infants even when the infant is not infected.
   C. **Classic cytomegalovirus inclusion disease** is rarely seen. It consists of intrauterine growth retardation, hepatosplenomegaly with jaundice, abnormal liver function tests, thrombocytopenia with or without purpura, severe central nervous system disease including microcephaly, intracerebral calcifications (most characteristically in the subependymal area), chorioretinitis, and progressive sensorineural hearing loss (10–20% of cases). Other symptoms include

hemolytic anemia and pneumonitis. By two years of age 5–15% of infants who are asymptomatic at birth may develop serious sequelae such as hearing loss or ocular abnormalities.

    D. Late sequelae. With subclinical infection, late sequelae such as mental retardation, learning disability, and sensorineural hearing loss have been attributed to CMV.

VI. Diagnosis

    A. Laboratory studies

        1. Culture for demonstration of the virus. The **"gold standard"** for CMV diagnosis is urine culture. Most urine specimens from infants with congenital CMV are positive within 48–72 hours. Many labs now use a shell vial tissue culture technique with detection of CMV induced antigens by monoclonal antibodies allowing for identification of virus within 18 hours. Recent studies evaluating a rapid assay for detection of CMV in saliva as a screening method for congenital infection has shown it to be at least as sensitive a method for detecting congenital infection as detection of viruria; given that saliva can be collected with less difficulty and expense, it may eventually replace the current use of urine screening.

        2. Serologic tests are available, but results may be hampered by the antigenic heterogeneity of the virus. A positive rheumatoid factor test is fairly specific but is positive in only 35–45% of cases. A complement fixation test that measures IgG will detect more than 75% of positive cases but also has a significant false-positive rate.

    B. Radiologic studies. Skull films or CT scans of the head may demonstrate characteristic intracranial calcifications.

VII. Management

    A. Antiviral agents. Ganciclovir has been shown in preliminary studies to be partially effective in the treatment of retinochoroiditis and pneumonitis in immunosuppressed patients, however, no controlled studies of treatment of congenital CMV infection are available. It is highly toxic and therefore unlikely to play an important role in congenital infection.

    B. Prevention. Affected infants may excrete the virus for months to years and are often a concern to personnel caring for them. In the nursery, they should be isolated, and those caring for them should use hand-washing, gowns, and gloves as protective measures. Seronegative pregnant women should not have contact with these infants.

HERPES SIMPLEX

    I. Definition. Herpes simplex virus (HSV) is a DNA virus related to cytomegalovirus, Epstein-Barr virus, and varicella virus, and is amongst the most prevalent of all viral infections encountered by humans.

   II. Incidence. Estimated rate of occurrence of neonatal HSV is 1 in 1000 to 1 in 5000 deliveries per year.

  III. Pathophysiology. Two serologic subtypes can be distinguished by antigenic and serologic tests: HSV-1 (orolabial) and HSV-2 (genital). Three quarters of neonatal herpes infections are due to HSV-2 with the remainder caused by HSV-1. HSV-1, however, is the cause of 7 to 50% of primary genital herpes infections. HSV infection of the neonate can be acquired at one of three times: intrauterine, intrapartum, or postnatal. Most infections are acquired in the intrapartum (80%) as ascending infections with ruptured membranes (4–6 hours is considered a critical period for this to occur) or by delivery through an infected cervix or vagina. The usual portals of entry for the virus are the skin, eyes, mouth, and respiratory tract. Once colonization occurs, the virus may spread by contiguity or via a hematogenous route. The incubation period is from 2 to 20 days. Three general patterns of neonatal HSV are: (1) disease localized to the skin, eyes, oral cavity, or central nervous system; (2) disseminated disease with or without central nervous system involvement; and (3) encephalitis with or without mucocutaneous lesions, but without visceral organ involvement. Fifty percent of infants born vaginally to mothers with a primary infection will themselves have HSV compared with only 4% of those born to mothers with recurrent infection. Maternal antibody is not necessarily protective in the fetus.

IV. **Risk factors.** The risk of genital herpes infection may vary with socioeconomic status and the number of sexual partners. Only approximately 40% of cases have signs or symptoms of genital herpes at the time of labor and delivery despite having active infection. The primary infection may be "active" for as long as 2 months.

V. **Clinical presentation.** Subclinical infections with HSV are very rare. The disease may be localized or disseminated. Humoral and cellular immune mechanisms appear important in preventing initial HSV infections or limiting its spread.

   A. **Localized infections** involving the skin, eyes, or oral cavity usually manifest at 10 to 11 days of age and account for approximately 20% of neonatal herpes. **Skin lesions** vary from discrete vesicles to large bullous lesions, and occasionally denude the skin. Assertive **mouth** lesions with or without cutaneous involvement can be seen. **Ocular** findings include keratoconjunctivitis and chorioretinitis. About 25% of this group will subsequently develop neurologic abnormalities even though there is no evidence of CNS involvement in the neonatal period.

   B. **Disseminated disease** involves the **liver and adrenal glands** as well as virtually any other organ. Approximately one half of these cases also have localized disease described above. Infants with disseminated HSV infection account for at least one-half of all neonatal herpes patients. Usually they present at 9 to 11 days of age. Presentation may include the signs and symptoms of localized disease as well as anorexia, vomiting, lethargy, fever, jaundice (with abnormal liver function tests), rash or purpura, apnea, respiratory distress, bleeding, and shock. Presentation with bleeding and cardiovascular collapse may be sudden and rapidly fatal. CNS involvement is present in two-thirds of these patients. Without antiviral therapy, 80% or more will die and most will have serious neurologic sequelae. Mortality rate is decreased to 15 to 20% with appropriate treatment, however, 40 to 55% of survivors will suffer long-term neurologic impairment.

   C. **Encephalitis.** CNS involvement with or without skin, eye, or mouth lesions. Clinical manifestations of encephalitis include seizures (focal and generalized), lethargy, irritability, tremors, poor feeding, temperature instability, bulging fontanelle, and pyramidal tract signs. These infants usually present at 15–17 days of age (one-third will have no herpetic skin lesions) and the mortality rate is about 17%; however, it may be as high as 50% in untreated patients. Of survivors, 40% have long-term neurologic sequelae, such as psychomotor retardation.

VI. **Diagnosis**

   A. **Laboratory studies**

      1. **Viral cultures.** The virus grows readily with preliminary results available in 24 to 72 hours. Cultures are usually obtained from conjunctiva, throat, feces, urine, nasal pharynx, and CSF. Surface cultures obtained before 24–48 hours of life may indicate exposure without infection. Recovery of virus from spinal fluid and characteristic lesions indicates infection regardless of the age of the infants.

      2. **Tzanck smear.** Cytologic examination of the base of skin vesicles with a Giemsa or Wright stain looking for characteristic but nonspecific giant cells and eosinophilic intranuclear inclusions.

      3. **Florescent antibody** test is becoming more available, however; it has a low sensitivity and perhaps increased false-positive results.

      4. **Serologic tests** are virtually useless in the diagnosis of neonatal infection, until a test for HSV IgM is available.

      5. **Lumbar puncture** should be performed in all suspected cases. Evidence of hemorrhagic central nervous system infection with increased white cells, red cells, and protein is found.

   B. **Radiologic studies. CT scan of the head** may be useful in the diagnosis of central nervous system disease, but MRI and an electroencephalogram (multiple independent foci of periodic slow and sharp wave discharge) are probably better for detecting earlier disease. In the neonate, central nervous system pathology is more diffuse than in older patients.

C. Other tests

1. **Brain biopsy** may be needed in certain cases to confirm the diagnosis; however, most people currently recommend a trial of treatment before considering brain biopsy.

2. **Parental examination.** The most valuable aid may be examination of the parents for lesions and questioning for a history of herpetic disease.

VII. Management

A. Antepartum. The American College of Obstetrics and Gynecology (ACOG) has revoked previous guidelines of weekly antenatal surveillance cultures of lower genital tract, beginning at 36 weeks gestation, as this has little correlation with virus spreading at time of delivery. Most infants with neonatal herpes are delivered to women with no history of infection and no lesions at time of delivery. Their current guidelines for management of genital herpes infection in pregnancy include most importantly that a history of genital herpes in pregnant women or in her partner(s) should be solicited and recorded in the prenatal record. If a positive history is obtained:

1. Cultures should be done when there is an active lesion during pregnancy to confirm the diagnosis. If there are no visible lesions at the onset of labor, vaginal delivery is acceptable.

2. Weekly surveillance cultures are not necessary if there are no visible lesions.

3. To identify potentially exposed neonates, cultures may be obtained from mother or neonate. Neonatal cultures should be done at greater than 24 to 48 hours, as earlier cultures may be surface contaminants. In women with herpetic lesions of the genital tract, when either labor or membrane rupture occurs, cesarean section should be done, preferably within 4 to 6 hours of membrane rupture. However, cesarean section may be of benefit in preventing neonatal herpes regardless of duration that membranes have been ruptured.

4. For patients with active HSV infection and premature rupture of membranes remote from term, the risk of extreme immaturity must be weighed against the risk of neonatal HSV infection.

B. Neonatal treatment

1. **Isolation.** The Committee on Infectious Diseases of the American Academy of Pediatrics currently recommends that infants with known infection or exposure to HSV be placed in contact isolation. (Herpesvirus is coated with a lipid layer and is easily killed with detergent soaps and water.) For possibly exposed infants or those at low risk of infection, isolation goals may be met by allowing infants to room-in with mothers if careful hand washing is observed. Many experts now advise early discharge of the low-risk exposed infant with frequent outpatient follow-up examinations.

2. **Pharmacologic therapy.** The first-line drug of choice is acyclovir with the second choice being Vidarabine (requires 12-hour infusion with a large volume of fluid). See Chapter 73 for doses.

3. **Feedings.** The infant may breast feed as long as no breast lesions are present on the mother, and the mother should be instructed in good hand washing technique.

VIRAL HEPATITIS

Hepatitis may be produced by many infectious and noninfectious agents. Typically, viral hepatitis refers to several clinically similar diseases that differ in etiology and epidemiology. These include hepatitis A, B, C, D (delta), and E. To date, perinatal transmission of hepatitis A, C, D, and E have not been well documented. It is unlikely that hepatitis A or E will prove to be a problem as they are not characterized by chronic carrier state. The risk of perinatal transmission of hepatitis C is unknown at present.

The differential diagnosis of a newborn liver disease includes: neonatal hepatitis (giant cell), biliary atresia, other infectious agents that cause hepatocellular injury (eg, CMV, rubella, varicella, toxoplasmosis, *Listeria,* syphilis, tuberculosis, as well as bacterial sepsis, which can cause nonspecific hepatic dysfunction). Table 61–1 outlines various hepatitis panel tests useful in the management of this disease.

HEPATITIS A

I. **Definition.** Hepatitis A **(infectious hepatitis)** is caused by RNA virus transmitted by the fecal-oral route. A high concentration of virus is found in stools of infected persons; it has not been found in urine or other body fluids. It causes the short-incubation form of viral hepatitis (15–50 days). There is no chronic carrier state.

II. **Pathophysiology.** Pregnant women with hepatitis A usually do not transmit the infection to their offspring. The risk of transmission is limited because the period of viremia is short and fecal contamination does not occur at the time of delivery.

III. **Clinical presentation.** Most infants are asymptomatic, with mild abnormalities of liver function.

IV. **Diagnosis**

A. **IgM antibody to hepatitis A virus** is present during the acute or early convalescent phase of disease. IgG (anti-HAV) appears in convalescent phase, and remains detectible.

B. **Liver function tests.** Characteristically, the transaminases (AST [SGOT], ALT [SGPT]) and serum bilirubin levels (total and direct) are elevated, while the alkaline phosphatase level is normal.

V. **Management**

A. **Maternal infection in the last trimester.** If the mother had acute hepatitis A infection in the last trimester, the infant should be treated with **immune globulin** (ISG) 0.02 mL/kg intramuscularly, at birth. Hepatitis A vaccine is currently being field-tested.

B. **Isolation.** The infant should be isolated with enteric precautions.

TABLE 61–1. HEPATITIS TESTING

HAV:	Hepatitis A virus	Etiologic agent of "infectious" hepatitis
Anti-HAV:	Antibody to HAV	Detectable at onset of symptoms, lifetime persistence
IgM Anti-HAV:	IgM class antibody to HAV	Indicates recent infection with HAV, positive up to 4–6 months postinfection
HBV:	Hepatitis B virus	Etiologic agent of "serum" hepatitis
HBsAg:	Hepatitis B surface antigen	Detectable in serum; earliest indicator of acute infection or indicative of chronic infection; several subtypes identified
Anti-HBs:	Antibody to HBsAg	Indicates past infection with and immunity to HBV, passive antibody from HBIG, or immune response from HBV vaccine
HBeAG:	Hepatitis Be antigen	Correlates with HBV replication, high titer HBV in serum, infectivity of serum
Anti HBe:	Antibody to HBeAg	Presence in carrier of HBsAg suggests lower titer of HBV and resolution of infection
HBcAg:	Hepatitis B core antigen	No commercial test available
Anti-HBc:	Antibody to HBcAg	Past infection with HBV at undefined time
IgM Anti-HBc:	IgM class antibody to HBcAg	Recent infection with HBV positive for 4–6 months after infection
HVC	Hepatitis C virus	Etiologic agent of hepatitis C
Anti-HCV	Antibody to hepatitis C	Serologic determinant of hepatitis C infection

HEPATITIS B

I. Definition. Hepatitis B (**serum hepatitis**) is caused by a double-shelled DNA virus. It has a long incubation period (45 to 160 days) after exposure.

II. Pathophysiology. If the mother is a chronic carrier, there is a substantial risk to the infant. In the fetus and neonate, transmission has been suggested by the following mechanisms.

   A. Transplacental transmission either during pregnancy or at time of delivery secondary to placental leaks.

   B. Natal transmission by exposure to HBsAg in amniotic fluid, vaginal secretions, or maternal blood.

   C. Post-natal transmission by fecal-oral spread, blood transfusion, breast-feeding, or other mechanisms.

III. Risk factors

   A. Factors associated with higher rates of HBV transmission to neonates include:

      1. Presence of HBe antigen and absence of anti-HBe in maternal serum—attack rates of 80 to 95% (if anti-HBe antigen present, rate decreases 25%) with over 85% of these infants being chronic carriers.

      2. Asian racial origin, particularly Chinese, with attack rates 40–70%.

      3. Maternal acute hepatitis in third trimester or immediately postpartum (70% attack rate).

      4. Higher titer HBsAg in maternal serum (attack rates parallel the titer).

      5. Antigenemia present in older siblings.

   B. Factors not related to transmission include:

      1. The particular HBV subtype in mother.

      2. Presence or absence of HB surface antigen in amniotic fluid.

      3. Presence or titer of anti-HBc in cord blood.

IV. Clinical presentation. Maternal Hepatitis B infection has not been associated with abortion, stillbirth, congenital malformations, or IUGR. Prematurity has occurred, especially with acute hepatitis during pregnancy. Fetus or newborns exposed to HBV present a wide spectrum of disease. The infants are rarely ill and usually asymptomatic with jaundice appearing less than 3% of the time. Various clinical presentations include:

   A. Mild transient acute infection.

   B. Chronic active hepatitis with or without cirrhosis.

   C. Chronic persistent hepatitis.

   D. Chronic asymptomatic HBsAg carriage.

   E. Fulminant fatal hepatitis B (rare).

V. Diagnosis

   A. Differential diagnosis. Major diseases to consider include biliary atresia and acute hepatitis due to other viruses (hepatitis A, CMV, rubella, and HSV).

   B. Transminases. AST (SGOT) and ALT (SGPT) levels may be markedly increased before the rise in bilirubin levels.

   C. Bilirubin (direct and indirect) levels may be elevated. The rise in direct bilirubin will occur later.

   D. Liver biopsy is occasionally indicated to differentiate biliary atresia from neonatal hepatitis.

   E. Hepatitis panel testing (Table 61–1).

      1. Mother. Test for HBsAg, HBeAg, anti-HBe, and anti-HBc.

      2. Infant. Test for HBsAg and anti-HBc. Most infants demonstrate antigenemia by six months of age with peak acquisition at three to four months. Cord blood is not a reliable indicator of neonatal infection (a) because contamination could have occurred with antigen-positive maternal blood or vaginal secretions and (b) because of the possibility of noninfectious antigenemia from the mother.

VI. Management

   A. HBsAg-positive mother. If the mother is HBsAg-positive, regardless of the status of her HBe antigen or antibody, the infant should be given hepatitis B immune globulin (HBIG), 0.5 mL intramuscularly, within 12 hours after delivery. Additionally, hepatitis B vaccine (plasma-derived or recombinant), 0.5 mL intramuscularly (anterolateral thigh), is given at birth and at 1 month and 6 months of age. If the first dose is given simultaneously with HBIG it should be administered at a separate site, preferably the opposite leg. HBIG and HB vaccinations do not interfere with routine childhood immunizations.

  B. **Isolation.** Precautions are needed in handling blood and secretions.
  C. **Breast-feeding.** HBsAg has been detected in breast milk of HBsAg-positive mothers, but only with special concentrating techniques. One study in Taiwan showed no difference in infection rates between bottle- and breast-fed infants. Given the efficacy of HBV vaccine with HBIG, even theoretical risk fo transmission through breast-feeding is of less concern.
  D. **Follow-up.** At 12 to 15 months of age, the infant should be screened for HBsAg and anti-HBs antibody to confirm immunity. If HBsAg is not detectible and anti-HBs is present, the child can be considered protected. Long-term effects in infants who become carriers of the virus may include cirrhosis, hepatocellular carcinoma, or chronic hepatitis.
  E. **Immunization program.** The CDC, the AAP, and the AFP have jointly mandated a comprehensive strategy for elimination of HBV transmission which includes routine immunization of all infants born to HBsAg negative mothers, integrated with other childhood immunizations. Two-dose schedules have been proposed, each includes three separate doses. In option #1, these are at birth, 2, and 6 months, and option #2 at 2, 4, and 6 months.

HEPATITIS C

  I. **Definition.** Non-A, Non-B hepatitis represents a composite of undefined infections probably caused by at least three different viruses.
 II. **Pathophysiology.** Primary infectious risk is associated with transfusion of blood or blood products. There is indirect evidence that maternal-to-infant transmission occurs.
III. **Clinical presentation.** Infants are asymptomatic, with elevation of liver function tests. Incubation period lasts approximately 45 days (range 14–115 days). Chronic carrier state develops frequently and may develop into significant chronic liver disease.
 IV. **Diagnosis.** An anti-HCV antibody has been developed to screen for hepatitis C and has been a reliable marker. Liver function tests may be elevated and fluctuate widely over time. The interval between exposure to HCV or onset of illness and detection of anti-HCV by serum enzyme immunoassay may be prolonged. In general, anti-HCV persists in patients who have chronic disease, it may disappear in those who have acute resolving hepatitis C. Polymerase chain reaction technology has been developed (unfortunately not yet clinically available) which allows for early detection of viremia in chronic hepatitis C.
  V. **Management.** If the mother was infected during the last trimester or at delivery, the risk of transmission to the infant is highest. The infant should be treated with **immune globulin** (ISG), 0.02 mL/kg intramuscularly, at birth; however, efficacy of this treatment is unknown. The infant should be followed by means of routine serum alanine aminotransferase (ALT [SGPT]) checks. It does not appear that a vaccine against hepatitis C will be available in the near future as homologous immunity is weak or absent.

HEPATITIS D

Hepatitis D, also known as *delta hepatitis,* is a defective RNA virus that cannot survive independently and requires the helper function of DNA virus hepatitis B. Therefore, it occurs either as co-infection with hepatitis B or superinfection of a hepatitis B carrier. It has been reportedly transmitted from mother to infant. Prevention of hepatitis B infection will prevent it. There are, however, no available treatments to prevent it in hepatitis B surface-antigen carriers before or after exposure. Management should be similar to that of hepatitis B infection (see above).

VARICELLA-ZOSTER INFECTIONS

Varicella-zoster (VZ) virus is a member of the herpesvirus family. There are 3 forms of varicella-zoster infections that involve the neonate: teratogenic, congenital, and postnatal. In the mother, infection is usually manifested as typical chicken pox or occasionally, as herpes zoster, or shingles (intrauterine infection less common than with maternal varicella).

TERATOGENIC VARICELLA-ZOSTER INFECTION

I. Definition. This form occurs when the mother has her first exposure to VZ virus during pregnancy. Viremia occurs prior to onset of rash, with fetal infection likely occurring during this time.

II. Incidence. This form is fortunately rare, since over 95% of women in the USA are immune to varicella (only 30 reported cases as of 1987).

III. Pathophysiology. Transmission of the virus probably occurs via respiratory droplets. The virus replicates in the oropharynx, and viremia results, with transplacental passage to the fetus. Almost all cases reported have involved exposure between the 8th to 20th weeks of pregnancy, except for one case at 28 weeks. The defects are the result of viral replication and destruction of developing fetal ectodermal tissue.

IV. Clinical presentation. Clinical examination may disclose defects in a number of organ systems, as outlined below.

    A. Limbs. Hypoplasia or atrophy of an extremity, paralysis with muscular atrophy, and hypoplastic or missing fingers are frequent findings. This is caused by invasion of the brachial and lumbar plexus.

    B. Eyes. Microphthalmos, chorioretinitis, cataracts, optic atrophy, Horner's syndrome (ptosis, miosis, enophthalmos).

    C. Skin. Findings are cicatricial skin lesions and the residua of infected bullous skin lesions.

    D. Central nervous system. Microcephaly, seizures, encephalitis, cortical atrophy, and mental retardation may be seen.

V. Diagnosis

    A. FAMA (fluorescent antibody to membrane antigen) test. This serologic test measures antibodies to VZ virus. Persistence of antibody beyond 6–8 months of age suggests intrauterine infection. This should be correlated with a maternal FAMA test to document a decrease.

    B. Serum VZ-specific IgM antibody. This documents infection in the infant.

VI. Management

    A. Mother. If the mother is exposed to VZ infection in the first or second trimester, some recommend treatment with **varicella-zoster immune globulin (VZIG)** if the history of varicella is negative or uncertain. This helps reduce complications in the mother but not the fetus. (See dosage in Chap 73.)

    B. Infant. Supportive care of the infant is required, since there is usually profound neurologic impairment. The infant often dies because of secondary infections. Survivors usually suffer profound mental retardation and major neurologic handicaps.

    C. Isolation. Isolation is not necessary.

CONGENITAL VARICELLA-ZOSTER INFECTION

I. Definition. This is the form of the disease that occurs when a pregnant women suffers chicken pox during the last 14 to 21 days of pregnancy, or within the first few days postpartum. Disease begins in the neonate within the first 10 days of life.

II. **Incidence.** Although the congenital form is more common than the teratogenic form, it is still rare, as only 0.7 per thousand pregnant women develop chicken pox.

III. **Pathophysiology.** One of 4 newborns will become infected when maternal varicella occurs during the last 3 weeks of pregnancy. If the infant is born within 5 days of the onset of rash in the mother, the disease will be more severe, since there is insufficient time for maternal antibody formation; the resulting death rate is 30% in affected infants. If the onset of maternal disease is more than 5 days before delivery or onset of neonatal disease is within the first four days, transplacental antibody transmission occurs, and fetal deaths are infrequent.

IV. **Clinical presentation.** There may only be mild involvement of the infant, with vesicles on the skin, or the following may be seen:

A. **Skin.** A centripetal rash (beginning on the trunk and spreading to the face and scalp, sparing the extremities) begins as red macules and progresses to vesicles and encrustation. Lesions are more common in the diaper area and skin folds. There may be 2 or 3 lesions or thousands of them. The main complication is staphylococcal and streptococcal secondary skin infections. Septicemia was seen in fewer than 0.5% of patients in one study.

B. **Lungs.** Lung involvement is seen in all fatal cases. It usually appears 2–4 days after the onset of the rash but may be seen up to 10 days after. Signs include fever, cyanosis, rales, and hemoptysis. Chest x-ray shows a diffuse nodular-miliary pattern, especially in the perihilar region.

C. **Other organs.** Focal necrosis may be seen in the liver, adrenals, intestines, kidneys, and thymus. Glomerulonephritis, myocarditis, encephalitis, and cerebellar ataxia are sometimes seen.

V. **Diagnosis**

A. **Tzanck smear.** This will demonstrate multinucleated giant cells with intracellular inclusions consistent with herpes virus infection. Diagnosis of VZ is usually based on clinical findings only and lab confirmation is seldom needed.

B. **Cultures.** VZ virus can be isolated from cultures of vesicular lesions during the first 3 days of the rash.

C. **Serum testing of VZ antibody.** Testing during the acute and convaslescent periods will document resolution.

VI. **Management**

A. **Varicella-zoster immune globulin**

1. **Perinatal infection.** Infants of mothers who develop VZ infection within 5 days before or 48 hours after delivery should receive 125 units VZIG as soon as possible and not later than 96 hours (see Chap 73). These infants should be placed in strict respiratory isolation for 28 days after receiving VZIG, since treatment will prolong the incubation period. VZIG does not reduce the clinical attack rate in treated newborns, however, they tend to develop milder infections than the untreated neonates.

2. **Maternal rash occurring more than 5 days before delivery.** Infants of mothers who develop a rash more than 5 days before delivery do not need VZIG. It is felt that infants will have received antibodies via the placenta.

B. **Vidarabine and acyclovir** may be used in severely affected infants to decrease the chance of dissemination and shorten the duration of skin lesions. Dosage information is in Chapter 73.

C. **Use antibiotics** if secondary bacterial skin infections occur.

D. **Serum test for varicella-zoster antibodies.** Performance of this test during the acute and convalescent periods deocuments resolution of the infection.

POSTNATAL VARICELLA-ZOSTER INFECTION

I. **Definition.** This form of the disease presents on days 10–28 of life. It does not represent transplacental infection from the mother.

II. **Pathophysiology.** Postnatal VZ infection occurs by droplet transmission. It is more common than congenital chicken pox. This disease is usually mild because of passive protection from maternal antibodies.

III. Clinical presentation. The typical chicken pox rash is seen with centripetal spread, beginning on the trunk and spreading to the face and scalp, and sparing the extremities. All stages of the rash may appear at the same time, from red macules to clear vesicles to crusting lesions. Complications of this form of the disease are rare but may include secondary infections and varicella pneumonia.

IV. Diagnosis. Same as for congenital varicella-zoster (p 356).

V. Management. This form of the disease is usually mild, and death is extremely rare.

   A. VZIG is recommended for infants less than 28 weeks gestational age or weighing 1000 g or less, regardless of the maternal history. It is also recommended in premature infants whose mothers do not have a history of chicken pox.

   B. Infants of greater than 28 weeks gestation should have sufficient transplacental antibodies if the mother is immune to protect them from the risk of complications.

   C. Isolation. Exposed infants should be placed in strict isolation for 10–21 days after the onset of the rash in the index case. Exposed infants who receive VZIG should be in strict respiratory isolation for 28 days.

SYPHILIS

I. Definition. Syphilis is a sexually transmitted disease caused by *Treponema pallidum*. **Early congenital syphilis** is when clinical manifestations occur before two years of age, **late congenital syphilis** is when manifestations occur at greater than two years of age. In 1990 a new surveillance case definition for congenital syphilis was adopted by the CDC to improve reporting of congenital syphilis by public health agencies. It calls for reporting all infants (and stillbirths) born to women with untreated or inadequately treated syphilis at delivery, regardless of neonatal symptoms or findings.

II. Incidence. Primary and secondary syphilis in the general population has increased significantly in the past few years, with a current rate of approximately 15 cases per 100,000 persons (highest since 1950). Along with this, there has been a fourfold rise in the number of cases of congenital syphilis reported. An estimated 2–5 infants are affected with congenital syphilis for every 100 women diagnosed with primary or secondary syphilis.

III. Pathophysiology. Treponemas appear able to cross the placenta at any time during pregnancy, thereby infecting the fetus. Syphilis can cause preterm delivery, stillbirth, congenital infection, or neonatal death, depending on the stage of maternal infection and duration of fetal infection prior to delivery. Untreated infection in the first and second trimester often leads to significant fetal morbidity, while with third trimester infection, many infants are asymptomatic. Infection can also be acquired by the neonate via contact of infectious lesions during passage through the birth canal. Virtually all infants born to untreated women with primary and secondary syphilis will have congenital infection, with 50% clinically symptomatic. Infection rate is only 40% with early latent disease and 6 to 14% with late latent stages. Mortality may be as high as 54% in infected infants.

IV. Clinical presentation. Generally neonates do not have signs of primary syphilis from in-utero-acquired infection. Their manifestations are systemic and similar to adults with secondary syphilis. There is an additional 40 to 60% chance for CNS involvement. Most common findings in neonatal period include hepatosplenomegaly, jaundice, and osteochondritis. Other signs include generalized lymphadenopathy, pneumonitis, myocarditis, nephrosis, pseudoparalysis (atypical erbs palsy), rash (vesicobullous, especially palms and soles), hemolytic anemia (normocytic, normochromic), leukemoid reaction, hemorrhagic rhinitis (snuffles). Late congenital syphilis manifests by Hutchinson's teeth, healed retinitis, eighth nerve deafness, saddle nose, mental retardation, arrested hydrocephalus, saber shins. Other clues to diagnosis of congenital syphilis include placentomegaly or congenital hydrops.

V. Diagnosis

A. Laboratory studies. Patients with congenital or acquired syphilis produce several different antibodies which are grouped as nonspecific, nontreponomal antibody (NTA) tests and specific antitreponomal antibody (STA) tests. NTA tests are inexpensive, rapid, and convenient screening tests that may indicate disease activity. They test patient's serum or CSF for its ability to flocculate a suspension of a cardiolipin-cholesterol lecithin antigen. They are used as initial screening tests and quantitatively to follow patient's response to treatment. False-positive reactions can be secondary to autoimmune disease, IV drug addiction, aging, pregnancy, and many infections such as hepatitis, mononucleosis, measles, and endocarditis.

1. Nonspecific reagin antibody tests. The two most used of these nonspecific reagin antibody tests include:

a. Venereal Disease Research Laboratory (VDRL) slide test. A VDRL titer at least two dilutions (fourfold) higher in the infant than in the mother signifies probable active infection. Titers should be followed and repeated. If titers decrease in the first 8 months of life, the infant is probably not infected.

b. Rapid plasma reagin (RPR) test. This is a nontreponemal test that detects antibodies cardiolipid and is a screening test for syphilis. It should not be used on spinal fluid. Normal test is negative and any positive test should be followed up with an FTA-ABS test. Titers can also be reported as for VDRL.

2. Specific treponomal tests. Specific STA tests verify diagnosis of current or past infection. These tests should be performed if nontreponomal tests are positive.

a. Fluorescent treponomal antibody absorption test (FTA-ABS test). This test may be positive in the infant secondary to maternal transfer of IgG. If positivity persists after 6–12 months, the infant is probably infected.

b. Microhemagglutination test for *T pallidum*. (MHTPA). This test uses less serum and is easier than FTA to perform; however, it may be less sensitive in early disease. It should be quantitative, as it can include IgG antibodies that crossed the placenta.

c. IgM FTA-ABS. This test measures antibody to the treponeme developed by the infant. It is not as specific as initially thought because false-positive results may occur. The test must be done at the Centers for Disease Control.

d. Newer serologic assays. Direct antigen tests for *T pallidum,* including an ELISA that uses monoclonal antibody to the organism's surface proteins, as well as a polymerase chain reaction that can detect the organism in CSF, amniotic fluid, and other specimens, are both being tested and could become commercially available obviating diagnosis of syphilis based on indirect evidence of antibody response.

3. Microscopic darkfield examination should be performed on appropriate lesions for spirochetes.

4. CBC and differential. Monocytosis is typically seen; look for hemolytic anemia or leukemoid reaction.

5. Lumbar puncture. Central nervous system disease may be detected by positive serologic tests, darkfield examination positive for spirochetes, elevated monocyte count, or elevated spinal fluid protein levels. FTA on CSF is not reliable.

B. Radiologic studies. X-ray studies of the long bones may show sclerotic changes of the metaphysis and diaphysis, with widespread osteitis and periostitis.

VI. Management

A. Treated mother. Infant born to mothers who received adequate penicillin treatment for syphilis during pregnancy are at minimal risk. The infant should be

treated if maternal treatment was inadequate, unknown, or given during the last 4 weeks of pregnancy or if a drug other than penicillin was used. In a pregnant women who has been treated for syphilis, quantitative NTA tests should be done monthly for the rest of her pregnancy.
  B. **VDRL-positive infant.** Infants with positive VDRL tests, even if this is only an indication of maternal transfer of IgG, should be treated if adequate follow-up cannot be obtained.
  C. **Definitive treatment.** See Chapter 73 for drug dosages. Due to reported treatment failures with benzathine penicillin G, current treatment guidelines recommend treating all infants born to women with untreated syphilis with aqueous crystalline penicillin G, 100,000–150,000 units/kg/24 hours IV or alternately 50,000 units/kg/day of procaine penicillin intramuscularly; duration of therapy should be 10–14 days in both instances.
  D. **Isolation procedures.** Precautions regarding drainage, secretions, and blood and body fluids are indicated for all infants with suspected or proven congenital syphilis until therapy has been given for 24 hours.
  E. **Follow-up care.** The infant should have repeated quantitative nontreponomal tests at 3, 6, and 12 months. Most infants will develop a negative titer with adequate treatment. A rising titer requires further investigation and retreatment.

GONORRHEA

  I. **Definition.** Infection with *Neisseria gonorrhoeae* (a gram-negative diplococcus) is a commonly reported communicable disease. Infection in pregnancy is important because of transmission to the fetus.
 II. **Incidence.** Prevalence of gonococcus infection among pregnant women varies from 0.6% or less to 7.6% or greater depending on the population. Approximately 30 to 35% of neonates acquire infection during vaginal delivery from infected mothers.
III. **Pathophysiology.** *N gonorrhoeae* primarily affects the endocervical canal. The infant may become infected during passage through an infected cervical canal or by contact with contaminated amniotic fluid if rupture of the membranes has occurred.
 IV. **Clinical presentations**
  A. **Ophthalmia neonatorum.** The most common clinical manifestation is gonococcal ophthalmia neonatorum. This occurs in fewer than 2% of cases of positive maternal gonococcal infection if appropriate eye prophylaxis is given. For a description of this disease, see Chapter 31.
  B. **Gonococcal arthritis.** The onset of gonococcal arthritis can be at any time from 1 to 4 weeks after delivery. It is secondary to gonococcemia. The source of bacteremia has been attributed to infection of the mouth, nares, and umbilicus. The most common sites are the knees and ankles, but any joint may be affected. The infant may present with mild or moderate symptoms. Drainage and antibiotics are necessary.
  C. **Amniotic infection syndrome.** This occurs when there is premature rupture of the membranes, with inflammation of the placenta and umbilical cord. The infant may develop clinical evidence of sepsis. Fluid obtained by gastric aspiration is usually positive for gonococci. This infection is associated with a high infant mortality rate.
  D. **Meningitis.**
  E. **Scalp abscess.** This is usually secondary to intrauterine fetal monitoring.
  F. **Stomatitis.**
  V. **Diagnosis**
  A. **Mother.** Endocervical scrapings should be obtained for culture.
  B. **Infant**

1. **Gram's stain** of any exudate, if present, should be obtained.
2. **Culture.** Material may be obtained by swabbing the eye or nasopharynx or the orogastric or anorectal areas. Blood should be obtained for culture.
3. **Spinal fluid studies.** Cell count, protein, culture, gram's stain, and others, should be ordered.

VI. Management
A. Antibiotic therapy
1. **Maternal infection.** Most infants born to mothers with gonococcal infection do not develop infection. However, since there have been some reported cases, it is recommended that full-term infants receive a single injection of penicillin G, 50,000 units intramuscularly, and that premature infants receive 20,000 units intramuscularly.
2. **Ophthalmia.** Give penicillin G, 50,000 units/kg intravenously every 12 hours for 7 to 10 days, plus saline irrigations. For penicillin-resistent strains give ceftriaxone 50 mg/kg/d once daily until cured.
3. **Arthritis and septicemia.** Give penicillin G, 75,000–100,000 units/kg/d intravenously in 4 doses for 7 days. (Alternatively, give ceftriaxone 50 mg IV or IM once a day for 7 to 10 days.)
4. **Meningitis.** Give penicillin G, 100,000–150,000 units/kg/d in four divided doses for at least 10 days.

B. Isolation. All infants with gonococcal infection should be placed in contact isolation until effective parenteral antimicrobial therapy has been given for 24 hours.

CHLAMYDIAL INFECTION

I. **Definition.** *Chlamydia trachomatis* is a highly specialized gram-negative bacterium which possesses a cell wall, contains DNA and RNA, and can be inactivated by several antimicrobial agents. However, due to its inability to generate adenosine triphosphate, it is an obligate intracellular parasite. It may cause urethritis, cervicitis, urethral symptoms, and salpingitis in the mother. In the infant, it may cause conjunctivitis and pneumonia.

II. **Incidence.** It is currently the most common sexually transmitted disease. The risk of infection to infants born to infected mothers is between 50 to 75%; conjunctivitis occurs in 20 to 50% and pneumonia in about 30%. Cervical chlamydial infection varies widely dependent on the population, with significant increase in young, low socioeconomic, and nonwhite populations (2–37%).

III. **Pathophysiology.** *C trachomatis* subtypes B–K cause the sexually transmitted form of the disease and the associated neonatal infection. They frequently cause a benign subclinical infection. The infant acquires infection during vaginal delivery through infected cervix. Infection after cesarean section is very rare, and usually only occurs with early rupture of amniotic membranes.

IV. **Clinical presentation.**
A. Conjunctivitis. See Chapter 31.
B. Pneumonia. This is one of the most common forms of pneumonia in the first three months of life. The respiratory tract may be directly infected during delivery. Approximately half of infants presenting with pneumonia will have concurrent or previous conjunctivitis. Pneumonia usually presents at 3–11 weeks of life. The infants experience gradual increase in symptoms over several weeks. Initially there is often one to two weeks of mucoid rhinorrhea followed by cough and increasing respiratory rate. Greater than 95% are afebrile. The cough is characteristic, paroxysmal and staccato, and it interferes with sleeping and eating. These infants may also have pulmonary congestion, and apnea may be present; however, this tends to be associated with secondary infection occurring together with chlamydia. Approximately one-third will have otitis media.

V. **Diagnosis**

A. Laboratory studies
1. **Rapid screening tests.** There are 2 rapid screening tests for **Chlamydia** that utilize direct smears of the conjunctiva or nasopharynx.
   a. **Fluorescent monoclonal antibody test (Microtrak).** This test takes only 30 minutes. Immunofluorescence requires considerable expertise in reading.
   b. **Enzyme immunoassay technique (Chlamydiazyme).** This test takes approximately 3 hours. Rate of false-negative and false-positive results may be a problem. Method is at present not recommended for conjunctival specimens.
2. **Culture of respiratory tract.** Material should be obtained for culture via nasopharyngeal aspiration or deep suctioning of the trachea and placed in special transport medium.
3. **IgM antibody to *C trachomatis* (pneumonia).** Either a significant rise in or high levels of the titer (1:64) indicate infection.
4. **Gram's stain** of eye discharge (see Chap 31).
5. **Other tests.** In cases of pneumonia, the white blood count is normal, but there is eosinophilia in 70% of cases. Blood gas measurements show mild to moderate hypoxia.
B. Radiologic studies. In cases of pneumonia, the chest x-ray may reveal hyperexpansion of the lungs, with bilateral symmetric interstitial or alveolar infiltrates.
VI. **Management**
   A. Prevention. In high-risk mothers, material should be obtained for culture and treatment should be given before delivery. Use of erythromycin eye drops instead of silver nitrate drops after birth will prevent conjunctivitis in the infant.
   B. Conjunctivitis. See Chapter 31.
   C. Pneumonia. Give erythromycin, 50 mg/kg/d in 3 divided doses for 14 days. This will not only shorten the clinical course but will decrease the duration of nasopharyngeal shedding. No isolation measures are necessary. See Chapter 73 for more details on dosing and pharmacologic information.

HUMAN IMMUNODEFICIENCY VIRUS (HIV)

I. **Definition.** AIDS was originally recognized as a clinical entity in 1981, and later found to be the end-stage of infection with human immunodeficiency virus (HIV), formerly known as HTLVIII, lymphadenopathy AIDS virus (LAV), and AIDS-associated retrovirus (ARV). It is a member of the lentivirus, or slow virus, subgroup of retroviruses. It is now appropriate to base a diagnosis solely on the presence of HIV infection. This allows the physician to determine when and what treatments should be used on an individual basis.

II. **Incidence.** With improved control of blood supply, the perinatal route will constitute nearly the sole route of acquisition of pediatric AIDS in the future. The World Health Organization has estimated that 10,000,000 adults and 1,000,000 children are infected with HIV worldwide. Between 1991–92 the number of children with HIV age 0–4 years old in the United States increased 16.6%, the largest increase in any age group. 95.8% of US children with HIV were 0–4 years old in 1992 and infected perinatally. Perinatal transmission accounts for the second largest proportionate increase in HIV second only to heterosexual contact resulting in HIV transmission. With many cases due to treatment of hemophilia or other blood disorders, improved screening of blood products will result in perinatal transmission being the sole cause of pediatric HIV infection in the future for this group.

III. **Pathophysiology.** HIV infects T_4 (helper) lymphocytes, the virus attaches to this cell via an interaction between the external viral glycoprotein and the region of the CD4 molecule present on the surface of T helper lymphocytes and some other cells. The virus selectively inhibits the growth of T_4 lymphocytes and eventually destroys these inducer and helper T cells, although it probably remains latent in a few cells. In children, the loss of T_4 lymphocytes leads initially to lack of direction to B cells which produce large amounts of nonspecific and ineffective immunoglobulins. As well, profound defects and cell-mediated immunity occur allowing a predisposition to opportunistic infections such as fungus, Pneumocystis carinii, and chronic diarrhea. The virus can also invade the CNS and produce psychosis and brain atrophy.

IV. **Risk factors**
   A. **High-risk mother.** Any infant born to a high-risk mother is at risk. High-risk mothers include intravenous drug users, hemophiliacs, spouses of bisexual males, women from areas where the disease is more prevalent in heterosexuals, and spouses of hemophiliacs. Both intrauterine and intrapartum transmission of the virus appear to be possible. Breast milk is probably also a transmission route. The risk of transmission appears to be greater if the mother's disease is advanced, her CD4 count is reduced or CD4/CD8 ratio is low, and/or P24 antigen is present. Transplacental infection is possible with the virus having been identified in 13 to 20 week abortus, as well as in the thymus of a 20-day-old infant who had been born at 28 weeks' gestation.
   B. **Blood transfusion.** Screening of blood donors has reduced but has not totally eliminated the risk, because some newly infected persons are viremic but seronegative for 2–4 months and because some infected persons (5–15%) are seronegative. The current risk for transmission of HIV per unit transfused is 1/225,000.
   C. **Breast milk.** The virus has been isolated in breast milk. In one case, the mother received a blood transfusion after delivery from a person who later developed AIDS. The mother breast-fed her infant, and both were seropositive for AIDS. Although the transmission via breast milk is felt to be rare, it is recommended that in developed countries with safe alternative nutrition that the infected mom should not breast-feed; however, in developing countries, where bottle-feeding is associated with significant mortality and morbidity, the risk of transmission of HIV via breast milk is much less than the risk of bottle-feeding itself.

V. **Clinical presentation.** The clinical presentation depends on the severity of disease.
   A. **Age.** Approximately one-third of children with vertically acquired HIV infection develop severe disease in the first year of life. The remainder have a more slowly progressive course, although nearly all show some manifestations of infections (clinical or immunological) by 12 months of age. The interval from HIV infection to the onset of symptoms or of AIDS is shorter in children infected congenitally than those infected by transfusion, and is shorter in children than in adults.
   B. **Symptoms and signs.** The patient may be asymptomatic or may have low birth weight, weight loss, failure to thrive, recurrent infections or episodes of otitis media, diarrhea, persistent candidiasis, hepatosplenomegaly, lymphadenopathy, neutropenia, thrombocytopenia, interstitial pneumonitis, chronic eczematoid dermatitis, or fever. The disease course is variable and long asymptomatic periods are sometimes present. In general the course is ultimately characterized by progressive immune dysfunction and clinical deterioration.
   C. **Characteristic craniofacial appearance.** Contrary to previous reports, there is no longer felt to be any characteristic craniofacial appearance present in infants infected with HIV.

VI. **Diagnosis.** Diagnosis is based on (1) suspicion of infection based on epidemiologic risk or clinical presentation, and (2) confirmation by serologic tests.
   A. **All other causes of immunodeficiency must be excluded.** These include both primary and secondary immunodeficiency states. Primary immunodeficiency diseases include DiGeorge's syndrome, Wiskott-Aldrich syndrome, ataxia-telangiectasia, agammaglobulinemia, severe combined immunodefi-

ciency, and neutrophil function abnormality. Secondary immunodeficiency states include those caused by immunosuppressive therapy, starvation, and lymphoreticular cancer.

B. Laboratory studies
    1. Positive test for HIV antibody. Diagnosis of HIV infection in children greater than 18 months of age is similar to adults, based on detection of anti-HIVgG antibodies in serum using enzyme-linked immunosorbent assay and Western blot. However, the use of IgG-based antibody tests has been problematic in the less-than-18-month age range due to the persistence of maternal transplacentally acquired antibodies in the child's serum. Recently available virologic tests permitting early diagnosis of HIV in infants in the first months of life include HIV culture, polymerase chain reaction (PCR), and P24 antigen detection. HIV culture and PCR are highly specific for HIV infection but sensitivity varies with age of infant. With these techniques, approximately 50% of infected infants can be identified at or near birth and greater than 95% can be diagnosed by 3–6 months of age. With respect to PCR test, if acid hydrolysis is used to disrupt antigen antibody complexes in serum, sensitivity of PCR antigen detection can be increased and is making this a promising tool for early diagnosis. All children with presumptively diagnosed HIV infection should have their infection status confirmed by repeating the original test or performing another virologic test. Children with two positive tests are considered HIV infected. Seropositive children who do not have a definitive virologic diagnosis should continue to be tested every 3 months by enzyme-linked immunosorbent assay and Western blot. A seropositive child of an HIV infected mother who is repeatedly HIV antibody negative by 18 months of age, and has never had a positive HIV culture/PCR/P24 antigen, is considered a seroconverter.

    2. Surrogate markers for disease. Immunological abnormalities including hyperimmunoglobulinemia, abnormal T lymphocytes subsets with low CD4 numbers, and an inverted CD4-CD8 ratio.

C. Presence of a "marker" disease that indicates cellular immunodeficiency. Marker diseases include candidiasis, cryptococcisis, Mycobacterium avium infection, Epstein-Barr virus infection, Pneumocystis carinii pneumonia, strongyloidiasis, and Kaposi's sarcoma. Cytomegalovirus infection and toxoplasmosis are included if toxoplasmosis occurs more than 1 month after birth and cytomegalovirus infection more than 6 months after birth.

VII. Management
  A. Prevention. Prevention is of paramount importance. An infected woman should avoid pregnancy. Testing of blood donors will help decrease the risk associated with transfusion. Transfusions should be avoided unless clinically indicated. Plasma protein fraction (Plasmanate) should be used instead of fresh-frozen plasma unless there is a documented clotting deficiency.

  B. General supportive care
    1. Intravenous immunoglobulin. HIV-infected infants are appropriate candidates for routine IVIG prophylaxis (400 mg/kg/dose q28 days.)

    2. Vaccines. Routine immunization schedules should be followed for DTP, MMR, HBV, Hib. Routine polio schedule is administered as IM inactivated polio vaccine (Salk). Pneumococcal vaccine is given at 2 years of age, and influenza vaccine is given annually.

    3. Nutrition. Close nutritional monitoring should be part of routine care for these children.

    4. Prophylaxis. It has become clear that very aggressive prophylaxis of these children will significantly improve their morbidity and mortality. Pneumocystis carini pneumonia prophylaxis should be instituted if CD4 values fall below age thresholds as recommended by Public Health Service guidelines. Drug of choice for this is trimethoprim-sulfamethoxazole (TMP/SMX). Alternates include Dapsone. Prophylaxis as needed for exposure to tuberculosis and varicella zoster virus (see Chap 73).

   5. **Other aspects of supportive care.** Neurodevelopmental supportive services include preschool early intervention programs and school-based developmental disability programs. Aggressive management and protocols for pharmacologic and nonpharmacologic pain management.
C. **Delivery.** The following procedures are recommended as standard "Universal Precautions" for delivery of a mother with proven infection or one who is a member of a high-risk group.
   1. Wear gown and gloves.
   2. If meconium aspiration occurs, perform intubation and suction with suction equipment or a DeLee apparatus.
   3. Items soiled by blood or amniotic fluid should be handled appropriately.
D. **Postdelivery management**
   1. Thoroughly clean off amniotic fluid and blood.
   2. Isolate the infant with the same precautions as for hepatitis B (blood and secretions precautions).
   3. Send serum for HIV antibody testing (state laws vary on requirements of consent for obtaining test as well as on confidentiality required).
   4. Make sure the infant has the best possible follow-up care.
   5. Perform and repeat HIV testing at 3 months and 6 months.
E. **Antiretroviral treatment.** The only antiretroviral drug currently available for treatment of children with HIV is zidovudine (formerly known as azidothymidine [AZT]), although dideoxyinosine (DDI) and dideoxycytosine (DDC) are being evaluated in Phase 1 studies in the United States. AZT inhibits viral reverse transcriptase activity or chain termination in viral DNA, and has been shown to prolong life in symptomatic adults. Phase 1 and Phase 2 studies in symptomatic children have suggested an increase in weight and well-being and improvement in HIV encephalopathy. Symptomatic children or children with low CD4 lymphocyte counts appear to be at highest risk for disease progression, and therefore early treatment of these children is of the utmost importance. This includes children less than 3 months of age. Ongoing multicenter trials continue in an attempt to establish appropriate regimens for these drugs. As well, efforts need to continue to make available for children agents that have already been shown to be effective in adults.

LYME DISEASE

Lyme disease is caused by the spirochete *Borrelia burgdorfi* and is transmitted by the bite of a deer tick. Over 90% of cases have been reported in the northeast coastal states. Diagnosis in the adult is made on clinical findings (flu-like symptoms, erythema chronicum migrans skin lesions, joint pain and swelling), as many diagnostic tests are often negative during the disease.

   Transplacental transmission has been reported, however the Centers for Disease Control has concluded that none of the adverse outcomes in these newborns could be definitively linked to Lyme disease. In the few cases of maternal-fetal transmission reported, problems in the infants have included stillbirths, heart diseases, and respiratory distress syndrome. Although prevention of maternal exposure is the best cure, many obstetricians will prescribe prophylactic antibiotics (amoxicillin, penicillin, erythromycin) (see Chap 73) for tick bites during pregnancy. If there is concern an infant has been born with Lyme disease, the CDC recommends treatment with the same regimen as for congenital syphilis (p 358).

REFERENCES

Balcarek KB: Neonatal screening for congenital cytomegalovirus infection by detection of virus in saliva. *J Inf Dis* 1993;**167**:1433.
Balfour HH et al: Antiviral drugs in pediatrics. *Am J Dis Child* 1989;**143**:1307.

Balisteri W: Viral hepatitis. *Pediatr Clin North Am* 1988;**35**:375.

Best JM: Rubella in: Greenough A, Osborne J, Sutherland S (eds) *Congenital, Perinatal and Neonatal Infections.* London, Churchill Livingstone 1992:171.

Boyer D, Gordon RC, Baker T: Lack of clinical usefulness of a positive latex agglutination test for Neissera meningitidis/Escherichia coli antigens in the urine. *J Pediatr Inf Dis* 1993;**12(9)**:779.

Chirico G et al: Intravenous gammaglobulin therapy for prophylaxis of infection in high-risk neonates. *J Peds* 1987;**110**:437.

Christensen RD et al: Granulocyte transfusions in neonates with bacterial infection, neutropenia, and depletion of mature marrow neutrophils. *Pediatr* 1987;**70**:1.

Donowitz LG: Practical infection control for human immunodeficiency virus infection in children. *J Pediatr Inf Dis* 1989;**8**:133.'

Edwards MS et al: Fibronectin levels in premature infants with late-onset sepsis. *J Perinatol* 1993;**13(1)**:8.

Falloon J et al: Human immunodeficiency virus infection in children. *J Peds* 1989;**114**:1.

Feigin RD et al: Diagnosis and management of meningitis. *J Pediatr Inf Dis* 1992;**11(9)**:785.

Feinkind L et al: HIV in Pregnancy. *Clin Perinatol* 1988;**15**:189.

Freij BJ: Herpesvirus infections in pregnancy: risks to embryo, fetus, and neonate. *Clin Perinatol* 1988;**15**:203.

Freij BJ et al: Maternal rubella and the congenital rubella syndrome. *Clin Perinatol* 1988;**15**:247.

Giacoia GP: New approaches for the treatment of neonatal sepsis. *J Perinatol* 1993;**13(3)**:223.

Grossman M: Human immunodeficiency virus infections in children: public health and public policy issues. *J Pediatr Inf Dis* 1987;**6**:113.

Hall RT et al: Characteristics of coagulase-negative staphylococci from infants with bacteremia. *J Pediatr Inf Dis* 1987;**6**:377.

Hammerschlag MR: Chlamydial infections. *J Pediatr* 1989;**114**:727.

Hill HR: Granulocyte transfusions in neonates. *Pediatr Rev* 1991;**12(10)**:298.

Hill HR: Intravenous immunoglubulin use in the neonate: role in prophylaxis and therapy of infection. *J Pediatr Inf Dis* 1993;**12(7)**:549.

Hodgman JE: Sepsis in the neonate. *Perinatol Neonatol* 1981;**5**:45.

Kinney JS et al: Should we expand the TORCH complex? *Clin Perinatol* 1988;**15**:727.

Jenkins M, Kohl S: New aspects of neonatal herpes. *Inf Dis Clin North Am* 1992;**6(1)**:57.

Koskiniemi M et al: Neonatal herpes simplex virus infection: a report of 43 patients. *J Pediatr Inf Dis* 1989;**8**:30.

Larson E: Trends in Neonatal Infections. *JOGNN* 1987;**Nov/Dec**:1404.

Lee RV: Parasites and pregnancy: the problems of malaria and toxoplasmosis. *Clin Perinat* 1988;**15**:351.

Lewis L: Congenital syphilis; serologic diagnosis in the young infant. *Inf Dis Clin North Am,* 1992;**6(1)**:31.

Manroe BL et al: The neonatal blood count in health and disease. Reference values for neutrophilic cells. *J Peds* 1979;**95**:85.

McDonald LK et al: Lack of toxicity in two cases of neonatal acyclovir overdose. *J Pediatr Inf Dis* 1989;**8**:529.

Oxtoby MJ: Human immunodeficiency virus and other viruses in human milk: placing the issues in broader perspective. *J Pediatr Inf Dis* 1988;**7**:825.

Perinatal herpes simplex virus infections. *ACOG Technical Bulletin;* No. 122, Nov 1988.

Pernoll ML et al: Chapter 25 in: *Diagnosis and management of the fetus and neonate at risk.* C.V. Mosby Company, 1986.

Pizzo PA: Emerging concepts in the treatment of HIV infection in children. *JAMA* 1989;**262**:14.

Pourcyrous M et al: Significance of serial C-Reactive Protein responses in neonatal infection and other disorders. *J Pediatr* 1993;**92(3)**:431.

Remington JS, Klein JO: Bacterial Sepsis and Meningitis. Chap 18, p 601 in: *Infectious Diseases of Fetus and Newborn Infant,* 3rd ed. Saunders, 1990.

Remington JS, Klein JO: Gonococcal Infection. Chap 26, p 848 in: *Infectious Diseases of the Fetus and Newborn Infant, 3rd ed. Saunders, 1990.*

Remington JS, Desmonts G: Toxoplasmosis. In: Remington JS, Klein JO (eds) *Infectious Diseases of the Fetus and Newborn Infant,* 3rd ed. Philadelphia, WB Saunders, 1990:89.

Rettig PJ: Perinatal infections with chlamydia trachomatis. *Clin Perinatol* 1988;**15**:321.

Rodriquez EM et al: Diagnostic methods for chlamydia trachomatis disease in neonates. *J Perinatol* 1987;**11**:232.

Sanchez PJ et al: Significance of a positive urine Group B Streptococcal latex agglutination test in neonates. *J Pediatr* 1990;**116**:601.

Scutchfield FD et al: AIDS update. *Post Grad Med* 1989;**85**:289.

Shapiro CN: Epidemioloxy of hepatitis B. *J Pediatr Inf Dis* 1993;**12(5)**:433.

Snyder JD: Expanding alphabet of viral hepatitis. *Semin Pediatr Gastroenterology and Nutrition,* 1991;**2(2)**:4.

Teberg AJ: Clinical manifestations of epidemic neonatal listeriosis. *J Pediatr Inf Dis* 1987;**6**:817.

Thore M et al: The role of commercial latex agglutination test in the diagnosis of Group B Streptococcal infection in neonates. *Acta Paediatr Scand* 1991;**80:**167.

Ukwu HN, Graham BS, Lambert JS: Perinatal transmission of human immunodeficiency virus infection and maternal immunization; strategies for prevention. *Obstet Gynecol* 1992;**80(3):**459.

Wendel GD: Gestational and congenital syphilis. *Clin Perinatol* 1988;**15:**287.

Whitley RJ: Neonatal herpes simplex virus infections. *Clin Perinatol* 1988;**15:**903.

Williams CL, Strobino BA: Lyme Disease transmission during pregnancy. *Contemp OB/GYN* 1990;**35:**48.

Working Group on Antiretroviral Therapy: National Pediatric HIV Resource Center. Antiretroviral therapy and medical management of the human immunodeficiency virus-infected child. *J Pediatr Inf Dis* 1993;**12(6):**513.

Zenker PN, Berman SM: Congenital syphilis; trends and recommendations for evaluation and management. *J Pediatr Inf Dis* 1991;**10(7):**516.

62 Intrauterine Growth Retardation (Small-for-Gestational-Age Infant)

I. Definition. The terms **intrauterine growth retardation (IUGR)** and **small for gestational age (SGA)** are used more or less interchangeably. There is considerable variability in the definition of what constitutes a growth-retarded infant. The term *IUGR* signifies an abnormality of the fetus itself or means that some insult to the fetus has interfered with normal growth. IUGR may also be defined as birth weight **below the 10th percentile** for gestational age or more than **2 standard deviations below the mean** for gestational age. The **ponderal index,** arrived at by the following formula,

$$\text{Ponderal index} = \frac{\text{Birth weight} \times 100}{\text{Crown–heel length}}$$

can be used to identify infants whose soft tissue mass is below normal for the stage of skeletal development (Battaglia, 1967). Thus, a ponderal index of below the 10th percentile may be used to identify IUGR infants.

   A. Term IUGR infants are those born at 37 weeks or later who are small for gestational age.

   B. Preterm IUGR infants are those who are delivered prematurely (before 37 weeks) who are small for gestational age.

II. Incidence. About 3–10% of all pregnancies are associated with IUGR, and 20% of stillborn infants are growth retarded. The perinatal mortality rate is 4–8 times higher for growth-retarded fetuses, and serious short- or long-term morbidity is noted in half of the affected surviving infants. It is estimated that one-third of infants with birth weights under 2800 g are in fact growth-retarded and not premature. In the USA, uteroplacental insufficiency is the leading cause of IUGR. An estimated 10% of cases are secondary to congenital infection. Chromosomal and other genetic disorders are reported in 5–15% of IUGR infants.

III. Pathophysiology. Fetal growth is influenced by fetal, maternal, and placental factors.

   A. Fetal factors (Table 62–1)

      1. Genetic factors. Potential for fetal growth is ultimately determined by genetic endowment. Racial and ethnic backgrounds influence size at birth irrespective of socioeconomic status. Males weigh an average of 150–200 g more than females at birth. This weight increase occurs late in gestation. Birth order affects fetal size; infants born to primiparous women weigh less than subsequent siblings. Genetic disorders such as achondroplasia, Russell-Silver syndrome, and leprechaunism also present with IUGR.

TABLE 62–1. FETAL FACTORS IN IUGR

Genetic factors
Racial, ethnic, and population differences
Genetic disorders
Chromosomal disorder
Female sex
Congenital anomalies
Congenital infections
Inborn errors of metabolism

2. **Chromosomal anomalies.** Chromosomal deletions or imbalances result in diminished fetal growth. Growth retardation is observed as a major feature of short-arm deletion of chromosome number 4, long-arm deletion of chromosome number 13, and trisomies 13, 18, and 21.

3. **Congenital malformations.** Anencephaly, gastrointestinal atresia, Potter's syndrome, and pancreatic agenesis are examples of congenital anomalies associated with IUGR.

4. **Fetal cardiovascular anomalies** (with the possible exception of transposition of the great vessels and tetralogy of Fallot). Abnormal hemodynamics are thought to be the basis of IUGR.

5. **Congenital infection.** TORCH infections are often associated with IUGR (see p 345). The clinical findings in different congenital infections are nonspecific and overlap considerably. IUGR with rubella causes damage during organogenesis and results in a decreased number of cells, whereas cytomegalovirus infection results in cytolysis and localized necrosis within the fetus.

6. **Inborn errors of metabolism.** Transient neonatal diabetes, galactosemia, and phenylketonuria are other disorders associated with IUGR.

B. **Maternal factors** (Table 62–2)

1. **Reduced uteroplacental blood flow.** Maternal disorders such as preeclampsia-eclampsia, chronic renovascular disease, and chronic hypertensive vascular disease often result in decreased uteroplacental blood flow and associated IUGR. Impaired delivery of oxygen and other essential nutrients is thought to limit organ growth and musculoskeletal maturation.

2. **Maternal malnutrition.** Maternal malnutrition leads to deficient substrate supply to the fetus. Total caloric consumption rather than protein or fat consumption appears to be the principal nutritional influence on birth weight. Famine causes a modest decline in birth weight, and in third-world countries, severe maternal malnutrition is the leading cause of IUGR. Negative effects on birth weight are most pronounced when starvation occurs in the last trimester.

3. **Multiple pregnancy.** Impaired growth results from failure to provide optimal nutrition for more than one fetus in utero. There is a progressive decrease in weight of singletons, twins, and triplets. In parabiotic twins, the smaller twin has decreased nutrient delivery secondary to abnormal placental blood flow resulting from arteriovenous communication in the chorionic plate.

4. **Drugs**

   a. **Cigarettes and alcohol.** Chronic abuse of cigarettes or alcohol is de-

TABLE 62–2. MATERNAL FACTORS IN IUGR

Pregnancy-induced hypertension (> 140/90 mm Hg)
Weight gain (< 0.9 kg/every 4 weeks)
Fundal lag (< 4 cm for gestational age)
Cyanotic heart disease
Heavy smoking
Residing at high altitude
Substance abuse and drugs
Short stature
Low socioeconomic class
Anemia (Hct < 30%)
Prepregnancy weight (< 50 kg)
Prior history of IUGR
Chronic hypertension
Renal disease
Severe maternal malnutrition
Multiple pregnancy
Low maternal age

monstrably associated with IUGR. The effects of alcohol and tobacco seem to be dose-dependent, with IUGR becoming more serious and predictable with heavy abuse.

   b. **Heroin.** Maternal heroin addiction is also often associated with IUGR.

   c. **Cocaine.** Cocaine use in pregnancy is associated with increased rates of IUGR (Orro, Dixon, 1987). The cause of IUGR may be mediated by placental insufficiency or direct toxic effect on the fetus.

   d. **Others.** Other drugs and chemical agents causing IUGR include known teratogens, antimetabolites, and therapeutic agents such as trimethadione, warfarin, and phenytoin. Each of these agents causes characteristic malformation syndromes.

   5. **Maternal hypoxemia.** Mothers with hemoglobinopathies, especially sickle cell disease, often have IUGR infants. Infants born at high altitudes tend to have lower mean birth weights for gestational age.

   6. **Other maternal factors.** Maternal short stature, young maternal age, low socioeconomic class, primiparity, grand multiparity, and low prepregnancy weight are associated with subnormal birth weight.

 C. **Placental factors** (Table 62–3)

   1. **Placental insufficiency.** In the first and second trimesters, fetal growth is determined mostly by inherent fetal growth potential. By the third trimester, placental factors—ie, an adequate supply of nutrients—assume major importance for fetal growth. When the duration of pregnancy exceeds the capacity of the placenta to nurture, placental insufficiency results, with subsequent impaired fetal growth. This phenomenon occurs mostly in postterm gestations but may occur at any time during gestation.

   2. **Anatomic problems.** Various anatomic factors such as multiple infarcts, aberrant cord insertions, umbilical vascular thrombosis, and hemangiomas are described in IUGR placentas. Premature placental separation may reduce the surface area exchange, resulting in impaired fetal growth. An adverse intrauterine environment is apt to affect both placental and fetal development; hence IUGR infants usually have small placentas.

IV. Classification

 A. **Symmetric IUGR.** (Hc = Ht = Wt, all < 10%.) The head circumference, length, and weight are all proportionately reduced for gestational age. Symmetric IUGR is due either to decreased growth potential of the fetus (congenital infection, genetic disorder) or to extrinsic conditions that are active early in pregnancy.

 B. **Asymmetric IUGR.** (Hc = Ht > Wt, all < 10%.) Fetal weight is reduced out of proportion to length and head circumference. The head circumference and length are closer to the expected percentiles for gestational age than is the weight. In these infants, brain growth is usually spared. The usual causes are uteroplacental insufficiency, maternal malnutrition, or extrinsic conditions appearing late in pregnancy.

V. Diagnosis

 A. **Establishing gestational age.** Determining the correct gestational age is imperative. The last menstrual period, size of the uterus, time of quickening (fluttering movements in the abdomen caused by fetal activity, appreciated by the

TABLE 62–3. PLACENTAL FACTORS IN IUGR

Abruptio placentae
Hemangioma
Single umbilical artery
Infarction
Aberrant cord insertion
Umbilical vessel thrombosis

mother for the first time), and early ultrasound measurements are used to determine gestational age.

B. Fetal assessment

1. Clinical diagnosis. The patient's history will raise the index of suspicion regarding suboptimal growth. Manual estimations of weight, serial fundal height measurements, and maternal estimates of fetal activity are simple clinical measures. Imprecision and inconsistency have prevented widespread confidence in these clinical methods.

2. Hormonal evaluation. Hormonal assays were at one time popular for assessment of IUGR but are rarely used today. Maternal urinary estriol and human placental lactogen levels tend to be low or falling in pregnancies with IUGR, though there is marked individual variation.

3. Ultrasonography. Currently, diagnostic ultrasound offers the greatest promise for diagnosis of IUGR. The following parameters used in combination will usually predict growth impairment with a high degree of accuracy:

a. Biparietal diameter (BPD). When serial measurements of BPD are less than optimal, 50–80% of infants will have subnormal birth weights.

b. Abdominal circumference. The liver is the first organ to suffer the effects of growth retardation. Reduced abdominal circumference is the earliest sign of asymmetric growth retardation and diminished glycogen storage.

c. Ratio of head circumference to abdominal circumference. The ratio normally changes as pregnancy progresses. In the second trimester the head circumference is greater than the abdominal circumference. At about 32–36 weeks' gestation, the ratio is 1:1, and after 36 weeks the abdominal measurements become larger. Persistence of a head:abdomen ratio greater than 1 late in gestation is predictive of asymmetric IUGR.

d. Femur length. Femur length appears to correlate well with crown-heel length and provides an early and reproducible measurement of length. Serial measurements of femur length are as effective as head measurements for detecting symmetric IUGR.

e. Placental morphology and amniotic fluid assessment may help in distinguishing a constitutionally small fetus from a growth-retarded fetus. For example, placental aging with oligohydramnios suggests IUGR and fetal jeopardy, whereas normal placental morphology with a normal amount of amniotic fluid suggests a constitutionally small fetus.

C. Neonatal assessment. (See also Chap 3.)

1. Reduced birth weight for gestational age is the simplest method of diagnosis.

2. Lubchenco charts (see Fig 3–2) may underestimate IUGR because they are based on observations made well above sea level.

3. The ponderal index can help identify neonates with IUGR whose birth weight is over 2500 g.

4. Ballard score. Gestational age can also be assessed by means of the Ballard scoring system. This examination is accurate within 2 weeks of gestation in infants weighing more than 999 g at birth and is most accurate at 30–42 hours of age. IUGR infants have a higher rating on this scale than premature infants with similar weights. See p 22 for Ballard examination and scoring.

VI. Complications (Table 62–4)

A. Hypoxia

1. Perinatal asphyxia. IUGR infants frequently have birth asphyxia, because they tolerate the stress of labor poorly.

2. Persistent pulmonary hypertension (persistent fetal circulation). Many IUGR infants are subjected to chronic intrauterine hypoxia, which results in abnormal thickening of the smooth muscles of the small pulmonary arterioles, which in turn reduces pulmonary blood flow and results in

TABLE 62–4. NEONATAL COMPLICATIONS OF IUGR

Metabolic disorders: hypoglycemia, hypocalcemia
Hypothermia
Hematologic disorders: polycythemia
Hypoxia: birth asphyxia, meconium aspiration, persistent fetal circulation
Congenital malformation

---

varying degrees of pulmonary artery hypertension. Because of this, IUGR infants are at risk of developing persistent fetal circulation. Hyaline membrane disease is less frequently seen in IUGR, since these infants tend to manifest advanced pulmonary maturity secondary to chronic intrauterine stress.

    3. Meconium aspiration. Postterm IUGR infants are at risk for meconium aspiration.

  B. Hypothermia. Thermoregulation is compromised in IUGR infants because of diminished subcutaneous fat insulation. Infants with IUGR secondary to fetal malnutrition late in gestation tend to be scrawny as a result of loss of subcutaneous fat. They tend to be more alert than their premature counterparts.

  C. Metabolic

    1. Hypoglycemia. Carbohydrate metabolism is seriously disturbed, and IUGR infants are highly susceptible to hypoglycemia as a consequence of diminished glycogen reserves and decreased capacity for gluconeogenesis. Hypothermia may potentiate the problem of hypoglycemia.

    2. Hypocalcemia. Idiopathic hypocalcemia may also occur in IUGR infants.

  D. Hematologic disorders. Hyperviscosity and polycythemia may result from increased erythropoietin levels secondary to fetal hypoxia associated with IUGR. Polycythemia may also contribute to hypoglycemia and lead to cerebral injury.

VII. Management. Antenatal diagnosis is the key to proper management of IUGR.

  A. History of risk factors. The presence of maternal risk factors should alert the obstetrician to the likelihood of fetal growth retardation. Ultrasonography confirms the diagnosis. Correctable causes of impaired fetal growth warrant immediate attention.

  B. Delivery and resuscitation. Appropriate timing of delivery is important. Delivery is usually undertaken when the lungs are mature or when biophysical data obtained by monitoring reveal fetal distress. Labor is particularly stressful to IUGR fetuses. Skilled resuscitation should be available, as birth asphyxia is common.

  C. Prevention of heat loss. Meticulous care should be taken to prevent heat loss (see Chap 5).

  D. Hypoglycemia. Close monitoring of blood glucose levels is essential for all IUGR infants. Hypoglycemia should be treated promptly with parenteral dextrose and early feeding, as outlined in Chapter 39.

  E. Hematologic disorders. A central hematocrit reading should be obtained to detect polycythemia.

  F. Congenital infection. IUGR infants should be examined for congenital malformations or signs of congenital infections. Many intrauterine infections are clinically silent, and screening for these should be done routinely in IUGR infants. (See TORCH infections, p 345.)

  G. Genetic anomalies. Screening of genetic anomalies should be done as indicated by the physical examination.

VIII. Outcome. The neurodevelopmental outcome depends mostly on the cause of the IUGR.

  A. Symmetric versus asymmetric IUGR. Infants with symmetric IUGR caused by decreased growth potential generally have a poor outcome, whereas infants with asymmetric IUGR in which brain growth is spared usually have a good outcome.

   B. Preterm IUGR infants have a higher incidence of abnormalities than the general population, as these infants are subjected to the risks of prematurity in addition to the risks of IUGR.
   C. Chromosomal disorders. IUGR infants with major chromosomal disorders have a 100% incidence of handicap.
   D. Congenital infections. Infants with congenital rubella or CMV infection with microcephaly have a poor outcome, with a handicap rate exceeding 50%.
   F. Learning ability. The school performance of IUGR infants is significantly influenced by social class, with children from higher social classes scoring better on achievement tests.

REFERENCES

Allen MC: Developmental outcome and follow-up of the small for gestational age infant. *Semin Perinatol* 1984;**8:**123.

Ballard JL, Novak KK, Driver M: A simplified score for assessment of fetal maturation of newly born infants. *J Pediatr* 1979;**95:**769.

Battaglia FC, Lubchenco LO: A practical classification of newborn infants by weight and gestational age. *J Pediatr* 1967;**17:**159.

Cassady G: The small for date infant. *Pathophysiol Manage Newborn* 1981;**15:**262.

Lockwood CJ, Weiner S: Assessment of fetal growth. *Clin Perinatology* 1986;**13:**3.

Lubchenco LO et al: Intrauterine growth and estimated from live born birthweight data. *Pediatrics* 1963;**32:**793.

Orro AS, Dixon SD: Perinatal cocaine and methamphetamine exposure. *J Pediatr* 1987;**111:**571.

Queenan JT: How to diagnose intrauterine growth retardation. *Contemp Obstet Gynecol* 1982;**19:**195.

Seeds JW: Impaired fetal growth: Definition and clinical diagnosis. *Obstet Gynecol* 1984:**64:**303.

Warshaw JB: Intrauterine growth retardation. *Pediatr Rev* 1986;**8:**107.

Williams RL et al: Fetal growth and perinatal viability in California. *Obstet Gynecol* 1982;**52:**624.

63 Multiple Gestation

I. **Incidence.** The incidence of multiple gestation is probably underestimated. Fewer than half of twin pregnancies diagnosed with ultrasonography during the first trimester are finally delivered as twins, a phenomenon that has been termed *vanishing twin*. Twins occur in 1–2% of deliveries after 20 weeks, and the triplet rate is about 0.1%. Two gestational sacs can be identified with ultrasonography by 6 weeks' gestation. In addition, routine screening for maternal alpha-fetoprotein (AFP) will identify about half of the pregnancies with multiple gestations at an early gestational age. About 12–20% of twins are identified after the onset of labor.

The incidence of monozygotic twinning is remarkably constant at 3–5 per 1000 pregnancies, while the rate for dizygotic twinning varies from 4 to 50 per 1000 pregnancies. About one-third of twins in the USA are monozygotic. The rate of monozygotic twinning is considered a chance phenomenon, whereas dizygotic twinning is due to multiple ovulation, shows wide ethnic variability, and may have a familial tendency.

II. **Risk factors.** The incidence of dizygotic twinning increases with a family history of twins, maternal age (peak at 35–39 years), previous twin gestation, increasing parity, maternal height, fecundity, social class, frequency of coitus, and exposure to exogenous gonadotropins (20–40% incidence) and clomiphene (6–8% incidence).

The risk of twinning decreases with undernourishment. Ethnic background (Black > Caucasian > Oriental) is a preconception risk factor for multiple gestation.

III. **Placentation**

A. **Classification.** Placental examination affords a unique opportunity to identify two-thirds to three-fourths of monozygotic twins at birth. Twin placentation is classified according to the placental disc (single, fused, or separate), number of chorions (monochorionic, dichorionic), and number of amnions (monoamniotic, diamniotic) (Fig 63–1.). Heterosexual (assuredly dizygotic) twins always have a dichorionic placenta, and monochorionic twins are always of the same sex. All monochorionic twins are believed to be monozygotic. In 70% of monozygotic twin pregnancies, the placentas are monochorionic, and the possibility exists for commingling of the fetal circulations. Fewer than 1% of twin pregnancies are monoamniotic.

B. **Complications.** Twin gestations are associated with an increased frequency of anomalies of the placenta and adnexa—eg, single umbilical artery or velamentous or marginal cord insertion (6–9 times more common with twin gestation). The cord is more susceptible to trauma from twisting. The vessels near the insertion are often unprotected by Wharton's jelly and are especially prone to thrombosis when compression or twisting occurs. Intrapartum fetal distress from cord compression and fetal hemorrhage from associated vasa previa are potential problems with velamentous insertion of the cord.

C. **Determination of zygosity.** The most efficient way to identify zygosity is as follows.

1. **Gender examination.** Male-female pairs are dizygotic. The dichorionic placenta may be separate or fused.

2. **Placental examination.** Twins with a monochorionic placenta (monoamniotic or diamniotic) are monozygotic. Care should be taken not to confuse apposed fused placentas for a single chorion. If doubt exists upon gross inspection of the dividing membranes, a transverse section should be studied. The zygosity of twins of the same sex with dichorionic membranes

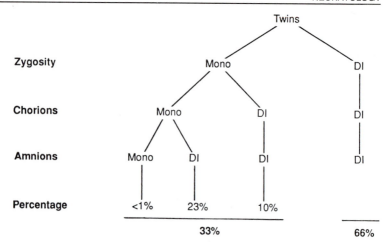

FIGURE 63–1. Percentage distribution of twins according to placental type.

cannot be immediately known. Genetic studies are needed (eg, blood typing, HLA typing, DNA markers, chromosome marking) to determine zygosity.

IV. **Mortality rates.** Although perinatal mortality rates for singleton pregnancies have continued to fall during the last decade, there has been little change in mortality rates for multiple pregnancies.

A. **Twins.** For twin gestations, the fetal mortality rate is 4%, the neonatal mortality rate is 7.6% (1.2% for singletons), and the perinatal mortality rate is 11.6% (2.2% for singletons). The perinatal death rate for twins is 9 times the rate for first-born singletons, and 11 times the rate for second-born singletons.

1. **Monoamniotic twins.** The mortality rate for monoamniotic twins is highest (50–60%), largely because of cord entanglement.

2. **Monozygotic twins.** Monozygotic twins have a perinatal mortality and morbidity rate that is 2–3 times that of dizygotic twins. Diamnionic monochorionic twins have a mortality rate of 25% and dichorionic twins a mortality rate of 8.9%.

3. **Prematurity in twins.** Approximately 10% of preterm deliveries are twin gestations, and they account for 25% of perinatal deaths in preterm deliveries.

4. **Fetal death.** Death of one fetus may affect the outcome of the survivor profoundly or minimally (Dudley, 1986). When the cause of death is intrinsic to one dichorionic fetus and does not threaten the other fetus, complications are rare. Hazardous intrauterine environments threaten both twins, whether monochorionic or dichorionic. With monochorionic placentas, the incidence of major complications or death in the surviving twin is approximately 50%.

B. **Triplets.** The neonatal mortality rate for triplets is 18.8%, and the perinatal mortality rate is 25.5%.

V. **Morbidity**

A. **Prematurity.** Prematurity and uteroplacental insufficiency are the major contributors to perinatal complications. The average twin delivery occurs at 37 weeks, and multiple gestation is complicated by preterm delivery (< 35 weeks) in 21.5% of patients.

B. **Intrauterine growth retardation.** The incidence of low birth weight in twins is approximately 50–60%, a figure that is 5–7 times higher than the incidence of low birth weight in singletons. In general, the more fetuses in a gestation, the smaller their weight for gestational age (Fig 63–2). Twins tend to grow at nor-

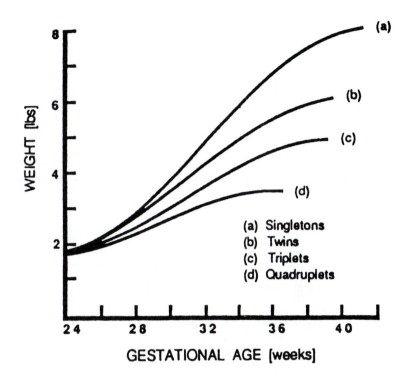

FIGURE 63–2. Growth curve showing mean weights of infants from single and multiple pregnancies by gestational age. (From Phelan MC. Twins. In Human malformations and related anomalies. Stevenson RE, Hall JG, Goodman RM, eds. Oxford University Press, 1993. Modified from McKeown T, Record RG: Observations of foetal growth in multiple pregnancy in man. J. Endocrin. 8:386, 1952.)

     mal rates up to about 30–34 weeks' gestation, when they reach a combined weight of 4 kg. Thereafter, they grow more slowly. Two-thirds of twins show some signs of growth retardation at birth.
  C. Uteroplacental insufficiency. The incidence of acute and chronic uteroplacental insufficiency is increased in multiple gestations. Five-minute Apgar scores of 0–3 are reported for 5–10% of twin gestations. These low scores may relate to acute stresses of labor, cord prolapse (1–5%), or trauma during delivery superimposed on chronic uteroplacental insufficiency.
VI. Congenital anomalies. Birth defects are two to three times more common in monozygotic twins than in singletons or dizygotic twins who have a 2–3% incidence of major defects diagnosed at birth. There are three mechanisms postulated for the increased frequency of structural defects in monozygotic twins: (1) deformations due to intrauterine space constraint, (2) disruption of normal blood flow due to placental vascular anastomoses, and (3) defects in morphogenesis. Such defects are usually discordant in monozygotic twins; however, in purely genetic conditions (eg, chromosomal abnormalities or single gene defects) concordance would be the rule.

A. **Anomalies unique to multiple pregnancies.** Certain anomalies, such as conjoined twins and acardia, are unique to multiple pregnancies.

B. **Deformations.** Twins are more likely to suffer from intrauterine crowding and restriction of movement leading to synostosis, torticollis, facial palsy, positional foot defects, and other defects (MacLennan, 1984).

C. **Vascular Disruptions.** Disruptions related to monozygotic vascular shunts may result in birth defects. Acardia occurs from an artery-to-artery placental shunt, in which reverse flow leads to the development of an amorphous recipient twin. In utero death of a cotwin may result in thromboembolic phenomenon, including DIC, cutis aplasia, porencephaly or hydranencephaly, limb reduction defects, intestinal atresias, or gastroschisis.

D. **Malformations.** Monozygotic twinning results in increased frequency of the following specific malformations: (1) sacrococcygeal teratoma, (2) sirenomelia sequence, including VACTERL association, (3) cloacal exstrophy sequence, (4) holoprosencephaly sequence, and (5) anencephaly.

VII. **Twin-twin transfusion syndrome**

A. **Vascular anastomoses.** The chorionic vascular bed of monozygotic (and usually monochorionic) twins seem to have limitless variations. However, almost all monochorionic placentas demonstrate vascular anastomoses, whereas dichorionic placentas rarely do. Vascular anastomoses may be superficial direct communications easily visible upon inspection between arteries (most common) or veins (uncommon); deep connections from arteries to veins via villi; or combinations of superficial and deep connections. This commonality of chorionic vasculature sets the stage for twin-twin transfusion syndrome.

B. **Incidence.** Despite the high frequency of vascular anastomosis in monochorionic placentation, the twin-twin transfusion syndrome is relatively uncommon (about 15% of monochorionic gestations).

C. **Clinical manifestations.** Clinically, the twin-twin transfusion syndrome is diagnosed when twins have a hemoglobin difference of more than 5 g/dL and is due to artery-to-vein anastamoses.

1. The **donor twin** tends to be pale and have a low birth weight, oligohydramnios, anemia, hypoglycemia, decreased organ mass, hypovolemia, and amnion nodosum. Donor twins often require volume expansion or red cell transfusion, or both.

2. The **recipient twin** is frequently plethoric and has a high birth weight, polyhydramnios, polycythemia/hyperviscosity, increased organ mass, hypervolemia, and hyperbilirubinemia. Recipient twins often require partial exchange transfusion with fresh-frozen plasma.

3. Rarely, either or both of the twins involved in a fetofetal transfusion may present with hydrops fetalis.

VIII. **Neonatal implications and management**

A. **Site of delivery.** When a complicated twin gestation has been identified, delivery should ideally be conducted at a high-risk perinatal center with 2 experienced pediatric delivery teams in attendance.

B. **Placental examination.** Examination of placenta(s) in the delivery room provides an early opportunity to determine zygosity and anticipate certain problems.

C. **Physical examination.** Infants should be examined for evidence of IUGR, congenital anomalies, and twin-twin transfusion syndrome. Central hematocrits should be obtained in both infants to look for anemia or polycythemia.

D. **Complications in newborn period.** The second-born twin is 2–4 times as likely to develop respiratory distress syndrome (Rokos, 1968), probably secondary to perinatal stress; however, the first-born twin may be at risk for developing necrotizing enterocolitis (Samm, 1986).

IX. **Risks beyond the neonatal period**

A. **Catch-up growth.** In monozygotic twins, birth weight differences may be as much as 20%, but the lighter twin has a remarkable ability to make up intrauterine growth deficits. However, if the birth weight of the lighter twin is less than the tenth percentile, the prognosis is guarded. With such marked discordance, the undersized twin often continues to be inferior in growth and intelligence into adult life.

B. **Acquired illnesses.** Illness in one twin increases the risk of illness in the other (Seigle, 1982). Epilepsy has an 85% concordance rate in identical twins. With acute lymphocytic leukemia or juvenile diabetes mellitus of one twin, the incidence in the other twin is 20% and 50%, respectively.

C. **Social problems.** Inadequate nurturing and child abuse are more likely with twins. Counseling for parents of twins may be invaluable (Seigel, 1982).

REFERENCES

Babson SG, Phillips DS: Growth and development of twins dissimilar in size at birth. *N Engl J Med* 1973;**289:**937.

Benirschke K: Multiple gestation: Incidence, etiology, and inheritance. Pages 511–526 in: *Maternal-Fetal Medicine.* Creasy RK, Resnik R (editors). Saunders, 1984.

Dudley DKL, Dalton ME: Single fetal death in twin gestation. *Semin Perinatol* 1986;**10:**65.

Hecht F, Hecht BK: Genetic and related biomedical aspects of twinning. *Pediatr Rev* 1983;**5:**179.

Johnson SF, Driscoll SG: Twin placentation and its complications. *Semin Perinatol* 1986;**10:**9.

Keet MP, Jaroszewica AM, Lombard CJ: Follow-up study of physical growth of monozygous twins with discordant within-pair birth weights. *Pediatrics* 1986;**77:**336.

Little J, Bryan E: Congenital anomalies in twins. *Semin Perinatol* 1986;**10:**50.

Macgillivray I: Epidemiology of twin pregnancy. *Semin Perinatol* 1986;**10:**4.

MacLennan AH: Multiple gestation: Clinical characteristics and management. Pages 527–538 in: *Maternal-Fetal Medicine.* Creasy RK, Resnik R (editors). Saunders, 1984.

Newton ER: Antepartum care in multiple gestation. *Semin Perinatol* 1986;**10:**19.

Rokos J et al: Hyaline membrane disease in twins. *Pediatrics* 1986;**42:**204.

Samm M et al: Necrotizing enterocolitis in infants of multiple gestation. *Am J Dis Child* 1986;**140:**937.

Seigle SJ, Seigle MM: Practical aspects of pediatric management of families of twins. *Pediatr Rev* 1982;**4:**8.

Smith DW: *Recognizable Patterns of Human Malformation,* 3rd ed. Saunders, 1982.

Wenstrom KD, Gall SA: Incidence, morbidity and mortality, and diagnosis of twin gestations. *Clin Perinatol* 1988;**15(1):**1.

64 Necrotizing Enterocolitis

I. **Definition.** Necrotizing enterocolitis (NEC) is an acquired neonatal disorder representing an end-expression of serious intestinal injury following a combination of vascular, mucosal, and toxic (and yet unidentified) insults to a relatively immature gut.

II. **Incidence**

  A. **NEC is predominantly a disorder of preterm infants,** with an incidence of 8–12% in infants under 1.5 kg. The incidence increases with decreasing gestational age. **Sixty to 80% of cases occur in high-risk premature infants,** while 10–25% occur in low-risk and full-term newborns. Infants with NEC represent 2–5% of NICU admissions.

  B. **NEC occurs sporadically or in epidemic clusters.**

III. **Pathophysiology.** Currently there is no single unifying theory for the pathogenesis of NEC that satisfactorily explains all of the clinical observations associated with this disorder. The generally accepted pathophysiologic sequence of events resulting in overt clinical disease is thought to involve an initial ischemic or toxic mucosal damage resulting in a loss of mucosal integrity. Then, with the availability of suitable substrate provided by enteral feedings, there is bacterial proliferation followed by invasion of the damaged intestinal mucosa by gas (hydrogen), producing organisms causing intramural bowel gas (pneumatosis intestinalis). This sequence of events may then progress to transmural necrosis or gangrene of the bowel and finally to perforation and peritonitis.

IV. **Risk factors**

  A. **Prematurity.** There is an inverse relationship between risk and gestational age. The lower the gestational age, the greater the risk, owing to the immaturity of the circulatory, gastrointestinal, and immune systems.

  B. **Asphyxia and acute cardiopulmonary distress** lead to low output states, resulting in redistribution of cardiac output away from the mesenteric circulation and causing episodic intestinal ischemia.

  C. **Enteral feedings.** NEC is rare in unfed infants. About 90–95% of infants with NEC have received at least one oral feeding.

   1. Enteral feeding provides necessary substrate for proliferation of enteric pathogens.
   2. Hyperosmolar formula or medications cause direct mucosal damage.
   3. There is a loss or lack of immunoprotective factors in enteral formula or in stored breast milk.

  D. **Polycythemia and hyperviscosity syndromes.** These have been shown to be definite risk factors both clinically and experimentally.

  E. **Exchange transfusions.** There has been a clinically observed association between NEC and exchange transfusions, which is probably due to intestinal ischemia secondary to wide variations in venous and/or arterial perfusion pressures.

  F. **Feeding volume and rapid increase in enteral feedings.** These play a role, but clinical evidence remains *controversial*.

  G. **Enteric pathogenic microorganisms.** Bacterial and viral pathogenesis, including *E coli, Klebsiella, Enterobacter, Pseudomonas, Salmonella, Staph epidermidis, Clostridia* sp, coronaviruses, rotaviruses, and enteroviruses, have all been implicated either directly or indirectly.

V. **Clinical presentation.** NEC usually presents within the first week of life and 3–7 days after initiating enteral feedings. During epidemic clustering of cases, age of onset is variable. The presentation may vary from a benign gastrointestinal abnormality such as abdominal distention (the most frequent early sign, noted in 70% of cases), ileus, and increased volume of gastric aspirate or bilious aspirate (two-thirds of cases) to frank signs of shock, blood per rectum, peritonitis, and perforation. It can also present with nonspecific signs such as labile temperature, apnea, bradycardia, or other signs that would make one suspect sepsis.

The clinical syndrome has been classified into stages by Bell et al (1978) and modified by Walsh and Kliegman (1986) to include systemic, intestinal, and radiographic findings.

A. Stage I: Suspected NEC
  1. **Systemic** findings are nonspecific, including apnea, bradycardia, lethargy, and temperature instability.
  2. **Intestinal** findings include gastric residuals and guiac positive stools.
  3. **Radiographic** findings are normal or nonspecific.
B. Stage IIA: Mild NEC
  1. **Systemic** findings are similar to stage I.
  2. **Intestinal** findings include prominent abdominal distention with or without tenderness, absent bowel sounds, and gross blood in the stools.
  3. **Radiographic** findings include ileus, with dilated loops with focal areas of pneumatosis intestinalis.
C. Stage IIB: Moderate NEC
  1. **Systemic** findings include mild acidosis and thrombocytopenia.
  2. **Intestinal** findings include abdominal wall edema, tenderness with or without a palpable mass.
  3. **Radiographic** findings include extensive pneumatosis and early ascites. Intrahepatic portal venous gas may be present.
D. Stage IIIA: Advanced NEC
  1. **Systemic** findings include respiratory and metabolic acidosis, assisted ventilation for apnea, decreasing blood pressure and urine output, neutropenia, and disseminated intravascular coagulation (DIC).
  2. **Intestinal** findings include spreading edema, erythema, and induration of the abdomen.
  3. **Radiographic** findings include prominent ascites and possibly persistent sentinel loop with no perforation.
E. Stage IIIB: Advanced NEC
  1. **Systemic** findings reveal deteriorating vital signs and laboratory indices, shock syndrome, and electrolyte imbalance.
  2. **Intestinal and radiographic** findings reveal evidence of perforation.
VI. Diagnosis. A high index of suspicion should be entertained for any infant with a history of a combination of the risk factors enumerated under **IV,** above.
  A. Clinical diagnosis. NEC is a tentative diagnosis in any infant presenting with the triad of feeding intolerance, abdominal distention, and grossly bloody stools (hematochezia) or acute change in stool character. Alternatively, the earliest signs may be identical to neonatal sepsis, that is, apnea, bradycardia, lethargy and abnormal white blood count indices, and thrombocytopenia.
  B. Laboratory studies. The following should be performed as baseline studies. If there is clinical progression of disease or if these laboratory tests are abnormal, the tests should be repeated every 8–12 hours.
  1. **Complete blood count and differential.** The white count may be normal but is more frequently either elevated, with a shift to the left, or low (leukopenia).
  2. **Platelet count.** Thrombocytopenia is seen. Fifty percent of patients with proven NEC have platelet counts less than 50,000/mL.
  3. **Blood culture** for aerobic and anaerobes.
  4. **Stool screening** for occult blood. Even though a clinical study has found that routine testing of stools for occult blood does not identify a population at greater risk for NEC, testing still continues on suspected patients so that changes in the stool can be followed.

5. **Stool screening** for reducing substances > 1% sugar or +2/+3 for reducing substances.

6. **Arterial blood gas measurements.** Metabolic or combined acidosis or hypoxia may be seen.

7. **Serum potassium level.** The serum potassium level may be high, secondary to hemolysis of red blood cells.

8. **Stool cultures for rotaviruses and enteroviruses** should be obtained if diarrhea is an epidemic in the nursery.

C. **Radiologic studies**

1. **Flat-plate x-ray studies of the abdomen**

   a. **Supportive for NEC.** Look for abnormal bowel gas patterns, ileus, or areas suspicious for pneumatosis intestinalis.

   b. **Confirmatory of NEC.** Look for (1) the presence of intramural bowel gas (pneumatosis intestinalis) and (2) the presence of intrahepatic portal venous gas (in the absence of an umbilical venous catheter).

2. **Lateral decubitus, cross-table lateral, or upright x-ray studies of the abdomen.** These studies may show free air with perforation.

Note: In the presence of pneumatosis intestinalis or portal venous gas, flat-plate and lateral decubitus or cross-table lateral x-ray studies of the abdomen should be obtained every 6–8 hours to check for the development of pneumoperitoneum signaling intestinal perforation. Serial x-ray studies may be discontinued with clinical improvement, usually after 48–72 hours. Perforation commonly occurs within 48–72 hours following pneumatosis or portal venous gas.

VII. **Management.** The main principle of management for confirmed NEC is to treat it as an acute abdomen with impending or septic peritonitis. The goal is to prevent progression of disease, intestinal perforation, and shock. If NEC occurs in epidemic clusters, cohort isolation has been shown to limit transmission.

A. **Basic NEC protocol.** Any infant with suspected NEC should be managed according to the following protocol.

1. **Nothing by mouth (NPO)** to allow gastrointestinal rest.

2. **Use of a nasogastric tube** (on low suction) to keep the bowel decompressed.

3. **Frequent monitoring of vital signs** (every 2–4 hours) and **abdominal circumference.**

4. **Removal of umbilical catheter and placement of peripheral venous (and possibly arterial) catheter,** depending on severity of illness.

5. **Antibiotics.** Start ampicillin and gentamicin or cefotaxime intravenously. Add anaerobic coverage (clindamycin or metronidazole [Flagyl]) if peritonitis or perforation is suspected (*controversial*). (See Chap 73 for dosages and other pharmacologic information.)

6. **Monitoring for gastrointestinal bleeding.** Check all gastric aspirates and stools for blood.

7. **Strict monitoring of fluid intake and output.** Try to maintain urine output of 1–3 mL/kg/h.

8. **Removal of potassium from intravenous fluids in the presence of hyperkalemia and or anuria.**

9. **Laboratory monitoring.** Check CBC, platelet count, potassium level, and blood gas levels frequently.

10. **Septic workup.** Culture blood, urine, and sputum. Some institutions routinely perform lumbar puncture for culture of cerebrospinal fluid prior to starting antibiotics (*controversial*).

11. **Radiologic studies.** Perform abdominal flat-plate x-ray studies every 6–8 hours.

B. **Management of stage 1.** Start the basic NEC protocol described above in **A.** If all cultures are negative and the infant has improved clinically, antibiotics can be stopped after 3 days. The infant can also be fed after 3 days if clinically improved.

C. **Management of stage IIA+B**
   1. **Basic NEC protocol,** including antibiotics for 10 days (see **A.5,** above).
   2. **NPO for 2 weeks.** Oral feedings may be started 7–10 days after radiographic demonstration of clearing of pneumatosis.
   3. **Total parenteral nutrition (TPN)** should be initiated. A caloric intake of at least 90–110 cal/kg/d should be attempted. TPN should be continued until full enteral feedings have been well established.
   4. **Supplemental oxygen.** Supplemental oxygen is indicated if there is evidence of hypoxia in arterial blood gas and/or pulse oximeter monitoring.
   5. **Thrombocytopenia,** if severe, can be treated with platelets.
   6. **Acidosis,** if progressive, can be treated with tromethamine (THAM) or sodium bicarbonate and mechanical ventilation.
   7. **Surgical consultation** is required.
   8. **Low dose dopamine infusion.** There is a theoretical benefit from low dose dopamine infusion (2–4 µg/kg/min) to improve intestinal blood flow in low flow states.

D. **Management of stage IIIA+B**
   1. **Basic NEC protocol,** as described in **A,** above.
   2. **Stage II management,** as described in **C,** above.
   3. **Respiratory support,** as indicated by blood gas levels and clinical status.
   4. **Blood pressure support.** Declining blood pressure and urine output, increasing nasogastric output, and increasing abdominal circumference suggest increasing third-space losses, perforation, or septic shock. Treatment includes replacement of ongoing fluid losses, volume expansion with colloids (see p 000) and vasopressors such as dopamine (see Chap 73 for dosage and other pharmacologic information). The goal is to maintain adequate mean blood pressure (see Appendix C, Fig C–1) and urine output (1–3 mL/kg/h).
   5. **Progressive leukopenia, granulocytopenia, and thrombocytopenia** usually parallel a deteriorating clinical status. Granulocyte transfusions are usually not indicated. Blood and platelet transfusion are frequently needed.

E. **Surgical management.** Surgical intervention is indicated if there is evidence of intestinal perforation. Perforations usually occur within 24–48 hours following the appearance of pneumatosis. Other indications (relative and not absolute) for surgical intervention in the absence of free intraperitoneal air include:
   1. **Deteriorating clinical condition** with failure to respond to appropriate medical management.
   2a. **Evidence of a persistent, fixed sentinel loop over 24 hours** suggesting a segment of gangrenous bowel. In these instances, paracentesis and peritoneal lavage to obtain peritoneal fluid for visual examination, Gram's staining, white blood count, and culture are helpful. The presence of brown-colored or particulate peritoneal fluid and bacteria on Gram's stain, a white count of more than 300/mm³, and positive culture results are strongly suggestive of gangrenous bowel. Introduction of air may confound later diagnosis of perforation.
   2b. **Metrizamide,** a water soluble contrast agent, has been used for the diagnosis of a silent perforation in selected cases.
   3. **Right lower quandrant mass.**
   4. **Abdominal wall erythema** suggests peritonitis and may also be an indication for operative intervention.
   5. **Spontaneous intestinal perforation** in the VLBW infant. As a recently recognized entity, it is also a cause of intestinal perforation in VLBW infants and appears to have several clinical features that distinguish it from classical NEC. The clinical course is of insidious onset without the usual GI signs of NEC. Instead, a bluish discoloration of the lower abdomen is often the only presenting early sign. Radiographic findings are limited to intraperitoneal air with no evidence of pneumatosis intestinalis, portal venous gas, or sentinel loop. At surgery, the perforations almost always are

in the distal ileum, well demarcated, and discrete. Management and treatment is standard for perforated bowel. Outcome and prognosis are better than for NEC with perforation.

VIII. Prognosis

A. **NEC with perforation** is associated with a mortality of 20–40%.

B. **Recurrent NEC** is a rare complication.

C. **Subacute or intermittent symptoms of bowel obstruction** due to stenosis or strictures of the colon and, less frequently, of the small bowel are seen in about 10–20%. A barium enema is usually confirmatory.

D. **Infants undergoing extensive surgical resection** require long-term parenteral nutrition, enterostomy care, and management of short gut syndrome. Chronic electrolyte imbalance and failure to thrive are common.

E. **In the absence of short gut syndrome,** growth, nutrition, and gastrointestinal function appear to catch up and are normal by the end of the first year.

REFERENCES

Abrams TJ et al: Occult blood in stools and necrotizing enterocolitis: Is there a relationship? *Am J Dis Child* 1988:**142(4)**:451.

Giacoia GP et al: Indomethacin and recurrent ileal perforations in a pre-term infant. *J Perinatol* 1993;**13(4)**:297.

Kliegman RM: Neonatal necrotizing enterocolitis: Bridging the basic science with the clinical disease. *J Pediatr* 1990;**117**:836.

McKeon RE et al: Role of delayed feeding and of feeding increments in necrotizing enterocolitis. *J Pediatr* 1992;**124**:764.

Nowicki P: Intestinal ischemia and necrotizing enterocolitis. *J Pediatr* 1990 Suppl; **117(1)**:S14.

Walsh MC, Kliegman RM: Necrotizing enterocolitis: Treatment based on staging criteria. *Pediatr Clin North Am* 1986;**33(1)**:179.

65 Neurologic Diseases

HYDROCEPHALUS

I. **Definition.** Hydrocephalus is defined as dilatation of the cerebral ventricular system. It is usually associated with large head circumference, but ventricular dilatation usually precedes head growth, so that head circumference may be normal. **Macrocephaly** is defined as a head circumference 2 or more standard deviations greater than the mean. Macrocephaly is not always associated with hydrocephalus.

II. **Pathophysiology and etiology**
   A. **Obstruction of cerebrospinal fluid flow.** Hydrocephalus is usually due to obstruction of cerebrospinal fluid flow.
      1. It is usually associated with increased intracranial pressure.
      2. It is termed *noncommunicating hydrocephalus* if obstruction occurs at the foramen of Monro, along the cerebral aqueduct (aqueduct of Sylvius), or at the base of the brain at the foramina of Magendie and Luschka. It is termed *communicating hydrocephalus* if cerebrospinal fluid passes through the foramen at the base of the brain but is improperly drained by the cerebral and cerebellar subarachnoid spaces.
   B. **Destructive process.** Less commonly, hydrocephalus is due to a destructive or atrophic process. This type is termed *hydrocephalus ex vacuo* and is *not* associated with increased pressure.
   C. **Increased cerebrospinal fluid production.** Rarely, hydrocephalus results from excessive production of cerebrospinal fluid, eg, due to papilloma of the choroid plexus.
   D. **Common causes**
      1. Congenital aqueductal stenosis. This disorder may be an X-linked recessive trait.
      2. Neural tube defects with Arnold-Chiari malformation.
      3. Posthemorrhagic obstruction (see Intraventricular Hemorrhage, p 385).
      4. Cerebral atrophy. This is the most common cause of hydrocephalus ex-vacuo.
   E. **Less common causes**
      1. Postinfectious.
      2. Dandy-Walker malformation.
      3. Aneurysm of vein of Galen.
      4. Tumors.
      5. Achondroplasia.
      6. Osteopetrosis.
   F. **Macrocephaly without hydrocephalus** is usually familial and benign, but it may be associated with neurocutaneous diseases (eg, neurofibromatosis, Sturge-Weber syndrome), metabolic storage diseases (eg, Hunter's or Hurler's syndrome), Beckwith-Wiedemann syndrome, or achondroplasia.
   G. **Multifactorial inheritance.** These cases result from an interaction between genetic and environmental factors.

III. **Risk factor.** The risk factor depends upon the underlying cause.

IV. **Clinical presentation**
   A. **Prenatal diagnosis**
      1. **Ultrasonographic** diagnosis in utero is common.
      2. **Polyhydramnios** is present in 10% of cases.

3. Breech presentation is reported in 30% of cases.
B. **Associated conditions** include an increased incidence of prematurity, postmaturity, and stillbirths.
C. **With neural tube defects**
   1. Eighty percent of infants with neural tube defects have hydrocephalus.
   2. The head circumference may be normal or nearly normal at birth.
D. **Due to posthemorrhagic obstruction**
   1. This form is usually detected by screening ultrasonography or CT scan of the head in high-risk preterm infants.
   2. Ventriculomegaly may be detected 2–3 weeks prior to onset of rapid head growth.
   3. With this form of hydrocephalus, the ventricles either return to normal size, arrest with mild hydrocephalus, or develop progressive hydrocephalus with signs of increased intracranial pressure.
E. **Signs of hydrocephalus.** If increased intracranial pressure is present, the infant may show signs of apnea, bradycardia, lethargy, vomiting, tense fontanelle, widely split sutures, dilated scalp veins, rapid head growth, and sclerae visible above the irises **(setting-sun sign).** Papilledema is rarely observed in neonates.

V. **Diagnosis**
A. **Intrauterine ultrasonographic screening** may detect hydrocephalus as early as 15–18 weeks' gestation. It is indicated when there is a family history of neural tube defect or congenital aqueductal stenosis.
B. **Physical examination.** The occipitofrontal head circumference should be carefully determined for all infants. The head circumference of the parents may be increased in up to 50% of cases when infants have macrocephaly. (Normal $[\pm 2\,SD]$ is 54 ± 3 cm for women and 55 ± 3 cm for men.) No further evaluation is required unless there are signs of increased intracranial pressure.
C. **CT scan or MRI of the head** is indicated if increased intracranial pressure is suspected or if the cause of macrocephaly is still uncertain.
D. **Neonatal screening**
   1. **Neural tube defects** are screened by CT scan or MRI of the head.
   2. **Premature infants** are screened with ultrasonography.
      a. **Indications**
         (1) Birth weight of less than 1500 g.
         (2) Larger, sick premature infants.
         (3) Rapidly enlarging head circumference.
         (4) Signs of increased intracranial pressure.
      b. **Yield.** Screening at 2 weeks of age will detect 98% of cases of posthemorrhagic hydrocephalus.
      c. **Follow-up.** Weekly follow-up examinations are indicated to observe for progression until there is definite stabilization or regression of the hydrocephalus.

VI. **Management**
A. **Prenatal diagnosis established**
   1. **With pulmonary maturity,** based on L:S ratio (see p 3), proceed to prompt delivery.
   2. **If the lungs are immature,** there are 3 options.
      a. Immediate delivery (with the risks of prematurity).
      b. Delayed delivery (with the risks of persistent increased intracranial pressure).
      c. In utero placement of a ventriculoamniotic shunt.
   3. **Consultation.** Ideal management calls for consultation with the obstetrician, neonatologist, neurosurgeon, ultrasonographer, geneticist, ethicist, and family members.
B. **Congenital aqueductal stenosis or neural tube defects.** Therapy for neonates with hydrocephalus associated with congenital aqueductal stenosis or neural tube defects is **decompression** by prompt placement of a ventricular

bypass shunt into an intracranial or extracranial compartment. **Ventriculoperitoneal shunts** are considered the method of choice. **Long-term complications of shunts** include infection (usually staphylococcal), occlusion, and organ perforation (due to intraperitoneal contact of a catheter with a hollow viscus).

  C. **Posthemorrhagic hydrocephalus**
    1. **Mild hydrocephalus** usually arrests or returns to normal size within the first few months of life.
    2. **Severe, rapidly progressive hydrocephalus**
      a. **Temporary measures** (unproved in randomized controlled trials)
        (1) Perform serial lumbar punctures.
        (2) Administer drugs to decrease cerebrospinal fluid production (eg, acetazolamide; see Chap 73).
        (3) Insert external ventricular drain.
      b. **Permanent management.** Perform a ventricular shunt procedure.

VII. **Prognosis**
  A. Previously the prognosis for infants with congenital hydrocephalus was poor, but with modern neurosurgical techniques, it has improved. **Long-term survival approaches 90%, and approximately two-thirds of infants who survive have normal or near-normal intellectual capabilities.**
  B. Once an infant has a ventricular bypass shunt placed, the infant will probably need a shunt for the rest of his life. Complications associated with shunts (see **VI.B,** above), are very common.
  C. The long-term outcome for preterm infants with posthemorrhagic hydrocephalus is strongly correlated with the severity of the hemorrhage and the degree of prematurity.

INTRAVENTRICULAR HEMORRHAGE

  I. **Definition.** Intraventricular hemorrhage (IVH) is an intracranial hemorrhage usually arising in the germinal matrix and periventricular regions of the brain. It is predominantly a disorder of preterm infants.
 II. **Incidence.** IVH occurs in 30–40% of infants weighing less than 1500 g at birth and in 50–60% of infants weighing less than 1000 g at birth. Although cases of prenatal IVH have been reported, the disorder usually occurs shortly after delivery: 60% in the first 24 hours, 85% in the first 72 hours, and 95% in the first week.
III. **Pathophysiology**
  A. **Subependymal germinal matrix.** The germinal matrix is present in premature infants but dissipates by 40 weeks' gestation. It is a weakly supported, highly vascularized area and is the site of production of neurons and glial cells of the cerebral cortex and basal ganglia.
  B. **Blood pressure changes.** Sudden elevations of arterial pressure cause hemorrhage into the germinal matrix.
  C. **Rupture** through the ependyma causes IVH in 80% of infants with germinal matrix hemorrhage.
  D. **Hydrocephalus.** Acute hydrocephalus may develop as a result of obstruction at the cerebral aqueduct or, less commonly, at the foramen of Monro. A more slowly progressive hydrocephalus sometimes develops as a result of obliterative arachnoiditis in the posterior fossa.
  E. **Periventricular hemorrhagic infarction.** Twenty percent of infants with IVH have associated intraparenchymal hemorrhage into an area of venous infarction and cortical ischemia.
IV. **Risk factors**
  A. **Strong risk factors**
    1. Extreme prematurity.
    2. Birth asphyxia.
    3. Respiratory distress syndrome.
    4. Pneumothorax.

     5. Sudden rise in arterial blood pressure.

  B. Other risk factors include administration of sodium bicarbonate, rapid blood volume expansion, patent ductus arteriosus, elevated central venous pressure, and disturbances of hemostasis.

V. Classification. Any method of classifying IVH must describe the location of the hemorrhage and the size of the ventricles. Numerous systems have been proposed, but the one developed by **Papile** is most often used. Although it was developed for CT scanning, it has also been applied to ultrasonography.

  Grade I. Subependymal, germinal matrix hemorrhage.

  Grade II. Intraventricular hemorrhage without ventricular dilatation.

  Grade III. Intraventricular hemorrhage with ventricular dilatation.

  Grade IV. Intraventricular hemorrhage with parenchymal extension.

VI. Clinical presentation. The clinical presentation is extremely diverse. IVH may be totally asymptomatic, or there may be subtle symptoms, eg, bulging fontanelle, sudden drop in hematocrit, apnea, bradycardia, acidosis, seizures, and changes in muscle tone or level of consciousness. A catastrophic syndrome is characterized by rapid onset of stupor or coma, respiratory abnormalities, seizures, decerebrate posturing, pupils fixed to light, eyes fixed to vestibular stimulation, and flaccid quadriparesis.

  A. Symptoms and signs may mimic those of other common neonatal disorders such as metabolic disturbances, asphyxia, sepsis, or meningitis.

  B. A diagnosis based upon clinical symptoms is inadequate.

    1. Of infants with IVH confirmed by CT scan, only 60% of cases were predicted on the basis of clinical criteria.

    2. Of infants with no IVH documented by CT scan, 25% had been judged to have hemorrhage by clinical criteria.

VII. Diagnosis

  A. Laboratory studies

    1. Examination of cerebrospinal fluid is normal in up to 20% of infants with IVH.

    2. The cerebrospinal fluid usually shows elevated red and white cells, with elevated protein concentration.

    3. It is frequently difficult to distinguish IVH from a "traumatic tap."

    4. Within a few days after hemorrhage, the cerebrospinal fluid becomes xanthochromic, with a decreased glucose concentration.

    5. Diagnosis by analysis of cerebrospinal fluid is often unreliable, and confirmatory imaging techniques are required.

    6. Often the cerebrospinal fluid shows a persistent increase in white cells and protein and a decreased glucose level, therefore making it difficult to rule out meningitis except by negative cultures.

  B. Radiologic studies. Ultrasonography is the usual method of diagnosis. Although CT scanning and MRI are acceptable alternatives, they are more expensive and require transport from the intensive care unit to the imaging device.

VIII. Management

  A. Prevention

    1. Avoidance of premature delivery and perinatal asphyxia will prevent many cases of IVH.

    2. General supportive care of premature infants should be given to maintain a stable acid-base status and avoid fluctuation of arterial and venous blood pressures.

    3. Pharmacologic prevention may be considered. None of the following regimens have been definitely proven to be safe and effective. All are considered experimental and *controversial*.

      a. Phenobarbital

        (1) Mother. Give 500 mg by slow intravenous infusion and then 100 mg orally every 24 hours until delivery or until labor ceases.

        (2) Infant. Give 2 doses of 10 mg/kg intravenously 12 hours apart and then 2.5 mg/kg every 12 hours intravenously, intramuscularly, or orally for 6 days.

    b. Pancuronium, 0.1 mg/kg intravenously as needed for paralysis for the first 72 hours of life.

    c. Indomethacin, 0.1 mg/kg intravenously every 12 hours for a total of 5 doses.

    d. Ethamsylate (125 mg/mL), 0.1 mL/kg intravenously within 2 hours of birth, then every 6 hours for 4 days. (Currently not available in USA.)

    e. Vitamin E. Dosage and route are *controversial.*

    f. Vitamin K, 10 mg intramuscularly, given to the mother every 5 days until delivery if still in labor.

B. Screening ultrasonography of head

    1. All infants weighing less than 1500 g at birth should be screened.

    2. Larger infants should be screened if risk factors are present or if there is evidence of increased intracranial pressure or hydrocephalus.

    3. The optimal age for diagnosis of IVH is 4–7 days, with follow-up at 14 days.

    4. The optimal age for diagnosis of hydrocephalus is 14 days, with follow-up at 2–3 months.

C. Acute hemorrhage

    1. General stabilization and supportive measures

        a. Maintain cerebral perfusion pressure by maintaining an adequate arterial blood pressure.

        b. Maintain normal blood volume and acid-base status.

    2. Follow-up serial imaging (ultrasonography or CT scanning) should be done to detect progressive hydrocephalus.

    Note: A randomized controlled trial of **lumbar punctures** to prevent hydrocephalus following IVH demonstrated no difference between a group of infants undergoing lumbar puncture with supportive care and a control group receiving supportive care only.

D. Hydrocephalus

    1. With mild hydrocephalus, ventricular enlargement will usually cease without additional therapy.

    2. For treatment of moderate or severe posthemorrhagic hydrocephalus, see p 385, **C.2.**

IX. Prognosis. The prognosis depends on the grade of hemorrhage.

    Grade I or II. Tnere is little or no increase in morbidity or mortality rates compared to those in infants with no IVH at 5 years of age.

    Grade III. Up to 75% of patients have severe developmental delays.

    Grade IV. Almost all (90%) die or suffer significant developmental delays.

NEONATAL SEIZURES

I. Definition. A seizure is defined clinically as a paroxysmal alteration in neurologic function, ie, behavioral, motor, or autonomic function, or all three (Volpe, 1989).

II. Incidence. Neonatal seizures are not uncommon. The incidence ranges from 1.5:1000 to 14:1000 live births.

III. Pathophysiology. The neurons within the central nervous system undergo depolarization as a result of inward migration of sodium. Repolarization occurs via efflux of potassium. A seizure occurs when there is excessive depolarization, resulting in excessive synchronous electrical discharge. Volpe has proposed the following 3 possible reasons for excessive depolarization: (1) failure of the sodium-potassium pump owing to a disturbance in energy production; (2) alteration in the neuronal membrane, causing a change in sodium permeability; and (3) a relative excess of excitatory versus inhibitory neurotransmitters. The basic mechanisms of neonatal seizures, however, are unknown.

    There are numerous causes of neonatal seizures but relatively few account for most cases (Table 65–1). Therefore, only common causes of seizures are discussed below.

TABLE 65–1. CAUSES OF NEONATAL SEIZURES

Perinatal asphyxia
Intracranial hemorrhage
  Subarachnoid hemorrhage
  Periventricular or intraventricular hemorrhage
  Subdural hemorrhage
Metabolic abnormalities
  Hypoglycemia
  Hypocalcemia
  Electrolyte disturbances: hypo- and hypernatremia
Amino acid disorders
Infections
  Meningitis
  Encephalitis
  Syphilis, cytomegalovirus infections, toxoplasmosis
  Cerebral abscess
Drug withdrawal
Toxin exposure (particular local anesthetics)
Inherited seizure disorders
  Benign familial epilepsy
  Tuberous sclerosis
  Zellweger's syndrome
Pyridoxine dependency

A. **Perinatal asphyxia** is the most common cause of neonatal seizures. These occur within the first 24 hours of life in most cases and may progress to overt status epilepticus. In premature infants, seizures are of the generalized tonic type, while in full-term infants they are of the multifocal clonic type. Accompanying subtle seizures are usually present in both types.

B. **Intracranial hemorrhage** whether subarachnoid, periventricular, or intraventricular, may occur as a result of hypoxic insults that can lead to neonatal seizures. Subdural hemorrhage, usually a result of trauma, can cause seizures.

  1. **Subarachnoid hemorrhage.** In primary subarachnoid hemorrhage, convulsions often occur on the second postnatal day, and the infant appears quite well during the interictal period.

  2. **Periventricular or intraventricular hemorrhage** arising from the subependymal germinal matrix is accompanied by subtle seizures, decerebrate posturing, or generalized tonic seizures, depending on the severity of the hemorrhage.

  3. **Subdural hemorrhage** over the cerebral convexities leads to focal seizures and focal cerebral signs.

C. **Metabolic disturbances**

  1. **Hypoglycemia** is frequently seen in infants with intrauterine growth retardation (IUGR) and in infants of diabetic mothers (IDMs). The duration of hypoglycemia and the time lapse before initiation of treatment determine the occurrence of seizures. Seizures are less frequent in IDMs, perhaps because of the short duration of hypoglycemia.

  2. **Hypocalcemia** has been noted in low birth weight infants, IDMs, asphyxiated infants, infants with DiGeorge's syndrome, and infants born to mothers with hyperparathyroidism. Hypomagnesemia is a frequent accompanying problem.

  3. **Hyponatremia** occurs because of improper fluid management or as a result of syndrome of inappropriate secretion of antidiuretic hormone (SIADH).

  4. **Hypernatremia** is seen with dehydration, excessive use of sodium bicarbonate, or incorrect dilution of concentrated formula.

  5. **Other metabolic disorders**

   a. **Pyridoxine dependency** leads to seizures resistant to anticonvulsants. Infants with this disorder experience intrauterine convulsions and are born with meconium staining. They resemble asphyxiated infants.

   b. **Amino acid disorders.** Seizures in infants with amino acid disturbances are invariably accompanied by other neurologic disorders. Hyperammonemia and acidosis are commonly present in amino acid disorders.

D. **Infections.** Intracranial infection due to bacterial or nonbacterial agents may be acquired by the neonate in utero, during delivery, or in the immediate perinatal period.

   1. **Bacterial infection.** Meningitis due to **group B streptococcus, *Escherichia coli,*** or ***Listeria monocytogenes*** infection is accompanied by seizures during the first week of life.

   2. **Nonbacterial infection.** Nonbacterial causes such as toxoplasmosis and infection with herpes simplex, cytomegalovirus, rubella, and coxsackie B viruses lead to intracranial infection and seizures.

E. **Drug withdrawal.** Three categories of drugs used by the mother lead to passive addiction and drug withdrawal (sometimes accompanied by seizures) in the infant. These are **analgesics** such as heroin, methadone, and propoxyphene (Darvon); **sedative-hypnotics** such as secobarbital; and **alcohol.**

F. **Toxins.** Inadvertent injection of local anesthetics into the fetus at the time of delivery (paracervical, pudendal, or saddle block anesthesia) may cause generalized tonic-clonic seizures. Mothers often notice the absence of pain relief during delivery.

IV. **Clinical presentation.** It is important to understand that **seizures in the neonate are different from those seen in older children.** The differences are perhaps due to the neuroanatomic and neurophysiologic developmental status of the newborn infant. In the neonatal brain, glial proliferation, neuronal migration, establishment of axonal and dendritic contacts, and myelin deposition are incomplete. **Four types of seizures,** based on clinical presentation, are recognized: subtle, clonic, tonic, and myoclonic.

   1. **Subtle seizures.** These seizures are not clearly clonic, tonic, or myoclonic and are more common in premature than in full-term infants. Subtle seizures are more commonly associated with an electroencephalographic seizure in premature infants than in full-term infants. They consist of tonic horizontal deviation of the eyes with or without jerking; eyelid blinking or fluttering; sucking, smacking, or drooling; "swimming," "rowing," or "pedaling" movements; and apneic spells. Apnea accompanied by electroencephalographic abnormalities has been called **convulsive apnea.** It is differentiated from nonconvulsive apnea, which is due to sepsis, lung disease, or metabolic abnormalities, by the absence of electroencephalographic abnormalities. Furthermore, during nonconvulsive apnea of 20 seconds' duration or longer, the heart rate decreases by 40% or more within 8 seconds, whereas in convulsive apnea, the heart rate does not change even when apnea lasts longer than 20 seconds. Apnea as a manifestation of seizures is usually accompanied or preceded by other subtle manifestations. In premature infants, apnea is unlikely to be a manifestation of seizures.

   2. **Clonic seizures** are more common in full-term infants than in premature infants and are commonly associated with an electroencephalographic seizure. There are 2 types of clonic seizures.

   a. **Focal seizures.** Well-localized, rhythmic, slow jerking movements involving the face and upper or lower extremities on one side of the body or the neck or trunk on one side of the body. Infants are usually unconscious during or after the seizures.

   b. **Multifocal seizures.** Several body parts seize in a sequential, non-Jacksonian fashion (eg, left arm jerking followed by right leg jerking).

   3. **Tonic seizures** occur primarily in premature infants. Two types of tonic seizures are seen.

    a. **Focal seizures.** Sustained posturing of a limb or asymmetric posturing of the trunk or neck, or both. Commonly associated with an electroencephalographic seizure.

    b. **Generalized seizures.** Most commonly, a tonic extension of both upper and lower extremities (as in decerebrate posturing) but may also present with tonic flexion of upper extremities with extension of the lower extremities (as in decorticate posturing). Uncommon to see electroencephalographic seizure disorders.

  4. **Myoclonic seizures** are seen in both full-term and premature infants and are characterized by single or multiple synchronous jerks. Three types of myoclonic seizures are seen.

    a. **Focal seizures.** Typically involve the flexor muscles of an upper extremity and not commonly associated with electroencephalographic seizure activity.

    b. **Multifocal seizures.** Asynchronous twitching of several parts of the body and not commonly associated with electroencephalographic seizure activity.

    c. **Generalized seizures.** Bilateral jerks of flexion of the upper and sometimes the lower extremities. More commonly associated with electroencephalographic seizure activity.

Note: It is important to distinguish **jitteriness** from seizures. Jitteriness is not accompanied by abnormal eye movements, and movements cease on application of passive flexion. In jitteriness, movements are stimulus-sensitive and are not jerky.

V. Diagnosis

  A. **History.** While it is often difficult to obtain a thorough history in infants transported to tertiary care facilities from other hospitals, the physician must make a concerted effort to elicit pertinent historical data.

    1. **Family history.** A positive family history of neonatal seizures is usually obtained in cases of metabolic errors and benign familial neonatal convulsions.

    2. **Maternal drug history** is critical in cases of narcotic withdrawal syndrome.

    3. **Delivery.** Details of the delivery provide information regarding maternal analgesia, the mode and nature of delivery, the fetal intrapartum status, and the resuscitative measures employed. Information regarding maternal infections during pregnancy point toward an infectious basis for seizures in an infant.

  B. **Physical examination**

    1. A thorough general physical examination should precede a well-planned neurologic examination. Determine the following:

      a. Gestational age.

      b. Blood pressure.

      c. Presence of skin lesions.

      d. Presence of hepatosplenomegaly.

    2. **Neurologic evaluation.** Neurologic evaluation should include assessment of the level of alertness, cranial nerves, motor function, primary neonatal reflexes, and sensory function. Some of the specific features to look for are the size and "feel" of the fontanelle, retinal hemorrhages, chorioretinitis, pupillary size and reaction to light, extraocular movements, changes in muscle tone, and the status of primary reflexes.

    3. **Notation of seizure pattern.** When seizures are noted, they should be described in detail, including site of onset, spread, nature, duration, and level of consciousness. Recognition of subtle seizures requires special attention.

  C. **Laboratory studies.** In selecting and prioritizing laboratory tests, one must utilize the information obtained by history taking and physical examination and look for common and treatable causes.

    1. **Serum chemistries.** Estimations of serum glucose, calcium, sodium, blood urea nitrogen and magnesium and blood gas levels must be performed. They may reveal the abnormality causing the seizures.

    2. **Spinal fluid examination.** Evaluation of the cerebrospinal fluid is essential,

since the consequences of delayed treatment or nontreatment of bacterial meningitis are grave.

3. **Metabolic disorders.** (See also Chap 59.) With a family history of neonatal convulsions, a peculiar odor about the infant, milk intolerance, acidosis, alkalosis, or seizures not responsive to anticonvulsants, other metabolic causes should be investigated.

   a. **Blood ammonia levels** should be checked.

   b. **Amino acids** should be measured in urine and plasma. The urine should be tested for reducing substances.

      (1) **Urea cycle disorders.** Respiratory alkalosis is seen as a result of direct stimulation of the respiratory center by ammonia.

      (2) **Maple syrup urine disease.** With 2,4-dinitrophenylhydrazine (2,4-DNPH) testing of urine, a fluffy yellow precipitate will be seen in cases of maple syrup urine disease (see Table 59–5).

D. **Radiologic studies**

   1. **Ultrasonography of the head** is performed to rule out intraventricular or periventricular hemorrhage.

   2. **CT scanning of the head** provides detailed information regarding intracranial disease. CT scanning is helpful in looking for evidence of infarction, hemorrhage, calcification, and cerebral malformations. Recent experience with this technique suggests that valuable information is obtained in term infants with seizures, especially when seizures are asymmetric.

E. **Other studies**

   1. **Electroencephalography.** EEGs obtained during a seizure will be abnormal. Interictal EEGs may be normal. However, an order to obtain an ictal EEG should not delay other diagnostic and therapeutic steps. The diagnostic value of EEG is greater when it is obtained in the first few days, since diagnostic patterns indicative of unfavorable prognosis disappear thereafter. Electroencephalography is valuable in confirming the presence of seizures when manifestations are subtle or when neuromuscular paralyzing agents have been given. EEGs are of prognostic significance in full-term infants with recognized seizures. For proper interpretation of EEGs, it is important to know the clinical status of the infant (including the sleep state) and any medications given.

VI. **Management.** Since repeated seizures may lead to brain injury, **urgent treatment is indicated. The method of treatment depends on the cause.**

A. **Hypoglycemia.** Hypoglycemic infants with seizures should receive 10% dextrose in water, 2–4 mL/kg intravenously, followed by 6–8 mg/kg/min by continuous intravenous infusion.

B. **Hypocalcemia** is treated with slow intravenous infusion of calcium gluconate (see dosage and other pharmacologic information in Chap 73). If serum magnesium levels are low (< 1.52 meq/L), magnesium should be given.

C. **Anticonvulsant therapy.** Conventional anticonvulsant treatment is employed when no underlying metabolic cause is found. Loading doses of phenobarbital and phenytoin control 70% of neonatal seizures.

   1. **Phenobarbital** is usually given first (see Chap 73 for dosage and other pharmacologic information). Neither gestational age nor birth weight seems to influence the loading or maintenance dose of phenobarbital. When phenobarbital alone fails to control seizures, another agent is employed. Gilman and associates (1989) found that sequentially administered phenobarbital controlled seizures in term and preterm newborns in 77% of cases. If seizures are not controlled at a serum phenobarbital level of 40 μg/mL, they recommend administering a second agent (eg, phenytoin [Dilantin]).

   2. **Phenytoin (Dilantin)** is employed next by many practitioners (see dosage and other pharmacologic information in Chap 73).

   3. **Diazepam (Valium)** has not been used extensively in control of neonatal seizures, and when utilized as a third agent, it did not improve seizure control. However, when used as a continuous intravenous infusion, 0.3 mg/kg/h,

it was quite effective in controlling seizures in 8 neonates, all of whom became somnolent but did not require artificial ventilation.

4. **Lorazepam (Ativan)** given intravenously has been quite effective and safe, even when repeated 4–6 times in a 24-hour period (see dosage and other pharmacologic information in Chap 73).

5. **Paraldehyde,** given rectally, has been used as an effective anticonvulsant (see Chap 73 for dosage and other pharmacologic information).

D. **Duration of anticonvulsant therapy.** The optimal duration of anticonvulsant therapy has not been established. While some recommend continuation of phenobarbital for a prolonged period, others recommend stopping it after seizures have been absent for 2 weeks.

VII. **Prognosis.** Since 1969, there has been some improvement in the neurologic outcome of infants experiencing seizures, but morbidity and mortality rates are still about 50%. As would be expected, the prognosis varies with the cause. Infants with hypocalcemic convulsions have an excellent prognosis, while those with seizures due to congenital malformations have a poor prognosis. Symptomatic hypoglycemia has a 50% risk of death or complications, while central nervous system infection carries a risk of 70%. Asphyxiated infants with seizures have a 60% chance of a poor outcome. Seventeen percent of patients with neonatal seizures have recurrent seizures later in life.

NEURAL TUBE DEFECTS

I. **Definition.** Neural tube defects (NTDs) are malformations of the developing brain and spinal cord, including:

A. **Open lesions** in chronological order of occurrence during the 3rd to 4th weeks of gestation.

1. **Craniorachischisis totalis** (neural plate-like structure without skeletal or dermal covering due to *complete* failure of neural tube closure).

2. **Anencephaly** (hemorrhagic and degenerated neural tissue is exposed through uncovered cranial opening extending from the lamina terminalis to the foramen magnum due to failure of *anterior* neural tube closure). Infants with anencephaly have a frog-like appearance when viewed face on.

3. **Myeloschisis** (rachischisis; spinal cord is exposed posteriorly without skeletal or dermal covering due to failure of *posterior* neural tube closure).

B. **Closed lesions** in chronological order of occurrence during the 4th to 7th weeks of gestation.

1. **Encephalocele** (herniation of brain tissue outside the cranial cavity due to mesodermal defect occurring at the time of or shortly after *anterior* neural tube closure). Approximately 80% occur in the occipital region.

2. **Myelomeningocele** (protrusion of spinal cord into a sac on the back through deficient axial skeleton with variable dermal covering). Approximately 80% occur in the lumbar region.

3. **Spina bifida occulta** are disorders of caudal neural tube which are covered by intact skin. Posterior dysraphic disturbances include myelocystocele (cystic dilation of central canal), diastematomyelia-diplomyelia (bifid spinal cord ± separation by a bony, cartilaginous or fibrous septum), meningocele (cystic dilation of the meninges not involving the spinal cord), lipomeningocele (cystic dilation with infiltration of fibro-fatty tissue), subcutaneous lipoma or tumors (eg, teratoma), dermal sinus with intradural extension, and tethered cord. Anterior dysraphic disturbances include neurenteric cyst, anterior meningocele, and the caudal regression syndrome.

II. **Incidence**

A. **Worldwide.** Approximately 1/1000 live births. Spina bifida occulta, anencephaly, and myelomeningocele are the more frequently encountered NTDs.

B. **Geographic variation, sex, race, and social class.**

1. East-west gradient.

2. Increased in whites and females.

3. Increased in infants of particularly young or particularly old mothers of lower socioeconomic class.

C. 95% of children with NTDs are born to couples with no family history.

D. Risk of occurrence is approximately

1. 0.3 to 1% if a close relative (sibling, niece, nephew) of either parent is affected.

2. 1% in women with insulin-dependent diabetes mellitus.

3. 1% in women with seizure disorders being treated with valproic acid or carbamazepine.

4. 3% with one affected parent.

E. Recurrence risk is:

1. 2–3% with one affected sibling.

2. Approximately 4–6% with two affected siblings.

F. Folic acid supplementation significantly reduces the occurrence and recurrence of NTDs.

III. Recognized causes of NTDs

A. Chromosome abnormalities.

1. Trisomy 13.

2. Trisomy 18.

3. Triploidy.

4. Unbalanced translocation.

5. Ring chromosome.

B. Single mutant genes.

1. Autosomal recessive (Meckel syndrome).

2. Autosomal dominant (median cleft face syndrome).

C. Teratogens.

1. Nitrates (cured meat, blighted potatoes, salicylates, and hard water).

2. Antifolates: aminopterin, methotrexate, phenytoin, phenobarbital, primidone, carbamazepine, and valproic acid.

3. Thalidomide.

4. Hyperglycemia in infants of diabetic mothers.

D. Nutritional and vitamin deficiency.

1. Folic acid.

2. Vitamin B12.

3. Zinc.

E. Maternal hyperthermia.

F. Multifactorial inheritance is involved in anencephaly, encephalocele, myelomeningocele, and meningocele.

G. Unknown causes.

IV. Management issues in infants with anencephaly.

A. Approximately 75% are stillborn, and the remainder die within the first two weeks of birth.

B. Supportive care: warmth, comfort, and enteral nutrition.

V. Management issues in infants with encephalocele

A. Look for associated malformations. Several syndromes with encephalocele are inherited in an autosomal recessive manner. Meckel's syndrome: occipital encephalocele, microcephaly, microphthalmia, cleft lip and palate, polydactyly, polycystic kidneys, ambiguous genitalia, and other deformities.

B. Prompt neurosurgical intervention is indicated to prevent ulceration and infection, except in those with massive lesions and marked microcephaly.

1. The encephalocele and its contents are excised as the brain tissue within is usually infarcted and distorted.

2. Operation can be deferred if adequate skin covering is present.

C. Ventriculoperitoneal shunt (VPS) placement may be required at a later time because as many as 50% of cases have secondary hydrocephalus.

D. Developmental deficits are determined by the extent of herniation; cerebral hemispheres from both sides or one side, cerebellum, and even brain stem can be involved.

1. **Visual deficits** are common with occipital encephalocele.
2. **Motor and intellectual deficits** are found in approximately 50% of patients.

VI. Management issues in patients with myelomeningocele: Team approach including primary care physician, geneticist, genetic counselor, neonatologist, urologist, neurosurgeon, orthopedic surgeon, and social worker.

A. **Correlate motor, sensory, sphincter function, and reflexes to functional level of lesion (Table 65–2).**
   1. Extent of neurologic dysfunction correlates with the level of the spinal cord lesion.
   2. Paraplegia *below the level of the defect.*
   3. Presence of the anal wink and anal sphincter tone suggests functioning sacral spinal segments.

B. **Closure of the back lesion within 24 or 48 hours** to prevent infection and further loss of function.

C. **Hydrocephalus is often noncommunicative secondary to Arnold-Chiari malformation** of the foramen magnum and upper cervical canal, with resultant downward displacement of the medulla, pons, and cerebellum and obstruction of cerebrospinal fluid.
   1. Risk of hydrocephalus is 95% for infants with thoracolumbar, lumbar, and lumbosacral lesions; 63% for those with occipital, cervical, thoracic, or sacral lesions.
   2. In most cases, hydrocephalus is not evident until after closure of the myelomeningocele, and placement of a VPS may be required at a later date.
   3. Aggressive treatment with early VPS placement may improve cognitive function.
   4. Serial ultrasound scans are necessary to follow progression of hydrocephalus because ventricular dilation may occur without rapid head growth or signs of increased intracranial pressure. The hydrocephalus usually becomes clinically overt two to three weeks after birth.
   5. Despite treatment of the myelomeningocele and hydrocephalus, approximately 50% of these infants may still succumb to death from aspiration, laryngeal stridor, and apnea attributable to the hindbrain anomaly.

D. **Urinary tract dysfunction** is one of the major causes of death after the first year of life.

TABLE 65–2. CORRELATION BETWEEN LEVEL OF MYELOMENINGOCELE, LEVEL OF CUTANEOUS SENSATION, SPHINCTER FUNCTION, REFLEXES, AND POTENTIAL FOR AMBULATION

Level of Lesion	Innervation	Cutaneous Sensation (Pin Prick)	Sphincter Function	Reflexes	Ambulation Potential
Thoracolumbar	T12–L2	Groin (L1) Anterior upper thigh (L2)	—	—	Full braces. Wheel-chair bound.
Lumbar	L3–L4	Anterior lower thigh and knee (L3) Medial leg (L4)	—	Knee jerk	May ambulate with braces and crutches.
Lumbosacral	L5–S1	Lateral leg & medial foot (L5) Sole of foot (S1)	—	Ankle jerk	May ambulate with or without short leg braces.
Sacral	S2–S4	Posterior leg and thigh (S2) Middle of buttock (S3) Medial buttock (S4)	Bladder and rectal function	Anal wink	May ambulate without braces.

Voluntary muscle movements are difficult to elicit in newborns with myelomeningocele and are therefore not helpful during initial evaluation. Furthermore, motor examination may be distorted initially by reversible spinal cord dysfunction above the level of the actual defect induced by exposure of the open cord.

1. More than 85% of myelomeningoceles located above S2 are associated with neurogenic bladder dysfunction, with urinary incontinence and ureteral reflux.
2. Without proper management, hydronephrosis develops with progressive scarring and destruction of the kidneys. Many of these infants succumb to urosepsis.
3. Renal ultrasound and voiding cystourethrogram may identify patients who could benefit from anticholinergic medication, clean and intermittent catheterization, prophylactic antibiotics, or early surgical intervention of the urinary tract.
4. Other associated renal anomalies: renal agenesis, horseshoe kidney, and ureteral duplications.

E. Orthopedic complications.
1. The lower extremities lack innervation and become atrophied.
2. Deformities of the foot, knee, hip, and spine are common as a result of muscle imbalance, abnormal in utero positioning, or teratologic factors.
3. Hip dislocation or subluxation is usually evident within the first year of life, especially in patients with mid-lumbar myelominingocele.
4. Treatment of orthopedic abnormalities takes place as soon as there is sufficient healing of the back wound.
5. Physical therapist assists with proper positioning of the extremities to minimize contractures and to maximize function.

F. Outcome of aggressive therapy (Table 65–2)
1. Overall mortality rate is now < 15% by 3 to 7 years of age.
2. Infants with sacral lesions have essentially no mortality.
3. Majority of children with lumbar myelomeningocele score within the normal range on intelligence and achievement tests, with the greatest and possibly progressive deficits on performance IQ, arithmetic achievement, and visual-motor integration, while keeping pace on reading and spelling.
4. IQ > 80 is found in essentially all patients with lesions below S1.
5. Approximately 50% of survivors with thoracolumbar lesions have IQ > 80.
6. Cognitive function is improved in the presence of favorable socioeconomic and environmental factors.

VII. Management issues in patients with spina bidifa occulta
A. Neonatal features.
1. Presence of spina bifida occulta is suggested by overlying abnormal collections of hair, hemangioma, pigmented macule, aplasia cutis congenita, skin tag, subcutaneous mass, cutaneous dimples or tracts.

B. Clinical presentations usually start later in infancy.
1. Delay in development of sphincter control.
2. Delay in walking.
3. Development of a foot deformity.
4. Recurrent meningitis.
5. Sudden deterioration may represent vascular insufficiency produced by tension on a tethered cord, angulation of the cord around fibrous or related structures, or cord compression from a tumor or cyst.

C. Diagnosis.
1. **Ultrasonography** is useful for screening.
2. **Metrizamide CT myelography and magnetic resonance imaging (MRI)** provide superior anatomical details. Advantages of MRI are that contrast is not needed and the infants are not exposed to radiation.

D. Surgical correction should take place in the newborn period before the onset of symptoms.

E. Surgical release of a tethered cord or decompression of the spinal cord within 48 hours of sudden deterioration may completely or partially reverse recently acquired deficits.

VIII. Diagnosis of NTDs
A. Prenatal screen using maternal serum alpha-fetoprotein (AFP) at 14–16

weeks of gestation. Elevated levels (≥ 2.5 multiples of the median corrected for gestational age) are indicative of open NTDs at a sensitivity of 90–100%, specificity of 96%, a negative predictive value of 99–100%, but a low positive predictive value.

  B. **Prenatal diagnosis.** Documentation of an elevated maternal serum AFP is followed by:

    1. Measurement of the **amniotic fluid acetylcholinesterase (AChE)** and **AFP** levels. If amniotic fluid AChE is elevated, prenatal diagnosis of open NTD is confirmed if the amniotic fluid AFP is also elevated. Amniocentesis is usually done at between 16–18 weeks of gestation, although it can technically be done as early as 14 weeks of gestation.

    2. The detection rate for anencephaly and open spina bifida is 100% when results of amniotic fluid AChE and AFP are combined, with a false-positive rate of only 0.04%.

    3. In skilled hands, a detailed ultrasonogram can be extremely sensitive and specific (close to 100% for both) at detection of NTDs. Ultrasonography should also be done when only the maternal serum AFP is elevated, even if the amniotic fluid AFP and AChE are normal, because there can be other major congenital defects besides NTDs.

IX. Prevention of NTDs.

  A. The **British Medical Research Council (MRC)** in 1991 demonstrated that **high-dose folate (4 mg daily), but not multivitamin without folate, reduced the recurrence risk of NTD by 72%.**

  B. Based on results from MRC, the **National Institute of Child Health and Human Development (NICHD)** recommends that

    1. "*Women who have had one or more affected offspring with NTD* should consume 4.0 mg of folic acid per day, from at least 1 month before conception through the first 3 months of pregnancy."

    2. Multivitamins should not be used because excess vitamin A and D would be ingested in taking a large enough dose to reach a dose of 4 mg of folic acid.

    3. Consumption of high-dose folic acid must be under a physician's supervision because there is still little information regarding its long-term effects and symptoms of pernicious anemia may be obscured, resulting in serious neurologic damage.

    4. Because 4 mg of folic acid did not prevent all NTDs in the MRC study, patients should be cautioned that folic acid supplementation does not preclude the need for counseling or consideration of prenatal testing for NTDs.

  C. The **American Academy of Pediatrics Committee on Genetics** has endorsed the **United States Public Health Services** recommendation that

    1. "*All women* of childbearing age in the United States who are capable of becoming pregnant should consume 0.4 mg of folic acid per day for the purpose of reducing their risk of having a pregnancy affected with spina bifida or other NTDs."

  D. **Sources of folic acid.**

    1. **Dietary.**

      a. The average diet in the United States contains 0.2 mg of folate, which is less bioavailable than folic acid.

      b. Folate intake ≥ 0.4 mg per day can be achieved thorough careful selection of folate-rich foods.

      c. Some breakfast cereals are fortified with folic acid.

    2. **Supplementation.**

      a. Folic acid is available over the counter in dosages up to 0.8 mg.

      b. Folic acid is also available by prescription in 1-mg tablets.

      c. Prenatal vitamins contain 0.8 or 1 mg of folic acid.

  E. Current epidemiological and biochemical evidence suggest that NTD is not primarily due to folate insufficiency but arises from changes in the metabolism of folate and possibly B_{12} in predisposed women. Amniotic fluid vitamin B_{12} levels have been found to be lower in pregnancies affected by NTD (Weekes et al, 1992).

F. Intestinal hydrolysis of dietary folate is not impaired in mothers who have had infants with NTD, although the response curve to a folate-enriched meal appears to differ significantly from mothers who have not had infants with NTD (Bower, 1993).

REFERENCES

Bergman I, Painter MJ, Crumine PK: Neonatal seizures. *Semin Perinatol* 1982;**6**:54.

Bower C et al: Absorption of pteroylpolyglutamates in mothers of infants with neural tube defects. *Br J Nutr* 1993;**69**:827.

Bower C, Stanley FJ, Nicol DJ: Maternal folate status and the risk for neural tube defects. The role of dietary folate. *Ann. NY Acad Science* 1993;**678**:146.

Brock DJH, Barron L, van Heyningen V: Prenatal diagnosis of neural tube defects with monoclonal antibody specific for acetylcholinesterase. *Lancet* 1985;**21**:5.

Committee on Genetics: Folic acid for the prevention of neural tube defects. *Pediatrics* 1993;**92**:493.

Dansky LV, Rosenblatt DS, Andermann E: Mechanisms of teratogenesis: folic acid and antiepileptic therapy. *Neurology* 1992;**42(suppl 5)**:32.

Dimmick JE, Kalousek DK: *Developmental pathology of the embryo & fetus.* Lippincott, 1992.

Donn SM, Goldstein GW, Roloff DW: Prevention of intraventricular hemorrhage with phenobarbital therapy: Now what? *Pediatrics* 1986;**77**:779.

Dykes FD et al: Posthemorrhagic hydrocephalus in high-risk preterm infants: Natural history, management and long-term outcome. *J Pediatr* 1989;**114**:611.

Dykes FD et al: Intraventricular hemorrhage: A prospective evaluation of etiopathogenesis. *Pediatrics* 1980;**66**:42.

Fraser RK et al: The unstable hip and mid-lumbar myelomeningocele. *J of Bone and Joint Surg* British Volume, 1992;**74(1)**:143.

Gilman JT et al: Rapid sequential phenobarbital treatment of neonatal seizures. *Pediatrics* 1989;**83**:674.

Glick PL et al: Management of ventriculomegaly in the fetus. *J Pediatr* 1984;**105**:97.

Hudgins RJ et al: Natural history of fetal ventriculomegaly. *Pediatrics* 1988;**82**:692.

Laurence KM et al: Double blind randomized controlled trial of folate treatment before conception to prevent recurrence of neural tube defects. *Br Med J* 1981;**282**:1509.

Lazzara A et al: Clinical predictability of intraventricular hemorrhage in preterm infants. *Pediatrics* 1980;**65**:30.

Lemire RJ: Neural tube defects: Clinical correlations. *Clin Neurosurg* 1983;**30**:165.

Lemire RJ et al: Neural tube defects. *JAMA* 1988;**259(4)**:558.

Main DM, Mennuti MT: Neural tube defects: Issues in prenatal diagnosis and counseling. *Obstet Gynecol* 1986;**67**:1.

McCullough DC, Balzer-Martin LA: Current prognosis in overt neonatal hydrocephalus. *J Neurosurg* 1982;**57**:378.

Michejda M, Queenan JT, McCullough D: Present status of intrauterine treatment of hydrocephalus and its future. *Am J Obstet Gynecol* 1986;**155**:873.

Mills JL, Raymond E: Effects of recent research on recommendations for periconceptional folate supplement use. *Ann. NY Acad Science* 1993;**678**:137.

Morrow JD, Wachs TD: Infants with myelomeningocele: Visual recognition memory and sensorimotor abilities. *Devel Med and Child Neur* 1992;**34(6)**:488.

MRC Vitamin Study Research Group. Prevention of neural tube defects: Results of the Medical Research Council Vitamin Study. *Lancet* 1991;**338**:131.

Myianthopoulos NC, Melnick M: Studies in neural tube defects: Epidemiologic and etiologic aspects. *Am J Med Genet* 1987;**26**:738.

Noetzel MJ: Myelomeningocele: Current concepts of management. *Clin Perinatol* 1989;**16(2)**:311.

Painter MJ, Berman I, Crumine PK: Neonatal seizures. *Pediatr Clin North Am* 1986;**63**:91.

Philip AGS et al: Intraventricular hemorrhage in preterm infants: Declining incidence in the 1980s. *Pediatrics* 1989;**84**:797.

Poland RL: Vitamin E for prevention of perinatal intracranial hemorrhage. *Pediatrics* 1990;**85**:865.

Rasmussen AG et al: A comparison of amniotic fluid alpha-fetoprotein and acetylcholinesterase in the prenatal diagnosis of open neural tube defects and anterior abdominal wall defects. *Prenat Diagn* 1993;**13**:93.

Recommendations for the use of folic acid to reduce the number of cases of spina bifida and other neural tube defects. *MMWR* 1992;**41(RR-14)**:1.

Robbin M et al: Elevated levels of amniotic fluid a-fetoprotein: Sonographic evaluation. *Radiology* 1993;**188**:165.

Sandovnick AD et al: Use of genetic counseling services for neural tube defects. *Am J Med Genet* 1987;**26**:811.

Schorah CJ et al: Possible abnormalities of folate and vitamin B12 metabolism associated with neural tube defects. *Ann. NY Acad Science* 1993;**678**:81.

Smithells RW et al: Further experience of vitamin supplementation for the prevention of neural tube defect recurrences. *Lancet* 1983;**1**:1027.

Verget RG et al: Primary prevention of neural tube defects with folic acid supplementation: Cuban experience. *Prenat Diagn* 1990;**10**:149.

Vintzileos AM, Ingardia CT, Nochinson DJ: Congenital hydrocephalus: Review and protocol for perinatal management. *Obstet Gynecol* 1983;**62**:539.

Volpe JJ: Intraventricular hemorrhage and brain injury in the premature infant. *Pediatr Clin North Am* 1989;**2**:361.

Volpe JJ: Neonatal seizures: Current concepts and revised classification. *Pediatrics* 1989;**84**:422.

Volpe JJ: *Neurology of the Newborn, Second Edition.* Saunders, 1987.

Warkany J: Hydrocephalus. Chap 25 in: *Conqenital Malformations.* Year Book, 1971.

Weekes EW et al: Nutrient levels in amniotic fluid from women with normal and neural tube defect pregnancies. *Biol Neo* 1992;**81(1)**:226.

Wills KE et al: Intelligence and acehivement in children with myelomeningocele. *J of Ped Psychol* 1990;**15(2)**:161.

66 Perinatal Asphyxia

I. **Definition.** Perinatal asphyxia exists when an antepartum event, labor, or a birth process diminishes the oxygen supply to the fetus, causing decreased fetal or newborn heart rate, which results in impairment of exchange of respiratory gases, oxygen, and carbon dioxide, and inadequate perfusion of the tissues and major organs. The **American Academy of Pediatrics and the American College of Obstetricians and Gynecologists** defined 4 clinical criteria in the *1992 Guidelines for Perinatal Care,* all of which must be present to diagnose perinatal asphyxia: (1) profound metabolic or mixed acidemia (pH < 7.00) on umbilical cord arterial blood sample; (2) persistence of an Apgar score of 0 to 3 for > 5 minutes; (3) clinical neurologic sequelae in the immediate neonatal period to include seizures, hypotonia, coma, or hypoxic-ischemic encephalopathy (HIE); and (4) evidence of multiorgan system dysfunction in the immediate neonatal period (see **V.D.,** below).

II. **Incidence.** Consensus on the incidence of perinatal asphyxia has been difficult to arrive at because of the non-uniform clinical criteria on which different institutions base their definitions. In a 1987 Finland study by Rantakallio, the overall incidence was 12.7% (diagnosis based on blood gas analysis and whether extra oxygen or assisted ventilation was needed, and including newborns with a low Apgar score alone). Cerebral palsy (CP) in term infants develops in 1 to 2 per 1000 live births and less than 10% of this subgroup is associated with evidence of perinatal asphyxia.

III. **Pathophysiology**

A. **Disorders associated with perinatal asphyxia**

1. **Antepartum period.** Maternal diabetes, preeclampsia, fetal malformation, postmaturity, prematurity, and intrauterine growth retardation.

2. **Intrapartum period.** Breech presentation, meconium staining, cephalopelvic disproportion, and cord compression.

3. **Other causes** include uterine malformation, precipitous labor, abruptio placentae, maternal shock, cord prolapse, and infection.

4. **Postnatal period.** Severe pulmonary disease, congenital heart disease, large patent ductus arteriosus, severe recurrent apneic spells, and sepsis with cardiovascular collapse.

B. **Pathophysiologic events** following perinatal asphyxia (Fig 66–1).

1. Altered carbohydrate and energy metabolism results in profound **disturbance of respiration and oxidative metabolism,** regional alterations in high energy compounds (eg, ATP), accumulation of extracellular potassium and intracellular calcium, intracellular **acidosis,** accumulation of hydrogen ions, steady decrease of pH to levels below 7.10, **decreasing heart rate and cardiac output,** and **altered neurotransmitters.** Metabolic acidosis develops as a result of anaerobic glycolysis with production of pyruvate and lactate.

2. **Loss of vascular autoregulation.** Initial circulatory effects of perinatal asphyxia include redistribution of cardiac output so that a larger proportion enters the brain. Cerebral blood flow is increased due to loss of cerebrovascular autoregulation. Within the brain, blood is focused to the brainstem at the expense of higher cerebral structures such as the cortex. In the cortex, end fields of perfusion are most susceptible to ischemia. If the asphyxia is severe, later effects include diminution of cardiac output, hypotension, and a corresponding fall in cerebral blood flow.

3. **Toxic effect of synaptically released excitatory amino acids.** Synaptic

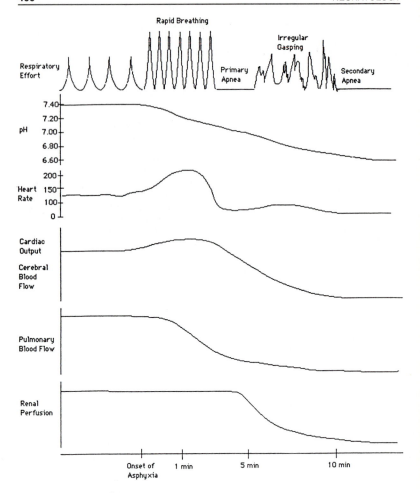

FIGURE 66–1. Pathophysiologic events following perinatal asphyxia.

release of glutamate, or failure of the glutamate re-uptake system in the face of ATP deficiency associated with oxygen deprivation, results in accumulation of extracellular glutamate, which causes immediate and delayed neuronal death. **Immediate neuronal death (minutes)** is due to sodium, chloride, and water influx, which results in an osmolar load and eventual lysis of the cell membrane. Cells can partially recover from immediate neuronal death then die some hours or days later. Timely intervention during recovery can allow rescue of some cells that would otherwise die. **Delayed neuronal death (hours)** is due to calcium influx. High intracellular free calcium results in activation of undesirable second messengers and enzymes, generation of free radicals, and disturbance of oxidative phosphorylation.

C. **Clinical events**

1. **The initial response** is hypertension and hyperpnea, followed by primary apnea, then gasping attempts to breathe.

2. **Unresolved hypoxia** leads to secondary apnea, bradycardia, and shock. In

general, brain injury occurs only when the asphyxia is severe enough to impair cerebral blood flow.

3. **Diminished cerebral blood flow** and loss of oxygen supply results in vessel injury.

4. **Cerebrovascular injury** leads to **cerebral edema.**

5. **Cerebrovascular hemorrhage** occurs upon reperfusion of ischemic and damaged areas of the brain. However, following prolonged and severe asphyxia, local tissue recirculation may not be restored upon reoxygenation due to collapsed capillaries in the presence of severe cytotoxic edema.

D. **Pathologic findings**

1. **Cortical changes.** Cortical edema, with flattening of cerebral convolutions, is followed by cortical necrosis until finally a healing phase results in gradual cortical atrophy. Cortical atrophy, if severe, may result in **microcephaly.**

2. **Other pathologic findings** common in term infants exposed to oxygen deprivation include selective neuronal necrosis (involving the Sommer's sector of the hippocampus and the Purkinje cells of the cerebellum), status marmoratus of the basal ganglia (the marbled appearance is due to the characteristic feature of hypermyelination), and parasagittal cerebral injury (bilateral and usually symmetrical, with the parietal-occipital regions affected more often than those regions anteriorly).

3. **Periventricular leukomalacia (PVL)** is necrosis of periventricular white matter, which has a predilection for premature infants. The incidence increases with length of survival and severity of postnatal cardiorespiratory disturbances; 25% of cases of PLV are complicated by hemorrhage into the lesion. PVL involving the pyramidal tracts usually results in spastic diplegic or quadriplegic cerebral palsy.

4. **Porencephaly or hydrocephaly** may follow cortical necrosis, intraventricular hemorrhage, or intracerebral hemorrhage.

5. **Brain-stem damage** is seen in the most severe cases of hypoxic-ischemic brain injury and results in permanent respiratory impairment.

IV. **Clinical presentation**

A. **Assessment at delivery.** Low Apgar scores identify newborns who need resuscitation and by themselves do not correlate with long-term outcome. The presence of meconium in amniotic fluid and Apgar scores have been inappropriately equated with "fetal distress" and "asphyxia" respectively, and both will be deleted in the 1993 revision of *International Classification of Diseases.*

B. **Syndrome of hypoxic-Ischemic encephalopathy.** This occurs in asphyxiated infants with Apgar scores of 0–3 for more than 5 minutes, onset of seizures at 12–24 hours of life, and onset of motor abnormalities by the end of the first week. Weakness in the full-term infant can be either a hemiparesis or involve the proximal limbs, upper more than lower. Weakness in the premature infant involves the lower limbs.

1. **Mild:** hyperalertness, uninhibited reflexes, sympathetic overactivity (duration of less than 24 hours).

2. **Moderate:** lethargy or stupor, hypotonia, suppressed primitive reflexes, seizures.

3. **Severe:** coma, flaccid tone, suppressed brain-stem function, seizures, increased intracranial pressure.

C. **Birth injury.** A diagnosis of hypoxic-ischemic encephalopathy secondary to birth injury is made when there is clinical evidence of birth trauma (eg, subdural hematoma) coexistent with Apgar scores of 0–3 within the first 5 minutes of life.

V. **Diagnosis.** None of the abnormalities listed below predict outcome well single-handedly. It is the occurrence of a sequence of indicators that carries predictive weight.

A. **Antepartum diagnosis**

1. **Fetal heart rate (FHR) monitoring.** Fetal bradycardia and late decelerations indicate a lack of oxygen supply to the fetus and suppression of the fetal myocardium.

2. **"Chronic fetal distress" pattern of FHR**
    a. Stable baseline heart rate between 120–160 beats/min.
    b. Persistently absent short-term variability.
    c. Intermittent, usually small, variable decelerations with overshoot, with amplitude less than 20 beats/min and duration less than 20 seconds.
    d. Absence of reactivity. Shields and Schifrin (1988) showed that almost all infants with this pattern had 1-minute Apgar scores of less than 7 and that almost 80% of the 5-minute Apgar scores were low.
3. **Real-time ultrasonography** shows decreased frequency of fetal activity, fetal breathing movements, decreased muscle tone (biophysical profile), pupillary dilatation in response to light, and abnormal fetal movement in response to external acoustic or vibrotactile stimuli.
4. **Aminiotic fluid volume.** An aminiotic fluid index (AFI) of 5 or less is associated with an increased incidence of meconium, fetal distress in labor, and a low 5-minute Apgar score.
5. **Assessment of fetoplacental blood flow using Doppler ultrasonography** shows that changes in the aortic blood flow velocity waveform may precede the development of pathologic fetal heart rate patterns and may provide an early warning of impending asphyxia.

B. **Intrapartum diagnosis**
1. **Fetal heart rate monitoring.**
2. **Sampling of fetal scalp capillary blood** to determine pH and Pao_2.
3. **Sampling of umbilical cord blood** for acid-base status.
4. **Observation of early passage of "heavy" meconium** (ie, at the time of rupture of membranes during active labor).

C. **Newborn asphyxia (asphyxia neonatorum).** There is no ideal measure of perinatal asphyxia in clinical practice.
1. **Apgar scores** have been shown to be not specific for hypoxia and have a weak relationship with other measures of perinatal compromise such as pH, meconium staining, and neurologic outcome. Most infants with low Apgar scores do not show evidence of biochemical asphyxia. Other factors that can account for low Apgar scores include gestational age, maternal medications, type of anesthetic administered, and the person who assigned the score. Fetal heart rate may diminish because of vagal influences unrelated to fetal hypoxia such as endotracheal, orogastric, or nasogastric suctioning.
2. **Acid-base analysis of umbilical cord blood** provides objective information about the acute and chronic respiratory and metabolic condition of the fetus at birth when maternal acid-base analysis is normal. A normal cord arterial pH may be useful in ruling out the diagnosis of birth asphyxia in the newborn with respiratory depression (Thorp, 1989).
3. **Base deficit calculation** is used as an index of severity of metabolic acidosis and the degree of compensation achieved by resuscitative efforts. A base deficit of 4 or more warrants further evaluation and correction. Neonatal acidosis is not specific for asphyxia. An important and more common etiology is sepsis.
4. Numerous abnormal **metabolites in blood and CSF** have been identified, possibly reflecting metabolic derangement associated with hypoxic-ischemic encephalopathy. Such research "markers" (not refined for use in clinical practice) include creatine kinase, hypoxanthine, lactate, lactate dehydrogenase, cord erythropoietin, and cord arginine vasopressin.

D. **Other organ systems requiring assessment.** Approximately 60% of "asphyxiated" newborn infants exhibit single- or multiple-organ injury.
1. **Cardiovascular system.** Hypotension, tachycardia, poor perfusion, tricuspid insufficiency, myocardial necrosis, and congestive heart failure may follow severe asphyxia.
    a. **Chest x-ray** may reveal an **enlarged heart.**
    b. **Electrocardiography** may show myocardial ischemia with ST segment depression and T wave inversion.

c. **Two-dimensional echocardiography with Doppler interrogation** shows both **right and left ventricular dysfunction** in 25% of severely asphyxiated infants. Left ventricular dilatation or dysfunction alone is infrequent (10%). Right ventricular dysfunction is more common (30%) and is manifested by a dilated right ventricle with high-velocity tricuspid regurgitation and atrial shunting. It is most frequently observed in infants with meconium-stained amniotic fluid.

d. **Serum creatinine phosphokinase levels** for myocardial damage (CPK-MB) have not been as diagnostically useful as previously reported.

2. **Renal function** may be depressed or transiently abolished following asphyxia, resulting in acute tubular or cortical necrosis or renal failure. **Oliguria** may be transient (present in the first 24 hours) or persistent (present for at least 36 hours). Poor outcome in term infants is associated with persistent oliguria, and in preterm infants, with both transient and persistent oliguria (Perlman, Tack, 1988). **Catheter drainage of the bladder** may be required as some asphyxiated infants may have acute urinary retention.

3. **Liver function.** Liver enzymes, especially gamma-glutamyl transpeptidase activity, clotting factors, serum ammonia, serum indirect bilirubin and total bile acid concentration are useful studies at 3–4 days' postnatal age in moderate to severe asphyxia.

4. **Gastrointestinal tract.** The GI tract may be compromised, and necrotizing enterocolitis is an associated delayed (5–7 days) complication. Caution with the first feeding is advised: isotonic or hypotonic feedings, small volumes, and close observation of gut tolerance to feedings are recommended.

5. **Lungs.** Observe for **respiratory distress syndrome** (see p 421) from surfactant deficiency or dysfunction and **persistent pulmonary hypertension,** especially in infants with a history of meconium-stained amniotic fluid (see p 291).

6. **Hematologic system. Thrombocytopenia** due to shortened platelet survival time when exposed to hypoxia may be present.

7. **Brain.** The neurologic examination provides **critical** information concerning the presence, site, extent of hypoxic-ischemic injury, and the prognosis.

a. Infants are usually **obtunded** if not comatose.

b. **Depressed reflexes,** loss of auditory and cranial reflexes, and cranial nerve palsies are the most common findings.

c. **Muscle tone is poor or flaccid.** Generalized hypotonia and paucity of spontaneous movements are common clinical features of severe hypoxic-ischemic encephalopathy.

d. **Hypoxic-ischemic spinal cord injury.** Ischemic injury to anterior horn cells within spinal cord gray matter is relatively common among hypotonic-hyporeflexic neonates following severe perinatal hypoxia-ischemia. Electromyographic examinations show injury to the lower motor neuron above the level of the dorsal root ganglion (Clancy, Sladky, Rorke, 1989).

e. **Serum osmolality and electrolytes** should be monitored for possible onset of syndrome of inappropriate antidiuretic hormone secretion (SIADH).

f. **Traumatic deliveries** may cause skull fracture, spinal cord injury, subdural hematoma, or subarachnoid hemorrhage.

g. Onset of **seizures** in 12–72 hours is not unusual. Serial EEG may be used to document severity and to follow progression of damage. Watch for seizures due to **low serum glucose levels.**

h. **Evoked electrical potentials** (auditory, cortical auditory, middle latency responses, visual, or somatosensory) may help to document levels of CNS damage.

i. **Intracranial pressure** (ICP) should be monitored in the severely asphyxiated term newborn. It is not a recognized feature in the preterm infant in the absence of hydrocephalus. ICP is normal initially and rises to a maximum at 24–72 hours of age; the cerebral perfusion pressures remain normal throughout this time period. The typical temporal profile of changes in ICP suggests that clinically recognizable brain swelling is a *consequence* of extensive cerebral necrosis rather than a cause of ischemic cerebral injury.

j. **Ultrasonography** is the **technique of choice for routine assessment of the brain in the premature newborn.** Although of major value for identification of IVH, major limitations in the first weeks of life exist for diagnosis of ischemic injury because of the inability of ultrasonography to reliably identify mild injury and to visualize lesions that are peripherally located and because of the poor specificity of increased echogenicity for distinguishing between hemorrhagic and ischemic injury in cerebral parenchyma.

k. **Doppler ultrasonography.** Higher cerebral blood flow velocity is found in asphyxiated infants during the first 4 days of life, coincidental with cerebral edema and neurologic abnormalities, thus suggesting that the changes in the cerebral circulation are at least partly caused by cerebral edema-induced increase of intracranial pressure following severe perinatal asphyxia (van Bel et al, 1987).

l. **CT scan.** The value of CT in the assessment of diffuse cortical neuronal injury is most apparent several weeks after severe asphyxial insults. During the first week after insult, the striking bilateral diffuse hypodensity reflects marked cortical neuronal injury, with associated edema corresponding closely to the occurrence of maximum intracranial pressure.

m. **Magnetic resonance imaging** (MRI) has become the **technique of choice for evaluation of hypoxic-ischemic cerebral injury in term and premature newborns.** It demonstrates superior anatomical detail, provides insight into the process of myelination and neuronal migration, the timing and evolution of cerebral injury, and does not expose the neonate to radiation. It may suggest other disorders, such as metabolic or neurodegenerative disorders, which may also present as obtundation or coma in the newborn period. The prolonged scanning time is still a problem for infants < 1800 g because of their vulnerability to hypothermia. Advances are being made to adapt the use of ferromagnetic life-support equipment in proximity of the scanner.

n. **Magnetic resonance spectroscopy (MRS)** provides a measure of "energy reserve." Using phosphorous-31 MRS, the absolute and relative quantities of phosphorous-containing compounds, such as phosphocreatine and ATP, can be used to characterize the progression to irreversible cell changes and death.

o. **Other potentially useful imaging techniques** include technetium scan (detects areas with disturbances of the blood-brain barrier), positron emission tomography (detects decreased parasagittal cerebral blood flow), cerebral hemodynamics using xenon-133 inhalation and single-photon emission computer tomography (Taudorf, Vorstrup, 1989), proton MRS, and near infrared spectroscopy (Wyatt et al, 1989).

VI. **Management**

A. **Optimal management is prevention** using the antepartum and intrapartum diagnostic modalities (see pp 401, 402).

B. **Immediate resuscitation**

1. **Maintenance of adequate ventilation and perfusion**

a. **Maintain tidal volumes between 5 and 7 mL/kg.**

b. **During the initial period of resuscitation, $Paco_2$ should be maintained between 25 and 30 mm Hg** to minimize cerebral edema. $Paco_2$ can then be normalized to 35–45 mm Hg after initial resuscitation.

c. **Maintain a pH of more than 7.35** with hyperventilation, sodium bicarbonate, or tromethamine (THAM), as acidic pH can potentiate pulmonary vasoconstriction.

d. Avoid hypoxemia ($PaO_2 < 40$ in premature infants and $PaO_2 < 50$ in term infants) **and hypercarbia** ($Paco_2 > 50$). Overcorrection of hypoxemia with resultant hyperoxemia may contribute to brain injury.

e. Avoid hypovolemia. Maintain adequate central venous pressure (6–8 cm H_2O). Capillary refill time of 5 seconds or less is consistent with poor perfusion. A small heart on the chest radiograph in the absence of excessive lung expansion is indicative of hypovolemia.

f. Inotropic support may be required to maintain the systemic mean blood pressure in the normal range appropriate for gestational age and birth weight. Do not treat just a low blood pressure value; evaluate the "whole" patient (ie, perfusion, renal output, oxygenation). Attempts should be made to maintain the systemic mean blood pressure above the pulmonary artery pressure to reverse the right-to-left shunt seen with persistent pulmonary hypertension.

g. Conversely, **avoid systemic hypertension** to prevent cerebral hemorrhagic injury.

h. Minimal handling of infant. Hypoxemia may result even from routine handling of the infant and endotracheal suctioning.

i. Partial exchange transfusion for significant polycythemia.

2. Control of seizures. Seizures associated with severe hypoxic-ischemic cerebral injury commonly occur on the first day of life and may be prolonged and refractory to anticonvulsant medication.

a. Phenobarbital is the **drug of choice** for the treatment of seizures in neonatal hypoxic-ischemic encephalopathy. Some centers start it before the onset of clinical seizures, based on the clinical impression that prophylaxis treatment reduces the likelihood of subsequent uncontrolled seizures by reducing catecholamines and cerebral edema and lowering overall metabolic activity at a time of great stress. Phenobarbital is discontinued after 7 days if no clinical seizures occur; otherwise, it is continued until the EEG and clinical observation show no seizure activity for at least 2 months.

b. Further anticonvulsant therapy must be considered if seizures occur despite adequate phenobarbital doses. Other agents that may be tried include diazepam, lorazepam, and phenytoin (see Chap 73 for dosages and other pharmacologic information).

3. Prevention of cerebral edema

a. Monitor intracranial pressures, if possible, in severely asphyxiated infants.

b. Avoid excessive volume expansion or rapid infusion of colloid solutions or sodium bicarbonate.

c. Maintain adequate oxygenation. Avoid aminophylline, as it may decrease cerebral blood flow and potentiate cerebral anoxia.

d. Maintain a normal range of Paco$_2$ (35–45 mm Hg). Hyperventilation to decrease Pco_2 to the range of 20–30 mm Hg may lower cerebral blood flow and is one way to minimize cerebral edema acutely, although further hyperventilation to Pco_2 less than 20 mm Hg may result in cerebral ischemia. Conversely, increased carbon dioxide levels may increase cerebral blood flow, cause vasodilatation, and risk new or extended intracranial hemorrhage.

e. Maintain a normal serum glucose level to provide adequate substrate for brain metabolism. Avoid hyperglycemia to prevent hyperosmolality or increased brain lactate levels.

f. Fluid and electrolyte management

(1) Maintain moderate to slight fluid restriction (eg, 60 mL/kg). If cerebral edema is severe, further restriction of fluid intake to 50 mL/kg is imposed.

(2) Monitor serum sodium and maintain normal levels.

(3) **Monitor urine output and specific gravity.** A urine output of 2.0–2.5 mL/kg/h and a urine specific gravity of 1.012–1.015 reflect adequate fluid management in the face of early cerebral edema.

(4) **Observe the infant for SIADH,** which is treated by stringent fluid restriction.

g. Glucocorticoids, mannitol, and phenobarbital are not proven therapeutic approaches to cerebral edema secondary to perinatal asphyxia.

C. **Potential new therapies**

a. **Prevention of free radical formation. Inhibitors of xanthine oxidase,** such as allopurinol and oxypurinol, can prevent formation of superoxide and hydrogen peroxide (Palmer and Roberts, 1991). **Iron chelators** like deferoxamine can reduce the amount of free iron which participate catalytically to form hydroxyl radicals (Rosenthal et al, 1992). **Prolonged suppression of nitric oxide production** *during recovery* can reduce brain injury (Trifiletti, 1992). However, complete inhibition of nitric oxide synthesis during cerebral hypoxia-ischemia could be deleterious.

b. **Free radical elimination. Exogenous administration of superoxide dismutase and catalase** can reduce superoxide formation and blood-brain barrier disruption (Armstead et al, 1992). **Vitamine E-like compounds** can prevent iron-dependent lipid peroxidation by scavenging peroxyl radicals (Hall et al, 1991).

c. **Excitatory amino acid antagonists** may protect against hypoxic-ischemic brain damage even when administered several hours following the insult to brain (McDonald et al, 1989).

d. **Calcium channel blockers** may prevent delayed neuronal injury, but recent trials have resulted in marked systemic hypotension (Levene et al, 1990).

VII. **Prognosis**

A. **Useful prognostic factors**

1. Data from electronic fetal monitoring, blood gas sampling, extended (out to 20 min) Apgar scores, imaging studies, and biochemical markers are helpful, but no single sign or symptom is a predictor of later outcome.

2. Normalization of tone by 15 minutes of life is a good prognostic sign.

3. Evidence of multisystem failure, particularly oliguria, increases the likelihood of disability.

4. Neonatal neurologic syndrome.

a. Severity.

b. Seizures.

(1) Early onset and difficult to control.

(2) Duration of more than 1–2 weeks.

c. Increased intracranial pressure.

d. Specific patterns of motor weakness may be predictive of the type of later cerebral palsy.

e. Persistent abnormalities of brain-stem function (generally incompatible with long-term survival).

5. Environmental, psychosocial, behavioral, and developmental variables are more predictive of 36-month outcome than are maternal, prenatal, and perinatal variables.

6. Microcephaly at 3 months of age is predictive of poor neurodevelopmental outcome (Shankaran, 1991).

B. Most infants who do experience hypoxic-ischemic insults do not exhibit abnormal neurologic features or subsequent evidence of brain injury. Peliowski and Finer (1992) showed that the overall risk of death for children with all stages of HIE combined was 12.5%, neurologic handicap 14.3%, and death plus handicap 25%.

1. Most children who had Stage 1 and 2 HIE do well.

2. Stage 3 HIE carries a mortality rate of approximately 80% and survivors

often have multiple disabilities including spastic cerebral palsy, severe/profound mental retardation, cortical blindness, and/or seizure disorder (Robertson, 1993).

3. Hearing deficits may develop with or without associated neurologic disability.

4. Girls who had HIE may have early sexual maturation (Robertson, 1990).

5. Nondisabled survivors of moderate HIE have delayed skills in reading, spelling, and/or arithmetic and have more difficulties with attention and short-term recall than survivors of mild HIE and normals.

C. The outcome of severe asphyxia neonatorum is always ominous, but efforts to resuscitate must always be undertaken as quickly as possible, with the expectation that every infant has the potential to respond and recover fully.

REFERENCES

American Academy of Pediatrics, American College of Obstetricians and Gynecologists: Relationship between perinatal factors and neurologic outcome. In: Poland RL, Freeman RK (eds), *Guidelines for Perinatal Care*, 3rd ed. American Academy of Pediatrics, 1992:221.

Armstead WM et al: Polyethyleneglycol superoxide dismutase and catalase attenuate increased blood-brain barrier permeability after ischemia in piglets. *Stroke* 1992;**23**:755.

Castle V et al: The effect of hypoxia on platelet survival and site of sequestration in the newborn rabbit. *Thromb Haemos* 1988;**59**:45.

Carter et al: The definition of acute perinatal asphyxia. *Clin Perinatol* 1993;**20**:287.

Clancy RR, Sladky JT, Rorke LB: Hypoxic-ischemic spinal cord injury following perinatal asphyxia. *Ann Neurol* 1989;**25**:185.

Clark GD: Role of excitatory amino acids in brain injury caused by hypoxia-ischemia, status epilepticus, and hypoglycemia. *Clin Perinatol* 1989;**16**:459.

Gilstrap III LC et al: Diagnosis of birth asphyxia on the basis of fetal pH, Apgar score, and newborn cerebral dysfunction. *Am J Obstet Gynecol* 1989;**161**:825.

Hall ED, Pazara KE, Braughler JM: U-78517F: A potent inhibitor of lipid peroxidation with activity in experimental brain injury and ischemia. *J Pharmacol Exp Ther* 1991;**258**:688.

Hill A: Assessment of the fetus: Relevance to brain injury. *Clin Perinatol* 1989;**16**:413.

Levene MI et al: The use of a calcium-channel blocker, nicardipine, for severely asphyxiated newborn infants. *Develop Med Child Neurol* 1990;**32**:567.

Lou HC: The "lost autoregulation hypothesis" and brain lesions in the newborn—an update. *Brain Devel* 1988;**10**:143.

Marlow N: Do we need an Apgar score. *Arch Dis Child* 1992;**67**:765.

McDonald JW, Silverstein FS, Johnston MW: Neuroprotective effects of MK-801, TCP, PCP, and CPP against N-methyl-D-aspartate induced neurotoxicity in an in vivo perinatal rat model. *Brain Res* 1989;**490**:33.

Painter MJ: Fetal heart rate patterns, perinatal asphyxia, and brain injury. *Pediatr Neurol* 1989;**5**:137.

Palmer C, Vannucci RC: Potential new therapies for perinatal cerebral hypoxia-ischemia. *Clin Perinatol* 1993;**20**:411.

Palmer C, Roberts RL: Reduction of perinatal brain damage with oxypurinol treatment after hypoxic-ischemic injury. *Pediatr Res* 1991;**29**:362A.

Peliowski A, Finer NN: Hypoxic-ischemic encephalopathy in the term infant. In: Sinclair J, Lucey J (eds), *Effective Care of Newborn Infant*. Oxford, Oxford University Press, 1992.

Perlman JM, Tack ED: Renal injury in the asphyxiated newborn infant: Relationship to neurologic outcome. *J Pediatr* 1988;**113**:875.

Robertson CMT, Finer NN: Long-term follow-up of term neonates with perinatal asphyxia. *Clin Perinatol* 1993;**20**:483.

Robertson CMT et al: Neonatal encephalopathy: An indicator of early sexual maturation in girls. *Pediatr Neurol* 1990;**6**:102.

Rosenthal RE et al: Prevention of post-ischemic brain lipid conjugated diene production and neurological injury by hydroxyethyl starch-conjugated deferoxamine. *Free Radic Biol Med* 1992;**12**:29.

Ruth VJ, Raivio KO: Perinatal brain damage: Predictive value of metabolic acidosis and the Apgar score. *Br Med J Clin Res* 1988;**297**:24.

Ruth VJ et al: Prediction of perinatal brain damage by cord plasma vasopressin, erythropoietin, and hypoxanthine values. *J Pediatr* 1988;**113**:880.

Shankaran S et al: Acute neonatal morbidity and long-term central nervous system sequelae of perinatal asphyxia in term infants. *Early Hum Dev* 1991;**25**:135.

Shields JR, Schifrin BS: Perinatal antecedents of cerebral palsy. *Obstet Gynecol* 1988;**71**:899.

Standards and guidelines for cardiopulmonary resuscitation (CPR) and emergency cardiac care (ECC). 6. Neonatal advanced life support. *JAMA* 1986;**255:**2969.

Taudorf K, Vorstrup S: Cerebral blood flow abnormalities in cerebral palsied children with a normal CT scan. *Neuropediatrics* 1989;**20:**33.

Thorp JA et al: Routine umbilical cord blood gas determinations? *Am J Obstet Gynecol* 1989; **161:**600.

Trifiletti RR: Neuroprotective effects of N^G-nitro-L-arginine in focal stroke in the 7-day old rat. *Eur J Pharmacol* 1992;**218:**197.

van Bel F et al: Cerebral blood flow velocity pattern in healthy and asphyxiated newborns: Controlled study. *Eur J Pediatr* 1987;**146:**461.

Volpe JJ: Hypoxic-ischemic encephalopoathy: Biochemical and physiological aspects. In: *Neurology of the Newborn,* 2nd ed. Saunders, 1987.

Williams CE et al: Pathophysiology of perinatal asphyxia. *clin Perinatol* 1993;**20:**305.

Wyatt JS et al.: Magnetic resonance and near infrared spectroscopy for investigation of perinatal hypoxic-ischemic brain injury. *Arch Dis Child* 1989;**64:**953.

67 Pulmonary Diseases

AIR LEAK SYNDROMES

I. Definition. The pulmonary air leak syndromes (pneumomediastinum, pneumo-thorax, pulmonary interstitial emphysema [PIE], and pneumopericardium) comprise a spectrum of disease with the same underlying pathophysiology. Over-distention of alveolar sacs or terminal airways leads to disruption of airway integrity, resulting in dissection of air into surrounding spaces.

II. Incidence. Although the exact incidence of the air leak syndromes is hard to determine, they are most commonly seen in infants with lung disease who are on ventilatory support in the NICU. In general, the more severe the lung disease, the higher the incidence of pulmonary air leak. Whereas air leak syndromes are seen most commonly in infants on ventilatory support, they all have been reported to occur spontaneously.

III. Pathophysiology. Overdistention of terminal air spaces or airways—the common denominator in all the pulmonary air leaks—can result from uneven alveolar ventilation; air trapping, or injudicious use of alveolar distending pressure in infants on ventilatory support. As lung volume exceeds physiologic limits, mechanical stresses occur in all planes of the alveolar or respiratory bronchial wall, with eventual tissue rupture.

    A. Barotrauma. The common denominator of the air leak syndromes is barotrauma. Barotrauma results whenever positive pressure is applied to the lung; it cannot be avoided in the ill newborn infant needing ventilatory support, but its effects should be minimized.

        1. Peak inspiratory pressure (PIP), positive end-expiratory pressure (PEEP), inspiratory time (IT), respiratory rate, and the inspiratory waveform all play an important role in the development of baro-trauma. It is difficult to determine which of these parameters is the most damaging and which plays the largest role in the development of the air leaks. Frequent and large oscillating pressures associated with intermittent positive-pressure ventilation (IPPV) may be more important than distend-ing pressure (PIP) or PEEP by themselves; the duration of positive pres-sure (IT) may be more important than the positive end-expiratory pressure (PEEP); distending pressure may be more important than either of the above.

        2. Inadvertent PEEP secondary to a very rapid rate and a short expiratory time may also be important.

    B. Other causes of lung overdistention. Barotrauma is not the only cause of lung overdistention. Gas trapping secondary to a ball-valve effect may occur with meconium aspiration or with the presence of other material such as mu-cous plugs in the airway. Other events, such as inappropriate intubation of the right main-stem bronchus, failure to wean following surfactant replacement therapy, or the development of high opening pressures with the onset of air breathing, can also lead to overdistention, with rupture of airway integrity at birth.

IV. Risk factors

    A. Ventilatory support. The infant on ventilatory support has an increased risk of developing one of the air leak syndromes. Some investigators report an incidence as high as 12% in infants on any type of ventilatory support.

    B. Meconium staining. Other infants at risk include those who are meconium stained at birth. In these infants, meconium may be plugged in the airways, with resultant air trapping. During inspiration, the airway expands allowing air to enter, but, during exhalation, there is airway collapse with resultant trapping of air behind meconium plugs.

   C. **Surfactant therapy.** Infants receiving surfactant replacement therapy may be at increased risk for the development of air leaks. With the return of pulmonary compliance, appropriate weaning must occur and may be necessary immediately following therapy. The clinician must watch for improvement in the infant's arterial blood gas levels and must wean ventilatory support as required.

  V. Clinical presentation. A high index of suspicion is necessary for the diagnosis of air leak syndromes. On clinical grounds, respiratory distress or a deteriorating clinical course strongly suggests air leak. See specific syndromes in **IX,** below.

 VI. Diagnosis. The definitive diagnosis of all of these syndromes is made radiographically. An anteroposterior chest x-ray film along with a cross-table lateral film is essential in diagnosing an air leak.

VII. Prevention. The best mode of treatment for all of the air leak syndromes is prevention—judicious use of ventilatory support, with close attention to distending pressure, PEEP inspiratory time, and appropriate weaning of ventilatory management, however, air leak syndromes will continue to be a problem in neonatal intensive care. Despite major advancement in ventilatory support and respiratory monitoring, barotrauma remains a prominent disadvantage to ventilatory support. The judicious use of ventilatory pressures and the adjustment of ventilator settings to provide a minimum of barotrauma is extremely important in the NICU.

VIII. Prognosis. The prognosis for the infant in whom an air leak develops depends on the underlying condition. In general, if the air leak is treated rapidly and effectively, the long-term outcome should not change. However, it must be remembered that early onset (PIE) (prior to 24 hours of age) is associated with a high mortality rate. Chronic lung disease of the newborn, or bronchopulmonary dysplasia (BPD), is also associated with severe pulmonary air leak syndromes.

 IX. Specific air leak syndromes.

   A. **Pneumomediastinum**

     1. **Definition.** Pneumomediastinum is air in the mediastinum from ruptured alveolar air that has traversed fascial planes.

     2. **Incidence.** The incidence of pneumomediastinum prior to the era of neonatal intensive care was approximately 2:1000 live births. The exact incidence is related to the degree of ventilatory support and is clearly higher today.

     3. **Pathophysiology.** Pneumomediastinum is preceded by PIE in almost every case. Following alveolar rupture, air traverses fascial planes and passes into the mediastinum.

     4. **Risk factors.** See p. 409.

     5. **Clinical presentation.** Unless accompanied by pneumothorax, pneumomediastinum may be totally asymptomatic. Spontaneous pneumomediastinum may develop in term infants not on ventilatory support and may be accompanied by mild respiratory distress. Physical findings in addition to respiratory distress may include an increase in anteroposterior diameter of the chest, and heart sounds may be difficult to auscultate.

     6. **Diagnosis.** On radiograph, pneumomediastinum may present in several different ways. The classic description is that of a "wind-blown spinnaker sail" (a lobe or lobes of the thymus being elevated off the heart). In other cases a halo may be seen around the heart in the anteroposterior projection, or evidence on this projection may be completely absent. Again, the cross-table lateral projection will show an anterior collection of air that may be difficult to distinguish from a pneumothorax.

     7. **Management.** There is no definitive treatment for pneumomediastinum. The temptation to insert a drain into the mediastinum should be resisted, as it will not be beneficial and may cause more problems than it will solve.

An oxygen-rich environment can be used in the term infant to attempt nitrogen washout if the pneumomediastinum is felt to be clinically significant.

    8. Prognosis. See p 410.

B. Pneumothorax.

    1. Definition. Pneumothorax is air between the visceral and parietal pleural surfaces.

    2. Incidence. Before the modern era of neonatal intensive care, the incidence of pneumothorax was 1–2%. With the advent of neonatal ventilator care, however, the incidence has risen dramatically. While the exact incidence is difficult to determine, it is directly related to the degree of ventilatory support delivered.

    3. Pathophysiology

        a. The term infant not on ventilatory support. Pneumothorax may develop spontaneously. It usually happens at the time of delivery, when a large opening pressure is initially necessary to inflate collapsed alveolar sacs.

        b. The infant on ventilatory support will have alveolar overdistention secondary to either injudicious use of distending pressure or failure to wean ventilatory pressure when compliance begins to return. Pneumothorax is usually preceded by rupture of the alveoli, with the interstitial air then traversing via fascial planes to the mediastinum. The pneumothorax is usually preceded by rupture of the alveoli, with the interstitial air then traversing via fascial planes to the mediastinum. The pneumomediastinum breaks through the mediastinal pleura to form a pneumothorax.

    4. Risk factors. See p 409.

    5. Clinical presentation. The clinical presentation of the neonate with pneumothorax depends on the setting in which it develops.

        a. The term infant with a spontaneous pneumothorax may be asymptomatic or only mildly symptomatic. These infants usually present with tachypnea and mild oxygen needs but may have the classic signs of respiratory distress (grunting, flaring, retractions, and tachypnea).

        b. The infant on ventilatory support will generally have a sudden, rapid clinical deterioration characterized by cyanosis, hypoxemia, hypercarbia, and respiratory acidosis. The most common time for the development of this complication is either immediately following the initiation of ventilatory support or when the infant begins to improve and compliance returns (eg, following surfactant therapy). In either case, other clinical signs may include decreased breath sounds on the involved side, shifted heart sounds, and asynchrony of the chest.

    6. Diagnosis. A high index of suspicion is necessary for the diagnosis of pneumothorax.

        a. Transillumination of the chest. With the aid of transillumination, the diagnosis of pneumothorax may be made without a chest x-ray study. A fiberoptic light probe placed on the infant's chest wall will illuminate the involved hemithorax. While this technique is beneficial in an emergency, it should not replace a chest x-ray study as the means of diagnosis.

        b. Chest x-ray study. Radiographically, pneumothorax is diagnosed on the basis of the following characteristics.

            (1) Presence of air in the pleural cavity separating the parietal and visceral pleura.

            (2) Collapse of the ipsilateral lobes.

            (3) Displacement of the mediastinum to the contralateral side.

            (4) Downward displacement of the diaphragm.

            In infants with respiratory distress syndrome (RDS), the compliance may be so poor that the lung may not collapse, with only minimal shift of the mediastinal structures. The anteroposterior x-ray film may not demonstrate the classic radiographic appearance if a large amount of the intrapleural air is situated just anterior to the sternum. In these situations, the cross-table lateral x-ray film will show a large lucent area immediately below the sternum, or the lateral decubitus x-ray film (with the suspected side up) will show free air.

   7. Management. Treatment of pneumothorax depends on the clinical status of the infant.

   a. Oxygen supplementation. In the term infant who is mildly symptomatic, an oxygen-rich environment is often all that is necessary. The inspired oxygen facilitates nitrogen washout of the blood and tissues and thus establishes a difference in the gas tensions between the loculated gases in the chest and those in the blood. This diffusion gradient results in rapid resorption of the loculated gas, with resolution of the pneumothorax. This mode of therapy is not appropriate in the preterm infant because of the risk of retinopathy of prematurity.

   b. Decompression. In the symptomatic neonate or the neonate on mechanical ventilatory support, immediate evacuation of air is necessary. The technique is described on p 239, **V.A.** Placement of a chest tube of appropriate size will eventually be necessary (see p 144).

C. Pulmonary interstitial emphysema (PIE)

   1. Definition. PIE is dissection of air into the perivascular tissues of the lung from alveolar overdistention or overdistention of the smaller airways.

   2. Incidence. This disorder arises almost exclusively in the very low birthweight infant on ventilatory support. If seen within the first 24 hours of life, it generally is associated with a poor prognosis. As time passes, its occurrence is less common, but it may be seen at any time during ventilatory management.

   3. Pathophysiology. PIE may be the precursor of all other types of pulmonary air leaks. With alveolar overdistention or overdistention of the conducting airways, or both, rupture may occur and there may be dissection of the air into the perivascular tissue of the lung. The interstitial air moves in the connective tissue planes and around the vascular axis, particularly the venous ones. Once in the interstitial space, the air moves along bronchioles, lymphatics, vascular sheaths, or directly through the lung interstitium to the pleural surface. The extrapulmonary air is trapped in the interstitium (PIE), or it may extend and cause pneumomediastinum, pneumopericardium, or pneumothorax.

   4. Risk factors. See p 409.

   5. Clinical presentation. The patient in whom PIE develops may have sudden deterioration, but more commonly, the onset of PIE will be heralded by a slow, progressive deterioration of arterial blood gas levels and the apparent need for increasing ventilatory support. Invariably a diffusion block develops in these patients, with the alveolar membrane becoming separated from the capillary bed by the interstitial air. The response to increased ventilatory support in the face of poor arterial blood gas levels may lead to worsening of PIE and sudden clinical deterioration. Infants with severe PIE may have sudden and rapid deterioration or may actually improve if the PIE progresses to pneumothorax.

   6. Diagnosis. In infants with PIE, the chest x-ray film will generally reveal radiolucencies that are either linear or cystlike in nature. The linear radiolucencies vary in length and do not branch; they are seen in the periphery of the lung as well as medially and may be mistaken for air bronchograms. The cystlike lucencies vary from 1.0 to 4.0 mm in diameter and can be lobulated.

   7. Management

   a. Lessening barotrauma. In general, once PIE is diagnosed, an attempt should be made to decrease ventilatory support and lessen barotrauma. Decreasing the peak inspiratory pressure, decreasing the PEEP, or shortening the inspiratory time may be required. All of these maneuvers will decrease barotrauma and possibly lessen PIE. During this time, some degree of hypercarbia and hypoxia may have to be accepted.

b. **Splinting of the affected side** has also proved beneficial in some cases of unilateral PIE.

c. **Other treatments.** More invasive measures include selective collapse of the involved lung on the side with the worse involvement, with selective intubation or even the insertion of chest tubes prior to the development of pneumothorax.

d. **High-frequency ventilation (HFV)** has proven useful in infants with severe PIE and with other types of pulmonary air leak. Both high frequency oscillatory ventilation and high frequency jet ventilation have both been used effectively in the treatment of PIE and other types of air leak syndromes. While these treatment modalities may improve survival of the infant with PIE, the long-term pulmonary outcome of these infants remains uncertain. However, randomized controlled trials have been completed and have revealed good results. The earlier HFV is begun following the onset of PIE or pulmonary air leak, the greater chance for survival.

8. **Prognosis.** See p 410.

D. **Pneumopericardium**

1. **Definition.** Pneumopericardium is air in the pericardial sac, which is usually secondary to passage of air along vascular sheaths. It is always a complication of mechanical ventilatory support.

2. **Incidence.** Pneumopericardium is a rare occurrence.

3. **Pathophysiology.** It is often said that pneumopericardium is always preceded by pneumomediastinum, but this is not universally true. The mechanism by which pneumopericardium develops is not well understood, but it is probably due to passage of air along vascular sheaths.

4. **Risk factors.** See p 409.

5. **Clinical presentation.** The clinical signs of pneumopericardium range from asymptomatic to the full picture of cardiac tamponade. The first sign of pneumopericardium may be a decrease in blood pressure or a decrease in pulse pressure. There may also be an increase in heart rate with distant heart sounds.

6. **Diagnosis.** Pneumopericardium has the most classic radiographic appearance of all the air leaks. A broad radiolucent halo completely surrounds the heart, including the diaphragmatic surface. This picture is easily distinguished from all the other air leaks by its extension completely around the heart in all projections.

7. **Treatment.** Treatment of pneumopericardium is essential and requires the placement of a pericardial drain or repeated pericardial taps. The procedure is described on p 161.

APNEA AND PERIODIC BREATHING

I. **Definitions.** Simply defined, apnea is the absence of respiratory gas flow for a period of 20 seconds, with or without a decrease in heart rate. There are several types.

A. **Central apnea** is of central nervous system origin and is characterized by the absence of gas flow with no respiratory effort.

B. **Obstructive apnea** is continued respiratory effort not resulting in gas flow.

C. **Mixed apnea** is a combination of central and obstructive.

D. **Periodic breathing,** defined as 3 or more periods of apnea lasting 3 seconds or more within a 20-second period of otherwise normal respiration, is also common in the newborn period. Currently it is not known whether or not there is an association between apnea and periodic breathing.

II. **Incidence.** The incidence of apnea and periodic breathing in the term infant has not been adequately determined. Approximately 50–60% of preterm infants have evidence of apnea: 35% present with central apnea, 5–10% with obstructive apnea, 15–20% with mixed apnea. Another 30% will have periodic breathing.

III. **Pathophysiology.** Apnea and periodic breathing probably have a common pathophysiologic origin, apnea being a step further along the continuum than periodic breathing. While the exact pathophysiology of these infants has not yet been elucidated, there are many theories.

    A. **Immaturity of respiratory control.** Since apnea is seen most commonly in the premature infant, some type of immaturity of the respiratory control mechanism is thought to play a role in most cases of apnea.

        1. **Hypoxic response.** The preterm infant is known to have abnormal biphasic response to hypoxia: a brief period of tachypnea followed by apnea. This response is unlike that seen in the adult or older child in whom hypoxia produces a state of prolonged tachypnea.

        2. **Carbon dioxide response.** The carbon dioxide response curve is shifted in the preterm infant, with higher levels of carbon dioxide required before respiration is stimulated.

    B. **Sleep-related response.** Sleep states may also play an important role in the development of apnea in the preterm infant. A shift from one sleep state to another is often characterized by instability of respiratory activity in the adult. The preterm infant spends about 80% of the time in sleep and has a difficult time making the transition between sleeping and waking states, which could lead to an increased risk for the development of apnea in these infants.

    C. **Protective reflexes** such as the apneic response to noxious substances in the airway may also play a role in the apneic episodes seen in the newborn infant.

    D. **Muscle weakness.** Overall muscle weakness (of both the muscles of respiration and the muscles that maintain airway patency) also plays an important role in pathophysiology.

    E. **All of the above point to an immature respiratory control mechanism in the preterm infant.** Whether the immaturity is operational at the level of the brain stem, the peripheral chemoreceptors, or the central receptors has yet to be determined. What is likely is that apnea results from a combination of immature afferent impulses to the respiratory control centers along with immature efferents from these same centers, giving rise to the poor ventilatory control.

    F. **Pathologic states can also lead to apnea in the infant.** The following disorders have all been associated with apnea in the neonatal period.

        1. **Hypothermia.**

        2. **Metabolic disturbances** such as hypoglycemia and hyponatremia.

        3. **Sepsis.**

        4. **Anemia.**

        5. **Hypoxemia.**

        6. **Central nervous system abnormalities** such as intraventricular hemorrhage.

        7. **Necrotizing enterocolitis.**

IV. **Risk factors**

    A. **Preterm infants.** The preterm infant is at the greatest risk for the development of apnea. Since apnea is believed to develop secondary to an immature or poorly developed respiratory control mechanism, this association should be obvious.

    B. **SIDS sibling.** The sibling of an infant who died from sudden infant death syndrome (SIDS) is also at great risk for having periods of apnea. Again, a poorly developed respiratory control mechanism is believed to be involved.

    C. **Neurologic disorders.** Since respiration depends on the integration of numerous central nervous system functions, the child with certain neurologic diseases may be at increased risk for the development of apnea.

V. **Clinical presentation**

    A. **Apnea within 24 hours after delivery.** Although apnea may be present at any time during the neonatal period, if it presents within the first 24 hours of life, it is usually not simple apnea of prematurity. Apnea during this time period is strongly associated with sepsis.

B. **Apnea after the first 3 days of life.** When apnea occurs after the first 3 days of life and is not associated with any other pathologic condition, it may be classified as apnea of prematurity. Apnea may also occur following weaning from ventilatory support and may be associated with intermittent hypoxia.

VI. **Diagnosis.** A high incidence of suspicion is necessary to diagnose apnea. If significant apnea is detected, an extensive workup is required in order to make an accurate diagnosis and develop a logical treatment plan.

A. **Monitoring of infants at risk.** All preterm infants should be closely monitored for the development of this often life-threatening condition. Close attention should be paid to the type of monitoring that is given to infants in intensive care units. Preterm infants are commonly on heart rate monitors only, and they will be identified as having apnea only if the heart rate drops below the monitor alarm limit (usually set at 80 beats/min). In this case, these infants may suffer profound hypoxia before bradycardia develops, or they may have apnea with significant hypoxemia but without a drop in heart rate. In order to detect apnea, these infants should have continuous monitoring of respiratory activity or monitoring of oxygenation, or both, using either transcutaneous oximetry or pulse oximetry.

B. **Physical examination.** Specific attention should be paid to physical findings such as lethargy, hypothermia, cyanosis, and respiratory effort. A good neurologic examination should also be performed.

C. **Laboratory studies**
   1. **Complete blood count with differential and platelet count** will help to rule out sepsis.
   2. **Arterial blood gas determinations** will screen for hypoxia.
   3. **Serum glucose, electrolyte, and calcium levels** will aid in the diagnosis of metabolic disturbances.

D. **Radiographic studies**
   1. **Chest x-ray study** to detect evidence of pathologic lung changes (eg, atelectasis, pneumonia, air leak).
   2. **Abdominal x-ray study** to detect signs of necrotizing entercolitis (see Chap 64).
   3. **Ultrasonography of the head** to detect intraventricular hemorrhage or other central nervous system abnormality.
   4. **CT scan of the head** may also be appropriate in infants with definite signs of neurologic disease.

E. **Other studies**
   1. **Electroencephalography.** An EEG may be necessary to complete the workup if there is any question about the neurologic status of the infant.
   2. **Pneumography.** A pneumogram is another essential tool in the diagnosis of apnea. Chest leads provide a tracing that gives a continuous recording of both heart rate and chest wall movement and can detect periods of central apnea and periodic breathing.
      a. **Abnormal pneumogram.** An abnormal pneumogram is defined as one in which one of the following patterns is demonstrated.
         (1) Periods of prolonged apnea (cessation of respiratory movement of > 20 seconds).
         (2) Short apnea (cessation of respiratory movement of < 20 seconds) if accompanied by bradycardia.
         (3) Episodes of periodic breathing lasting more than 5% of the total quiet or sleep time.
      b. **Four-channel pneumogram.** A more accurate instrument for the diagnosis of apnea is a 4-channel pneumogram, in which a nasal thermistor to detect air flow and a pulse oxymeter are added to the standard heart-rate and chest-wall channels. With the addition of thermistor, central apnea can easily be distinguished from obstructive apnea. The addition

of the pulse oxymeter helps in determining if there are significant oxygen desaturations during periods of apnea or heart rate drops. This distinction carries more than academic interest, since treatment of the disorder should be directed specifically to the type of apnea that is detected.

c. **Polysomnography.** In research-oriented centers, a polysomnogram (a study that monitors specific EEG leads and muscle movement) can be used for a more thorough workup of apnea. This study will not only determine the type of apnea that occurs but can also relate it to the sleep stage of the infant. While polysomnography is certainly not indicated in all infants with apnea, its use may be beneficial in determining the exact pathogenesis of this enigmatic condition. Only after a thorough diagnostic evaluation, can adequate therapy for apnea be instituted.

VII. **Management.** Treatment for apnea must be individualized.

A. **Specific therapy.** If an identifiable cause of apnea is determined, it should be treated accordingly. For example: sepsis should be treated with antibiotics (see Chap 73); hypoglycemia with glucose infusion; electrolyte abnormalities (see specific abnormality in On-Call Problems) and anemia should be corrected.

B. **General therapy.** If a cause cannot be identified or if one can be identified but is not amenable to treatment (eg, intraventricular hemorrhage), there are several approaches to treatment.

1. **Supplemental oxygen.** Merely increasing the ambient oxygen concentration will often alleviate apneic spells. The mechanism of action is probably secondary to decreasing the number of unidentified hypoxic spells.

2. **Continuous positive airway pressure (CPAP)** is used with some success, probably acting by the same mechanism as supplemental oxygen. This method is an invasive therapeutic modality and should be used only when other methods have failed.

3. **Oscillating water bed.** Placing the infant on an oscillating waterbed has been used with some success. This procedure is felt to increase the tactile stimulation the infant is receiving and thereby increase output from efferent nerves in the respiratory centers. Randomized, controlled trials have shown that it may not be effective therapy, but some centers may use it in selected cases.

4. **Pharmacologic therapy.** If the above methods fail, the next line of approach is to begin administration of respiratory stimulants.

a. **Theophylline** is the drug used most commonly in the treatment of apnea. The exact mechanism of action is open to debate, but it probably works through direct stimulation of the respiratory centers as well as by lowering the threshold to carbon dioxide. Some clinicians think it may act by direct stimulation of the diaphragm. (See Chap 73 for dosage and other pharmacologic information.)

b. **Caffeine** can also be used in the treatment of apnea, and since it has a longer half-life than theophylline, it may be a better drug. If caffeine is used, it is imperative that caffeine levels be monitored. (See Chap 73 for dosage and other pharmacologic information.)

c. **Doxapram.** Doxapram, a potent respiratory stimulant, has recently been shown to be effective when theophylline and caffeine have failed. The duration of treatment with doxapram has been limited to 5 days, but the drug may be used longer if indicated. Benzyl alcohol is the preservative used in doxapram. Duration of therapy depends on the cumulative dose of benzyl alcohol.

5. **Mechanical ventilation.** Some infants continue to have apneic spells despite adequate treatment. If the apnea is severe and is associated with hypoxia or significant bradycardia, intubation and mechanical ventilation may be indicated.

C. **Discharge planning and follow-up.** A major issue in the management of infants with apnea is deciding when to stop administration of theophylline and whether or not the infant needs to be discharged on theophylline, a home monitor, or both.

1. **Discontinuing medications.** Consider stopping theophylline therapy when the apnea has resolved and the infant weighs between 1800 and 2000 g. If the infant remains asymptomatic following the discontinuation of theophylline therapy, the child may be discharged without further therapy.

2. **Reinstituting medications.** If symptomatic apnea recurs after discontinuing therapy, theophylline therapy should be reinstituted and a decision made to discharge the infant on this medication or to keep the infant hospitalized longer. The use of home monitors in addition to theophylline therapy is *controversial.* Therapeutic theophylline levels are maintained until the child reaches 52 weeks of postconception age; then theophylline therapy is discontinued and pneumography is performed. If the pneumogram is normal, therapy can be stopped. If the pneumogram is abnormal, the infant needs to be restarted on theophylline and monitoring continued. Another attempt can be made to discontinue theophylline in 4 weeks.

3. **Home apnea monitoring.** Even though home monitoring has not been proved to prevent morbidity and mortality associated with apnea and remains *controversial,* most neonatologists and pediatricians feel that until a better understanding of this condition is reached, home monitoring is the best approach available. The use of home monitors with theophylline remains *controversial.* If an infant is discharged on theophylline and a monitor, the guidelines are the same as in **C.2,** above.

VIII. Prognosis. In most infants, apnea resolves without the occurrence of long-term deficiencies. Once the child is weaned from medication or a monitor, or both, outcome is no different from gestational age-matched counterparts.

BRONCHOPULMONARY DYSPLASIA

I. **Definition.** Bronchopulmonary dysplasia (BPD) has become a general term for various forms of chronic lung disease that develop in premature infants treated with mechanical ventilation for respiratory distress syndrome (RDS). The term *bronchopulmonary dysplasia* was coined by Northway in 1967 to denote a chronic pulmonary syndrome associated with the use of mechanical ventilation in premature infants with RDS. He noted an orderly progression of clinical, pathologic, and radiologic changes from the early findings of severe RDS (stage 1) to severe, chronic pulmonary insufficiency (stage 4). However, these infants with RDS were more mature and larger at birth than are many survivors of RDS today. Two more recent definitions of BPD have been suggested. In the first, the diagnosis of BPD is made in the infant who requires positive-pressure ventilation in the first week of life and has clinical signs of chronic respiratory disease, an oxygen requirement, and an abnormal chest x-ray film at 28 days of age. More recently, it has been shown that an abnormal pulmonary outcome is better predicted by a requirement for oxygen at 36 weeks' postconceptional age. The terms *BPD* and *chronic lung disease* are often used interchangeably to refer to a variety of chronic respiratory disorders.

II. **Incidence.** The reported incidence of BPD is variable, depending on how BPD is defined and on the patient population under study. In babies with birth weights under 1000 g, the incidence of BPD has been reported to be as low as 3–4% when defined as Northway stage 3 or 4 disease or as high as 70% when defined as the need for supplemental oxygen at 28 days of age. Exogenous surfactant replacement therapy has not yet been shown to consistently decrease the incidence of BPD.

III. **Pathophysiology.** BPD is a multifactorial disorder. It begins with acute lung injury in a susceptible host. Continued lung injury and abnormal repair lead to structural changes and chronic pulmonary dysfunction.

A. **Lung injury** can occur as a result of:

1. **Surfactant deficiency.** Collapse of saccules, with distention of distal alveolar ducts and further maldistribution of ventilation, may lead to injury.
2. **Pulmonary edema.** RDS is almost always accompanied by pulmonary edema, which may be worsened by hypoproteinemia and increased pulmonary blood flow (as occurs in infants with patent ductus arteriosus).
3. **Oxygen exposure.** Prolonged exposure to high concentrations of oxygen can have multiple adverse effects, including epithelial and endothelial cell damage and/or death, ciliary dysfunction, decreased lung lymph flow, alteration of surfactant synthesis, and inhibition of lung growth.
4. **Mechanical ventilation.** Positive distending pressure, the presence of an endotracheal tube, tracheal suctioning, and improperly warmed or humidified inspired gases may all lead to lung injury.
5. **Inflammation.** Neutrophils are capable of releasing a variety of toxic substances including proteases, oxygen free radicals, and a host of mediators of inflammation. The presence of neutrophils in the tracheal aspirates of infants with RDS who subsequently develop BPD, suggests that they may contribute to the pathogenesis of BPD.

B. **Pathologic changes.** The pathology of BPD varies with the stage of the disease. Early pathologic lung changes include areas of atelectasis filled with proteinaceous fluid alternating with areas of overexpansion. Airway injury is seen as loss of epithelium and cilia or, in a more severe form, as necrotizing tracheobronchitis. Late findings may include interstitial fibrosis, cystic dilatation, atelectasis, interstitial edema, and lymphatic distention.

IV. **Risk factors.** The risk of developing BPD increases with decreasing gestational age and birth weight. Prematurity, white race, male sex, and a family history of reactive airway disease have all been associated with an increased risk of BPD.

V. **Clinical presentation**

A. **General presentation.** Typically, BPD occurs in infants weighing less than 2000 g and of less than 34 weeks' gestation at birth who have required supplemental oxygen and mechanical ventilation for RDS. Infants who develop BPD often fail to demonstrate the rapid improvement in the first week of life that is common in uncomplicated RDS. Instead, they frequently have a prolonged course of ventilator and oxygen dependency. This course may be accompanied by poor growth, intermittent pulmonary edema, or airway reactivity, or all three.

B. **Physical examination**

1. **General signs.** Tachypnea, tachycardia, retractions, and nasal flaring are common. Upon breathing room air, these signs may worsen and cyanosis may occur.
2. **Pulmonary examination.** Retractions and diffuse rales are also common. Wheezing or prolongation of expiration may also be noted. The presence of digital clubbing indicates long-standing hypoxemia.
3. **Cardiovascular examination.** A right ventricular heave, single S_2, or prominent P_2 may accompany cor pulmonale.
4. **Abdominal examination.** The liver may be enlarged secondary to right heart failure or may be displaced downward into the abdomen secondary to pulmonary hyperinflation.

VI. **Diagnosis**

A. **Laboratory studies.** Laboratory studies reflect the chronic nature of the disease.

1. **Arterial blood gas levels** frequently reveal carbon dioxide retention. However, if the respiratory difficulties are chronic and stable, the pH is usually normal.
2. **Electrolytes.** Abnormalities of electrolytes may result from chronic carbon dioxide retention (elevated serum bicarbonate), diuretic therapy (hyponatremia, hypokalemia, hypochloremia), or fluid restriction (elevated urea nitrogen and creatinine), or all three.

B. **Radiologic studies**

1. **Chest x-ray study.** Radiographic findings may be quite variable. They may appear only as diffuse haziness and hypoinflation in infants who were very immature at birth and have persistent oxygen requirements, while in other infants, they may be more similar to those originally described by Northway—streaky interstitial markings, atelectasis, cysts, and hyperinflation. It is often difficult to distinguish new x-ray findings from chronic changes without the benefit of comparison to previous x-ray films.

2. **Abdominal ultrasonography or x-ray study.** Radiologic studies of the abdomen may demonstrate the presence of renal or, less commonly, biliary tract stones secondary to long-term use of diuretics (eg, furosemide).

C. **Other studies. Electrocardiography** and **echocardiography** may show right ventricular hypertrophy and elevation of pulmonary artery pressure with right axis deviation, increased right systolic time intervals, thickening of the right ventricular wall, and abnormal right ventricular geometry.

VII. Management

A. **Prevention.** Much recent attention has been focused on the development of ways to prevent the occurrence of both RDS and BPD.

1. **Prevention of prematurity.** Therapies directed toward decreasing the risk of prematurity and the incidence of RDS include improving prenatal care and the use of tocolytic agents, antenatal corticosteroids, and exogenous surfactants.

2. **Prevention of BPD.** Management of the infant with RDS is directed toward reducing the risk of subsequent BPD.

   a. **Established modalities** include minimizing exposure to oxygen and barotrauma, restricting fluids, and aggressively treating patent ductus arteriosus.

   b. **Other modalities**

      (1) **Antioxidant therapy.** Treatment with the dietary antioxidant, **vitamin E,** has been attempted, with variable results. However, there was an unacceptably high incidence of side effects in infants receiving parenteral vitamin E. Extensive therapeutic trials of other antioxidants have not been performed.

      (2) **Dexamethasone.** There is evidence that dexamethasone may be effective in preventing or ameliorating BPD when started early in the course and tapered very gradually. Little work has been done to either identify optimal dosing regimens or compare corticosteroid preparations.

      (3) **Vitamin A.** Vitamin A is known to be important in epithelial cell differentiation and repair. When administered intramuscularly, it has been shown to decrease the incidence of BPD in very low birth weight infants. Although this study was small, the results are promising and await confirmation in a larger trial.

B. **Treatment of BPD.** The management of infants with BPD is often complex and time-consuming. It requires recognition of the gradual transition from RDS to BPD and corresponding changes in the therapeutic approach. Once BPD is present, the goal of management is to prevent further injury, augment pulmonary function, prevent cor pulmonale, and aid growth and development.

1. **Respiratory management**

   a. **Supplemental oxygen.** In contrast to RDS—for which the emphasis is on minimizing exposure to oxygen—maintaining adequate oxygenation is important in the infant with BPD in order to prevent complications such as cor pulmonale and growth failure. Supplemental oxygen is required. Monitoring of oxygenation is most easily accomplished with a pulse oximeter that measures arterial oxygen saturation (Sao_2), although transcutaneous oxygen monitoring is also useful. The infant should be studied during its various activities, including rest, sleep, and feeding. Blood gas measurements are important for the assessment of pH and $Paco_2$ but are of limited use in monitoring oxygenation, since they provide information about only one point in time. For infants with fully vascularized retinas (usually about 40 weeks' postconceptional age), it is probably optimal to maintain $Sao_2 > 95\%$ or $Pao_2 \geq 70$ torr. For less mature infants, Sao_2 should probably be maintained in the 90–94% range.

b. **Positive-pressure ventilation.** Prolonged mechanical ventilation is frequently required. Problems with air trapping can be significant and may be reduced by decreasing ventilator rate and increasing the time for exhalation. Weaning is a gradual process that can be facilitated by tolerating $Paco_2$ in excess of 50 torr. Nasal continuous positive airway pressure (CPAP) can be useful as an adjunctive therapy following extubation.

c. **Bronchodilators.** A response to bronchodilators has been demonstrated in very young and very immature infants. A variety of agents are available for the treatment of airway reactivity. (See also Chap 73 for detailed pharmacologic information.)

   (1) **Beta-2 agonists.** Several beta-2 agonists have been shown to produce measurable improvements in lung mechanics and gas exchange in infants. Among those available as inhaled agents are **metaproterenol** (0.25–0.5 mg/kg, every 2–8 hours), **albuterol** (0.05–0.15 mg/kg every 2–8 hours), **isoetharine** (0.1–0.2 mg/kg every 2–8 hours) and **terbutaline** (0.1–0.3 mg/kg every 2–8 hours).

   (2) **Theophylline.** Theophylline has potentially beneficial actions, including smooth muscle dilation, improvement of diaphragmatic contractility, central respiratory stimulation, and mild diuretic effects. It appears to improve lung function in BPD when levels are maintained at more than 10 µg/mL. Side effects are fairly common and may include CNS irritability, gastroesophageal reflux, and GI irritation.

   (3) **Cromolyn sodium.** The precise mechanism of action is unknown, but this drug is believed to reduce the mediators of inflammation released into the airways following both antigenic and nonspecific stimuli. There is some evidence to suggest that it may be of benefit in infants with BPD when given as an aerosol in doses of 20 mg every 6–8 hours.

   (4) **Anticholinergic agents. Aerosolized atropine** (0.08 mg/kg) has been shown to improve lung function, similarly to metaproterenol, in infants with BPD. Systemic absorption occurs, and side effects, including flushing, urinary retention, tachycardia, dryness of the skin and mouth, and mental status changes, may occur with repeated doses.

   (5) **Corticosteroids.** The benefits of inhaled corticosteroids and short courses of oral or parenteral corticosteroids in the treatment of asthma in pediatric and adult patients are well established. However, their use for treatment of reactive airway disease in BPD has not been studied.

2. **Management of pulmonary edema**

   a. **Fluid restriction.** Restricting fluid to 150 mL/kg/d or less is often required. It can be accomplished by concentrating proprietary formulas to 24 cal/oz. Increasing the caloric density further, to 27–30 cal/oz, requires the addition of fat (eg, MCT oil, corn oil) and carbohydrate (eg, Polycose) to avoid excessive protein intake.

   b. **Diuretic therapy**

   (1) **Chlorothiazide and spironolactone.** This combination is ideal for chronic management. It has been shown to improve lung function and has relatively few side effects. When used in doses of 20 mg/kg/d (chlorothiazide) and 2 mg/kg/d (spironolactone), a good diuretic re-

sponse can often be obtained without the need for electrolyte supplementation.

    (2) Furosemide. Furosemide is a more potent diuretic than chloro-
thiazide and spironolactone and is particularly useful acutely for
rapid diuresis. It is associated with side effects such as electrolyte
abnormalities, calciuria with bone demineralization and renal stone
formation, and ototoxicity, thereby limiting its usefulness as a
chronic medication.

  3. Corticosteroids. The use of corticosteroids in established BPD remains
controversial. Long courses of dexamethasone in gradually tapering doses
appear to benefit some patients. Possible side effects include infection,
hypertension, gastric ulcer, and hyperglycemia. Alternate delivery methods
(eg, aerosols) and dosing strategies have not been thoroughly studied.

  4. Nutrition. Because growth is essential for recovery from BPD, adequate
nutritional intake is crucial. Infants with BPD frequently have high caloric
needs (120–150 kcal/kg/d or more) due to increased metabolic expendi-
tures. Concentrated formula is often necessary to provide sufficient calories and prevent pulmonary edema.

  5. Discharge planning. Oxygen can often be discontinued prior to NICU discharge. However, home oxygen therapy can be a safe alternative to long-
term hospitalization. The need for home apnea and bradycardia monitoring
must be decided on an individual basis but is generally recommended for
infants discharged home on oxygen. All parents should be instructed in
CPR.

  6. General care. Care plans for older infants with BPD should include adapt-
ing their routine for home life and involving the parents in their care. Immunizations should be given at the appropriate chronologic age. Periodic
screening for chemical evidence of rickets and echocardiographic evidence of right ventricular hypertrophy is recommended. Assessment by a
developmentalist and occupational or physical therapist, or both, can be
useful for prognostic and therapeutic purposes.

VIII. Prognosis. The prognosis for infants with BPD depends on the degree of pulmonary dysfunction and the presence of other medical conditions. Most deaths
occur in the first year of life as a result of cardiorespiratory failure, sepsis or respiratory infection or as sudden, unexplained death.

  A. Pulmonary outcome. The short-term outcome of infants with BPD, including
those requiring oxygen at home, is surprisingly good. Weaning from oxygen is
usually possible prior to their first birthday, and they demonstrate catch-up
growth as their pulmonary status improves. However, in the first year of life,
rehospitalization is necessary for about 30% of patients for treatment of
wheezing or respiratory infections, or both. Although upper respiratory infections are probably no more common in infants with BPD than in normal infants, they are more likely to be associated with significant respiratory symptoms. The 10-year outcome, assessed in children who were more mature and
larger at birth than many infants today, is characterized by increased airway
resistance and reactivity.

  B. Neurodevelopmental outcome. Children with BPD appear to be at increased risk for adverse neurodevelopmental outcome compared to comparable infants without BPD. Neuromotor and cognitive dysfunction appear to
be more common. In addition, children with BPD may be at higher risk for
significant hearing impairment and retinopathy of prematurity. They are also
at risk for later problems, including learning disabilities, attention deficits, and
behavior problems.

HYALINE MEMBRANE DISEASE (RESPIRATORY DISTRESS SYNDROME)

  I. Definition. Hyaline membrane disease (HMD) is also called *respiratory distress* *syndrome (RDS).* This clinical diagnosis is warranted in a preterm newborn with respiratory difficulty—including tachypnea (60/min), chest retractions, and cyanosis on room air—that persists or progresses over the first 48–96 hours of life and with a characteristic chest x-ray film (uniform reticulogranular pattern and air bronchograms). The clinical course of the disease varies with the size of the infant, the severity of the disease, the presence of infection, the degree of shunting of blood through a patent ductus arteriosus, and whether or not assisted ventilation was initiated (Stark, 1986).

II. **Incidence.** HMD severe enough to require assisted ventilation occurs in about 25% of infants born at 30 weeks' gestation. The incidence increases with increasing prematurity. In the United States, 40,000 newborns are affected annually. Although survival is over 90%, RDS accounts for 20% of all neonatal deaths.

III. **Pathophysiology.** The infant with HMD exhibits dependency on supplemental oxygen and increased work of breathing. Both are due to progressive atelectasis from lack of surfactant and an overly compliant chest wall. Surfactant is a surface-active material produced by airway epithelial cells called **type II pneumocytes.** This cell line differentiates, and surfactant synthesis begins at 24–28 weeks' gestation. Type II cells are sensitive to and decreased by asphyxial insults in the perinatal period. The maturation of this cell line is delayed in the presence of fetal hyperinsulinemia. The maturity of type II cells is enhanced by chronic intrauterine stress such as pregnancy-induced hypertension, intrauterine growth retardation (IUGR), and twin gestation. Surfactant, composed chiefly of phospholipid (75%) and protein (10%), is produced and stored in the characteristic **lamellar bodies** of type II pneumocytes. This lipoprotein is released into the airways, where it functions to decrease surface tension and maintain alveolar expansion at physiologic pressures.

A. **Lack of surfactant.** In the absence of surfactant, the small air spaces collapse, with each expiration resulting in progressive atelectasis. Exudative proteinaceous material and epithelial debris, resulting from progressive cellular damage, collect in the airway and directly decrease total lung capacity. In pathologic specimens, this material stains typically as **eosinophilic hyaline membranes**—thus the pathologic diagnosis of hyaline membrane disease.

B. **Presence of an overly compliant chest wall.** In the presence of a chest wall with weak structural support owing to prematurity, the large negative pressures generated to open the collapsed airways cause retraction and deformation of the chest wall instead of inflation of the poorly compliant lungs.

C. **Shunting.** The presence or absence of a cardiovascular shunt through a patent ductus arteriosus or foramen ovale, or both, may change the presentation or course of the disease process. The course of HMD results in acidosis and hypoxia, which can increase pulmonary vascular resistance. When pulmonary (right) pressure exceeds systemic (left) pressure, right-to-left shunting results. The clinical course is often complicated by cardiomegaly and pulmonary edema, owing to a large left-to-right shunt through the patent ductus or foramen ovale.

D. **Decreased intrathoracic pressure.** The infant with HMD who is less than 30 weeks' gestational age often presents with immediate respiratory failure due to inability to generate the intrathoracic pressure necessary to inflate the lungs without surfactant.

IV. **Risk factors.** Factors that increase or decrease the risk of HMD are listed in Table 67–1.

V. **Clinical presentation**

A. **History.** The infant is **preterm,** either by dates or by gestational examination, *or* has a **history of asphyxia in the perinatal period.** It presents with some **respiratory difficulty at birth that becomes progressively more severe.** The classic worsening of the atelectasis, as seen on chest x-ray film, and increasing oxygen requirement for 48–72 hours with subsequent diuresis and improvement (or death), have been modified by the increased ability to provide respiratory support for these infants.

TABLE 67–1. RISK FACTORS THAT INCREASE OR DECREASE THE RISK OF HYALINE MEMBRANE DISEASE

Increased Risk	Decreased Risk
Prematurity	Chronic intrauterine stress
Male sex	Prolonged ruptured membranes
Familial predisposition	Maternal hypertension
Cesarean without labor	Narcotic/cocaine use
Perinatal asphyxia	IUGR or SGA
Chorioamnionitis	Corticosteroids
Hydrops	Thyroid hormone
	Tocolytic agents

B. Physical examination. The infant exhibits **cyanosis on room air, nasal flaring, tachypnea, grunting on expiration,** and **retractions** of the chest wall. The infant grunts to prolong expiration, and this mechanism actually improves alveolar ventilation. The retractions occur and increase as the infant is forced to develop high transpulmonary pressure to reinflate atelectatic air spaces.

VI. Diagnosis

A. Laboratory studies

1. **Blood gas sampling** is essential in the management of HMD. Usually intermittent arterial sampling is performed. Although there is no consensus, most neonatologists agree that **arterial oxygen tensions of 50–70 mm Hg and arterial carbon dioxide tensions of 45–60 mm Hg are acceptable.** Most would maintain the pH at or above 7.25 and the arterial oxygen saturation at 88–95%. *Note:* In addition, continuous transcutaneous oxygen and carbon dioxide monitors or oxygen saturation monitors, or both, are proving invaluable in the minute-to-minute monitoring.

2. **Hemoglobin or hematocrit measurements** are needed early to guide the choice of plasma volume expanders if the infant has evidence of shock.

3. **Serum glucose levels** may be high or low initially and must be followed closely to assess the adequacy of dextrose infusion.

4. **Septic workup.** A partial septic workup, including complete blood count, platelet count, blood culture, amniotic fluid culture, urine culture, and latex agglutination test of the infant's urine for group B streptococcal antigen, should be considered for each infant with a diagnosis of HMD, since early-onset sepsis, eg, infection with group B streptococcus or *Haemophilus influenzae,* can be indistinguishable from HMD on clinical grounds alone.

5. **Serum electrolyte levels** should be followed every 12–24 hours for management of parenteral fluids.

6. **Serum calcium levels** should be followed daily, since hypocalcemia is common in sick, nonfed, preterm, or asphyxiated infants.

7. **Blood type, Rh, and Coombs' test determinations** are needed because:
   a. Transfusion may be indicated to correct hypotension, persistent poor perfusion, or falling blood hematocrit resulting from routine phlebotomy.
   b. The possibility of significant hyperbilirubinemia and the need for exchange blood transfusions exists in these infants, owing to prematurity, acidosis, and delayed feeding and stooling.

B. Chest x-ray study.
An anteroposterior chest x-ray film should be obtained for all infants with respiratory distress of any duration. If the infant is close to term, a cross-table lateral view may be considered to search for evidence of free air between the chest wall and lung parenchyma. The typical radiographic finding is a **uniform reticulogranular pattern, referred to as a "ground glass" appearance accompanied by air bronchograms.** During the clinical course, sequential x-ray films may reveal air leaks secondary to ventilatory intervention as well as the onset of changes compatible with bronchopulmonary dysplasia.

C. Echocardiography
is a valuable diagnostic tool in the evaluation of an infant with hypoxemia and respiratory distress. Significant congenital heart disease

can be excluded by this technique. Vascular shunts either away from or toward the lungs may be demonstrated and appropriate therapy instituted.

VII. Management

A. Prevention.
The following preventive measures have resulted in improved survival of infants at risk for RDS.

1. **Antenatal ultrasonography** for more accurate assessment of gestational age and fetal well-being.
2. **Continuous fetal monitoring** to document fetal well-being during labor or to signal the need for intervention when fetal distress is discovered.
3. **Prevention and intervention of premature labor,** using both tocolytic agents and corticosteroids to induce lung maturation.
4. **Assessment of fetal lung maturity** prior to delivery (lecithin:sphingomyelin ratio and phosphatidyl glycerol). (See p. 3.)

B. Respiratory support

1. **Endotracheal intubation and mechanical ventilation** are the mainstays of therapy for infants with respiratory distress syndrome in whom apnea or hypoxemia with respiratory acidosis develops. Mechanical ventilation usually begins with rates of 30–60 breaths/min and inspiratory:expiratory ratios of 1:2. An initial peak inspiratory pressure (PIP) of 18–30 cm water is used, depending on the size of the infant and the severity of the disease. A positive end-expiratory pressure (PEEP) of 4 cm water results in improved oxygenation probably due to increased airway pressure, which is kept as low as possible while still maintaining ventilation and oxygenation. The lowest possible pressures and inspired oxygen concentrations are maintained in an attempt to minimize damage to parenchymal tissue.
2. **Continuous positive airway pressure (CPAP).** Nasal prong or nasopharyngeal CPAP (NPCPAP) may be used early to delay or prevent the need for endotracheal intubation. It works best on larger infants with mild to moderate disease and good respiratory effort. NPCPAP may be used upon extubation and it may decrease the chance of reintubation. Nasopharyngeal tubes plug frequently. Therefore, their use must be accompanied by routine replacement of the tube each 6–8 hours.
3. **Complications.** Pulmonary air leaks, such as pneumothorax, pneumomediastinum, pneumopericardium, and pulmonary interstitial emphysema, may occur. Chronic complications include respiratory problems such as bronchopulmonary dysplasia and tracheal stenosis.

C. Fluid and nutritional support.
In the very ill infant, it is now possible to maintain nutritional support with parenteral nutrition for an extended period. The specific needs of preterm and term infants are becoming better understood, and the nutrient preparations available reflect this understanding (see Chap 8).

D. Drug therapy.
Sedation with **phenobarbitol, pentobarbitol,** and **chloral hydrate** is commonly used to control ventilation in these sick infants. In some institutions morphine or fentanyl is used for its analgesic, as well as sedative, effect. Muscle relaxation with pancuronium in infants with RDS remains *controversial.* Sedation might be indicated for infants with respiratory patterns that increase the likelihood of an air leak. These infants "fight" the ventilator support and consistently exhale on the inspiratory part of the ventilator cycle. Sedation or muscle paralysis of infants with fluctuating cerebral blood flow velocity theoretically decreases the risk of intraventricular hemorrhage.

E. Surfactant replacement.
(See also Chap 6.) Surfactant replacement is now typically used in the treatment of HMD. Double-blind randomized trials have proved that exogenous surfactant given either as a preventilatory dose or within 6 hours of birth in "rescue" studies dramatically reduces the number of cases of severe RDS (80% oxygen and mean airway pressures of more than 10 cm water). Two products (**Exosurf Pediatric** and **Survanta**) are available and there is no clear advantage between them. Surfactant replacement, although proved to be immediately effective in reducing the severity of RDS, has not clearly been shown to decrease the long-term oxygen requirements

or the development of chronic lung changes. Currently, long-term follow-up studies have not shown significant differences between surfactant-treated patients and nontreated control groups with regard to PDA, IVH, ROP, NEC, BPD, and long-term mortality. In 4- to 6-year follow-up studies, no adverse effects attributable to surfactant therapy have been identified. Studies are in progress to see if these products are effective in the treatment of respiratory distress of other etiologies where acquired surfactant deficiency may be part of the pathophysiology, ie, infectious pneumonia or meconium aspiration syndrome.

VIII. Prognosis. The prognosis for infants with HMD is highly dependent on birth weight (see Table 67–2).

MECONIUM ASPIRATION

I. Definition. Normally, meconium is the first intestinal discharge of the newborn infant and is composed of epithelial cells, fetal hair, mucus, and bile. However, intrauterine stress may cause in utero passage of meconium into the amniotic fluid. Subsequent to passage, the meconium-stained amniotic fluid may be aspirated by the fetus in utero or by the newborn during labor and delivery. If meconium is aspirated, it can cause airway obstruction and an intense inflammatory reaction, resulting in severe respiratory distress. The presence of meconium in amniotic fluid is a **warning sign of fetal distress,** calling for careful supervision of labor and assessment of fetal well-being.

II. Incidence. The incidence of meconium-stained amniotic fluid varies from 8% to 20% of all deliveries. The passage of meconium in an asphyxiated infant under 34 weeks' gestation is unusual; thus, meconium aspiration affects chiefly **term and postmature infants.**

III. Pathophysiology

A. In utero passage of meconium. Asphyxia and other forms of intrauterine stress may cause increased intestinal peristalsis, with relaxation of the external anal sphincter and passage of meconium. The effect of intrauterine hypoxia on peristalsis and sphincter tone seems to increase with gestational age, so that a premature infant with meconium-stained fluid at birth may have suffered a more severe insult than a postmature infant.

B. Aspiration of meconium. After passage of meconium into the amniotic fluid, gasping respirations of the asphyxiated fetus, either in utero or during labor and delivery, can cause aspiration of the meconium-stained amniotic fluid into the large airways of the lung. (Normal fetal respiratory activity results in movement of lung secretions from the airways into the amniotic fluid.) The thick meconium causes airway obstruction, resulting in respiratory distress.

1. Airway obstruction. With aspiration of meconium distally, total or partial airway obstruction may occur. In areas of total obstruction, atelectasis develops; but in areas of partial obstruction, a ball-valve phenomenon occurs,

TABLE 67–2. PROGNOSIS AND OUTCOMES IN PATIENTS WITH HYALINE MEMBRANE DISEASE BASED ON BIRTH WEIGHT

Birth Weight (g)	Survival Percentage	Risk of BPD[a]	Risk of Stage III/IV ROP[b]
501	5	All	Very high
501–750	40	Most	Moderate
751–1000	75	Half	Present
1001–1500	98	Few	Low

[a] Bronchopulmonary dysplasia, patients on oxygen at 28 days.
[b] Retinopathy of prematurity.

resulting in air trapping and hyperexpansion. Air trapping increases the risk of air leak to 21–50%.

   2. Chemical pneumonitis. Ultimately, interstitial and chemical pneumonitis develops, with resulting bronchiolar edema and narrowing of the small airways. Uneven ventilation due to areas of partial obstruction and superimposed pneumonitis causes severe carbon dioxide retention and hypoxemia. Pulmonary vascular resistance increases as a direct result of hypoxia, acidosis, and hyperinflation of the lungs. The increase in pulmonary vascular resistance may lead to atrial or ductal right-to-left shunting and further desaturation.

IV. Risk factors. The following factors have been associated with an increased risk of meconium passage and subsequent aspiration.
   A. Postterm pregnancy.
   B. Preeclampsia-eclampsia.
   C. Maternal hypertension.
   D. Maternal diabetes mellitus.
   E. Abnormal fetal heart rate.
   F. Small-for-gestational-age infants.
   G. Biophysical profile ≤ 6.
   H. Maternal heavy smoking, chronic respiratory disease, or cardiovascular disease.

V. Clinical presentation. The presentation of an infant with meconium-stained amniotic fluid who has aspirated meconium in the trachea is variable. Symptoms depend on the severity of the hypoxic insult and the amount and viscosity of the meconium aspirated.
   A. General features
      1. The infant. Infants with meconium-stained amniotic fluid often exhibit signs of postmaturity: they are small for gestational age with long nails and peeling skin stained with yellow or green pigment. These infants may have respiratory depression at birth, with poor respiratory effort and decreased muscle tone if there has been significant perinatal asphyxia associated with the passage of meconium.
      2. The amniotic fluid. The meconium present in amniotic fluid varies in quantity, appearance, and viscosity, ranging from a small to a copious amount and from a thin green-stained fluid to a thick "pea soup" consistency. It appears that heavily stained fluid is more clearly associated with severe respiratory distress and higher morbidity and mortality rates than lightly stained fluid.
   B. Airway obstruction. If a large amount of thick meconium is aspirated, the infant presents with acute airway obstruction manifested by deep gasping respirations, cyanosis, and poor air exchange. The airway must be rapidly cleared by endotracheal suctioning.
   C. Respiratory distress. The infant who has aspirated meconium into the distal airways but does not have total airway obstruction manifests signs of respiratory distress secondary to increased airway resistance and air trapping, ie, **tachypnea, nasal flaring, rib retraction, and cyanosis.** Some infants who do not experience acute airway obstruction **may have a delayed presentation,** with only mild initial respiratory distress, which becomes more severe hours after delivery as chemical pneumonitis develops.
   Note: Although many infants with meconium-stained amniotic fluid appear normal at birth and exhibit no signs of respiratory distress, a short episode of asphyxia may well have induced passage of meconium.
   D. Other pulmonary abnormalities. There may be a noticeable increase in the anteroposterior diameter of the chest if air trapping develops. With air trapping, auscultation reveals decreased air exchange, ie, variable rales, rhonchi, and wheezing.

VI. Diagnosis
   A. Laboratory studies. Arterial blood gas levels characteristically reveal

hypoxemia. Hyperventilation may result in respiratory alkalosis in mild cases, but infants with severe disease usually manifest respiratory acidosis with carbon dioxide retention due to airway obstruction and pneumonitis. If the patient has suffered severe perinatal asphyxia, combined respiratory and metabolic acidosis are present.

B. Radiologic studies. A **chest x-ray film** typically reveals hyperinflation of the lung fields and flattened diaphragms. There are coarse, irregular patchy infiltrates with increased lung fluid. Pneumothorax or pneumomediastinum may be present. The severity of x-ray findings may not always correlate with the clinical disease.

VII. Management

A. Prenatal management. The key to management of meconium aspiration lies in prevention during the prenatal period.

1. **Identification of high-risk pregnancies.** The approach to prevention begins with recognition of predisposing maternal factors that may cause uteroplacental insufficiency and subsequent fetal hypoxia during labor (see 426).

2. **Monitoring.** During labor, careful observation and fetal monitoring should be performed. Any signs of fetal distress (eg, appearance of meconium-stained fluid with membrane rupture, loss of beat-to-beat variability, deceleration patterns) warrant assessment of fetal well-being by scrutiny of fetal heart tracings and fetal scalp pH. If assessment indicates a compromised fetus, delivery by the most appropriate route should be accomplished as soon as possible.

B. Delivery room management. Delivery room management of the meconium-stained infant is discussed on p 15.

C. Management of the newborn with meconium aspiration. Infants who have meconium suctioned from the trachea are at risk for pneumonitis and air leak syndromes and must be observed closely for signs of respiratory distress. In addition, infants with meconium-stained fluid and low Apgar scores may have suffered asphyxial injury and should be examined for signs of end-organ damage.

1. **Respiratory management**

   a. **Pulmonary toilet.** If suctioning the trachea does not result in clearing of secretions, it may be advisable to leave an endotracheal tube in place for pulmonary toilet. Chest physiotherapy every 30 minutes to 1 hour, as tolerated, will aid in clearing the airway.

   b. **Arterial blood gas levels.** On admission to the NICU, the infant requires arterial blood gas measurements to assess ventilatory compromise and supplemental oxygen needs. If the patient requires more than 40% FiO_2, an arterial line should be placed.

   c. **Oxygen monitoring.** A transcutaneous oxygen monitor or pulse oximeter may provide information regarding the patient's ability to tolerate stress and will assist in preventing hypoxemia.

   d. **Chest x-ray films** should be obtained after delivery if the infant is in distress. It may help determine which patients will develop respiratory distress.

   e. **Antibiotic coverage.** Meconium promotes the growth of bacteria in vitro. Since it is impossible to differentiate meconium aspiration from pneumonia radiographically, infants with infiltrates on chest x-ray film should be started on broad-spectrum antibiotics (ampicillin and gentamicin; see Chap 73 for dosages and other pharmacologic information) after appropriate cultures have been obtained.

   f. **Supplemental oxygen.** If oxygen requirements continue to increase and acceptable oxygenation cannot be maintained, a trial of continuous positive airway pressure (CPAP) may be considered. CPAP may help with oxygenation in certain patients, but it may also aggravate preexisting air trapping and increase the risk of air leak. If possible, arterial oxygen tension should be maintained in the range of 80–90 mm Hg to prevent hypoxic pulmonary vasoconstriction, which may result in development of persistent pulmonary hypertension (PPH).

g. **Mechanical ventilation.** Patients with severe disease who are in impending respiratory failure with hypercapnia and persistent hypoxemia require mechanical ventilation.

(1) **Rate settings.** Ventilation must be tailored to the individual patient. These patients typically require higher inspiratory pressures than patients with hyaline membrane disease, and they do better with rates of 60 breaths/min or greater. Relatively short inspiratory times allow for adequate expiration in patients with preexisting air trapping.

(2) **Complications.** The clinician must maintain a high index of suspicion for air leak. For any unexplained deterioration of clinical status, a chest x-ray study should be done to rule out air leak. With the development of edema, exudation, air trapping and the resulting decrease in lung compliance, high mean airway pressures may be required in a patient who is at risk for air leak. The approach to ventilation must be directed at preventing hypoxemia and providing adequate ventilation at the lowest mean airway pressure possible to reduce the risk of catastrophic air leak.

h. **Extracorporeal membrane oxygenation (ECMO).** Patients who cannot be ventilated by conventional means may be candidates for ECMO (see Chap 11).

i. **High-frequency jet ventilation.** Reports suggest that high-frequency jet ventilation may offer an alternative ventilatory mode for selected patients.

2. **Cardiovascular management.** Persistent pulmonary hypertension is frequently associated with meconium aspiration. The development of pulmonary hypertension may be a result of hypoxic pulmonary vasoconstriction, abnormal muscularization of the pulmonary microcirculation, or both. To minimize the risk of PPH, aggressive resuscitation and stabilization are essential.

3. **General management.** Infants who have aspirated meconium and require resuscitation often develop metabolic abnormalities such as hypoxia, acidosis, hypoglycemia, hypocalcemia, and hypothermia. Because these patients may have suffered perinatal asphyxia, surveillance for any end-organ damage is essential (see Chap 66).

VIII. **Prognosis.** Complications are common, and the mortality rate may exceed 50%. In patients surviving severe meconium aspiration, bronchopulmonary dysplasia may result from oxygen toxicity and prolonged mechanical ventilation. Those with significant asphyxial insult may demonstrate neurologic sequelae.

TRANSIENT TACHYPNEA OF THE NEWBORN

I. **Definition.** Transient tachypnea of the newborn (TTN) is also known as *"wet lung"* and *"type II respiratory distress syndrome."* It is a benign disease of near-term, term, or large premature infants who have respiratory distress shortly after delivery that usually resolves within 3 days.

II. **Incidence.** The incidence of TTN is estimated at 1–2% of all newborns.

III. **Pathophysiology**

A. **Delayed resorption of fetal lung fluid.** TTN is thought to occur because of delayed resorption of fetal lung fluid from the pulmonary lymphatic system. The increased fluid volume causes a reduction in lung compliance and increased airway resistance. This results in tachypnea and retractions. Infants delivered by elective cesarean section are at risk because of lack of the normal vaginal thoracic squeeze, which forces lung fluid out.

B. **Pulmonary immaturity.** One study noted that a mild degree of pulmonary immaturity is a central factor in the cause of TTN. They found a mature L:S ratio but negative phosphatidylglycerol (the presence of phosphatidylglycerol means completed lung maturation). Infants who were closer to 36 weeks' gestation than 38 weeks had an increased risk of TTN.

C. **Mild surfactant deficiency.** One hypothesis is that TNN may represent a mild surfactant deficiency in these infants.

IV. **Risk factors**
    A. Elective cesarean delivery.
    B. Male sex.
    C. Macrosomia.
    D. Excessive maternal sedation.
    E. Prolonged labor.
    F. Negative amniotic fluid phosphatidylglycerol.
    G. Birth asphyxia.
    H. Fluid overload to mother, especially with oxytocin infusion.
    I. Maternal asthma.
    J. Delayed clamping of umbilical cord. Optimal time is 45 seconds.
    K. Breech delivery.
    L. Fetal polycythemia.
    M. Infant of diabetic mother.

V. **Clinical presentation.** The infant is usually near-term, term, or large and premature and shortly after delivery has tachypnea (> 60 breaths/min). The infant may also have grunting, nasal flaring, rib retraction, and varying degrees of cyanosis. The chest often appears to have the classic "barrel chest" secondary to the increased anteroposterior diameter. There are usually no signs of sepsis. Some may have edema and a mild ileus on physical examination.

VI. **Diagnosis**
    A. **Laboratory studies**
        1. **Prenatal testing.** A mature L:S ratio with presence of phosphatidylglycerol in the amniotic fluid may help to rule out hyaline membrane disease.
        2. **Postnatal testing**
            a. **Arterial blood gas** on room air will show some degree of hypoxia. Hypercarbia, if it exists, is usually mild (pCO_2 < 55 torr).
            b. **Complete blood count and differential** is normal in TTN but should be obtained if considering an infectious process. The hematocrit will also rule out polycythemia.
            c. **Urine Antigen test** may help rule out group B streptococcal pneumonia.
    B. **Radiologic studies**
        1. **Chest x-ray study.** The typical findings in TTN are:
            a. Hyperexpansion of the lungs.
            b. Prominent perihilar streaking (secondary to engorgement of periarterial lymphatics).
            c. Mild to moderately enlarged heart.
            d. Depression (flattening) of the diaphragm.
            e. Fluid in the minor fissure, and perhaps fluid in the pleural space.
    C. **Other tests.** Any infant who is hypoxic on room air must have a **100% oxygen test** to rule out heart disease. (This test is described on p 282.)

VII. **Management**
    A. **General**
        1. **Oxygenation.** Initial management consists of providing adequate oxygenation. Start with hood oxygen and deliver enough to maintain normal arterial saturation. These infants typically require only hood oxygen, usually less than 60%. If the oxygen needs to be increased and 100% hood oxygenation does not work, change to nasal CPAP. If these maneuvers do not work, intubate the infant and proceed with mechanical ventilation. If the

infant requires 100% oxygen or endotracheal intubation with ventilator support, another disease process should be suspected.

2. **Feeding.** Because of the risk of aspiration, an infant should not be fed by mouth if the respiratory rate is over 60 min. If the respiratory rate is less than 60 breaths/min, oral feeding is permissible. If the rate is 60–80 breaths/min, feeding should be by nasogastric tube. If the rate is over 80/min, intravenous nutrition is indicated.

3. **Diuretics.** Two randomized trials using Furosemide showed an increase in weight loss in the treated group but no difference in decrease or duration of respiratory symptoms or length of hospital stay.

B. **Confirm the diagnosis.** TTN is often a diagnosis of exclusion and other causes of tachypnea should be excluded first. The usual causes of tachypnea are:

1. **Pneumonia.** If the infant has pneumonia, the prenatal history will usually suggest infection. There may be maternal chorioamnionitis, premature rupture of membranes, and fever. The blood count may show evidence of infection (neutropenia or leukocytosis with abnormal numbers of immature cells. The urine antigen test may be positive if the infant has group B streptococcal infection. Remember, it is better to give broad-spectrum antibiotics if there is any suspicion or evidence of infection. The antibiotics can always be discontinued if the cultures are negative in 3 days.

2. **Heart disease.** The 100% oxygen test should be done to rule out heart disease (see p 282). Cardiomegaly may be seen.

3. **Hyaline membrane disease.** The infant will normally be premature or have some reason for delayed lung maturation, such as maternal diabetes. The chest x-ray film is helpful because it shows the typical HMD reticulogranular pattern with air bronchograms and underexpansion (atelectasis) of the lungs.

4. **Cerebral hyperventilation.** This disorder is seen when CNS lesions cause overstimulation of the respiratory center, resulting in tachypnea. The CNS lesions can include meningitis or hypoxic-ischemic insult. Arterial blood gas measurements show respiratory alkalosis.

5. **Metabolic disorders.** Infants with hypothermia, hyperthermia, or hypoglycemia may all have tachypnea.

6. **Polycythemia/Hyperviscosity.** This syndrome may present with tachypnea with or without cyanosis.

VIII. **Prognosis.** TTN is self-limited and usually lasts only 1–3 days with no risk of further pulmonary dysfunction.

REFERENCES

Allen RW, Jung AL, Lester PD: Effectiveness of chest tube evacuation of pneumothorax in neonates. *J Pediatr* 1981;**99**:629.

Alpan G et al: Doxapram in the treatment of idiopathic apnea on prematurity unresponsive to aminophylline. *J Pediatr* 1984;**104**:634.

Ballard J, Musial MJ, Myers MG: Hazards of delivery room resuscitation using oral methods of endotracheal suctioning. *Pediatr Infect Dis* 1986;**5**:198.

Bancalari E, Gerhardt T: Bronchopulmonary dysplasia. *Pediatr Clin North* 1986;**33**:1.

Bednarek FJ, Roloff DW: Treatment of apnea of prematurity with aminophylline. *Pediatrics* 1973;**55**:335.

Blanchard PW, Brown TM, Coates AL: Pharmacotherapy in bronchopulmonary dysplasia. *Clin Perinatol* 1987;**14**:881.

Brooks JG et al: Selective bronchial intubation for the treatment of severe localized pulmonary emphysema in newborn infants. *J Pediatr* 1977;**91**:648.

Carson BS: Prevention of meconium aspiration syndrome. *Neonatal Grand Rounds* 1986;**3**:3.

Creasy RK, Resnik R: *Maternal-Fetal Medicine: Principles and Practice.* Saunders, 1984.

Escobedo MB, Gonzales A: Bronchopulmonary dysplasia in the tiny infant. *Clin Perinatol* 1986;**13**:315.

Fanaroff AA, Martin RJ: *Neonatal-Perinatal Medicine: Diseases of the Fetus and Infant,* 4th ed. Mosby, 1987.

Fiascone JM et al: Bronchopulmonary dysplasia: Review for the pediatrician. *Curr Probl Pediatr* 1989;**19:**169.

Ficheux H et al: Simultaneous determination of hemoglobin and coproporphyrin by second derivative differential spectrophotometry: Application to the diagnosis of meconium aspiration. *Clin Chim Acta* 1989;**189(1):**53.

Goetzman BW: Understanding bronchopulmonary dysplasia. *Am J Dis Child* 1986;**140:**332.

Goldsmith JP, Klarotkin EH. Pages 189–199 in: *Assisted Ventilation of the Neonate.* Saunders, 1981.

James DL et al: Non specificity of surfactant deficiency in neonatal respiratory disorders. *Brit Med J* 1984;**288:**1635.

Jobe AH, Taeusch HW (editors): *Surfactant Treatment of Lung Disease.* Report of the Ninety-Sixth Ross Conference on Pediatric Research. Ross Laboratories, 1988.

Kattwinkel J: Neonatal apnea: Pathogenesis and therapy. *J Pediatr* 1977;**90:**342.

Kattwinkel J et al: Apnea of prematurity. *J Pediatr* 1985;**86:**588.

Keszler M et al: Combined high-frequency jet ventilation in a meconium aspiration model. *Crit Care Med* 1986;**14(1):**34.

Linder N et al: Need for endotracheal intubation and suction in meconium-stained neonates. *J Pediatr* 1988;**112(4):**613.

Mansfield PB et al: Pneumopericardium and pneumomediastinum in infants and children. *J Pediatr Surg* 1973;**8:**691.

Merritt TA et al: Immunologic consequences of exogenous surfactant administration. *Semin Perinatol* 1988;**12:**221.

Merritt TA, Northway WH Jr, Boynton BR: *Contemporary Issues in Fetal and Neonatal Medicine (4): Bronchopulmonary Dysplasia.* Blackwell Scientific, 1989.

Miller MJ, Carlo WA, Martin RJ: Continuous positive airway pressure selectively reduces obstructive apnea in preterm infants. *J Pediatr* 1985;**106:**91.

Murphy JD, Vawter GF, Reid LM: Pulmonary vascular disease in fatal meconium aspiration. *J Pediatr* 1984;**104:**758.

O'Brodovich HM, Mellins RB: Bronchopulmonary dysplasia: Unresolved neonatal acute lung injury. *Am Rev Respir Dis* 1986;**132:**694.

Perleman EJ, Moore GW, Hutchins GM: Pulmonary vasculature in meconium aspiration. *Hum Pathol* 1989;**20(7):**701.

Philips III JB: Management of the meconium-stained infant. *Neonatal Grand Rounds* 1986;**3:**1.

Reynolds MS, Wallander KA: Use of surfactant in the prevention and treatment of neonatal RDS. *Clin Pharmacol* 1989;**8:**559.

Schatz M et al: Increased transient tachypnea of the newborn in infants of asthmatic mothers. *Am J Dis Child* 1991;**145(2):**156–58.

Shapiro DL, Notter RH: Controversies regarding surfactant replacement therapy. *Clin Perinatol* 1988;**15:**891.

Spillman T et al: Detection frequency by thin layer chromatography of phosphatidylglycerol in amniotic fluid with clinically functional pulmonary surfactant. *Clin-Chem* 1988;**34(10):**1976.

Spitzer AR, Fox WW: Infant apnea. *Pediatr Clin North Am* 1986;**33:**561.

Stark AE, Frantz III ID: Respiratory distress syndrome. *Pediatr Clin North Am* 1986;**33:**533.

Stevens JC, Eigen H, Wysomierski D: Extracorporeal membrane oxygenation as treatment of severe meconium aspiration syndrome. *South Med J* 1989;**82(6):**696.

Taylor GA, Short BL, Kriesemer P: Extracorporeal membrane oxygenation: Radiographic appearance of the neonatal chest. *Am J Radiol* 1986;**146(6):**1257.

Thibeault DW, Gregory GA: Pages 499–519 in: *Neonatal Pulmonary Care.* Appleton-Century-Crofts, 1986.

Trento A, Griffith BP, Hardesty RL: Extracorporeal membrane oxygenation experience at the University of Pittsburgh. *Am Thorac Surg* 1986;**42(1):**56.

Trindade O et al: Conventional vs. high-frequency jet ventilation in a piglet model of meconium aspiration: Comparison of pulmonary and hemodynamic effects. *J Pediatr* 1985;**107(1):**115.

Vance J: Antenatal and neonatal management of meconium staining. *MO Perinatal Prog* 1984;**7:**1.

Van Golde LMG et al: The pulmonary surfactant system: Biochemical aspects and functional significance. *Physiol Rev* 1988;**68:**374.

68 Renal Diseases

ACUTE RENAL FAILURE

I. **Definition.** In neonates, acute renal failure is defined as the absence of urinary output (anuria) or as urine output of less than 0.5 mL/kg/24 h (oliguria) with an associated increase in serum creatinine. Ninety-nine percent of infants void by 48 hours (see Table 44–1 for average times from birth to first voiding).

II. **Incidence.** In some studies, as many as 23% of neonates have some form of renal failure, with prerenal factors identified as the cause in 73%.

III. **Pathophysiology.** Normal urine output is about 1–3 mL/kg/h in newborns, and the normal newborn kidney has poor concentrating ability. Renal failure leads to problems with volume overload, hyperkalemia, acidosis, hyperphosphatemia, and hypocalcemia. Acute renal failure is traditionally divided into 3 categories, as follows.

   A. **Prerenal failure.** Prerenal failure is due to decreased renal perfusion. Causes include dehydration (poor feeding, increased insensible losses referable to radiant warmers), perinatal asphyxia, and hypotension (septic shock, hemorrhagic shock, cardiogenic shock due to congestive heart failure).

   B. **Intrinsic renal failure.** If poor renal perfusion persists, acute tubular necrosis with intrinsic renal failure may result. Other causes are nephrotoxins such as aminoglycosides and methoxyflurane anesthesia, congenital anomalies (eg, renal agenesis, polycystic kidney disease), disseminated intravascular coagulation (DIC), renal vein or renal artery thrombosis, and isolated cortical necrosis.

   C. **Postrenal failure.** All the causes involve obstruction to urinary outflow. These include bilateral ureteropelvic obstruction, bilateral ureterovesical obstruction, posterior urethral valves, urethral diverticulum or stenosis, large ureterocele, neurogenic bladder, blocked urinary drainage tubes, and extrinsic tumor compression.

IV. **Risk factors.** Dehydration, sepsis, asphyxia, and administration of nephrotoxic drugs to the neonate are risk factors for acute renal failure. Maternal diabetes may increase the risk for renal vein thrombosis and subsequent renal insufficiency.

V. **Clinical presentation**

   A. **Decreased or absent urine output.** Low or absent urine output is usually the presenting problem. Ninety-nine percent of infants void by 48 hours (see Table 44–1).

   B. **Family history.** A history of urinary tract disease in other family members should be sought, a history of oligohydramnios, which frequently accompanies urinary outflow obstruction or severe renal dysplasia or agenesis.

   C. **Physical examination.** The following abnormalities on physical examination are significant.

   1. **Abdominal mass,** suggesting a distended bladder, polycystic kidneys, or hydronephrosis.
   2. **Potter's facies,** associated with renal agenesis.
   3. **Meningomyelocele,** associated with neurogenic bladder.
   4. **Pulmonary hypoplasia,** due to severe oligohydramnios in utero secondary to inadequate urinary output.
   5. **Urinary ascites,** which may be seen with posterior urethral valves.
   6. **Prune belly** (hypoplasia of the abdominal wall musculature and cryptorchidism), associated with urinary abnormalities.

VI. Diagnosis

A. Bladder catheterization. Perform bladder catheterization, using a 5F or 8F feeding tube to confirm inadequate urine output (see Chap 16 for details of procedure). Immediate passage of large volumes of urine suggests obstruction (eg, posterior urethral valves) or a hypotonic (neurogenic) bladder.

B. Laboratory studies

1. **Serum urea nitrogen and creatinine levels**

   a. **Urea nitrogen level** > 15–20 mg/dL suggests dehydration or renal insufficiency.

   b. **Creatinine level.** Normal serum creatinine values are 0.8–1.0 mg/dL at 1 day, 0.7–0.8 mg/dL at 3 days, and less than 0.6 mg/dL by 7 days of life. Higher values suggest renal disease except in low birth weight infants; a creatinine level of < 1.6 mg/dL is considered normal in them. (Rule of thumb: If the creatinine doubles, then 50% of the renal function has been lost.)

2. **Urinary indices** of acute renal failure are listed in Table 68–1. Order a spot urine osmolality, a serum and spot urine sodium, and serum and urine creatinine and calculate the fractional excretion of sodium and the renal failure index. These indices are of limited value if measured while the effect of diuretics such as furosemide are present.

$$\text{Fractional excretion of sodium (FeNa)} = \frac{\text{Urine Na}}{\text{Urine Cr}} \times \frac{\text{Plasma Cr}}{\text{Plasma Na}} \times 100$$

$$\text{Renal failure index (RFI)} = \frac{\text{Urine Na}}{\text{Urine Cr}} \times \text{Plasma Cr}$$

3. **Complete blood count and platelet count** may reveal thrombocytopenia, seen with sepsis or renal vein thrombosis.

4. **Serum potassium levels** should be followed to rule out hyperkalemia.

5. **Urinalysis** may reveal hematuria (associated with renal vein thrombosis, tumors, DIC; see Hematuria, p 434), or pyuria, suggesting urinary tract infection that is either the cause of renal insufficiency (sepsis) or the result of mechanical obstruction.

C. Diagnostic fluid challenge. If the patient does not have clinical volume overload or congestive failure, give a fluid challenge. Give normal saline or colloid solution, 5–10 mL/kg as IV bolus; repeat once PRN. If there is no response, give furosemide, 1 mg/kg. If there is still no increase in urine output, obstruction above the level of the bladder must be ruled out by ultrasound examination. If there is no evidence of obstruction and the patient does not respond to these maneuvers, the most likely cause of anuria or oliguria is intrinsic renal failure.

D. Radiologic studies

1. **Abdominal ultrasonography** can delineate hydronephrosis, dilated ureters, abdominal masses, a distended bladder, or renal vein thrombosis.

2. **Intravenous urography** has limited usefulness in the neonatal period, owing to the poor concentrating ability of the kidney, and is of limited value in the setting of renal failure.

TABLE 68–1. RENAL FAILURE INDICES IN THE NEONATE

	Prerenal	Renal
Urine osmolality (mosm)	> 400	< 400
Urine Na (meq/L)	31 ± 19	63 ± 35
Urine/plasma Cr	29 ± 16	10 ± 4
Fractional excretion of Na	< 2.5	> 2.5
Renal failure index (RFI)	< 3.0	> 3.0

3. **Abdominal x-ray studies** may show spina bifida or an absent sacrum, which can cause neurogenic bladder.
4. **Radionuclide scanning** can delineate functioning renal parenchyma (dimercaptosuccinic acid [DMSA]) and give some indication of renal flow and function (diethyltriamine pentaacetic acid [DTPA]).

VII. Management
A. General management
1. **Replace insensible fluid losses** (preterm, 50–70 mL/kg/d; term, 30 mL/kg/d) plus fluid output (urine, gastrointestinal tract).
2. **Keep strict intake and output and frequent weight records.**
3. **Follow serum sodium and potassium levels** frequently, and replace losses cautiously as needed. Infants with renal failure should never be given intravenous fluids containing potassium, since hyperkalemia, if it occurs, may be lethal. If hyperkalemia does occur, treat as outlined in Chapter 37.
4. **Restrict protein** to less than 2 g/kd/d and ensure adequate nonprotein caloric intake. Formulas such as breast milk PM 60/40 are frequently used for infants with renal failure.
5. **Hyperphosphatemia and hypocalcemia frequently coexist, and phosphate binders such as aluminum hydroxide,** 50–150 mg/kg/d orally, **should be used to normalize the phosphate.** Once the phosphate is normal, calcium with or without vitamin D supplements is usually needed.

   For tetany/convulsions, acute IV calcium replacement with 10% calcium gluconate 40 mg/kg or 10% calcium chloride will increase the serum calcium 1 mg/dL. Follow ionized calcium if available in your lab.
6. **Metabolic acidosis may require chronic oral bicarbonate supplementation. Blood pressures should be followed serially,** because these infants are always at risk for developing chronic hypertension. IV bicarbonate therapy should be given if the pH < 7.25 or the serum bicarbonate < 12 meq. HCO_3 deficit = (24 – observed) × 0.5 body wt in kg.

B. Definitive management
1. **Prerenal failure** is treated by correcting the specific cause (see section above).
2. **Postrenal failure.** Acute management involves bypassing the obstruction with a bladder catheter or by percutaneous nephrostomy drainage, depending on the level of the obstruction. Surgical correction is usually indicated at some point.
3. **Intrinsic renal disease.** If renal disease is caused by toxins or acute tubular necrosis, renal function may recover to some extent with time.
4. **Dialysis.** If recovery of renal function is expected or if renal transplantation is considered an option when the child is older, peritoneal dialysis is the treatment most commonly used in the neonate. On occasion hemodialysis, ultrafiltration, and CAVH (continuous arterio-venous hyperfiltration) may be required.

HEMATURIA

I. **Definition.** Hematuria is the presence of gross or microscopic blood in the urine. More than 3 red cells per high-power field is usually considered abnormal. A red-stained diaper usually signifies hematuria but may be due to bile pigments, porphyrins, or urates.
II. **Incidence.** Hematuria is not a common problem in newborns.
III. **Pathophysiology.** Hematuria in the newborn may be caused by perinatal asphyxia, cortical or medullary necrosis, infection, trauma (birth or iatrogenic, such as bladder aspiration or catheterization), renal vein or renal artery thrombosis, hyperosmolar infusions into umbilical catheters, neoplasms (rhabdomyosarcoma, nephroblastoma), urinary tract obstruction (urolithiasis following Lasix administration) or infection, coagulopathy, and neonatal glomerulonephritis (most commonly caused by syphilis).

IV. **Risk factors** include coagulopathy, urinary tract infection, obstruction, maternal diabetes (renal vein thrombosis), indwelling urinary catheters, and traumatic delivery.

V. **Clinical presentation**

    A. **History.** A maternal history of diabetes may arouse a suspicion of renal vein thrombosis. The birth history and Apgar scores may suggest perinatal asphyxia.

    B. **Physical examination.** Examination may reveal the presence of an abdominal mass (obstruction, neoplasm, renal vein thrombosis). The presence of an umbilical or bladder catheter should be noted.

VI. **Diagnosis**

    A. **Laboratory studies**

        1. **Urinalysis.** Microscopic examination and dipstick testing will confirm the presence of blood or other causes of "red urine." **Red cell casts** are seen with intrinsic renal disease such as glomerulonephritis. **Bacteria or white cells** suggest urinary tract infection.

        2. **Urine culture.** Collection of urine by bladder aspiration or catheterization is preferred and is outlined in Chapters 15 and 16.

        3. **Serum urea nitrogen and creatinine levels** may reveal renal insufficiency.

        4. **Coagulation studies.** PT, PTT, and thrombin time may provide clues to DIC or hemorrhagic disease of the newborn. Thrombocytopenia suggests renal vein thrombosis.

    B. **Radiologic studies**

        1. **Ultrasonography** will show neoplasms, renal vein thrombosis, or obstruction in the urinary tract.

        2. **Ancillary testing** such as intravenous urography, arteriography, and nuclear scans may be indicated.

VII. **Management.** Treatment is directed at the underlying cause.

URINARY TRACT INFECTION

I. **Definition.** Urinary tract infection (UTI) is the presence of pathogenic bacteria or fungus in the urinary tract with or without symptoms of infection. A definitive diagnosis is made by culture of any organism in a urine specimen that has been properly collected by suprapubic bladder aspiration, ideally, or by gentle catheterization.

II. **Incidence.** Various series report an incidence of 0.5–1.0% in term infants weighing more than 2500 g and higher rates (3–5%) in premature infants or infants weighing less than 2500 g. (***Note:*** male > female incidence in neonatal period.)

III. **Pathophysiology.** When urinary tract infection is present in an infant less than 1 year of age, an associated urinary tract abnormality is found in about 50% of neonates. Associated anomalies that may give rise to urinary tract infection include neurogenic bladder, urethral valves, vesicoureteral reflux, and ureteropelvic junction obstruction. The predominant organisms are gram-negative rods, with *E coli* the most common. In neonates, UTIs are most frequently acquired by hematogenous spread.

IV. **Risk factors** include indwelling urinary catheters, systemic sepsis with hematogenous seeding of the urinary tract, urinary tract obstruction, neurogenic bladder (myelodysplasia), and male newborns. Recent evidence suggests that uncircumsized males may be at higher risk for UTI.

V. **Clinical presentation**

    A. **Signs of sepsis.** The infant may present with frank signs of sepsis (respiratory distress, apnea, bradycardia, hypoglycemia, poor perfusion).

    B. **Nonspecific findings.** The signs are often subtle and may include poor feeding, vomiting, jaundice, or failure to thrive.

VI. **Diagnosis**

    A. **Laboratory studies**

1. **Urine culture.** Suprapubic aspiration or catheterization is mandatory for a good urine culture in a neonate. "Bag" urine is felt by some to be inadequate to achieve reliable culture results.
2. **Blood cultures** should be obtained before starting antibiotic therapy.
3. **Urinalysis.** Microscopic examination may show white blood cells, but the presence of bacteria is a more reliable sign of UTI in the neonate, especially when urine is collected by suprapubic aspiration.
4. **Complete blood count** may show leukocytosis.
5. **Serum bilirubin** may be elevated.
   B. No other studies are indicated.
VII. **Management**
   A. **Initial antibiotic treatment.** Initial antibiotic therapy usually consists of intravenous ampicillin and gentamicin until definitive urine and blood culture results are reported. (See Chap 73 for dosages and other pharmacologic information.)
   B. **Further investigations.** To rule out anatomic abnormalities in the neonate, renal/bladder ultrasound, contrast voiding cystourethrogram (VCUG), and renal scan are indicated and at times, an IVP for complex problems. Urologic consultation is usually recommended.
VIII. **Prognosis.** Up to one-fourth of infants can have recurrent UTI within the first year of life. Effective use of long-term suppressive antibiotics (in the presence of vesicoureteral reflux) along with any indicated corrective surgery has dramatically reduced the long-term incidence of renal scarring and renal insufficiency.

REFERENCES

Edelmann CM (ed): *Pediatric Kidney Disease* 2nd ed. Little, Brown & Co., Boston, 1992.

Ginsburg CM, McCracken GH: Urinary tract infections in young infants. *Pediatrics* 1982;**69:**409.

Greenhill A, Gruskin AP: Laboratory evaluation of renal function. *Pediatr Clin North Am* 1976;**23:**661.

Matthew OP et al: Neonatal renal failure: Usefulness of diagnostic indices. *Pediatrics* 1980;**65:**57.

Norman ME, Asadi FK: A prospective study of acute renal failure in the newborn infant. *Pediatrics* 1979;**63:**475.

69 Retinopathy of Prematurity

I. **Definitions**
  A. **Retinopathy of prematurity (ROP)** is a disorder of the developing retinal vasculature due to interruption of normal progression of newly forming retinal vessels. Vasoconstriction and obliteration of the advancing capillary bed is followed in succession by neovascularization extending into the vitreous, retinal edema, retinal hemorrhages, fibrosis, and traction on, and eventual detachment of, the retina. In most cases, the process is reversed before fibrosis occurs. **Advanced stages may lead to blindness.**
  B. **Retrolental fibroplasia.** As originally described, the condition was seen only in its most advanced form, after extensive fibrosis and scarring had already occurred behind the lens. It was therefore termed *retrolental fibroplasia*. It is now understood that several recognizable changes occur in the developing vasculature before end-stage fibrosis occurs, making this condition a true retinopathy because it is found chiefly in prematures, it is now called *retinopathy of prematurity (ROP)*.
  C. **Cicatricial ROP.** The term *cicatricial ROP* refers to fibrotic disease.
II. **Incidence.** About 400–600 children per year may be blinded by ROP, representing 20% of blindness in preschool children. Of particular concern are the increasing numbers of survivors weighing less than 1000 g who have the highest incidence of ROP and who may account for much of the current epidemic. The NIH sponsored CRYO-ROP study, carried out in 1986–1987, showed that 65.8% of infants < 1251 g developed ROP of any stage. 2% of infants 1000–1250 g developed threshold, stage III+, disease eligible for treatment while 15.5% of infants < 750 g did so. Threshold disease occurred at a median postconceptional age of 37 weeks regardless of gestational age at birth or chronologic age.
III. **Pathophysiology**
  A. **Historical perspective.** Retrolental fibroplasia (RLF) was first described by Terry in the 1940s and was associated with the use of oxygen in newborn infants by Patz and associates (1984). The **first epidemic,** estimated to be responsible for 30% of cases of blindness in preschool children by the end of the 1940s, occurred during a period of relatively liberal oxygen administration. After this association was recognized, oxygen use in nurseries was curtailed. Although the incidence of RLF fell, infant mortality rates in newborn infants increased. In the 1960s, improved oxygen monitoring techniques made possible the cautious reintroduction of oxygen into the nursery. Despite improved oxygen monitoring, however, a **second epidemic** of retrolental fibroplasia (retinopathy of prematurity) appeared in the late 1970s and has continued into the 1990s.
  B. **Normal embryology of the eye.** In the normally developing retina, there are no retinal vessels until about 16 weeks' gestation. Until then, oxygen diffuses from the underlying choroidal circulation. At 16 weeks, in response to an unknown stimulus (relative hypoxia as the retina thickens has been suggested), cells derived from mesenchyme traveling in the nerve fiber layer emanate from the optic nerve head. These cells, called *spindle cells* are the precursors of the retinal vascular system. A fine capillary network advances through the retina to the ora serrata, or retinal edge. More mature vessels form behind this advancing network. Vascularization on the nasal side of the ora serrata is complete at about 8 months' gestation, whereas that on the temporal side is ordinarily complete at term. Once completely vascularized, the retinal vasculature is no longer susceptible to insults of the type that lead to ROP.

C. Etiology

1. There appear to be 2 phases in the development of ROP, as described by Patz.

   a. Early vasoconstriction and obliteration of the capillary network in response to high oxygen concentrations noted experimentally.

   b. Vasoproliferation, which follows the period of high oxygen exposure, perhaps in response to an **angiogenic factor** released by the hypoxic retina. Considerable evidence has been developed to support this hypothesis. Phelps and Rosenbaum (1984) studied kittens made hyperoxic and then allowed to recover in room air (21% oxygen) or 13% oxygen. Those recovering in the hypoxic environment had worse retinopathy than those recovering in room air, suggesting that retinal hypoxia may play a role.

2. Alternatively, Kretzer et al (see McPherson [1986] reference) have proposed that the mesenchymal spindle cells form intercellular gap junctions in response to increased oxygen tensions. These increased gap junctions then form a barrier to ongoing mesenchymal migration into the retina, and the normal progression of vascularization ceases. These authors postulate further that the spindle cells produce an angiogenic substance that leads secondarily to abnormal vasoproliferation. They have reported experimental evidence that the administration of vitamin E decreases gap junction formation although this remains *controversial.*

IV. Risk factors.
The association of ROP with oxygen alone is now not so clear. There have been many recorded instances of ROP in premature infants not exposed to elevated oxygen concentrations. Many other factors such as extreme prematurity, maternal complications, apnea, sepsis, hyper- and hypocapnia, vitamin E deficiency, intraventricular hemorrhage, anemia, exchange transfusion, hypoxia, lactic acidosis, and bright light have been implicated. The pathophysiology of ROP is still unclear. Experimental studies have focused chiefly on the role of oxygen although extreme prematurity is now known to be the most significant risk factor.

V. Clinical presentation.
Several methods of classification of ROP have been used. With development of the **International Classification of ROP,** there is now general agreement on staging of active disease.

Stage I. A thin **demarcation line** develops between the vascularized region of the retina and the avascular zone.

Stage II. This line develops into a **ridge** protruding into the vitreous, in which there is histologic evidence for an arteriovenous shunt.

Stage III. Extraretinal fibrovascular proliferation occurs with the ridge. Neovascular tufts may be found just posterior to the ridge. (Fig 69–1).

Stage IV. Fibrosis and scarring occur as the neovascularization extends into the vitreous. Traction occurs on the retina, resulting in **retinal detachment.**

Plus disease (eg, stage III+) may occur when vessels posterior to the ridge become dilated and tortuous.

VI. Diagnosis. Ophthalmoscopic examination
by an experienced examiner usually confirms the diagnosis. Various protocols are used, depending on the institution.

A. **The American Academy of Pediatrics** recommends ophthalmoscopic examination at 5–7 weeks or discharge for all oxygen-exposed premature infants who weigh less than 1800 g or are delivered at less than 35 weeks' gestation. Infants less than 1300 g or 30 weeks' gestation require examination regardless of oxygen exposure.

B. Screening criteria suggested by Brown et al (1987) and based on examinations of 2986 neonates, attempt to decrease unnecessary examinations by limiting them to those who weigh less than 1600 g, examining those over 1600 g only if they have been exposed to oxygen for more than 50 days.

C. In the recently completed trial of cryopexy for ROP, examinations for infants who weigh less than 1251 g were begun at 4–6 weeks of age and repeated every 2 weeks until maturity or until eyes were prethreshold, just prior to eligibility for treatment. Because rapid progression can occur, they were then ex-

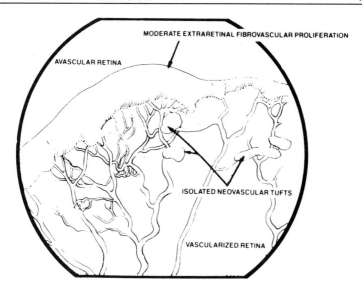

FIGURE 69–1. Schematic drawing of moderate stage III retinopathy of prematurity. Optic nerve head is at the bottom of drawing, and periphery of the retina is at the top. (*Reproduced, with permission, from Garner A: International classification of retinopathy of prematurity. Pediatrics 1984;74:127.*)

amined every week until eligible for treatment at stage III+ or until regression occurred. Overall, an initial examination between 4–6 weeks in smaller infants is advised. In the absence of disease, examinations should be repeated every 2–4 weeks until the retina is mature.

VII. Management

    A. Circumferential cryopexy is now the treatment of choice for progressive (stage III+) disease in an attempt to prevent further progression by destroying cells that may be releasing angiogenic factors. Results of the recent large collaborative NIH-sponsored trial indicate that cryopexy carried out at state III+ can reduce the incidence of severe visual impairment by 50% if performed within 72 hours of detecting threshold disease. If both eyes are involved, cryopexy is usually performed in one eye only as there are some risks with the procedure, such as vitreal hemorrhage. If there are enough risk factors for retinal detachment, however, cryopexy may be performed in both eyes. It is imperative that an ophthalmologist skilled in cryopexy perform the procedure.

    B. Laser photocoagulation. Preliminary data suggest that this technique is equally effective and safer than cryopexy. Further trials are in progress.

    C. Vitamin E. The administration of pharmacologic doses of vitamin E for ROP is *controversial;* currently there is no proof of clear benefit. Reported side effects include sepsis, necrotizing enterocolitis, and intraventricular hemorrhage. Even so, maintenance of normal serum vitamin E levels is a prudent management objective.

    D. Decreased lighting intensity. Glass et al (1985) reported a decreased incidence of ROP in infants cared for in an area of reduced light intensity. A subsequent study (Ackerman et al, 1989) showed no effect. A collaborative study is now under way.

    E. Retinal reattachment. Stage IV disease has been treated by attempts at retinal reattachment without significant success to date. Reattachment of late retinal detachments in childhood has met with more success.

    F. Vitrectomy has not substantially improved the outcome in cicatricial disease.

G. Follow-up eye examinations are advocated every 1–2 years for infants with fully regressed ROP and every 6–12 months for infants with cicatricial ROP.

VIII. Prognosis. Ninety percent of cases of stage I and stage II disease regress spontaneously. Current information suggests that 50% of cases of stage III+ disease regress spontaneously. Of those that do progress to stage III+, the incidence of severe visual impairment can be reduced by approximately 50% if circumferential cryopexy is carried out by a skilled ophthalmologist. Sequelae of regressed disease such as myopia, strabismus, amblyopia, glaucoma, and late detachment require regular follow-up.

REFERENCES

Ackerman B, Sheruonit E, Williams J: Reduced incidental light exposure: Effect on the development of retinopathy of prematurity in low birth weight infants. *Pediatrics* 1989;**83**:958.

American Academy of Pediatrics. Clinical considerations in the use of oxygen. In: *Guidelines for Perinatal Care,* 3rd ed. AAP and ACOG, 1992.

Committee Report: Vitamin E and the prevention of retinopathy of prematurity. *Pediatrics* 1985;**76**:315.

Cryotherapy for Retinopathy of Prematurity Cooperative Group. Multicenter trial of cryotherapy for retinopathy of prematurity: Preliminary results. *Pediatrics* 1988;**81**:697.

Flynn JT: Retinopathy of prematurity. *Pediatr Clin North Am* 1987;**34**:1847.

Garner A: International classification of retinopathy of prematurity. *Pediatrics* 1984;**74**:127.

Glass P et al: Effect of bright light in the hospital nursery on the incidence of retinopathy of prematurity. *N Engl J Med* 1985;**313**:401.

Graeber JE, Schwartz TL: Retinopathy of prematurity: diagnosis, treatment and outcome. In: *Textbook of Prematurity.* Witter F, Keith L (eds). Little, Brown and Co., Boston, 1993.

Lucey JF, Dangman BD: A reexamination of the role of oxygen in retrolental fibroplasia. *Pediatrics* 1984;**82**:73.

McNamara JA, Tasman W, Brown GC et al: Laser photocoagulation for stage 3+ retinopathy of prematurity. *Ophthalmol* 1991;**98**:576.

McPherson AR, Hittner HM, Kretzer FL: *Retinopathy of Prematurity: Current Concepts and Controversies.* Decker, 1986.

Palmer EA, Flynn JT, Hardy RJ et al: for the Cryotherapy for Retinopathy of Prematurity Cooperative Group. Incidence and early course of retinopathy of prematurity. *Ophthalmol* 1991;**98**:1628.

Patz A: Current concepts of the effect of oxygen on the developing retina. *Curr Eye Res* 1984;**3**:159.

Phelps DL: Retinopathy of prematurity: An estimate of vision loss in the United States—1979. *Pediatrics* 1981;**67**:924.

Phelps DL: Role of vitamin E therapy in high-risk neonates. *Clin Perinatol* 1988;**15**:955.

Phelps DL, Rosenbaum AL: Effects of marginal hypoxemia on recovery from oxygen-induced retinopathy in the kitten model. *Pediatrics* 1984;**73**:1.

70 Rickets and Disorders of Calcium and Magnesium Metabolism

RICKETS

I. **Definition.** Rickets is a chronic disorder of calcium metabolism characterized by x-ray evidence of bone demineralization and elevated serum alkaline phosphatase levels.

II. **Incidence.** The incidence of rickets in low birth weight infants is approximately 30%.

III. **Pathophysiology**

A. **Chronic diseases.** Infants with chronic debilitating diseases (notably **bronchopulmonary dysplasia [BPD]**) are at greatest risk for rickets. Typically, these infants require high caloric intake to sustain good weight gain. Bone demineralization can progress despite intakes of calcium, 50–60 mg/kg/d; phosphorus, 25 mg/kg/d; and vitamin D, 400 IU/d. These infants also have an increased incidence of rib fractures secondary to severe bone demineralization, with peak occurrence at about 2 months of age. Most infants with rickets also have received intermittent or routine doses of furosemide.

B. **Very low birthweight infants** (< 1250 g). Prenatal placental insufficiency leads to low plasma phosphate concentrations in VLBW infants. Concomitant reduced renal tubular reabsorption of phosphate in this population exacerbates the phosphate deficiency. If untreated, 42% of these infants have been shown to develop radiological evidence of rickets. Careful attention to appropriate phosphate supplementation prevents rickets in this group of infants.

C. **Diuretics. Furosemide** has marked calciuric effect, and the increased calcium loss exacerbates calcium efflux from bones. **Thiazide diuretics** (eg, hydrochlorothiazide) tend to reduce urinary calcium losses and therefore can ameliorate bone demineralization.

IV. **Risk factors**

A. Very low birthweight.

B. Chronic diseases, especially BPD.

C. Chronic stress.

D. Malnutrition.

E. Administration of inappropriate quantities of calcium, phosphorus, or vitamin D.

F. Diuretics.

V. **Clinical presentation**

A. **Poor weight gain** despite very high caloric intake is often seen in these infants.

B. **Rib and other bone fractures** may be seen in advanced stages of rickets.

C. **Respiratory distress** is occasionally seen.

VI. **Diagnosis**

A. **Laboratory studies**

1. **Alkaline phosphatase levels** are usually more than 280 IU/L and can be over 500 IU/L.

2. **Serum calcium levels** are usually normal.

3. **Serum phosphorus levels** may be low (< 3 mg/dL).

4. **Vitamin D levels.** Infants with rickets typically have increased levels of 1,25-hydroxyvitamin D, which reverts to normal when the disease resolves. 25-Hydroxyvitamin D levels may be depressed with active rickets, which resolves after treatment. See Fig. 70–1.

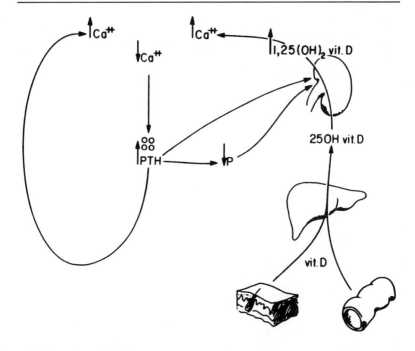

FIGURE 70–1. Vitamin D metabolism. *(From Tsang RC, et al. "Pediatric Parathyroid Disorders" PCNA, 26:223, 1979, Reproduced with permission)*

    B. Radiologic studies. Sequential x-ray studies demonstrate gradual bone demineralization ("washed-out bones"). Some centers utilize the more sensitive bone mineral analyzer to follow smaller changes in bone density, but this instrument is not widely available. X-ray films provide evidence of progressive bone demineralization. Serial films may also show lucency at the metaphyses of long bones and loss of the normal opaque line at the metaphyseal end. In advanced stages, metaphyseal fraying and cupping can be seen—most markedly at the knees and wrists. Poor mineralization at the anterior aspects of the ribs (rachitic rosary) and rib fractures may also be seen.

VII. Management and prognosis

    A. Nutrition. In order to sustain adequate weight gain, infants with rickets usually have an increased need for calories and for additional calcium, vitamin D, and phosphate. A formula such as one of the special care formulas for premature infants (Similac Special Care, Enfamil Premature), which contain 1.2–1.4 g/L of calcium and have a calcium:phosphate ratio of 2:1 with 400–800 IU vitamin D per day, has been shown to stimulate bone mineralization and resolution of rickets. **Alkaline phosphatase levels** should be monitored every 1–2 weeks until normal levels are obtained.

    B. Calcium supplementation. Infants who are NPO should be given about 45 mg/kg/d of elemental calcium intravenously with a calcium:phosphate ratio of 2–3:1 and 400–800 IU vitamin D per day. Rarely, additional benefit can be achieved with higher doses of vitamin D.

    C. Prognosis. This condition is completely reversible with careful management. Depending on the severity of the disease, most infants should fully recover within weeks to months of detection and treatment.

HYPOCALCEMIA

I. **Definition.** In infants in intensive care nurseries, disorders of calcium metabolism frequently develop; hypocalcemia is the most common. Hypocalcemia is defined as total serum calcium (tCa) levels less than 6 mg/dL, tCa levels of less than 7 mg/dL with symptoms, or ionized calcium (iCa) levels of less than 3 mg/dL (1.0 mM). Some authors have suggested that iCa levels greater than 2.5 mg/dL (0.8 mM) are adequate in some infants.

II. **Pathophysiology.** Ionized calcium is the biologically important form of calcium. Total serum calcium levels have repeatedly been shown not to be predictive of serum ionized calcium levels. Therefore, tCA levels are unreliable as criteria for true hypocalcemia. In premature infants, it has been shown that tCa levels as low as 6 mg/dL or less correspond to iCa levels greater than 3 mg/dL.

A. **Early-onset neonatal hypocalcemia (ENH).** During the third trimester of pregnancy, the human fetus receives at least 140 mg/kg/d of elemental calcium via the umbilical cord. Most of this calcium is readily incorporated into the newly forming bones. Following delivery, this massive supply of calcium is suddenly stopped, and calcium must be given enterally.

1. **A full-term infant** receiving 100–120 mL of normal formula would be receiving 50–60 mg/kg/d of calcium orally. Despite this drop in supply, full-term infants tolerate the change well and do not become hypocalcemic.

2. **Premature or sick infants** often become hypocalcemic during the first 3 days of life. Total serum calcium levels can drop to less than 7 mg/dL and occasionally fall below 6 mg/dL.

3. **Calcium levels** (both iCa and tCa) usually return to normal within 48–72 hours whether or not supplemental calcium is given. It has also been shown that immunoreactive parathyroid hormone (iPTH) is often low at birth but rises to higher levels within 24–72 hours after delivery. Intravenous calcium supplementation has been shown to suppress this increase in iPTH.

B. **Hypocalcemia secondary to prolonged poor enteral intake.** After 3 days of life, infants tolerating enteral feedings usually do not need calcium supplementation. Normal formula supplies adequate calcium for bone mineralization in full-term infants. Calcium-rich formula—formula with an elemental calcium concentration of 1.2–1.4 g/L and a calcium:phosphate ratio of 2:1—is usually sufficient for bone growth in premature infants. However, if feedings cannot be advanced rapidly or if the infant must be maintained NPO, parenteral calcium supplementation is needed to prevent bone demineralization. These infants often maintain normal iCa and tCa levels at the expense of bone calcium. Furthermore, magnesium deficiency secondary to malnutrition can suppress iPTH levels and thus cause hypocalcemia.

C. **Hypocalcemia secondary to maternal diabetes.** After infants of diabetic mothers are born, their serum glucose levels rapidly decline as a result of **hyperinsulinemia.** These infants also secrete higher amounts of **calcitonin,** which inhibits calcium mobilization from bone. iPTH may also be lower in these infants and may not increase as rapidly following delivery. Therefore, these infants can have a relative intolerance to phosphate and have an increased risk of developing hypocalcemia.

D. **Hypocalcemia secondary to perinatal stress.** Stressed neonates who have suffered from perinatal sepsis, asphyxia, TORCH infections, compromised placental blood flow, or meconium aspiration also have an increased risk of hypocalcemia. This is believed to be due to the effects of corticosteroids and catecholamines during stress.

E. **Hypocalcemia secondary to alkalosis.** The amount of tCa that is ionized is inversely proportionate to serum pH. Infants who are acidotic have higher than expected iCa levels, and alkalotic infants can likewise be clinically hypocalcemic even if their tCa level is greater than 7 mg/dL. This is a direct pH effect.

F. **Hypocalcemia secondary to blood transfusions.** Citrate, a normal component of stored blood, forms a neutral soluble complex with calcium and thus reduces the amount of calcium that is ionized. Citrate is metabolized to bicarbonate within a few hours after administration and may induce a mild metabolic alkalosis that will also tend to decrease the amount of iCa. The amount of citrate administered with periodic blood replacement usually does not lead to clinical hypocalcemia. However, the amount of citrate given as a result of exchange transfusion—especially repeated transfusions—is much higher and may reduce serum iCa.

G. **Hypocalcemia secondary to furosemide therapy.** Due to its action on the ascending loop of Henle and the proximal tubule, furosemide causes hypercalciuria, which can lead to hypocalcemia, bone demineralization, or both. This effect can be most severe with chronic use of this medication.

III. **Risk factors.** There is an increased incidence of hypocalcemia within the first 3 days of life in premature or sick neonates. The risk of hypocalcemia increases with the degree of prematurity. Infants who also have an increased risk of hypocalcemia are:

   A. Infants with poor enteral intake.
   B. Infants of diabetic mothers.
   C. Infants stressed during the perinatal period.
   D. Infants receiving blood transfusions.
   E. Infants with alkalosis.
   F. Infants receiving furosemide.
   G. Infants receiving excessive phosphate intake.
   H. Infants with insufficient magnesium intake.
   I. Infants with congenital hypoparathyroidism (eg, DiGeorge's syndrome).

IV. **Clinical presentation**

   A. **Acute hypocalcemia.** Infants who are acutely hypocalcemic may present with apnea, irritability, slight tremors of the extremities, profound tetany, or seizures. Cardiac dysfunction may also occur, characterized by prolonged QT intervals and arrhythmias.

   B. **Chronic hypocalcemia.** Infants who are chronically hypocalcemic may develop rickets characterized by apnea, bone demineralization, elevated alkaline phosphatase levels, and rib and long bone fractures.

V. **Diagnosis**

   A. **Laboratory studies**

      1. **Total and ionized calcium.** Serum iCa levels of less than 3 mg/dL are diagnostic of hypocalcemia. In the absence of iCa levels, serum tCa levels of less than 6 mg/dL or tCa levels of less than 7 mg/dL with clinical symptoms can be considered diagnostic of hypocalcemia.

      2. **Serum magnesium levels** of less than 1.5 mg/dL indicate hypomagnesemia, which can accompany hypocalcemia.

      3. **Alkaline phosphatase levels** greater than 225 IU/L are elevated and can be an early sign of rickets.

      4. **Urinary calcium losses** can be estimated either by **random spot or 24-hour urine collections.** Calcium:creatinine ratios (measured in spot urine specimens) greater than 0.21–0.25 are indicative of hypercalciuria. Twenty-four-hour urinary calcium levels greater than 4 mg/kg/24h also indicate hypercalciuria.

   B. **Radiologic studies.** Bone demineralization can be grossly estimated by reviewing sequential x-ray films of ribs and long bones. Rickets can be suggested by metaphyseal lucency accompanied by metaphyseal fraying and cupping. These findings are best seen at the knees and anterior rib ends (rachitic rosary). Rib fractures can also be seen in severe cases.

   C. **Other studies.** Electrocardiography may show prolonged QT intervals or arrhythmias as a result of hypocalcemia or hypomagnesemia.

VI. **Management.** Parenteral calcium therapy may be associated with significant untoward effects. These include nephrolithiasis, cardiac arrhythmias, subcutaneous calcium deposition endangering joint mobility, peripheral skin sloughs, and the recently recognized possibility of metastatic calcifications in the brains of very sick neonates. **Expectant nonintervention** is therefore suggested for early-onset neonatal hypocalcemia, reserving treatment with parenteral calcium therapy for cases in which profound or clinical (symptomatic) hypocalcemia exists.

A. **Early-onset neonatal hypocalcemia (ENH).** If treatment is necessary based on iCa or tCa levels or symptoms, intravenous **10% calcium gluconate** (containing 9 mg elemental calcium per mL) should be given (for dosage, see Chap 73). This is usually more than adequate to maintain normal ionized calcium levels. Excessive treatment can suppress iPTH levels and for that reason should be avoided. There is no real benefit to continuous drip infusion compared to bolus administration in the treatment of ENH. When calcium gluconate is given without phosphate, most of the calcium is rapidly excreted in the urine. But in the acute stage and during the first 3 days of life, calcium can be given every 6 hours because it is impractical to give phosphate at this time.

B. **Hypocalcemia secondary to poor enteral intake.** Parenteral nutrition is usually started on days 3–4 of life, and calcium and phosphate must be started both for maintenance and to support bone growth. The intrauterine dose of 140 mg/kg/d of elemental calcium cannot be achieved by the intravenous route because of precipitation with phosphate. **An intravenous dosage of 45 mg/kg/d of elemental calcium with a calcium:phosphate ratio ranging from 1.3:1.0 to 2:1 has been shown to be optimal in promoting both calcium and phosphate retention.** Supplementation with intravenous calcium can cause hypercalciuria. If intravenous calcium is given without phosphate, most of the calcium is released in the urine and thus is not utilized for bone formation. Although phosphate is needed, excessive phosphate can lead to hypocalcemia. **Vitamin D supplements** of 400 IU/d should also be provided. Parenteral supplementation of calcium and phosphate may be hampered by precipitation in parenteral nutrition solutions. Factors that tend to increase the risk of precipitation include: elevated pH of the solution, excessively high concentrations of calcium and phosphate, low concentrations of amino acids, high temperature, prolonged standing times, addition of calcium salts first or prior to final dilution, and use of the chloride salt as the source of calcium.

C. **Hypocalcemia secondary to maternal diabetes.** Since these infants are at greater risk for developing hypocalcemia, serum calcium levels must be closely monitored. The treatment criteria are the same as those outlined above for ENH.

D. **Hypocalcemia secondary to perinatal stress.** The treatment criteria are the same as those for ENH except when the infant is maintained alkalotic (see below).

E. **Hypocalcemia secondary to alkalosis.** Since alkalotic infants (eg, infants being treated for persistent pulmonary hypertension) can be clinically hypocalcemic with tCa levels greater than 7 mg/dL, maintenance calcium therapy should be started when blood pH levels reach 7.5.

F. **Hypocalcemia secondary to blood transfusions.** The amount of citrate administered with periodic blood replacement usually does not lead to clinical hypocalcemia. However, the rate of citrate given as a result of exchange transfusion is much higher and may reduce serum iCa. Hypocalcemia secondary to blood transfusion can be treated prophylactically (with calcium gluconate) or if symptoms of hypocalcemia are noted (see Chap 73 for dosages and other pharmacologic information). Low iCa levels and clinical symptoms of hypocalcemia are rarely encountered even when extra calcium is not given.

G. **Hypocalcemia secondary to furosemide therapy.** Infants receiving furosemide have an increased urinary loss of calcium. This loss can be demonstrated by measurement of calcium:creatinine ratios in spot urines or tCa in 24-hour urine collections. If hypercalciuria exists, an attempt should be made to **substitute a thiazide diuretic (most commonly chlorothiazide) for furosemide.** However, if furosemide is thought to be essential, a lower dose of furosemide in combination with a thiazide should be used (1 mg furosemide to 10 mg chlorothiazide 3 times daily). Thiazides tend to cause calcium retention and can overcome the hypercalciuric effect of furosemide. These efforts will reduce the risk of nephrocalcinosis, which is directly related to the amount of calcium excreted in the urine. However, this combination can cause significant diuresis and increase urinary potassium loss. Fluids and electrolytes must therefore be carefully monitored if combination therapy is chosen. If more than 5 meq/kg/d of potassium supplementation is required after diuretics are started, **spironolactone** therapy should also be started (see Chap 73). Spironolactone has little or no effect on urinary calcium loss but helps to reduce the severity of hypokalemia in infants receiving either furosemide or thiazide therapy.

VII. Prognosis. Hypocalcemia can be effectively controlled with close monitoring of calcium, phosphate, and vitamin D intake, and urinary calcium losses.

HYPERCALCEMIA

I. Definition. Hypercalcemia is defined as total serum calcium levels greater than 11 mg/dL and ionized calcium levels greater than 5 mg/dL (1.7 mM). tCa is not predictive of iCa levels and thus is not a reliable measure of hypercalcemia. Acidotic infants may have iCa levels greater than 5 mg/dL even though tCa levels are 10 mg/dL or less.

II. Pathophysiology. Hypercalcemia may be due to parathyroid-related causes or to mechanisms unrelated to the parathyroid.

   A. Congenital primary hyperparathyroidism (rare).
   B. Congenital secondary hyperparathyroidism due to maternal hypoparathyroidism (rare).
   C. Subcutaneous fat necrosis (if extensive, may lead to hypercalcemia when large amounts of calcium are released from subcutaneous fat).
   D. Fanconi's syndrome.
   E. Benign familial hypercalcemia.
   F. Iatrogenic hypercalcemia due to excessive calcium supplements.
   G. Hypervitaminiosis D.
   H. Hypoproteinemia.
   I. Excessive thiazide treatment.

III. Risk factors

   A. Excessive supplemental calcium.
   B. Excessive vitamin D supplement.
   C. Rare congenital hypercalcemia.

IV. Clinical presentation. Clinical symptomatology is important in establishing significant hypercalcemia. Symptoms include poor feeding with poor weight gain, depressed tone, lethargy, polyuria, and shortening of the QT interval as evidenced by eletrocardiography. Seizures can also be seen in severe cases.

V. Diagnosis

   A. Laboratory studies
      1. Total and ionized calcium. Ideally, iCa levels greater than 5 mg/dL establish hypercalcemia. If iCa levels are not available, tCa levels greater than 11 mg/dL can be considered abnormal. Infants who are acidotic or hypoproteinemic may have iCa levels greater than 5 mg/dL even though tCa is 10 mg/dL or less. Therefore, clinical symptoms are important in establishing the diagnosis of hypercalcemia.
      2. Intakes of calcium, phosphate, and vitamin D should be checked. The calcium:phosphate ratio should be 2:1, and vitamin D dosage should be 400–800 IU/d.
      3. Serum total protein and the **albumin:globulin ratio** should also be obtained.
      4. Tubular resorption of phosphate is usually reduced when hyperparathyroidism exists.
      5. Immunoreactive parathyroid hormone (iPTH) can be measured to establish hyperparathyroidism.

6. **Vitamin D levels.** Hypervitaminosis D can usually be determined by careful review of vitamin intake. However, if this is not clear, **25-hydroxyvitamin D** can be measured. This value would be elevated if excess vitamin D has been given.

B. **Radiologic studies.** X-rays are helpful in establishing the cause of hypercalcemia. Bone demineralization is typical of hyperparathyroidism, and osteosclerotic lesions are seen with hypervitaminosis D. Hypercalciuria can be very severe with excessive calcium intake or with normal calcium intake plus inadequate phosphate intake.

VI. Management

A. **General.** Treatment depends on the cause, but in general the calcium intake should be reduced and vitamin D supplements withheld. Some authors recommend avoidance of sunlight. After hypercalcemia has resolved, the actual calcium, phosphate, and vitamin D needs can be estimated based on normal bone mineralization without recurrence of hypercalcemia. If the infant is receiving a thiazide diuretic (which increases calcium retention in the kidneys), the drug should be discontinued.

B. **Acute symptomatic hypercalcemia**

   1. When acute symptomatic hypercalcemia exists, **furosemide** may be effective in reducing serum calcium due to its marked hypercalciuric effect (see dosage in Chap 73). Fluid and electrolyte intake must be monitored closely if furosemide is used.

   2. In older children and adults, calcitonin has been used for hypercalcemia associated with immobilization (patients in traction) and for acute hypercalcemic states at a dosage of 5–8 units/kg/dose intravenously or intramuscularly every 12 hours. It is unlikely that calcitonin therapy would be needed in neonates.

C. **Surgical intervention.** Very rarely, when severe hyperparathyroidism exists, parathyroidectomy may be needed.

VII. Prognosis. Complete resolution of hypercalcemia occurs rapidly if it is treated promptly.

HYPOMAGNESEMIA

I. **Definition.** Hypomagnesemia is defined as a serum magnesium level less than 1.52 meq/L (0.75 mmol/L).

II. **Pathophysiology.** Magnesium is required as a catalyst for many intracellular enzymatic reactions. Calcium homeostasis cannot be maintained if serum magnesium levels are low. The usual cause of low magnesium levels is inadequate intake following delivery.

III. **Risk factors**

   A. Hypocalcemia.

   B. Inadequate intake of magnesium.

IV. **Clinical presentation.** The most common manifestation of hypomagnesemia is hypocalcemia that fails to respond to calcium therapy.

V. **Diagnosis.** Serum magnesium levels should be checked in all severely stressed infants. If the level is adequate and there is normal magnesium intake, repeated checks are not necessary unless hypocalcemia occurs.

VI. **Management.** Acute hypomagnesemia should be treated with **magnesium sulfate** until the magnesium level is normalized or symptoms resolve. The route may be intramuscular or intravenous; however, with intravenous administration, careful electrocardiographic monitoring is indicated, owing to the risk for arrhythmias (see Chap 73 for dosage and other pharmacologic information). If feedings are started early, parenteral magnesium is unnecessary; however, if the infant has poor enteral intake, parenteral nutrition should include magnesium.

VII. **Prognosis.** This condition often goes unrecognized. However, when detected, complete resolution occurs with treatment.

HYPERMAGNESEMIA

I. Definition. Hypermagnesemia is defined as serum magnesium levels in excess of 2.3 meq/L (1.15 mmol/L).

II. Pathophysiology. Increased serum magnesium levels depress the central nervous system and decrease skeletal muscle contractility. These effects can be reversed by increased serum iCa levels. The most common cause of hypermagnesemia in neonates is treatment of the mother with magnesium sulfate. Less commonly, it can occur with administration of a magnesium-containing antacid, especially when urine output is decreased. Hypermagnesemia can also be caused by magnesium sulfate enemas, which are absolutely contraindicated in neonates.

III. Risk factors

   A. Administration of magnesium sulfate to mother prior to delivery.

   B. Administration of magnesium-containing antacids to neonate, especially when urinary output is decreased.

   C. Magnesium sulfate enemas (absolutely contraindicated in neonates).

IV. Clinical presentation. The symptoms of hypermagnesemia are very similar to those of hypercalcemia. These include poor feeding, lethargy, depressed tone, hyporeflexia, apnea, and decreased gastrointestinal motility with abdominal distention.

V. Diagnosis

   A. Laboratory studies. Elevated **serum magnesium levels** are diagnostic.

   B. Electrocardiography. A shortened QT interval is seen on ECG.

VI. Management

   A. Fluids and electrolytes. If enteral feedings are not tolerated, maintenance intravenous fluids should be provided, with careful monitoring of serum electrolytes and pH.

   B. Respiratory care. In rare cases of severe apnea, intubation and mechanical ventilation are needed.

   C. Exchange transfusion can effectively reduce serum magnesium levels; but this should be reserved for extreme cases.

VII. Prognosis. Hypermagnesemia usually resolves spontaneously, provided renal function is maintained.

REFERENCES

Aiken G, Lenney W: Calcium and phosphate content of intravenous feeding regimens for very low birthweight infants. *Arch Dis Child* 1986;**61**:495.

Brown DR, Steranka BH, Taylor FH: Treatment of early-onset neonatal hypocalcemia: Effects on serum calcium and ionized calcium. *Am J Dis Child* 1981;**135**:24.

Chesney RW: Requirements and upper limits of vitamin D intake in the term neonate, infant, and older child. *J Pediatr* 1990;**116**:159.

Cooper LJ, Anast CS: Circulating immunoreactive parathyroid hormone levels in premature infants and the response to calcium therapy. *Acta Paediatr Scand* 1985;**74**:669.

Greer FR, Steichen JJ, Tsang RC: Effects of increased calcium, phosphorus, and vitamin D intake on bone mineralization in very low-birth-weight infants fed formulas with Polycose and medium-chain triglycerides. *J Pediatr* 1982;**100**:951.

Holland PC, Wilkinson AR, Diez J, Lindsell DRM: Prenatal Deficiency of phosphate, phosphate supplementation and rickets in very low birthweight infants. *Lancet* 1990;**335**:697.

Knight P, Heer D, Abenour G: CaxP and Ca/P in the parenteral feeding of preterm infants. *JPEN* 1983;**7**:110.

Koo WWK: Calcium, phosphorus, and vitamin D requirements of infants receiving parenteral nutrition. *J Perinatol* 1989;**8**:263.

Macmahon P, Blair ME, Treweeke P, Kovar IZ: Association of mineral composition of neonatal intravenous feeding solutions and metabolic bone disease of prematurity. *Arch Dis Child* 1989;**64**:489.

Rudloff S, Lonnerdal B: Calcium retention from milk-based infant formulas, whey-hydrolysate formula, and human milk in weanling rhesus monkeys. *Am J Dis Child* 1990;**144**:360.

Steichen JJ et al: Elevated serum 1,25-dihydroxyvitamin-D concentrations in rickets of very low-birth-weight infants. *J Pediatr* 1981;**99**:293.

Vileisis RA: Furosemide effect on mineral status of parenterally nourished neonates with chronic lung disease. *Pediatrics* 1990;**85**:316.

71 Surgical Diseases of the Newborn

ALIMENTARY TRACT OBSTRUCTION

VASCULAR RING

I. **Definition.** *Vascular ring* denotes a variety of anomalies of the aortic arch and its branches that create a "ring" of vessels around the trachea and esophagus.

II. **Pathophysiology.** Partial obstruction of the trachea or the esophagus, or both, may result from extrinsic compression by the encircling ring of vessels.

III. **Clinical presentation.** Dysphagia or stridor (respiratory insufficiency), or both, are the modes of presentation.

IV. **Diagnosis** is by **barium swallow,** which identifies extrinsic compression of the esophagus in the region of the aortic arch.

V. **Management** consists of surgical division of a portion of the constricting ring of vessels. The specific surgical plan must be tailored to the particular type of aortic arch anomaly present.

ESOPHAGEAL ATRESIA

I. **Definition.** The esophagus ends blindly about 10–12 cm from the nares. In 85% of cases, the distal esophagus communicates with the posterior trachea (distal tracheoesophageal fistula [TEF]).

II. **Pathophysiology.** Complete esophageal obstruction results in inability of the infant to handle his own secretions, producing "excess salivation" and aspiration of pharyngeal contents. More importantly, the direct communication between the stomach and the tracheobronchial tree via the distal TEF allows the crying newborn to greatly distend the stomach with air; embarrassment of diaphragmatic excursion promotes basilar atelectasis and subsequent pneumonia. Additionally, the distal TEF permits reflux of gastric secretion directly into the tracheobronchial tree, causing chemical pneumonitis, which may be complicated by bacterial pneumonia.

III. **Clinical presentation.** The pregnancy may have been complicated by polyhydramnios. After delivery, the infant typically is unable to swallow saliva, which drains from the corners of the mouth and requires frequent suctioning. Attempts at feeding will result in prompt regurgitation, coughing, choking, and cyanosis.

IV. **Diagnosis** is established by **attempting to pass a nasogastric tube and meeting resistance at 10–12 cm from the nares** followed by **chest x-ray** for confirmation. Chest x-ray will show the tube to end or coil in the region of the thoracic inlet. The x-ray film should also be examined for possible skeletal anomalies, pulmonary infiltrates, cardiac size and shape, and abdominal bowel gas patterns. The absence of gas in the gastrointestinal tract implies esophageal atresia without TEF (10% of cases), for which surgical management will probably differ from that for the more common esophageal atresia with TEF. Careful contrast x-ray study of the proximal esophageal pouch can also be performed to delineate the precise length of the proximal pouch and to rule out the rare proximal TEF.

V. **Management**
   A. **Preoperative treatment** should focus on protecting the lungs by evacuating the proximal esophageal pouch with an **indwelling Replogle tube or frequent suctioning,** and by **placing the baby in a relatively upright position (45**

degrees) to lessen the likelihood of reflux of gastric contents up the distal esophagus into the trachea. **Broad-spectrum antibiotics** should be administered.

B. **Surgical therapy.** The steps and timing of surgical therapy must be individualized. Some surgeons perform preliminary gastrostomy to decompress the stomach and provide additional protection against reflux. Ligation of the tracheoesophageal fistula and esophageal anastomosis are the essential steps in total surgical correction.

DUODENAL OBSTRUCTION

I. **Definition.** Obstruction of the lumen of the duodenum may be either complete or partial, preampullary or postampullary, and may be caused by either intrinsic or extrinsic problems.

II. **Pathophysiology**

A. **Duodenal atresia** results in complete obstruction of the lumen of the duodenum, whereas symptoms of partial obstruction will result from a stenotic lesion.

B. **Annular pancreas** is a congenital anomaly of pancreatic development, which results in an encircling "napkin ring" of pancreatic tissue about the descending duodenum. It can result in either complete or, more commonly, partial duodenal obstruction.

C. **Malrotation** may cause complete or partial duodenal obstruction in 1 of 2 ways. In uncomplicated malrotation, peritoneal attachments (Ladd's bands) may compress the duodenum, resulting in total or, more commonly, partial obstruction. Midgut volvulus may complicate nonrotation and nonfixation of the intestine. The entire midgut may twist on the pedicle of its blood supply, the superior mesenteric artery, resulting in duodenal obstruction and eventual nonviability of the midgut.

III. **Clinical presentation**

A. **General.** Infants with duodenal obstruction typically present with **vomiting (often bilious).** Abdominal distention is not usually a prominent feature. Polyhydramnios may have been present.

B. **Duodenal atresia.** The presence of **Down's syndrome, esophageal atresia,** or **imperforate anus** suggests duodenal atresia.

C. **Midgut volvulus** typically presents with symptoms of **duodenal obstruction (bilious vomiting)** and evidence of **intestinal ischemia (mucoid bloody stools),** usually in an infant who for days or weeks has eaten and stooled normally.

IV. The **differential diagnosis** includes duodenal atresia (stenosis), annular pancreas, and malrotation with or without the complication of midgut volvulus.

V. **Diagnosis.** The exact cause of the obstruction may not be known until laparotomy.

A. **Abdominal x-ray study.** In complete duodenal obstruction, the pathognomonic x-ray finding is a **"double-bubble."** Two large gas collections, one in the stomach and the other in the first portion of duodenum, are the only lucencies in the GI tract.

B. **Radiologic contrast studies**

1. **Partial obstructions** will probably require an **upper GI series** to identify the site of difficulty.

2. **Malrotation.** It is important to eliminate malrotation as a possibility since its complication, midgut volvulus, is a true surgical emergency. This is best done by an **upper GI series,** identifying a transverse portion of the duodenum leading to a fixed ligament of Treitz, or by **barium enema,** localizing the cecum to its normal, right lower quadrant position.

VI. **Management**

A. **Duodenal atresia or annular pancreas.** In cases of atresia or annular pancreas, **gastric suction** will control vomiting and allow "elective" surgical correction.

B. **Malrotation** mandates **immediate surgical intervention,** because the viability of the intestine from the duodenum to the transverse colon may be at risk from midgut volvulus.

PROXIMAL INTESTINAL OBSTRUCTION

I. **Definition.** Proximal intestinal obstruction is obstruction of the jejunum.
II. **Pathophysiology.** Jejunal obstruction typically results from atresia of that segment of the bowel, usually as a result of a vascular accident in utero.
III. **Clinical presentation.** Infants with jejunal obstruction usually present with **bilious vomiting associated with minimal abdominal distention** since few loops of intestine are involved in the obstructive process.
IV. **Diagnosis.** A plain **abdominal x-ray study** reveals only a few dilated small bowel loops with no gas distally.
V. **Management.** Surgical correction is required.

DISTAL INTESTINAL OBSTRUCTION

I. **Definition.** The term *distal intestinal obstruction* denotes partial or complete obstruction of the distal portion of the gastrointestinal tract. It may be either small bowel (ileum) or large bowel obstruction. The list of causes includes:
   A. **Ileal atresia.**
   B. **Meconium ileus**
      1. **Uncomplicated (simple) obstruction of the terminal ileum** by pellets of inspissated meconium.
      2. **Complicated meconium ileus,** implying compromise of bowel viability either prenatally or postnatally.
   C. **Colonic atresia.**
   D. **Meconium plug–hypoplastic left colon syndrome.**
   E. **Hirschsprung's disease (congenital aganglionic megacolon).**
II. **Clinical presentation.** Infants with obstructing lesions in the distal intestine all have similar signs and symptoms. They typically have **distended abdomens, fail to pass meconium,** and **vomit bilious material.**
III. **Diagnosis**
   A. **Abdominal x-ray studies** show multiple dilated loops of intestine; the site of obstruction (distal small bowel vs colon) cannot be determined on plain x-ray films.
   B. **Contrast radiologic studies.** The preferred diagnostic test is contrast enema. It may identify colonic atresia, outline microcolon (which may signify complete distal small bowel obstruction), or suggest a transition zone (which may signify Hirschsprung's disease). The procedure can identify and treat meconium plug–hypoplastic left colon syndrome. If the test is normal, ileal atresia, meconium ileus, and Hirschsprung's disease are possibilities.
   C. **Sweat test.** A sweat test may be needed to document cystic fibrosis in cases of meconium ileus (unlikely to be helpful in the first few weeks of life).
   D. **Mucosal rectal biopsy** for histologic detection of ganglion cells is the safest and most widely available screening test for Hirschsprung's disease. However, **laparotomy** is often necessary to determine the exact nature of the problem in infants with normal results of barium enema.
IV. **Management**
   A. **Nonoperative management** is "curative" in cases of meconium plug and hypoplastic left colon.
      1. Passage of time and **colonic stimulation by digital examination and rectal enemas** promote return of effective peristalsis.
      2. **In infants who achieve apparently normal bowel function,** one must rule out Hirschsprung's disease by **mucosal rectal biopsy;** a small percentage of patients with meconium plug will prove to have aganglionosis.
      3. Interestingly, **uncomplicated meconium ileus,** if identified, can often be treated by nonoperative means. **Repeated enemas with Hypaque or**

acetylcysteine (Mucomyst) may disimpact the inspissated meconium in the terminal ileum and relieve the obstruction.

B. **Surgical therapy.** Surgical intervention is required for atresia of the ileum or colon, for complicated meconium ileus, and when the diagnosis is in doubt. Hirschsprung's disease is treated in the neonatal period by colostomy through ganglionic bowel.

IMPERFORATE ANUS

I. **Definition.** Imperforate anus is the lack of an anal opening of proper location or size. There are 2 types: high and low.

A. **In high imperforate anus,** the rectum ends above the puborectalis sling, the main muscle responsible for maintaining fecal continence. There is never an associated fistula to the perineum. In males there may be a rectourinary fistula, and in females, a rectovaginal fistula.

B. **In low imperforate anus,** the rectum has traversed the puborectalis sling in correct position. Variants include anal stenosis, imperforate anus with perineal fistula, and imperforate anus without fistula.

II. **Diagnosis** is by **inspection and calibration of any perineal opening.** All patients with imperforate anus should have **x-ray studies of the lumbosacral spine and urinary tract,** because there is a high incidence of dysmorphism in these areas.

III. **Management.** Surgical therapy in the neonate consists of colostomy for high anomalies and perineal anoplasty or dilation of fistula for low lesions. If the level is not known, colostomy is preferable to blind exploration of the perineum. If colostomy is done, a contrast x-ray study of the distal limb should be performed to ascertain the level at which the rectum ends and to determine the presence or absence of an associated fistula.

CAUSES OF RESPIRATORY DISTRESS

CHOANAL ATRESIA

I. **Definition.** Choanal atresia is a congenital blockage of the posterior nares, caused by persistence of a bony septum (90%) or a soft tissue membrane (10%).

II. **Pathophysiology.** Unilateral or bilateral obstruction at the posterior nares may be due to soft tissue or bone. Choanal atresia, which is complete and bilateral, is one of the causes of respiratory distress immediately following delivery. The effects of upper airway obstruction are compounded because neonates are obligate nose-breathers and will not "think" to breathe through the mouth.

III. **Clinical presentation.** Respiratory distress due to partial or total upper airway obstruction is the mode of presentation.

IV. **Diagnosis** is made by **inability to pass a catheter into the nasopharynx** via either side of the nose.

V. **Management.** Simply **making the infant cry and thereby breathe through its mouth** will temporarily improve breathing. Insertion of an **oral airway** will maintain the ability to breathe until surgical correction of the atresia is performed.

PIERRE-ROBIN SYNDROME

I. **Definition.** This anomaly consists of mandibular hypoplasia in association with cleft palate.

II. **Pathophysiology.** Airway obstruction is produced by posterior displacement of the tongue associated with the small size of the mandible.

III. **Clinical presentation.** Severity of symptoms varies, but most infants manifest a high degree of partial upper airway obstruction.

IV. **Management**
   A. **Infants with mild involvement** can be cared for in the **prone position** and fed through a special **Breck nipple.** Adjustment to the airway compromise will take place over days or weeks.
   B. **More severe cases** require **nasopharyngeal tubes or surgical procedures** to hold the tongue in an anterior position. **Tracheostomy** is generally a last resort.

VASCULAR RING

Airway compromise is rarely severe and is usually manifested by stridor.

LARYNGOTRACHEAL CLEFT

   I. **Definition.** Laryngotracheal cleft is a rare congenital anomaly in which there is incomplete separation of the larynx (and sometimes the trachea) from the esophagus, resulting in a common channel of esophagus and airway. This communication may be short or may extend almost the entire length of the trachea.
   II. **Pathophysiology.** The persistent communication between the larynx (and occasionally a significant portion of the trachea) and the esophagus results in recurring symptoms of aspiration and respiratory distress with feeding.
   III. **Clinical presentation.** Respiratory distress during feeding is the presenting symptom.
   IV. **Diagnosis. Contrast swallow** may suggest the anomaly, but **endoscopy** is essential in firmly establishing the diagnosis and delineating the extent of the defect.
   V. **Management.** Laryngotracheal cleft is treated by surgical correction, which is difficult and often unsuccessful.

H-TYPE TRACHOESOPHAGEAL FISTULA

   I. **Definition.** This anomaly is the third most common type of tracheoesophageal fistula (TEF), making up 5% of cases. Esophageal continuity is intact, but there is a fistulous communication between the posterior trachea and the anterior esophagus.
   II. **Pathophysiology.** If the fistula is small, as is usually the case, "silent" aspiration takes place during feedings with resulting pneumonitis. If the fistula is unusually large, coughing and choking may accompany each feeding.
   III. **Clinical presentation.** Symptoms, as noted above, depend on the size of the fistula.
   IV. **Diagnosis. Barium swallow** is the initial diagnostic study and may identify the fistula. The most accurate procedure, however, is **bronchoscopy** (perhaps combined with esophagoscopy); this should allow discovery and perhaps cannulation of the fistula.
   V. **Management.** Surgical correction is required. The approach (neck or chest) is determined by location of the fistula.

INTRINSIC ABNORMALITIES OF THE AIRWAY

   I. **Definition.** Abnormalities of, or within, the airway that cause partial obstruction fall into this category. Examples include laryngomalacia, paralyzed vocal cord, subglottic web, and hemangioma.
   II. **Pathophysiology.** These lesions result in partial obstruction of the airway and cause stridor and respiratory distress of varying severity.
   III. **Clinical presentation.** See II, above.
   IV. **Diagnosis.** The diagnosis is established by **endoscopy** of the airway.
   V. **Management** is individualized. Some problems, such as laryngomalacia, will be outgrown if the child can be supported through the period of acute symptoms. Other lesions, such as subglottic webs, may be amenable to endoscopic resection or laser therapy.

CONGENITAL LOBAR EMPHYSEMA

I. **Definition.** *Lobar emphysema* is a term used to denote hyperexpansion of the air spaces of a segment or lobe of the lung.

II. **Pathophysiology.** Inspired air is trapped in an enclosed space. As the cyst of entrapped air enlarges, normal lung is increasingly compressed. Cystic problems are more common in the upper lobes.

III. **Clinical presentation.** Small cysts may cause few or no symptoms and are readily seen on x-ray film. Giant cysts may cause significant respiratory distress, with mediastinal shift and compromise of the contralateral lung.

IV. **Diagnosis.** Usually the cysts are easily seen on plain **chest x-ray films.** However, the radiologic findings may be confused with that of tension pneumothorax.

V. **Management.** Therapeutic options include **observation** for small asymptomatic cysts, **repositioning of the endotracheal tube** to selectively ventilate uninvolved lung for 6–12 hours, **bronchoscopy** for endobronchial lavage, and operative resection of the cyst with or without the segment or lobe from which it arises.

CYSTIC ADENOMATOID MALFORMATION

I. **Definition.** The term *cystic adenomatoid malformation* encompasses a spectrum of congenital pulmonary malformation involving varying degrees of adenomatosis and cyst formation.

II. **Pathophysiology.** Severity of symptoms is related to the amount of lung involved and particularly to the degree to which normal ipsilateral and contralateral lung is compressed.

III. **Clinical presentation.** Signs of respiratory insufficiency such as **tachypnea** and **cyanosis** are modes of presentation.

IV. **Diagnosis.** The characteristic pattern on **chest x-ray film** is multiple discrete air bubbles, occasionally with air fluid levels, involving a region of the lung. The radiographic appearance can mimic that of congenital diaphragmatic hernia.

V. **Management.** Treatment is surgical resection of involved lung, allowing reexpansion of compressed normal pulmonary tissue.

CONGENITAL DIAPHRAGMATIC HERNIA

I. **Definition.** A patent pleuroperitoneal canal through the foramen of Bochdalek is the essential defect in congenital diaphragmatic hernia (CDH).

II. **Pathophysiology**

  A. **Prenatal.** The abnormal communication between the peritoneal an pleural cavities allows herniation of intestine into the pleural space as the developing gastrointestinal tract returns from its extracoelomic phase at 10–12 weeks' gestation. Depending on the degree of pulmonary compression by herniated intestine, there may be marked diminution of bronchial branching, limited multiplication of alveoli, and persistence of muscular hypertrophy in pulmonary arterioles. These anatomic abnormalities are most notable on the side of the CDH (usually the left); they are also present to some degree in the contralateral lung.

  B. **Postnatal.** After delivery, the anatomic anomaly may contribute to the development of one or both of the following pathologic conditions.

    1. **Pulmonary parenchymal insufficiency.** Infants with CDH have an abnormally small functional lung mass. Some have so few conducting air passages and developed alveoli—a condition known as *pulmonary parenchymal insufficiency*—that survival is unlikely.

    2. **Pulmonary hypertension.** Infants with CDH are predisposed anatomically to pulmonary hypertension, also known as *persistent fetal circulation (PFC).* In this condition, blood is shunted around the lungs through the foramen ovale and patent ductus arteriosus. Shunting promotes acidosis and hypoxia, both of which are potent stimuli to additional pulmonary vasoconstriction. Thus, a vicious cycle of clinical deterioration is established.

III. Clinical presentation. Most infants with CDH exhibit significant respiratory distress within the first few hours of life.

IV. Diagnosis. Afflicted babies tend to have scaphoid abdomens since there is a paucity of the gastrointestinal tract located in the abdomen. **Auscultation** reveals diminished breath sounds on the affected side. Diagnosis is established by a **chest x-ray film** that reveals a bowel gas pattern in one hemithorax, with shift of mediastinal structures to the other side and compromise of the contralateral lung.

V. Management

    A. Indwelling arterial catheter. Blood gas levels should be monitored by an indwelling arterial catheter.

    B. Supportive care. Appropriate **respiratory and metabolic support** should be provided.

    C. Nasogastric intubation should be done to lessen gaseous distention of the stomach and intestine. For the same reason, any positive-pressure ventilation must be delivered by endotracheal tube, never by mask.

    D. Surgical correction is by reduction of intrathoracic intestine and closure of the diaphragmatic defect. Surgical intervention is obviously an essential element of treatment, but it is not the key to survival.

    E. Extracorporeal membrane oxygenation (ECMO) is being employed at an increasing number of centers in the treatment of neonates with severe respiratory failure. Exposure of venous blood to the extracorporeal circuit allows correction of pO_2 and pCO_2 abnormalities, as well as recovery of the lungs from the trauma associated with positive pressure ventilation. Most centers now report survival in 50–80% of neonates. (see Chap 11).

VI. Prognosis. With conventional therapy, mortality rates for infants with CDH are still in the range of 50–80%. This high rate has prompted a search for other modes of treatment in addition to the expensive, labor-intensive modality ECMO.

    A. Fetal surgery has been done successfully on a limited basis, with the idea that in utero intervention will lessen the risk for development of pulmonary hypoplasia, which may be incompatible with life after delivery.

    B. Medications. Another major area of research is the attempt to develop a pharmacologic agent to selectively decrease pulmonary vascular resistance. Such an agent would help solve the problem of PFC.

ABDOMINAL MASSES

RENAL MASSES

In most clinical series, the majority of abdominal masses in neonates are renal in origin. They may be unilateral or bilateral, solid or cystic. After physical examination, evaluation begins with ultrasonography, which is simple and safe to perform. Ultrasonography should define the solid or cystic nature of the mass, the presence or absence of normal kidneys, and yield information on other intra-abdominal abnormalities. Intravenous pyelography (IVP) may be helpful but is not necessary in every case. In selected instances, more involved procedures such as renal scan, CT scan, retrograde pyelography, venography, and arteriography may be needed to define the problem and plan appropriate therapy.

    I. Multicystic kidney. This is a form of renal dysplasia and the most common renal cystic disease of the newborn. Fortunately, it is usually unilateral. Ultrasonography can define the nature of the disorder, and IVP is useful in assessing the remainder of the urinary system. Nephrectomy is appropriate treatment.

    II. Hydronephrosis. Urinary obstruction, depending on its location, can cause unilateral or bilateral flank and abdominal masses. Treatment is by correction of the obstructing lesion or decompression proximal to it. A kidney rendered nonfunctional by back pressure is usually best removed. Obstructive uropathy is one category of lesion suitable for in utero intervention. Surgery on the developing fetus to decompress the obstructed urinary system may improve the postnatal status and increase survival.

III. **Infantile polycystic kidney disease.** Inherited in an autosomal recessive fashion, this entity involves both kidneys and carries a grim prognosis.

IV. **Renal vein thrombosis.** The typical presentation is flank mass(es) and hematuria, usually within the first 3 days of life. Risk factors are maternal diabetes and dehydration. In general, conservative nonoperative management is recommended.

V. **Wilms' tumor.** See p 457.

OVARIAN MASSES

Simple ovarian cyst has been called the most frequently palpated abdominal mass in the female neonate. It presents as a relatively mobile smooth-walled abdominal mass. It is not associated with malignancy, and excision with preservation of any ovarian tissue is curative.

HEPATIC MASSES

The liver can be enlarged, often to grotesque proportions, by a variety of problems. When physical examination, ultrasonography, and other x-ray studies suggest hepatic origin, angiography should be performed. This study may be diagnostic and will aid in surgical planning. Lesions include:

I. **Hepatic cysts.**

II. **Solid, benign tumors.**

III. **Vascular tumors.**

   A. **Hemangiomas** of the liver may cause heart failure, thrombocytopenia, and anemia. Therapeutic options include digitalis, corticosteroid administration, embolization, hepatic artery ligation, and liver resection.

   B. **Hemangioendothelioma.**

IV. **Malignant tumors. Hepatoblastoma** is by far the most common liver cancer in the neonate. Serum alpha-fetoprotein may be elevated. While surgical resection remains the key to achieving cure, new chemotherapeutic protocols (cisplatin [Platinol] and doxorubicin [Adriamycin]) may significantly improve the formerly dismal prognosis for infants with this tumor.

GASTROINTESTINAL MASSES

Palpable abdominal masses that arise from the gastrointestinal tract are unusual and tend to be cystic, smooth-walled, and mobile (depending on size). Causes include intestinal duplication and mesenteric cyst.

RETROPERITONEAL TUMORS

NEUROBLASTOMA

I. **Definition.** Neuroblastoma is a primitive malignant neoplasm that arises from neural crest tissue. It is probably the most common congenital tumor and is usually located in the adrenal gland.

II. **Clinical presentation.** This tumor typically presents as a firm, fixed, irregular mass extending obliquely from the costal margin, occasionally across the midline and into the lower abdomen.

III. **Diagnosis**

   A. **Laboratory studies.** A **24-hour urine collection** should be analyzed for VMA and other metabolites.

   B. **Radiologic studies.** A plain **abdominal x-ray film** may reveal calcification within the tumor. **IVP** and **CT scan** typically show extrinsic compression and inferolateral displacement of the kidney. Search for possible metastatic deposits involves **bone marrow aspiration and biopsy, bone scan, chest x-ray study,** and **chest CT scan.**

IV. Management. Planned therapy should take into account the well-recognized but poorly understood fact that neuroblastoma is notably less aggressive in the young infant than in the older child.

WILMS' TUMOR (NEPHROBLASTOMA)

 I. **Definition.** Wilms' tumor is an embryonal renal neoplasm in which blastemic, stromal, and epithelial cell types are present. Renal involvement is usually unilateral but may be bilateral (5% of cases).

 II. **Clinical presentation.** Palpable abdominal mass extending from beneath the costal margin is the usual mode of presentation.

 III. **Risk factors** include aniridia, hemihypertrophy, certain genitourinary anomalies, and a family history of nephroblastoma.

 IV. **Diagnosis**
   A. **Laboratory studies.** There is no tumor marker for Wilms' tumor.
   B. **Radiologic studies.** Ultrasonography is followed by IVP or CT scan, or both, which reveal intrinsic distortion of the calyceal system of the involved kidney. The possibility of tumor thrombus in the renal vein and inferior vena cava should be evaluated by ultrasonography and venography, if necessary.

 V. **Management**
   A. **Unilateral renal involvement.** Nephrectomy is the first step in treatment. Surgical staging determines the administration of radiotherapy and chemotherapy; both are very effective.
   B. **Bilateral renal involvement.** Treatment of bilateral Wilms' tumor is highly individualized.

TERATOMA

 I. **Definition.** Teratoma is a neoplasm containing elements derived from all 3 germ-cell layers: endoderm, mesoderm, and ectoderm. Teratomas in the neonate are primarily sacrococcygeal in location and are believed to represent a type of abortive caudal twinning.

 II. **Clinical presentation.** This tumor is usually grossly evident as a large external mass in the sacrococcygeal area. Occasionally, however, it may be presacral and retroperitoneal in location, and it may present as an abdominal mass.

 III. **Diagnosis.** See II, above. **Digital rectal examination** of the presacral space is important.

 IV. **Management.** Because the incidence of malignancy in these tumors increases with age, **prompt surgical excision** is required.

ABDOMINAL WALL DEFECTS

GASTROSCHISIS

 I. **Definition.** Gastroschisis is a centrally located, full-thickness abdominal wall defect with 2 distinctive anatomic features.
   A. **The extruded intestine never has a protective sac covering it.**
   B. **The umbilical cord is an intact structure at the level of the abdominal skin, just to the left of the defect.** Typically, the opening in the abdominal wall is 2–4 cm in diameter, and the solid organs (liver and spleen) reside in the peritoneal cavity.

 II. **Pathophysiology.** Exposure of unprotected intestine to irritating amniotic fluid in utero results in its edematous, indurated, foreshortened appearance. Because of these intestinal abnormalities, development of appropriate peristalsis and effective absorption is significantly delayed, usually by several weeks. Fortunately, associated congenital anomalies are rare in patients with gastroschisis.

III. Clinical presentation. See **I** and **II,** above.

IV. Diagnosis. The key differential diagnosis is ruptured omphalocele, although the **diagnosis is readily apparent in most cases.** Increasingly, **prenatal ultrasonography** identifies gastroschisis.

V. Management

  A. General considerations. All agree that infants with gastroschisis should be delivered at a neonatal center equipped and staffed to provide definitive care. Less certain is the recommended mode of delivery. Some have argued that abdominal wall defect is an indication for cesarean section. However, recent articles note that in the absence of other factors, vaginal delivery does not increase the mortality, morbidity, or length of hospital stay for newborns with gastroschisis.

  B. Specific measures

  1. Temperature regulation. Immediate attention should be directed toward maintenance of normal body temperature. The tremendous intestinal surface area exposed to the environment puts these infants at great risk of hypothermia.

  2. Protective covering. It is best not to keep replacing moist, saline-soaked gauze over the exposed intestine, because doing so promotes evaporative heat loss. It is better to **apply a dry (or moist) protective dressing and then wrap the abdomen in layers of cellophane.** A warm, controlled environment should be provided.

  3. Nasogastric decompression is helpful.

  4. Broad-spectrum antibiotic coverage is appropriate, given the unavoidable contamination.

  5. Total parenteral nutrition (TPN). A protracted ileus is to be expected, and appropriate intravenous nutritional support must be provided.

  6. Surgical correction. As soon as the infant's condition permits, operative correction should be undertaken. Complete reduction of herniated intestine, with primary closure of the abdominal wall, or placement of unreduced intestine in a protective prosthetic silo, with subsequent staged reduction over 7–14 days, is usually performed.

OMPHALOCELE

  I. Definition. An omphalocele is a herniation of abdominal contents into the base of the umbilical cord. The gross appearance of omphalocele differs from that of gastroschisis in 2 important respects.

  A. A protective membrane encloses the malplaced abdominal contents (unless rupture has occurred, eg, during the birth process).

  B. Elements of the umbilical cord course individually over the sac and come together at its apex to form a normal-appearing umbilical cord.

  II. Associated anomalies. Significant associated congenital anomalies occur in about 25–40% of infants with omphalocele. Problems include chromosomal abnormalities, congenital diaphragmatic hernia, and a variety of cardiac defects.

  III. Clinical presentation. There are different sizes of omphaloceles. The smaller ones typically contain only intestine; large or giant omphaloceles contain liver and spleen as well as the gastrointestinal tract. The peritoneal cavity in infants with large or giant omphaloceles is very small, as growth has proceeded without the solid organs in proper position.

  IV. Diagnosis. The anomaly is **usually apparent.** Ruptured omphalocele may be confused with gastroschisis; both defects are characterized by exposed intestine, but infants with omphalocele do not possess an intact umbilical cord at the level of the abdominal wall, to the left of the defect. Careful studies to identify associated congenital anomalies should be carried out.

  V. Management. Reduction, even in stages over a lengthy period of time, may be very difficult to achieve. Therapeutically, infants with omphalocele fall into 2 main groups.

  A. Ruptured sac. Infants with ruptured sacs resemble those with gastroschisis. The unprotected intestine should be cared for as described for gastroschisis (see p 458, **B.2**) and the problem should be corrected surgically on an emergent basis.

  B. Intact sac. Intact omphalocele is a less urgent surgical problem. The protective membrane conserves heat and in most cases allows effective peristalsis. This sac should be carefully protected. Some surgeons favor daily dressing changes with gauze pads impregnated with povidone iodine until the sac toughens and desiccates. The timing of surgery is influenced by a number of factors, including the dimensions of the defect, the size of the infant, and the presence of other anomalies.

EXSTROPHY OF THE BLADDER

  I. Definition. Exstrophy of the bladder is a congenital malformation of the lower anterior abdominal wall. In this defect, the internal surface of the posterior wall of the urinary bladder extrudes through the abdominal wall defect. The problem occurs in varying degrees of severity, ranging from epispadias to complete extroversion of the bladder, with exposure of the ureteral orifices.

  II. Clinical presentation. The lower abdominal wall defect is obvious; exposed bladder mucosa is markedly edematous and friable.

  III. Diagnosis. Diagnosis is by **inspection. Radiologic evaluation of the proximal urinary tract** is advisable.

  IV. Management

  A. Protective covering. The bladder should be carefully protected with **Vaseline gauze or cellophane wrap.** Attention should also be paid to protection of the surrounding skin.

  B. Surgical repair. In most centers, primary closure of the bladder is attempted within the first 48–72 hours of life, while the sacroiliac joints are still pliable and the pelvis can be "molded" to allow better approximation of the pubic rami.

CLOACAL EXSTROPHY

  I. Definition. Cloacal exstrophy is a rare but devastating complex of anomalies, including imperforate anus, exstrophy of the bladder, omphalocele, and vesicointestinal fistula, frequently with prolapse of bowel through the fistula onto the bladder mucosa.

  II. Clinical presentation. See **I,** above.

  III. Diagnosis. Diagnosis is by **inspection.** Evaluation of the genitourinary system and gastrointestinal tract is appropriate.

  IV. Management

  A. Protective covering. Exposed mucosa, both bladder and intestine, should be protected with **Vaseline gauze or cellophane wrap.** Ointments should be applied to the surrounding skin to prevent maceration.

  B. Surgical care. Prompt operation to separate the fecal and urinary streams is imperative.

MISCELLANEOUS SURGICAL CONDITIONS

NECROTIZING ENTEROCOLITIS

In most centers, necrotizing enterocolitis (NEC) is the most common indication for operation in neonates (see also Chap 64). Abdominal exploration is usually reserved for infants with full-thickness necrosis of the intestine, usually manifested by pneumoperitoneum (best identified by serial left lateral decubitus x-ray films). Other less common indications for surgery include cellulitis and induration of the abdominal wall and an unchanging abdominal mass. Delayed stricture formation, which is most common on the left side of the colon, complicates NEC in 15–25% of cases.

HYPOSPADIAS

 I. **Definition.** Hypospadias is a developmental anomaly in which the external opening of the urethra is present on the underside of the penis or on the perineum rather than in its normal position at the end of the penile shaft.
 II. **Clinical presentation.** There are different anatomic classifications, depending on the location of the meatal opening and on the degree of chordee (curvature of the penis). There is a high incidence of associated **cryptorchidism** in the patients. Severe cases of hypospadias may be confused with ambiguous genitalia.
 III. **Diagnosis.** The anomaly is **readily apparent** (see I and II, above). **Radiologic evaluation of the urinary system** is appropriate.
 IV. **Management.** Surgical correction should usually not be attempted in the newborn. Because foreskin tissue may be needed for later surgical correction, **circumcision must be avoided** in infants with hypospadias.

HERNIA AND HYDROCELE

 I. **Definition.** Persistence of a patent processus vaginalis (related to testicular descent) is responsible for inguinal hernia-hydrocele in the neonate.
   A. **Inguinal hernia.** The opening of the patent processus at the internal ring is large enough to allow a loop of intestine to extrude from the abdominal cavity with an increase in intra-abdominal pressure.
   B. **Hydrocele.** The patent processus is too narrow to permit egress of intestine; peritoneal fluid drips down along the course of the narrow patent processus and accumulates in the scrotum.
 II. **Diagnosis**
   A. **Inguinal hernias** tend to present as lumps or bulges that come and go at the pubic tubercle. Less commonly, they descend into the scrotum.
   B. **Hydroceles** are typically scrotal in location, transilluminate, and are not reducible.
 III. **Management**
   A. **Inguinal hernia** carries a 15–20% risk of incarceration during the first year of life. Accordingly, they are usually surgically repaired when the infant's general medical condition permits.
   B. **Hydrocele** frequently resolves without specific treatment, as the obliteration of the narrow patent processus continues after birth. Persistence of hydrocele for 6–12 months is an indication for surgical repair.

UNDESCENDED TESTICLES (CRYPTORCHIDISM)

Undescended testicles occur in about 33% of premature and 3% of term male infants. Many undescended testes will descend in the first few months after birth. Unless there is an associated inguinal hernia, surgical correction is usually not performed until the infant is between 1 and 2 years of age, although some surgeons favor earlier correction.

POSTERIOR URETHRAL VALVES

 I. **Definition.** Posterior urethral valves are abnormal valves in the urethra at the verumontanum. They represent the most common cause of congenital obstructive uropathy in males.
 II. **Pathophysiology.** The high degree of bladder outlet obstruction caused by posterior urethral valves results in proximal dilatation. The urinary bladder enlarges, the ureters become dilated and tortuous, and back pressure in the collecting systems compromises developing renal parenchyma.
 III. **Clinical presentation**

    A. Prenatal ultrasonography is currently identifying many infants with posterior urethral valves.

    B. After birth, neonates with this anomaly present with bilateral flank masses, distended bladder, and poor urinary stream (with dribbling).

IV. Diagnosis. Voiding cystourethrography documents the abnormal valves.

V. Management. The goal of therapy is preservation of renal function and avoidance of renal failure.

    A. Evaluation of renal function and the infant's general status should be carried out.

    B. Stabilization, rehydration, correction of electrolyte abnormalities, and treatment of urinary tract infection should be accompanied by transurethral drainage of the bladder, using a 5F infant feeding tube.

    C. Surgical therapy

        1. Ablation of valves is the initial operative procedure favored by most pediatric urologists.

        2. Urinary diversion may be indicated.

REFERENCES

Arensman RM, Cornish JD (eds): *Extracorporeal Life Support.* Blackwell, 1993.

Bethel CAI, Szashore JH, Touloukian RJ: Caesarean section does not improve outcome in gastroschisis. *J Pediatr Surg* 1989;**24:**1.

Fallis JC, Filler RM, Lemoine G (eds): *Pediatric Thoracic Surgery.* Elsevier, 1991.

King LR (editor): *Urologic Surgery in Neonates and Young Infants.* Saunders, 1988.

Pierro A et al: Preoperative chemotherapy in "unresectable" hepatoblastoma. *J Pediatr Surg* 1989;**24:**24.

Powell DM, Othersen HB, Smith CD: Malrotation of the intestine in children: Effect of age on presentation and therapy. *J Pediatr Surg* 1989;**24:**777.

Welch J et al (editors): *Pediatric Surgery,* 4th ed. Year Book, 1986.

72 Thyroid Disorders

Disorders of thyroid function in infants often present a diagnostic dilemma. Signs of thyroid dysfunction are rarely present at birth and initial signs and symptoms are often subtle or misleading. A good understanding of the unique thyroid physiology and the assessment of thyroid function in neonates is necessary in order to recognize, diagnose, and treat thyroid disorders.

GENERAL CONSIDERATIONS

I. **Fetal and neonatal thyroid function**
   A. **Embryogenesis** occurs during the first 10 to 12 weeks of gestation. Thyroid activity remains low until mid-gestation and then increases slowly until term.
   B. **Thyroid hormones** undergo rapid and dramatic changes in the immediate postnatal period.
      1. An acute release of thyrotropin-stimulating hormone (TSH) occurs within minutes after birth. Peak values of 60 to 80 μU/mL are seen at 30 to 90 minutes. Levels decrease to less than 5 μU/mL by 3 to 5 days.
      2. Stimulated by the TSH surge, thyroxine (T_4), free T_4 (FT_4), and triiodothyronine (T_3) rapidly increase, reaching peak levels by 24 hours. Levels decrease slowly over the first few weeks of life.
   C. **Thyroid function in the premature infant.** Identical changes in TSH, T_4, and T_3 are seen in premature infants, however, absolute values are lower. TSH levels return to normal by 3 to 5 days of life, regardless of gestational age.

II. **Physiologic action of thyroid hormone**
   Thyroid hormones have profound effects on growth and neurologic development. They also influence O_2 consumption, thermogenesis, and the metabolic rate of many processes.

III. **Assessment of thyroid function.** Thyroid tests are intended to measure the level of thyroid activity and to identify the cause of thyroid dysfunction.
   A. **T_4 concentration** is the most important parameter in the evaluation of thyroid function. Greater than 99% of T_4 is bound to thyroid hormone-binding proteins. Therefore, changes in these proteins may affect T_4 levels.
   B. **Free T_4** reflects the availability of thyroid hormone to the tissues.
   C. **TSH measurement** is one of the most valuable tests in evaluating thyroid disorders, particularly primary hyperthyroidism.
   D. **T_3 concentration** is particularly useful in the diagnosis and treatment of hyperthyroidism.
   E. **Thyroid-binding globulin (TBG)** can be measured directly by RIA. T_3 resin uptake provides an indirect measure of TBG and is now considered an outdated test. TBG may be decreased in preterm infants, malnutrition, and chronic illness. It is increased by estrogens and heroin. Drugs such as dilantin, diazepam, heparin, and furosemide compete with T_4 for TBG-binding sites resulting in falsely low T_4 levels.
   F. **TRH stimulation test** can assess pituitary and thyroid responsiveness. It is used to differentiate between secondary and tertiary hypothyroidism.
   G. **Thyroid imaging**
      1. **Thyroid scan** is used to identify functional thyroid tissue. [123]I is the preferable isotope for children.
      2. **Ultrasound** is useful in evaluating anatomy but is not a reliable alternative to a scan.

CONGENITAL HYPOTHYROIDISM

I. **Definition.** Congenital hypothyroidism is defined as a significant decrease in, or the absence of, thyroid function present at birth.

II. **Incidence.** The overall incidence is 1 in 3500 to 1 in 4500 births. It is more prevalent in females than males by a ratio of 2:1. It is more common in Hispanic and Asian infants (1 in 3000 births) and less common in blacks (1 in 32,000 births). Incidence is significantly increased in Down syndrome (1 in 140).

III. **Etiologic classification**

   A. Primary hypothyroidism

   1. Developmental defects such as ectopic thyroid (most common), thyroid hypoplasia, or agenesis.

   2. Inborn errors of thyroid hormone synthesis.

   3. Maternal exposure to radioiodine, propylthiouracil, or methimazole during pregnancy.

   4. Iodine deficiency (endemic cretinism).

   B. Secondary hypothyroidism—TSH deficiency.

   C. Tertiary hypothyroidism—TRH deficiency.

IV. **Clinical presentation.** Symptoms are usually absent at birth, however, subtle signs may be detected during the first few weeks of life.

   A. **Early manifestations.** Signs at birth include prolonged gestation, LGA, large fontanelles, and RDS. Manifestations which may be seen by 2 weeks include hypotonia, lethargy, hypothermia, prolonged jaundice, and feeding difficulty.

   B. **Late manifestation.** Classic features usually appear after 6 weeks and include puffy eyelids, coarse hair, large tongue, myxedema, and hoarse cry.

V. **Diagnosis**

   A. **Screening.** Newborn screening for congenital hypothyroidism is mandatory in most states.

   1. **Method.** Most programs use a twofold process using the filter paper spot technique. A T_4 measurement is followed by a measurement of TSH in specimens with low T_4 values ($T_4 \leq 10^{th}$ percentile).

   2. **Timing.** The ideal time for screening is between day 2 and 6 of life. Babies discharged before 48 hours should be screened prior to discharge. However, this increases the number of false-positive results due to the TSH surge occurring at birth.

   3. **Results.** A low T_4 level (less than 7 µg/mL) and TSH concentrations greater than 40 µU/mL is indicative of congenital hypothyroidism. Borderline TSH levels (20–40 µU/mL) should be repeated.

   B. **Diagnostic Studies**

   1. Serum for confirmatory measurements of T_4 and TSH concentrations should be done. If an abnormality of TBG is suspected, FT_4 and TBG concentrations should also be done.

   2. Thyroid scan remains the most accurate diagnostic modality to determine the cause of congenital hypothyroidism.

VI. **Management**

   A. **Consultation** with a pediatric endocrinologist is recommended.

   B. **Treatment.** Sodium-L-Thyroxine is the drug of choice because of its uniform potency and reliable absorption. The average starting dose is 10–15 µg/kg/d. Usually term infants receive a 50 µg tablet daily and preterm infants 25 µg daily. The goal of therapy is to maintain T_4 concentration in the upper normal range (10–16 µg/dL) and TSH below 10 µU/mL.

   C. **Follow-up.** Frequent T_4 and TSH measurements are required to ensure optimal treatment. Recommended follow-up:

   1. At 2 and 4 weeks after initiation of therapy.

   2. Every 1–2 months for the first year.

   3. Two weeks after changing dosage.

VII. **Prognosis** is dependent on the age at onset of therapy.

NEONATAL THYROTOXICOSIS

I. **Definition.** Neonatal thyrotoxicosis is defined as a hypermetabolic state resulting from excessive thyroid hormone activity in the newborn.

II. **Etiology.** This disorder usually results from transplacental passage of thyroid-stimulating immunoglobulin (TSI) from a mother with Grave's disease.

III. **Incidence.** Rare disorder occurring only in about 1 of 70 thyrotoxic pregnancies. (The incidence of thyrotoxicosis in pregnancy is 1 to 2 per 1000 pregnancies.)

IV. **Clinical presentation.** Fetal tachycardia in the third trimester may be the first manifestation. Signs are usually apparent within hours after birth unless the mother was taking antithyroid medications, in which case the presentation may be delayed 2 to 10 days. Thyrotoxic signs include irritability, tachycardia, flushing, temor, poor weight gain, thrombocytopenia, and arrhythmias. A goiter is usually present and may be large enough to cause tracheal compression.

V. **Diagnosis**
   A. **History and physical.** A maternal history of Grave's disease and the presence of a goiter is suggestive of thyrotoxicosis.
   B. **Laboratory studies.** Diagnosis is confirmed by demonstrating increased levels of T_4, FT_4, and T_3 with suppressed levels of TSH.

VI. **Management.** Although the disorder is usually self-limited, therapy depends on the severity of the symptoms.
   A. **Mild**—close observation. No therapy.
   B. **Moderate**—administration of one of the following antithyroid medications.
      1. Lugol's solution (iodine), 1 drop every 8 hours.
      2. Propylthiouracil (PTU), 10 mg/kg/d in 3 divided doses.
      3. Methimazole, 0.5 to 1 mg/kg/d in 3 divided doses.
   C. **Severe**—in addition to antithyroid medication, propranolol, 1 to 2 mg/kg/d in 2 to 4 divided doses may be used.

VII. **Prognosis.** The disorder is usually self-limited and disappears spontaneously within 2 to 4 months. Mortality in affected infants is about 15% if the disorder is not recognized and treated properly.

TRANSIENT DISORDERS OF THYROID FUNCTION IN THE NEWBORN

I. **Euthyroid sick syndrome**
   A. **Definition.** Transient alteration in thyroid function associated with severe nonthyroidal illness.
   B. **Incidence.** Frequently seen in premature infants due to their increased susceptibility to neonatal morbidity. Preterm infants with RDS have been the most frequently reported patients with this disorder.
   C. **Diagnosis.** A low T_3 level is usually present associated with low or normal T_4 and normal TSH. Infants are euthyroid (normal TSH).
   D. **Treatment.** No treatment is required. Abnormal thyroid functions return to normal as the sick infant improves.

II. **Transient hypothyroxinemia**
   A. **Incidence.** All preterm infants have some degree of hypothyroxinemia (> 50% have levels < 6.5 μg/dL).
   B. **Pathophysiology.** Presumed to be related to immaturity of the hypothalamic-pituitary axis.
   C. **Diagnosis.** Low T_4 and FT_4 with normal TSH and normal response to TRH stimulation test.
   D. **Treatment.** No treatment is required. This disorder corrects spontaneously with progressive maturation, usually in 4 to 8 weeks.

RERERENCES

American Academy of Pediatrics AAP Section on Endocrinology and Committee on Genetics, on Genetics, and American Thyroid Association Committee on Public Health: Newborn screening for congenital hypothyroidism: recommended guidelines. *Pediatrics* 1993;**9(6)**:1203–09.

Bertrand J, Rappaport R, Sizonenko PC: Assessment of endocrine functions. Chap 47, p 658 in:

Pediatric Endocrinology, Physiology, Pathophysiology and Clinical Aspects, 2nd ed. Williams & Wilkins, 1993.

The California Newborn Screening Program: Primary congenital hypothyroidism revisited. Spring 1993.

Czernichow P: Thyrotropin and thyroid hormones. Chap 6, p 79 in: *Pediatric Endocrinology, Physiology, Pathophysiology and Clinical Aspects,* 2nd ed. Williams & Wilkins, 1993.

DeLange F, Czernichow P: Hypothyroidism. Chap 18, p 252 in: *Pediatric Endocrinology, Physiology, Pathophysiology and Clinical Aspects,* 2nd ed. Williams & Wilkins, 1993.

Fisher DA: Euthyroid low thyroxine (T_4) and triiodothyronine (T_3) states in premature and sick neonates. *Pediatric Clin North Am* 1990;**37:**1297.

Fisher DA, Klein AH: Thyroid development and disorders of thyroid function in the newborn. *N Engl J Med* 1981;**304:**702–08.

Gruters A: Congenital hypothyroidism. *Pediatric Ann* 1992;**21(1):**15, 18–21, 24–28.

Polk DH, Fisher DA: Fetal and neonatal thyroid physiology. Chap 185, p 1842 in: *Fetal and Neonatal Physiology* Vol 2. Saunders, 1992.

Polk DH, Fisher DA: Disorders of the thyroid gland. Chap 109, p 954 in: *Schaffer and Avery's Diseases of the Newborn,* 6th ed. Saunders, 1991.

Sobel EH, Saenger P: Hypothyroidism in the newborn. *Pediatrics Rev* 1989;**11:**15.

Zimmerman D, Gan-Gaisano M: Hyperthyroidism in children and adolescents. *Pediatric Clin North Am* 1990;**37:**1273.

73 Commonly Used Medications

Acetaminophen (APAP, Liquiprin, Tempra, Tylenol)

Indications and use: Analgesic-antipyretic.

Actions: Mechanism of analgesic effect is unclear. Reduction of fever is produced by direct action on the hypothalamic heat-regulating center.

Supplied: Suppositories, elixir, liquid, drops (preferred).

Route: PO, PR.

Dosage: 5–10 mg/kg/dose q4–6 h as needed.

Adverse effects: Hepatic necrosis with overdosage, rash, fever, blood dyscrasias (neutropenia, pancytopenia, leukopenia, thrombocytopenia). May be hepatotoxic with chronic use.

Acetazolamide (Diamox)

Indications and use: For use as a mild diuretic or as an anticonvulsant in refractory neonatal seizures. To decrease CSF production in posthemorrhagic hydrocephalus; also used in the treatment of renal tubular acidosis.

Actions: Carbonic anhydrase inhibitor. Appears to retard abnormal discharge from CNS neurons. Beneficial effects may be related to direct inhibition of carbonic anhydrase or may be due to the acidosis produced. Also produces urinary alkalosis useful in the treatment of renal tubular acidosis.

Supplied: Injection, tablets. (Suspension can be compounded by pharmacist.)

Route: IV, PO.

Dosage:

- Diuretic: 5 mg/kg/dose qd–qod.
- Anticonvulsant: 8–30 mg/kg/day PO divided q6–8h.
- Alkalinize urine: 5 mg/kg/dose 2 to 3 times over 24 hours.
- Decrease CSF production: 50–100 mg/kg/day divided q6–8h.

Elimination: Unchanged in urine; half-life is 4–10 hours.

Adverse effects: Gastrointestinal irritation, anorexia, transient hypokalemia, drowsiness, paresthesias.

Comments: Limited clinical experience in neonates. Used as an adjunct to other medications in refractory seizures. Tolerance to diuretic effect with long-term use.

Acyclovir (Zovirax)

Classification: Antiviral agent.

Action and spectrum: Indicated in herpes simplex and varicella-zoster viral infections. Virostatic activated in virally infected cells, inhibits viral DNA polymerase, and is a viral chain terminator. Good activity against herpes simplex (types 1 and 2) and varicella-zoster viruses. Poor activity against Epstein-Barr virus and cytomegalovirus. CSF concentrations are 50% those of plasma.

Supplied: Injection, topical, suspension.

Route: Topical, IV, PO.

Dosage:
- Topical: Apply sufficient amount to cover lesion q3h.
- IV: 30–40 mg/kg/day divided q8h for 10–14 days (dilute to final concentration of 7 mg/mL and infuse over 60 minutes).

Adverse effects: Transient elevation of serum creatinine, thrombocytosis, jitters, rash, hives.

Comments: Drug of choice for documented or suspected herpes encephalitis (suggest 40 mg/kg/day IV in divided doses for 14 days).

Adenosine (Adenocard)

Indications and use: Conversion to sinus rhythm of paroxysmal supraventricular tachycardia.

Actions: Adenosine is a purine nucleoside naturally occurring in all human cells. It slows conduction time through the AV node, interrupts reentry pathways through the AV node to restore normal sinus rhythm. Its electrophysiologic effects are mediated by depression of calcium slow channel conduction, an increase in potassium conductance, and possibly indirect antiadrenergic effects.

Supplied: Injection, 6 mg/2 mL.

Route: IV.

Dosage: 37.5 mcg/kg by rapid IV push over 1–2 seconds. Increase by 37.5 mcg/kg increments at 1 minute intervals until effect observed. (Range 37.5–250 mcg/kg).

Adverse effects: Do not use in second- or third-degree AV block. May produce a short lasting first-, second-, or third-degree heart block, hypotension, brief dyspnea, and facial flushing. Half-life: less than 10 seconds; duration: 20–30 seconds. Carbamazepine increases the degree of heart block caused by adenosine. Methylxanthines (caffeine, theophylline) are competitive antagonists; larger adenosine doses may be required.

Albumin, Human (various)

Indications and use: Plasma volume expander. Treatment of hypoproteinemia.

Actions: Maintains plasma colloid oncotic pressure. Intravenous administration causes a shift of fluid from the interstitial spaces into the circulation. Serves as a carrier for many substances such as bilirubin. Limited nutritional value.

Supplied: Injection, 50 mg/mL (5%), 250 mg/mL (25%) (contains 130–160 meq sodium/L.

Route: IV.

Dosage: 0.5–1 g/kg IV (or 10–20 mL/kg of 5% IV bolus) repeated as necessary. Maximum 6 g/kg/day.

Adverse effects: Infrequent. Rapid infusion may cause vascular overload and precipitation of congestive heart failure. Hypersensitivity reactions may include chills, fever, nausea, and urticaria.

Comments: More purified than plasma protein fraction and thus less likely to cause hypotension.

Alprostadil (Prostaglandin E$_1$, Prostin VR)

Indications and use: Any state in which blood flow must be maintained through the ductus arteriosus to sustain either pulmonary or systemic circulation until corrective or palliative surgery can be performed. Examples are pulmonary atresia, pulmonary stenosis, tricuspid atresia, transposition of the great arteries, aortic arch interruption, coarctation of the aorta, and severe tetralogy of Fallot.

Actions: Vasodilator, platelet aggregation inhibitor. Smooth muscle of the ductus arteriosus is especially sensitive to its effects, responding to the drug with marked dilatation. Decreased response after 96 hours of infusion. Maximal improvement in PaO$_2$, usually within 30 minutes in cyanotic infants, 1.5–3 hours in acyanotic infants.

Supplied: Injection.

Route: IV.

Dosage: 0.05 mcg/kg/min. Decrease to lowest rate that will maintain response.

Adverse effects: Cutaneous vasodilation, seizure-like activity, jitteriness, temperature elevation, hypocalcemia, apnea, thrombocytopenia, hypotension.

Comments: Use cautiously in infants with bleeding tendencies.

Amikacin Sulfate (Amikin)

Classification: Aminoglycoside.

Action and spectrum: Primarily bactericidal against gram-negative organisms by inhibiting protein synthesis. Active against gram-negative bacteria, including most *Pseudomonas* and *Serratia.* No activity against anaerobic organisms.

Supplied: Injection.

Route: IM or IV (infuse over 30 minutes).

Dosage: Dosage should be monitored and adjusted by use of pharmacokinetics. Initial empiric dosing based on body weight:

- < 1.2 kg, 0–4 weeks postnatal age: 7.5 mg/kg/dose q18–24h
- 1.2–2 kg:
    0–7 Days: 7.5 mg/kg/dose q12–18h
    > 7 Days: 7.5 mg/kg/dose q8–12h
- > 2 kg:
    0–7 Days: 10 mg/kg/dose q12h
    > 7 Days: 10 mg/kg/dose q8h

Elimination: Renal (glomerular filtration); half life is 4–8 hours; volume of distribution is 0.6 L/kg.

Comments: Lowest overall resistance of all the aminoglycosides and thus should be reserved for infections with organisms resistant to other aminoglycosides. Adjust dosage according to serum peak and trough levels. Draw serum levels at about the fourth maintenance dose (draw serum trough sample 30 minutes to just before dose and serum peak sample 30 minutes after infusion is complete). Therapeutic peak level 25–35 mcg/mL and trough level 10 mcg/mL. Nephrotoxicity associated with serum trough concentrations >10 mcg/mL; ototoxicity with serum peak concentrations > 35–40 mcg/mL (more cochlear damage than vestibular).

Amphotericin B (Fungizone)

Classification: Antifungal agent.

Action and spectrum: Acts by binding to sterols and disrupting the fungal cell membranes. Broad spectrum of activity against *Candida* and other fungi.

Supplied: Injection.

Route: IV.

Dosage:

- Initially: Test dose of 0.25 mg/kg IV over 4 hours. Use 0.1 mg/mL concentration in 5% dextrose. Incompatible with sodium chloride.
- Increment: Increase daily dosage by 0.25 mg/kg/day qd–qod as tolerated to maximum daily or alternate-day dosage 0f 0.75–1.5 mg/kg. A total dosage of 30–35 mg/kg should be given over 6 weeks or longer, though a lower dose may suffice. In general, infusions should be given over 2–6 hours, though infusion over 1–2 hours may be used if tolerated.
- Intrathecal or intraventricular: Reconstitute with sterile water at 0.25 mg/mL; dilute with CSF fluid and reinfuse. Usual dose: 0.25–0.5 mg.

Elimination and metabolism: Slow renal excretion.

Adverse effects: Few adverse effects in neonates as opposed to adults. May cause fever, chills, vomiting, thrombophlebitis at injection sites, renal tubular acidosis, renal failure, hypomagnesemia, hypokalemia, bone marrow suppression with reversible decline in hematocrit, hypotension, hypertension, wheezing, and hypoxemia.

Comments: Irritation at infusion site may be reduced by addition of heparin (1 unit/mL). Protect solution from light. Monitor serum potassium, magnesium, urea nitrogen, creatinine, alkaline phosphatase, and AST (SGOT) qd–qod until the dosage is stabilized, then every week. Monitor CBC every week. Discontinue if BUN > 40 mg/dL or if serum creatinine > 3 mg/dL or if liver function tests are abnormal.

Ampicillin (Polycillin, others)

Classification: Semisynthetic penicillinase-sensitive penicillin.

Action and spectrum: The penicillins are bactericidal and act by inhibiting the late stages of cell wall synthesis. Ampicillin is as effective as penicillin G in pneumococcal, streptococcal, and meningococcal infections and is active also against many strains of *Salmonella, Shigella, Proteus mirabilis, Escherichia coli, Listeria,* and most strains of *Haemophilus influenzae.* It is inactivated by staphylococcal and *H influenzae* beta-lactamases.

Supplied: Powder to make pediatric drops, oral suspension, and injection.

Route: PO, IM, IV.

Dosage:

- Meningitis
  Age 0–7 days: 100–200 mg/kg/day IV or IM divided q12h.
  Age > 7 days: 200–300 mg/kg/day IV or IM divided q6–8h: maximum dose 400 mg/kg/day.
- Other indications:
  Age 0–7 days: 50 mg/kg/day PO, IV, or IM divided q12h.
  Age > 7 days: 75 mg/kg/day PO, IV, or IM divided q12h.

Elimination and metabolism: 90% excreted unchanged in urine. Half-life in neonates is 2 hours.

Adverse effects: Hypersensitivity, rubella-like rash, abdominal discomfort, nausea, vomiting, diarrhea, eosinophilia. Very large doses may cause CNS excitation or convulsions.

Comments: Ampicillin is the penicillin of choice in combination with an aminoglycoside in the prophylaxis and treatment of infections with group B streptococci, group D streptococci (enterococci), and *Listeria* monocytogenes. Contains 3 meq of sodium per gram.

Ampicillin/Sulbactam (Unasyn)

Classification: Combination beta-lactamase inhibitor and beta-lactam agent.

Action and spectrum: The bactericidal spectrum of ampicillin is extended by the addition of sulbactam, a beta-lactamase inhibitor, to include beta-lactamase-producing strains of *S aureus, S epidermidis,* enterococcus, *H influenzae, B catarrhalis,* and *Klebsiella* spp, including *K pneumoniae.* Also has good activity against *B fragilis,* making it a suitable choice for single drug treatment of intra-abdominal and pelvic infections caused by susceptible organisms.

Supplied: Injection.

Route: IV or IM.

Dosage:

  Age 0–7 days: 50 mg/kg/day IV or IM q12h.
  Age > 7 days: 75 mg/kg/day IV or IM q12h.
- Meningitis:
  Age 0–7 days: 100–200 mg/kg/day IV q12h.
  Age > 7 days: 200–300 mg/kg/day IV or IM q6–8h.
  Maximum dose 400 mg/kg/day.

Elimination: See Ampicillin, above.

Adverse effects: See Ampicillin, above.

Comments: See Ampicillin, above.

Atropine Sulfate

Indications and use: Sinus bradycardia, cardiopulmonary resuscitation, reversal of neuromuscular blockade. Used preoperatively to inhibit salivation and reduce excessive secretions of the respiratory tract.

Actions: A competitive antagonist of acetylcholine at smooth muscle, cardiac muscle, and various glandular cells, leading to increased heart rate, reduced gastrointestinal motility and tone, urinary retention, cycloplegia, and decreased salivation and sweating.

Supplied: Injection, ophthalmic ointment, ophthalmic solution.

Route: IV, IM, SC, PO, Intratracheal (IT).

Dosage:

- Bradycardia in infants and children: 0.02–0.03 mg/kg/dose q2–3 min prn.
- Preanesthetic: 0.03 mg/kg/dose.

Adverse effects: Xerostomia, blurred vision, mydriasis, tachycardia, palpitations, constipation, urinary retention, ataxia, tremor, hyperthermia. Toxic effects especially likely in children receiving low doses.

Comments: Contraindicated in thyrotoxicosis, tachycardia secondary to cardiac insufficiency, and obstructive gastrointestinal disease. In low doses, may cause paradoxical bradycardia secondary to its central actions.

Aztreonam (Azactam)

Classification: Monobactam antibiotic.

Action and spectrum: Antibacterial activity due to inhibition of mucopeptide synthesis in cell wall. Bactericidal against most *Enterobacteriaceae* and *Pseudomonas aeruginosa* but little or no activity against gram-positive aerobic bacteria or anaerobic bacteria.

Supplied: Injection.

Route: IV.

Dosage:

- Premature infants: 50 mg/kg/dose q12h.
- Term infants: 50 mg/kg/dose q8h.

Elimination: Renal (glomerular filtration and secretion). Half-life is approximately 6–10 hours. Volume of distribution 0.26–0.36 L/kg.

Adverse effects: Diarrhea, nausea, vomiting, rash irritation at infusion site, increased prothrombin time, transient eosinophilia.

Comments: Used primarily for Pseudomonas infections.

Beractant (Survanta)

Indications and use: Prevention and treatment of respiratory distress syndrome of preterm infants.

Actions: Beractant is natural bovine lung extract containing phospholipids, neutral lipids, fatty acids, and surfactant-associated proteins to which dipalmitoylphosphatidylcholine (DPPC), palmitic acid, and tripalmitin are added to mimic the surface-tension lowering properties of natural lung surfactant. Surfactant lowers surface tension on alveolar surfaces during respiration and stabilizes the alveoli against collapse.

Supplied: Suspension in single use vials containing 25 mg phospholipids/mL, 8 mL. Refrigerate.

Route: Intratracheal using a 5 French end-hole catheter.

Dosage: 4 mL/kg (100 mg of phospholipids/kg) birth weight. Give in four increments, repositioning the infant with each dose. Inject each quarter-dose gently into the catheter over 2–3 seconds. Ventilate the infant after each quarter-dose for at least 30 seconds or until stable. Four doses of 4 mL/kg can be given in the first 48 hours of life, no more frequently than every 6 hours.

Adverse effects: Most adverse effects are associated while administering the beractant to the infant: transient bradycardia, oxygen desaturation. Less frequent adverse effects: Endotracheal tube reflux, pallor, vasoconstriction, hypotension, endotracheal tube blockage, hypertension, hypocarbia, hypercarbia, apnea. In two studies the rate of intracranial hemorrhage was significantly higher in infants who received beractant than in controls. When all study results were pooled, however, there was no difference in intracranial hemorrhage.

Bumetanide (Bumex)

Indications and use: Management of edema associated with congenital heart disease, congestive heart failure, hepatic or renal disease.

Actions: Inhibition of the active chloride and, possibly, sodium transport systems of the loop of Henle. Urinary excretion of sodium, chloride, potassium, hydrogen, calcium, magnesium, ammonium, phosphate, and bicarbonate increases with bumetanide induced diuresis. Renal blood flow increases substantially due to renovascular dilation.

Supplied: Injection, 0.25 mg/mL, tablets.

Route: PO, IV, IM.

Dosage: 0.015 mg/kg/dose up to 0.1 mg/kg/daily.

Adverse effects: Hypokalemia, hypochloremia, hyponatremia, metabolic alkalosis, hypotension.

Comments: Patients refractory to furosemide may respond to bumetanide for diuretic therapy. Although patient may respond differently, bumetanide is approximately 40 times more potent on a milligram per milligram basis than furosemide.

Caffeine Citrate

Indications and use: Apnea of prematurity.

Actions: Similar to those of other methylxanthine drugs (theobromine and theophylline). Caffeine appears to be more active on and less toxic to the CNS and the respiratory system. Proposed mechanisms of action include increased production of cAMP and alterations of intracellular calcium concentrations. Stimulates the CNS and exerts a positive inotropic effect on the myocardium. Stimulates voluntary skeletal muscle and gastric acid secretion. Increases renal blood flow and GFR. Stimulates glycogenolysis and lipolysis.

Supplied: Injection and oral solution are extemporaneously compounded by the pharmacy; not commercially available.

Route: IV (not IM), PO.

Dosage:

- Loading dose: 20 mg caffeine citrate (10 mg caffeine base) IV or PO.
- Maintenance dose (caffeine base): 2.5–5.0 mg/kg/day as a single daily dose.

Adverse effects: Nausea, vomiting, gastric irritation, agitation, tachycardia, and diuresis. Symptoms of overdosage include arrhythmias and tonic-clonic seizures.

Comments: Contraindicated in hypersensitivity to the drug. Therapeutic levels are 5–25 mcg/mL; severe toxicity is associated with levels > 50 mcg/mL. Initial half-life in neonates is 90–100 hours, decreasing to 6 hours at approximately 60 weeks postconceptual age. Serum levels should be monitored.

Calcium Chloride

Indications and use: Symptomatic hypocalcemia such as neonatal tetany. Last-resort agent in cardiac arrest when other agents have failed to improve myocardial contraction. Overdose of calcium channel blocker.

Actions: Calcium is essential for the functional integrity of the nervous, muscular, skeletal, and cardiac systems and for clotting function.

Supplied: Injection, 100 mg/mL (10%, 10 mL) contains 27 mg (1.35 meq) elemental calcium and 1.35 meq chloride per milliliter.

Route: IV, PO.

Dosage:

- Cardiac arrest (as last resort): 20–30 mg/kg/dose (10% solution) IV every 10 minutes prn.
- Maintenance in infants: 70 mg/kg/day IV divided q6h, or as infusion.

Adverse effects: Arrhythmias (eg, bradycardia) and deterioration of cardiovascular function. Extravasation may cause skin sloughing. May potentiate digoxin-related arrhythmias.

Comments: Contraindicated in ventricular fibrillation or hypercalcemia. Use with caution in digitalized patients. Chloride salt is preferred to gluconate form (see below) during cardiac arrest because the calcium in the chloride is already ionized and the gluconate requires metabolism to release the calcium ion. Precipitates when mixed with sodium bicarbonate.

Calcium Gluconate

Indications and use: Treatment of asymptomatic hypocalcemia, prevention of hypocalcemia in susceptible neonates, and prevention of hypocalcemia during exchange transfusion.

Actions: See Calcium Chloride. Calcium gluconate must be metabolized to release calcium ion.

Supplied: Injection 10% = 100 mg/mL (9 mg {0.45 meq} elemental calcium per milliliter).

Dosage:

- Maintenance IV: 200–700 mg/kg/day divided q6h, or as infusion; maximum rate = 200 mg/kg over 10 minutes.
- Maintenance PO: 200–800 mg/kg/day divided q6h mixed in feedings.
- Exchange transfusion: 0.45 meq (1 mL 10%)/dL of citrated blood.

Adverse effects and comments: See Calcium Chloride. Oral form may cause constipation.

Captopril (Capoten)

Indications and use: Congestive heart failure and hypertension.

Actions: Competitive inhibitor of angiotensin-converting enzyme; causes fall in angiotensin II and aldosterone levels, decrease in systemic vascular resistance, and augmentation of cardiac output.

Supplied: Tablets. (Tablets can be dissolved in water and administered orally within 1 hour, or an oral liquid can be compounded by the pharmacist.)

Route: PO.

Dosage:

- Neonates: 0.1–0.4 mg/kg/dose, 1 to 4 times daily.
- Infants: 0.5–6.0 mg/kg/day divided q6–24h.

Adverse effects: Hypotension, rash, fever, eosinophilia, neutropenia, gastrointestinal disturbances.

Comments: Use with caution in patients with low renal perfusion pressure. Reduce dose with renal impairment.

Cefazolin Sodium (Ancef, Kefzol)

Classification: First-generation cephalosporin.

Action and spectrum: A broad-spectrum semisynthetic beta-lactam antibiotic bactericidal by virtue of its inhibition of cell wall synthesis. Good activity against gram-positive cocci (except enterococci), including penicillinase-producing staphylococci. Gram-negative coverage includes *E coli,* most *Klebsiella,* many *Haemophilus influenzae,* and indole-positive *Proteus.* Organism resistance is primarily due to elaboration of beta-lactamases, which inactivate the antibiotic through hydrolysis.

Supplied: Injection.

Route: IM or IV (infuse over 20–30 minutes).

Dosage:

- Newborn and premature infants:
  < 2000 g: 40 mg/kg/day divided q12h.
  > 2000 g: and age > 7 days: 60 mg/kg/day divided q12h.
- Age 1 month and older: 25–100 mg/kg/day divided q6–8h.

Elimination and metabolism: 100% excreted unchanged in urine. Half-life is 1.5–4 hours.

Adverse effects: Infrequent except for allergic reactions, including fever, rash, and urticaria. May cause leukopenia, thrombocytopenia, and a positive Coombs test reaction. Excessive dosage (especially in renal impairment) may result in CNS irritation with seizure activity.

Comments: Use with caution in patients with a history of severe allergic reactions to penicillins. Dosage reduction is required in moderate to severe renal failure. Contains 2 meq sodium per gram.

Cefotaxime Sodium (Claforan)

Classification: Third-generation cephalosporin.

Action and spectrum: Mechanism of action is identical to that of other beta-lactam antibiotics and is bactericidal. Active chiefly against gram-negative organisms (except *Pseudomonas* sp), including *E coli, Enterobacter* sp, *Klebsiella* sp, *Haemophilus influenzae* (including ampicillin-resistant strains), *Proteus mirabilis* and indole-positive *Proteus, Serratia marcescens, Neisseria gonorrhoeae,* and *Neisseria meningitidis.* Generally poor activity against gram-positive aerobic organisms.

Supplied: Injection.

Route: IM or IV (infuse over 30 minutes).

Dosage:

> < 7 days old: 100 mg/kg/day divided q12h.
> > 7 days old: 150 mg/kg/day divided q8h.
- Meningitis: 200 mg/kg/day divided q6h.

Elimination and metabolism. Excreted principally unchanged in the urine. Half-life in neonates is 1–4 hours.

Adverse effects: Hypersensitivity reactions, thrombophlebitis, serum sickness-like reaction with prolonged administration, diarrhea, and, rarely, blood dyscrasias, hepatic dysfunction, or renal damage.

Comments: Cefotaxime should be reserved for suspected or documented gram-negative meningitis or sepsis. When used as empiric therapy, should combine with ampicillin or aqueous penicillin G to provide gram-positive coverage (ie, group B streptococci, pneumococci, *Listeria monocytogenes*). High degree of stability to beta-lactamases. Third-generation cephalosporins have been proved to induce the emergence of multi-drug-resistant bacteria when used excessively and without proper clinical indications. Contains 2.2 meq sodium per gram.

Cefoxitin (Mefoxin)

Indications and use: Treatment of infections from gram-negative enteric organisms, ampicillin-resistant *Haemophilus influenzae,* and anaerobic bacteria, including *Bacteroides fragilis* species.

Actions: A second-generation cephalosporin. A beta-lactam antibiotic bactericidal by inhibiting cell wall synthesis.

Supplied: Powder for injection, 1, 2, and 10 g vials.

Route: IV, IM.

Dosage: Infants weighing < 2 kg and > 7 days postnatal: 90 mg/kg/day divided q8h. ≥ 3 months old: 80–160 mg/kg/day divided q4–6h.

Adverse effects: Usually well tolerated. May cause rash, thrombophlebitis, positive direct Coombs test, eosinophilia, and increase in liver enzymes.

Ceftazidime (Fortaz, Tazidime)

Classification: Third-generation cephalosporin.

Action and spectrum: A broad-spectrum gram-negative semisynthetic beta-lactam antibiotic bactericidal by virtue of its inhibition of cell wall synthesis. Poor gram-positive activity as compared to first-generation cephalosporins but has good activity against gram-negative aerobic bacteria including *Neisseria meningitidis, Haemophilus influenzae,* and most of the *Enterobacteriacea.* It has excellent activity against *Pseudomonas aeruginosa* (the best of all third-generation cephalosporins) Ceftazidime has little activity against *Listeria monocytogenes* and enterococcus.

Supplied: IV.

Route: IM, IV over 20–30 minutes.

Dosage:

- < 2000 g < 7 days 30 mg/kg/dose IV q12h.
- > 2000 g < 7 days 30 mg/kg/dose IV q8h.
- > 2000 g > 7 days 30 mg/kg/dose IV q8h.

Elimination: Renal (glomerular filtration) 100% excreted unchanged; half-life 2.2–4.7 hours.

Adverse effects: Infrequent except for allergic reactions including fever, rash, and urticaria. May cause transient leukopenia, neutropenia, and thrombocytopenia, direct positive Coombs' test, and transient elevation in liver function test.

Comments: Penetrates well into CSF; concentrations approximate 25–50% of serum concentrations. Ceftazidime in combination with ampicillin (for *Listeria*) can be used to treat suspected gram-negative meningitis in the neonate. It is also an alternative to aminoglycosides for *P aeruginosa* therapy, particularly in patients with renal failure.

Ceftriaxone Sodium (Rocephin)

Classification: Third-generation cephalosporin.

Action and spectrum: Mechanism of action identical to that of other beta-lactam antibiotics. High degree of stability to beta-lactamases and good activity against both gram-negative and gram-positive organisms except for *Pseudomonas* sp, enterococci, methicillin-resistant staphylococci, and *Listeria monocytogenes.* Has longest serum half-life of all currently available cephalosporins.

Supplied: Injection.

Route: IM or IV (infuse over 30 minutes).

Dosage:

- Meningitis: 100 mg/kg/day divided q12h.
- Other infections: 50 mg/kg/day divided q12–24h.

Elimination and metabolism: Both biliary and renal excretion. Half-life is 5.2–8.4 hours.

Adverse effects: Mild diarrhea and eosinophilia are most common. May also cause neutropenia, rash, thrombophlebitis, and bacterial (gastrointestinal) or fungal overgrowth. Rare reports of increased prothrombin times. Increases free and erythrocyte-bound bilirubin in premature infants with hyperbilirubinemia; use with caution in infants with hyperbilirubinemia.

Comments: Many clinical studies support once-a-day dosing. Do not use as sole drug in infections due to staphylococci or pseudomonas. Combine with ampicillin for initial empirical therapy of meningitis (Ceftriaxone has poor activity against *Listeria*). Generally no dosage reduction is required in renal or hepatic dysfunction. Contains 2.4 meq sodium per gram.

Cefuroxime (Kefurox, Zinacef)

Classification: Second-generation cephalosporin.

Action and spectrum: Mechanism of action identical to that of other, beta-lactam antibiotics. Active against both gram-positive and gram-negative organisms, including streptococci (except enterococci), both penicillinase-producing and nonpenicillinase-producing staphylococci (not including methicillin-resistant staphylococci), *Escherichia coli, Haemophilus influenzae* (including ampicillin-resistant strains), *Klebsiella* sp, *Neisseria gonorrhoeae* and *N meningitidis, Proteus mirabilis, Salmonella* sp, *Shigella* sp, and *Enterobacter* sp.

Supplied: Injection.

Route: IM or IV (IV preferred; infuse over 30 minutes).

Dosage: 100 mg/kg/day divided q12h.

Elimination and metabolism: Primarily excreted unchanged in the urine. Half-life is 5–8 hours in infants < 4 days and 1.6–3.8 hours in infants > 8 days.

Adverse effects: Generally free of adverse effects but may cause hypersensitivity reactions, thrombophlebitis, elevated serum transaminases, mildly elevated BUN, diarrhea, and, rarely, blood dyscrasias (transient neutropenia, leukopenia, thrombocytopenia).

Comments: Cefuroxime is the only first- or second-generation cephalosporin that crosses the blood-brain barrier. It provides no activity against *Listeria,* so ampicillin should be added in initial empirical therapy. Cefuroxime has added gram-negative coverage over first-generation cephalosporins while retaining very good gram-positive coverage. Decrease dosage in renal failure. Contains 2.4 meq sodium per gram. Limited experience in neonates.

Cephalothin Sodium (Keflin)

Classification: First-generation cephalosporin.

Action and spectrum: Mechanism of action identical to that of other beta-lactam antibiotics. Active against both gram-positive and gram-negative organisms, including streptococci (except enterococci), both penicillinase-producing and nonpenicillinase-producing staphylococci (but not methicillin-resistant staphylococci), *Escherichia coli, Proteus mirabilis, Klebsiella* sp, *Haemophilus influenzae, Salmonella* sp, and *Shigella* sp.

Supplied: Injection.

Route: IV (infuse over 30 minutes).

Dosage:

- < 2000 g and 0–7 days old: 40 mg/kg/day divided q12h.
- < 2000 g and > 7 days old: 60 mg/kg/day divided q8h.
- > 2000 g and 0–7 days old: 60 mg/kg/day divided q8h.
- > 2000 g and > 7 days old: 80 mg/kg/day divided q6h.

Elimination and metabolism: 75% excreted unchanged in the urine.

Adverse effects: Hypersensitivity reactions, thrombophlebitis, serum sickness-like reaction with prolonged use, diarrhea, neutropenia, leukopenia, transient elevation of AST (SGOT). May falsely elevate serum creatinine.

Comments: Generally better activity against gram-positive organisms than second- or third-generation drugs. Dosage adjustment required in renal failure. Contains 2.8 meq sodium per gram.

Chloral Hydrate (Aquachloral Supprettes, Noctec)

Indications and use: Sedation.

Actions: CNS depressant. Mechanism of action not completely understood. Usual doses produce mild CNS depression and quiet, deep sleep; higher doses can result in general anesthesia with concurrent respiratory depression.

Supplied: Syrup, suppositories.

Route: PO, PR.

Dosage: 20–30 mg/kg/dose PO or rectally q6–8h prn. Maximum dose is 50 mg/kg/dose.

Adverse effects: Gastrointestinal irritation resulting in nausea, vomiting, and diarrhea, paradoxical excitation, respiratory depression, particularly if administered with opiates and barbiturates. Direct hyperbilirubinemia with chronic use. Overdose can be lethal.

Comments: Contraindicated with marked renal or hepatic impairment.

Chlorothiazide (Diuril)

Indications and use: Fluid overload, pulmonary edema, and hypertension.

Actions: The thiazide diuretics enhance the excretion of sodium chloride and water by interfacing with transport of sodium ions across the renal tubular epithelium in the cortical nephron. Potassium, bicarbonate, magnesium, phosphate, and iodide excretion are also enhanced, whereas calcium excretion is decreased. Duration of action of chlorothiazide and hydrochlorothiazide is 6–12 hours; onset of action is within 2 hours, and peak action is at 3–6 hours.

Supplied: Suspension; Injection, 500 mg (as sodium) per 20-mL vial.

Route: PO, IV.

Dosage: 20–40 mg/kg/day divided q12h.

Adverse effects: Hypokalemia, hypochloremic alkalosis, prerenal azotemia, hyperuricemia, hyperglycemia, hypermagnesemia, volume depletion, and dilutional hyponatremia may occur in situations of excessive fluid intake.

Comments: Do not use in patients with anuria or hepatic dysfunction.

Cholestyramine Resin (Questran)

Classification: Resin-binding agent.

Indications and use: For use as a resin-binding agent in patients with chronic diarrhea and short gut syndrome to decrease fecal output.

Action: Cholestyramine resin releases chloride ion and absorbs bile acid in the intestine, forming a nonabsorbable complex preventing enterohepatic recirculation of bile salts.

Supplied: Powder.

Route: PO.

Dosage: 1–2 g/dose bid to qid.

Elimination: Not absorbed, excreted in the feces.

Adverse effects: Constipation. High doses can cause hyperchloremic acidosis and increase urinary calcium excretion.

Comments: May bind concurrent oral medications.

Chloramphenicol (Chloromycetin)

Action and spectrum: A broad-spectrum agent. Interferes with or inhibits protein synthesis. Bactericidal for *Haemophilus influenzae* and *Neisseria meningitis;* bacteriostatic for *Escherichia coli, Klebsiella, Serratia, Enterobacter, Salmonella, Shigella, Neisseria gonorrhoeae,* staphylococci, *Streptococcus pneumoniae,* and groups A, B, C, nonenterococcal D, and G streptococci. Drug of choice for *Salmonella typhi* infection.

Supplied: Injection, oral suspension, ophthalmic solution.

Route: PO, IM, or IV (infuse over 5–15 minutes).

Dosage:

- < 2000 g and 0–7 days old: 25 mg/kg/day q24h.
- < 2000 g and > 7 days old: 25 mg/kg/day q24h.
- > 2000 g and 0–7 days old: 25 mg/kg/day q24h.
- > 2000 g and > 7 days old: 50 mg/kg/day divided q12h.
- Ophthalmic solution: 1 drop in each eye q6–12h.

Elimination and metabolism: Metabolized by the liver. Half-life is 9–27 hours.

Adverse effects: Idiosyncratic reactions result in aplastic anemia (irreversible and rare), reversible bone marrow suppression (dose-related), allergy (rash, fever), diarrhea, vomiting, stomatitis, glossitis, *Candida* superinfection, "gray baby" syndrome (early signs are hyperammonemia and unexplained metabolic acidosis; other signs are abdominal distention, hypotonia, gray skin color, cardiorespiratory collapse).

Comments: Avoid use where possible. Must monitor serum levels. Desired peak is 10–25 mcg/mL, levels > 50 mcg/mL are strongly associated with "gray baby" syndrome. Monitor CBC with differential, platelet count, and reticulocyte count every 3 days.

Cimetidine (Tagamet)

Indications and use: Duodenal and gastric ulcers, hypersecretory conditions (eg, Zollinger-Ellison syndrome).

Actions: A histamine (H2) receptor antagonist; competitively inhibits the action of histamine on the parietal cells, decreasing gastric acid.

Supplied: Oral liquid, injection.

Route: IV, PO.

Dosage: 20 mg/kg/day IV or PO divided q6h.

Adverse effects: CNS toxicity such as alterations in consciousness, cholestatic jaundice, increased serum concentrations of hepatic-metabolized drugs. Reduce theophylline dose 50% if used concurrently.

Comments: Limited use in neonates.

Clindamycin (Cleocin)

Action and spectrum: Bactericidal activity by inhibiting protein synthesis. Active against both aerobic and anaerobic streptococci (except enterococci), most staphylococci (except methicillin-resistant strains), *Bacteroides* sp (except *B melaninogenicus*), *Fusobacterium varium, Actinomyces israelii, Clostridium perfringens,* and *Clostridium tetani.* It is chiefly used against the above anaerobes. Not effective against gram-negatives or many clostridial species.

Supplied: Injection, oral solution.

Route: PO, IM, or IV (infuse over 10–20 minutes).

Dosage:

- < 2000 g and 0–7 days old: 15 mg/kg/day divided q8h.
- < 2000 g and > 7 days old: 15 mg/kg/d divided q8h.
- > 2000 g and 0–7 days old: 15 mg/kg/day divided q8h.

- > 2000 g and > 7 days old: 20 mg/kg/day divided q6h.

Elimination and metabolism: Primarily hepatic metabolism.

Adverse effects: Sterile abscess formation at IM injection site. Vomiting and diarrhea occur frequently. Pseudomembranous colitis due to suppression of normal flora and overgrowth of *Clostridium difficile* is uncommon but potentially fatal (treated with oral vancomycin or metronidazole). Rash, glossitis, and pruritus occur occasionally. Serum sickness, anaphylaxis, hematologic (granulocytopenia, thrombocytopenia), and hepatic abnormalities occur rarely.

Comments: Does not cross the blood-brain barrier; therefore, do not use to treat meningitis.

Cosyntropin (Cortrosyn)

Indications and use: Aid in diagnosis of adrenocortical insufficiency.

Actions: Stimulates the adrenal cortex to secrete cortisol (hydrocortisone) and other substances.

Dosage: 0.015 mg/kg (one dose only).

Supplied: Injection: 0.25 mg/vial; dilution = 0.25 mg/mL.

Route: IM, IV (infuse initial dilution over 2 minutes).

Comments: For rapid diagnostic screening of adrenocortical insufficiency, plasma cortisol concentrations should be measured prior to and 60 minutes after administration of cosyntropin; 0.25 mg is equivalent to 25 USP units of corticotropin.

Curare: See Tubocurare.

Dexamethasone (Decadron, Various)

Indications: Resistant neonatal hypoglycemia; airway edema. Used in weaning infants with bronchopulmonary dysplasia (BPD) from the ventilator.

Actions: Primarily used as an antiinflammatory or immunosuppressive agent; due to its minimal mineralcorticoid activity, is not indicated for replacement therapy in adrenocortical insufficiency; a long-acting, potent glucocorticoid lacking sodium-retaining activity with low to moderate doses; increases urinary calcium excretion.

Supplied: Injection; Solution; Inhalation (Aerosol): 200 mcg/spray.

Route: IV, IM, PO, Inhalation.

Dosage:

- BPD: (dosage not well established) 0.5 mg/kg/day IV divided q12h × 3 days then 0.3 mg/kg/day divide q12h × 72h, decrease dose by 0.1 mg/kg/day q72h until 0.1 mg/kg/day is reached, then give on alternate days for 1 week and discontinue.
- Neonatal Hypoglycemia: (dose not well established) 0.25 mg/kg/dose repeated q12h prn.
- Airway edema: 0.25 mg/kg/dose q12h generally beginning 24 hrs before planned extubation and continued × 2–4 doses after.

Adverse effects: With long-term use: increased susceptibility to infection, osteoporosis, growth retardation, hyperglycemia, fluid and electrolyte disturbances, cataracts, myopathy, and acute adrenal insufficiency.

Diazepam (Valium)

Indications: Status epilepticus, convulsions refractory to other combined anticonvulsant agents; hyperglycinemia.

Actions: Exact action is unknown; appears to act at the CNS to produce sedative, hypnotic, skeletal muscle relaxant, and anticonvulsant effects.

Dosage:

- Status epilepticus: 0.1–0.3 mg/kg/dose IV q15–30 min to maximum total dose of 2–5 mg

- Continuous refractory convulsions: 0.1–0.3 mg/kg/dose IV bolus followed by 0.3 mg/kg/h as continuous IV (dilute in saline to 0.1 mg/mL)
- Hyperglycinemia: 1.5–3.0 mg/kg/day PO divided q6–8h (in combination with sodium benzoate, 125–200 mg/kg/day PO divided q6–8h).
- Drug withdrawal: see p 307, Table 57–3.

Adverse effects: May cause drowsiness, ataxia, rash, vasodilation, respiratory arrest, and hypotension.

Comments: Observe for and be prepared to manage respiratory arrest.

Diazoxide (Hyperstat IV, Proglycem)

Indications and use: Hypertension and persistent neonatal hypoglycemia.

Actions: Nondiuretic thiazide with antihypertensive and hyperglycemic effects. Reduces total peripheral vascular resistance by direct relaxation of arteriolar smooth muscle. Inhibits pancreatic insulin release.

Supplied: Oral suspension, 50 mg/mL; injection, 300 mg/20 mL.

Route: IV, PO.

Dosage:

- PO: 8–15 mg/kg/d in 2 or 3 divided doses q8–12h.
- IV: 3–5 mg/kg/dose; repeat in 20 min if no effect.

Adverse effects: When given for short periods, adverse effects rare. May cause bilirubin displacement from albumin, hypotension, hyperglycemia, hyperuricemia, rash, fever, leukopenia, thrombocytopenia, and ketosis.

Digoxin (Lanoxin)

Indications and use: Congestive heart failure, atrial fibrillation or flutter, and paroxysmal AV nodal tachycardia.

Actions: Digoxin exerts a positive inotropic effect on the myocardium. Antiarrhythmic actions are due to an increase in AV nodal refractory period produced by increased vagal activity and by a sympatholytic effect.

Supplied: Pediatric injection, 100 mcg/mL; elixir, 50 mcg/mL.

Route: IV, PO, IM.

Dosage:

- (TDD = total digitalizing dose, to be divided ½, ¼, ¼ q8h.)
  (**Note:** Oral doses (elixir) are approximately 20% higher than IV doses listed below.)
- Premature infants (up to 2.5 kg): TTD = 10–20 mcg/kg IV; maintenance = 2.5 mcg/kg/dose q12h IV.
- Term infants: TDD = 30 mcg/kg IV; maintenance = 4 mcg/kg/dose q12h IV.
- Infants 1–12 months: TDD = 35 mcg/kg IV; maintenance = 4–5 mcg/kg/dose q12h IV.
- Reduce dose in renal dysfunction.

Therapeutic levels: 0.5–2.0 ng/mL, up to 3 ng/mL. Considerable overlap exists between toxic and therapeutic serum levels.

Adverse effects: Persistent vomiting is usually the most common sign of digoxin toxicity in infants. Other adverse effects are anorexia, nausea, dysrhythmias (paroxysmal ventricular contractions, blocks, tachycardia, other), and delirium. Toxicity is markedly enhanced by hypokalemia.

Management of toxicity: Give Fab fraction of specific digoxin antibody (digoxin immune fab [ovine] [**Digibind**] intravenously in equimolar amounts (ie, 60 mg Fab/1 mg digoxin). Give potassium chloride if hypokalemic.

Comments: Digoxin is contraindicated in second- and third-degree block, idiopathic hypertrophic subaortic stenosis (IHSS), and atrial flutter or fibrillation with slow ventricular rates.

Dobutamine (Dobutrex)

Indications and use: To increase cardiac output during states of depressed contractility such as septic shock, organic heart disease, or cardiac surgical procedures.

Actions: A direct $beta_1$ agonist; actions on $beta_2$- and alpha-adrenergic receptors are much less marked than those of dopamine. Unlike dopamine, dobutamine does not cause release of endogenous norepinephrine nor does it have any effect on dopaminergic receptors.

Supplied: Injection, 250 mg/20 mL.

Route: IV.

Dosage: 2–10 mcg/kg/min by continuous infusion. Maximum dosage is 40 mcg/kg/min.

Adverse effects: Generally dose-related. Chiefly ectopic heart beats, increased heart rate, and blood pressure elevations.

Comments: Contraindicated in idiopathic subaortic stenosis and atrial fibrillation.

Dopamine (Dopastat, Intropin)

Indications and use: To increase tissue perfusion after adequate fluid volume replacement in septic states; improve cardiac output and stroke volume with severe congestive heart failure refractory to digoxin and diuretics; and increase cardiac output, blood pressure, and urine flow in patients in shock.

Actions: Actions are dose-dependent. Low doses act directly on dopaminergic receptors to produce renal and mesenteric vasodilation; in moderate doses, $beta_1$-adrenergic effects become prominent, resulting in a positive inotropic effect on the myocardium; high doses stimulate alpha-adrenergic receptors, producing increased peripheral resistance and renal vasoconstriction.

Supplied: Injection, 40, 80, 160 mg/mL.

Route: IV by continuous infusion.

Dosage: (**Note:** Dose-effect relationship is speculative in neonates.)

- Low dose: 0.5–5 mcg/kg/min causes increased renal perfusion.
- Moderate dose: 5–10 mcg/kg/min causes increased cardiac output.
- High dose: 10–40 mcg/kg/min causes systemic vasoconstriction.
- Suggested drip administration:

$$\frac{(6 \times \text{Infant's weight [kg]} \times \text{Desired dose [mcg/kg/min]})}{\text{Rate in mL/h}}$$
= mg dopamine per 100 mL of solution

Adverse effects: Dopamine may cause ectopic heart beats, tachycardia, hypotension, hypertension, and excessive diuresis. Gangrene of the extremities has occurred with high doses over prolonged periods. Extravasation may cause tissue necrosis and sloughing of surrounding tissues; if this occurs, inject phentolamine 0.1 to 0.2 mg/kg diluted to 1 mL saline throughout the affected area.

Comments: Administration of phenytoin intravenously to patients receiving dopamine may result in severe hypotension and bradycardia; therefore, use with extreme caution.

Doxapram (Dopram)

Indications and use: Apnea of prematurity resistant to methylxanthine therapy.

Actions: Analeptic agent with potent respiratory and CNS stimulant properties.

Supplied: Injection, 20 mg/mL.

Route: IV.

Dosage: 0.5–1.5 mg/kg/h (Max: 2.5 mg/kg/h) by continuous IV infusion; decrease infusion rate when control of apnea is achieved.

Therapeutic range: < 5 mcg/mL. At a dose of 1.5 mg/kg/h, the mean serum concentration reported was 3.2 mcg/mL (assay not available in most centers).

Adverse effects: Increase in blood pressure, heart rate, cardiac output, and skeletal muscle hyperactivity may occur. Abdominal distention, increased gastric residuals, vomiting, jitteriness, hyperglycemia, glycosuria, and seizures have been reported in neonates.

Comments: Efficacy of doxapram in premature neonates with severe idiopathic apnea resistant to theophylline has been documented. Use cautiously because of its side effects. Should not be given during the first few days of life, when hypertensive episodes may be associated with an increased risk of intraventricular hemorrhage. Doxapram has a narrow therapeutic range, and its use warrants serum drug level monitoring. It is contraindicated in cardiovascular and seizure disorders. Benzyl alcohol is contained in the formulation, which may accumulate to toxic levels after prolonged use.

Epinephrine

Indications and use: Bradycardia, cardiac arrest, cardiogenic shock, anaphylactic reactions, bronchospasm.

Actions: Acts directly on both alpha- and beta-adrenergic receptors, with beta$_2$ effects predominating at lower doses. Exerts both positive chronotropic and inotropic effects on the heart and relaxes bronchial smooth muscle. Alpha adrenergic stimulation produces an increase in systolic blood pressure and constriction of renal blood vessels.

Supplied: Injection, 0.1 mg/mL (1:10,000) and 1 mg/mL (1:1000).

Route: IV or ET.

Dosage: (1:10,000 used IV).

- IV bolus: 0.1–0.3 mL/kg/dose q5min prn.
- IV infusion: Start with 0.1 mcg/kg/min. Maximum dose is 1.5 mcg/kg/min (titrate).
- Intratracheal: 0.1–0.3 mL/kg/dose diluted 1:1 with normal saline.

Adverse effects: Hypertension, tachycardia, nausea, pallor, tremor, cardiac arrhythmias, increased myocardial oxygen consumption, and decreased renal and splanchnic blood flow.

Epinephrine Hydrochloride (Sus-Phrine)

Indications and use: Relaxation of bronchial smooth muscle, cardiac stimulation, and dilation of skeletal muscle vasculature.

Actions: Direct action on both alpha-adrenergic and beta-adrenergic receptors. Alpha-adrenergic effects are thought to occur from production of cAMP, whereas beta-adrenergic effects result from inhibition of adenyl cyclase activity.

Supplied: Injection; Suspension 1:200 (5 mg/ml), 0.3mL amps.

Route: SC.

Dosage: Suspension (1:200) give 0.005 mL/kg/dose (0.025 mg/kg) to a maximum of 0.15 mL q8–12h.

Adverse effects: Tremor, tachycardia, hypertension, increased myocardial oxygen consumption, decreased renal and splanchnic blood flow, and cardiac arrhythmias.

Comments: Longer-acting form of epinephrine useful in patients who require chronic therapy such as those with bronchopulmonary dysplasia (BPD).

Erythromycin (Ilosone, others)

Classification: Macrolide antibiotic.

Action and spectrum: Acts by suppression of protein synthesis. Action may be bactericidal or bacteriostatic at normal therapeutic concentrations. Spectrum of activity is broad and includes the streptococci (except enterococci), *Staphylococcus aureus*, *Clostridia*, *Corynebacterium diphtheriae*, *Listeria monocytogenes*, *Haemophilus influenzae*, *Bordetella pertussis*, *Brucella*, *Campylobacter fetus*, *Branhamella catar-*

rhalis, Neisseria gonorrhoeae, Legionella micdadei and *Legionella pneumophilia, Rickettsia, Mycoplasma pneumoniae, Chlamydia trachomatis, Treponema pallidum,* and some *Bacteroides* sp. Ophthalmic form is routinely instilled into the eyes of newborn infants as prophylaxis against ophthalmia neonatorum.

Supplied: Oral suspension, oral drops, erythromycin base (Ilotycin Ophthalmic) ointment, injection.

Route: PO, IV over 60 minutes, ophthalmic.

Dosage:

- 0–7 days old: 20 mg/kg/day divided q12h.
- > 7 days old: 30 mg/kg/day divided q8h.
- > 2000 g: 30–40 mg/kg/day divided q8h.
- Ophthalmic as prophylaxis: Instill 2 inches in each eye once.
- Ophthalmic for acute infection: Instill 2 inches in each eye q6h.

Elimination and metabolism: Hepatic metabolism, excreted via the bile and kidneys. Half-life is 1.5–3 hours (prolonged in renal failure).

Adverse effects: Stomatitis, epigastric distress, oral or perianal candidiasis. Transient cholestatic hepatitis and allergic reactions occur rarely. May cause increased serum levels of theophylline, digoxin, and carbamazepine.

Comments: Parenteral forms are painful and irritative; dilute to 5 mg/mL and infuse over 30–60 min. Do not use IM. Lactobionate formulation contains 180 mg of benzyl alcohol per gram of erythromycin.

Ethacrynic Acid (Edecrin)

Indications and use: When prompt diuresis is needed in patients refractory to other diuretics. Other diuretics should be tried first because ethacrynic acid is more toxic.

Actions: Loop diuretic. Inhibits reabsorption of sodium and chloride in the proximal and distal tubules and the loop of Henle. Ethacrynic acid inhibits sodium reabsorption to a greater degree than other diuretics. Ethacrynic acid does not appear to have direct effect on the pulmonary vasculature as furosemide does.

Supplied: Injection, 50 mg in 50 mL vials for reconstitution; tablet, 25 mg (scored). (No oral liquid is available.)

Route: PO, IV.

Dosage: 0.5 to 1 mg/kg/dose qd in preterm infants; q12h in full-term neonates; more frequently, if needed in older infants. Max: 2mg/kg IV or 6 mg/kg PO.

Adverse effects: Inject IV dose slowly over several minutes. May cause dehydration, electrolyte depletion, diarrhea, GI upset, GI bleeding, hearing loss, rash, local irritation and pain, hematuria. Hypoglycemia and neutropenia (rare).

Fentanyl Citrate (Sublimaze)

Indications and use: Analgesia, anesthesia, sedation.

Actions: A synthetic opiate agonist. Acts similarly to morphine and meperidine but without cardiovascular effects of those drugs and with shorter-lasting respiratory depressant effects.

Supplied: Injection, 50 mcg/mL.

Route: IV.

Dosage:

- Analgesia: 2 mcg/kg/dose q2–4h prn or by continuous infusion at 0.1–3 mcg/kg/h.
- Anesthesia: Major surgery, 30–50 mcg/kg/dose; minor surgery, 2–10 mcg/kg/dose.
- Sedation: 2 mcg/kg/dose q2–4h prn or by continuous infusion of 0.5–1.0 mcg/kg/h (titrate).

Adverse effects: Bradycardia, muscular rigidity with reduced pulmonary compliance or apnea, bronchoconstriction, laryngospasm.

Comments: Limited experience in neonates, 0.1 mg of fentanyl is equivalent to 10 mg of morphine or 75 mg of meperidine. Concurrent ventilatory assistance is suggested with its use. Tachyphylaxis occurs after several days of therapy. Adheres to ECMO filter membranes; may have to adjust dose.

Ferrous Sulfate (20% Elemental Iron) (various)

Indications and use: Treatment and prevention of iron deficiency anemia.

Actions: Iron is needed for the production of heme proteins. The use of iron-fortified formulas during the first year of life will usually prevent iron deficiency anemia in both the preterm and term infant. Iron-fortified formulas can be fed safely to preterm infants. Of the ferrous salts available (sulfate, fumarate, gluconate), sulfate is preferred.

Supplied: Drops (preferred), 75 mg/0.6 mL (15 mg elemental iron); elixir, 220 mg/5 mL (44 mg elemental iron); syrup, 90 mg/5 mL (18 mg elemental iron).

Route: PO.

Dosage: (Recommendations of the American Academy of Pediatrics; dosages are for elemental iron.)

- Term infants: 1 mg/kg/day starting no later than 2 months of age.
- Preterm infants: 2 mg/kg/day starting no later than 2 months of age.
- Iron deficiency anemia: 6 mg/kg/day in 4 divided doses.

Adverse effects: GI irritation (vomiting, diarrhea, constipation, darkens stool color).

Comments: Caution parents to guard against iron poisoning from accidental ingestion. Antidote is chelation with deferoxamine; consult specialized references and regional poison control center for further information.

Flucytosine (Ancobon)

Classification: Antifungal agent.

Action and spectrum: Flucytosine penetrates fungal cells, where it acts as antimetabolite, ultimately interfering with protein synthesis. It is active in vivo against some strains of *Cryptococcus* and *Candida*. May be synergistic with amphotericin B.

Supplied: Capsules. (Pharmacist can compound aqueous solution.)

Route: Oral.

Dosage: 50–100 mg/kg/day divided q6h.

Dosage in renal impairment: 12.5–25 mg/kg/day divided as follows:

- q12h for creatinine clearance of 20–40 mL/min.
- q24h for creatinine clearance of 10–20 mL/min.
- q24–48 for creatinine clearance of < 10 mL/min.

Serum concentrations: 24–120 mcg/mL.

Pharmacokinetics: Volume of distribution—0.68 L/kg; half-life, 3 to 5 hours; renal elimination.

Adverse effects: Vomiting, diarrhea, rash, anemia, leukopenia, thrombocytopenia, elevated liver function tests, increased BUN and creatinine, CNS disturbances.

Furosemide (Lasix)

Indications and use: Fluid overload, pulmonary edema, congestive heart failure, hypertension.

Actions: Inhibits active chloride transport in the ascending limb of the loop of Henle. Furosemide-induced diuresis results in enhanced excretion of sodium chloride, potassium, calcium, magnesium, bicarbonate, ammonium, hydrogen, and possibly phosphate. Intravenous administration increases venous capacitance independently of its diuretic effect, resulting in rapid improvement of pulmonary edema.

Supplied: Oral solution, 10 mg/mL; injection, 10 mg/mL.

Route: PO, IV, IM.

Dosage:

- PO: 1–2 mg/kg/dose q12h as initial dose and increase slowly if needed, since more may be required due to highly variable bioavailability.
- IV or IM: 1 mg/kg/dose q12–24h slowly. If there is not an increase in urine output, double the above doses and repeat.

Adverse effects: Hypokalemia, hypocalcemia, hyponatremia. With prolonged use, nephrocalcinosis, hypochloremic metabolic alkalosis.

Gamma Globulin Intravenous (IV IgG) (Gamimune N, Sandoglobulin, Gammagard)

Indications and use: Immunodeficiency syndromes, suspected sepsis (*controversial*). Sandoglobulin is also indicated for treatment of idiopathic thrombocytopenic purpura (ITP).

Actions: Establishes immediate (passive) IgG antibody serum levels.

Supplied: Injection, 50 mg/mL (Gamimune N 10 and 50 mL) or powder for injection (Sandoglobulin 1 g/vial).

Route: IV only.

Dosage:

- Suspected sepsis: IV IgG 400–500 mg/kg/dose × 1–2 dose; repeat weekly.
- Immunodeficiency syndrome:
  Sandoglobulin: 200 mg/kg (as initial dilution at rate of 0.5–1.0 mL/min once per month. If desired clinical response or level of IgG insufficient then increase dose to 300 mg/kg or repeat dose more frequently.
  Gamimune N: 100 mg/kg or 2 mL/kg (at initial flow rate of 0.01–0.02 mL/kg/min for 30 minutes, may dilute in 5% dextrose) once per month. If no adverse effects observed, then increase rate to 0.02–0.04 mL/kg/min. If desired clinical response not achieved or level of IgG insufficient, increase dose to 200 mg/kg (4 mL/kg) or repeat dose more frequently than once per month.
  Gammagard: 100 mg/kg once per month (initial rate of 0.5 mL/kg/h). If desired clinical response not achieved or level of IgG insufficient, increase dose to 200–400 mg/kg to maintain serum IgG level > 500 mg/dL.
- Idiopathic thrombocytopenia purpura:
  Sandoglobulin: 400 mg/kg/day for 5 consecutive days. (See above administration rate for immunodeficiency syndrome.)

Adverse effects: Hypotension and anaphylaxis. If either occurs, the rate of infusion should be decreased or stopped until resolved, then resumed at a slower rate as tolerated. Preparations contain antibodies to group B streptococcus and *E coli*. Substantial variation among lots and manufacturers.

Gentamicin Sulfate (Garamycin, others)

Classification: Aminoglycoside.

Action and spectrum: Bactericidal activity by inhibition of bacterial protein synthesis. Active chiefly against gram-negative aerobic bacteria, including most *Pseudomonas, Proteus* sp, and *Serratia*. Some activity against coagulase-positive staphylococci but ineffective against anaerobes and streptococci. Provides some synergistic effect against group D streptococci (enterococci) when used in combination with a penicillin.

Supplied: Injection, intrathecal injection, ophthalmic solution.

Route: IM, IV (infuse over 30 minutes), Intrathecal (not recommended).

Dosage: Base initial dose on body weight, then monitor levels and adjust using pharmacokinetics.

- IV (preferred), IM:
  <7 days postnatal age:
  <1 kg and < 28 weeks gestational age: 2.5 mg/kg/dose q24h.
  <1.5 kg and < 34 weeks gestational age: 2.5 mg/kg/dose q18h.

>1.5 kg and > 34 weeks gestational age: 2.5 mg/kg/dose q12h.
>7 days postnatal age:
<1.2 kg: 2.5 mg/kg/dose q18–24h.
>1.2 kg: 2.5 mg/kg/dose q8h.
- Intrathecal or intraventricular: 1–2 mg qd.
- Ophthalmic solution: Instill one drop into each eye q4–12h.

Elimination and metabolism: Renal excretion by glomerular filtration. Half-life is 4–8 hours initially.

Adverse effects: Irreversible vestibular injury, proteinuria, uremia, oliguria, macular rash.

Comments: Desired serum peak is 4–10 mcg/mL (sample obtained 30 minutes after infusion completed) and desired serum trough is < 2 mcg/mL (sample obtained 30 minutes to just prior to next dose). In general, a set of peak and trough levels should be obtained at about the 4th maintenance dose. Monitor serum creatinine every 3–4 days. Excessive serum peak levels are associated with ototoxicity and excessive trough levels with nephrotoxicity. May be given orally in nursery epidemics of entero-pathogenic *E coli* or NEC. The aminoglycosides should not be used alone against gram-positive pathogens.

Glucagon

Indications and use: Hypoglycemia as seen in infants of diabetic mothers (IDM); hypo-glycemia due to other causes unresponsive to routine treatment. Bowel spasm during barium enema.

Actions: Glucagon, a hormone produced by the alpha cells of the pancreas, causes increased breakdown of glycogen to form glucose and inhibition of glycogen syn-thetase. Blood glucose elevation occurs. Produces relaxation of the smooth muscle in the gastrointestinal tract when the drug is administered parenterally.

Supplied: Injection, 1-mg (1-unit) vials.

Route: SC, IM, IV.

Dosage: 0.025–0.3 mg/kg/dose; may repeat in 20 min prn. Infant of diabetic mother (IDM): 0.3 mg/kg/dose. Max: 1 mg.

Adverse effects: Hypersensitivity, nausea, and vomiting.

Comments: Incompatible with electrolyte-containing solutions; compatible with dex-trose solutions. **Caution:** Do not delay initiation of glucose infusion while observing for glucagon effect.

Heparin Sodium

Indications and use: Primary role is as an anticoagulant. Used to diagnose and treat disseminated intravascular coagulation (DIC) and to maintain patency of arterial or venous lines.

Actions: In combination with antithrombin III (heparin cofactor), heparin inactivates co-agulation factors IX, X, XI, XII, and thrombin, inhibiting conversion of fibrinogen to fibrin.

Supplied: Injection, 10, 100, 1000, 5000 units/mL.

Route: SC, IV.

Dosage:
- Loading dose: 50 units/kg as IV bolus.
- Maintenance dosage: 10–20 units/kg/h as continuous infusion.
- To maintain line patency: 0.5–1 unit/mL of fluid.
- Antidote: Protamine sulfate, 1 mg for each 100 units of heparin given in the pre-ceding 3–4 hours up to a maximum dose of 50 mg.

Hepatitis B Immune Globulin (H-BIG, others)

Indications and use: Prophylaxis of hepatitis B exposure.

Actions: Passive immunization agent. Immune serum provides protection against the hepatitis B virus by directly providing specific antibody to hepatitis B surface antigen (HBsAg). The immunity is transient, usually lasting about 30 days.

Supplied: Injection, 1-, 4-, and 5-mL vials.

Route: IM only.

Dosage: 0.5 mL administered within 12 hours after delivery. (Repeat at 3 months and 6 months if vaccine was not given.)

Adverse effects: Swelling, warmth, erythema, and soreness at injection site. Rarely, rash, fever, and urticaria.

Comments: Do not use in IgA deficiency, thrombocytopenia, coagulopathy. Administer into gluteal or deltoid muscle region. Do not administer intravenously.

Hepatitis B Vaccine (Haptavax-B, Recombivax HB, Engerix B)

Indications and use: Prophylaxis for infants at increased risk for hepatitis B.

Actions: Induces protective antibody formation to hepatitis B virus (anti-HBs).

Supplied: Injection: Recombivax 10 mcg/mL, Heptavax 20 mcg/mL, Engerix 20 mcg/mL and 10 mcg/0.5 mL.

Route: IM only.

Dosage: 0.5 mL IM (equivalent to Recombivax 2.5 mcg, Heptavax 10 mcg, Engerix B 10 mcg).

Adverse effects: Swelling, warmth, erythema, and soreness at injection site. Rarely, vomiting, rash, low-grade fever.

Comments: Do not give intravenously or intradermally. A single booster may be needed in 5 years. Administer in anterolateral thigh.

Hyaluronidase (Wydase)

Indications and use: Treatment of extravasation injuries.

Actions: Hyaluronidase is an enzyme that temporarily breaks down hyaluronic acid (tissue cement) and thereby allows the infiltrated drug or solution to be absorbed over a larger surface area. This speeds absorption and reduces tissue contact time with irritant substance.

Supplied: Injection, 150 units/mL as a lyophilized powder or a stabilized solution. The solution must be refrigerated.

Route: SC.

Dosage: Dilute to 15 units/mL in normal saline. Inject 0.2 mL into the needle that was used to infuse the IV before it is removed, and four 0.2 mL injections into the leading edge of the extravasation. Elevate the extremity. Do not apply heat. May repeat if necessary.

Adverse effects: Usually well tolerated. Urticaria (rare). Administer hyaluronidase within one hour of the extravasation, if possible.

Hydralazine (Apresoline)

Indications and use: For hypertension and as an afterload reducing agent to treat congestive heart failure.

Actions: Direct-acting vasodilator that reduces peripheral resistance and blood pressure and relaxes venous capacitance vessels. Reflex increase in heart rate, cardiac output, and stroke volume is probably produced in response to the decrease in peripheral vascular resistance.

Supplied: Injection, 20 mg/mL tablets, 10 mg (oral liquid can be compounded by the pharmacist).

Route: IM, IV, PO.

Dosage:

- IV or IM: 0.1–0.5 mg/kg/dose q6h (maximum of 2 mg/kg/dose).
- PO: 0.5–7.0 mg/kg/day divided q6–8h.

Adverse effects: Most frequent are headache, palpitations, and tachycardia; most serious is a reversible lupuslike syndrome. Tachyphylaxis often occurs on chronic therapy.

Comments: Contraindicated in mitral valve rheumatic heart disease.

Hydrochlorothiazide (various)

Indications and use: Hypertension, pulmonary edema.

Actions: See Chlorothiazide.

Supplied: Solution 50 mg/5 mL and 100 mg/mL.

Route: PO.

Dosage: Up to 3.3 mg/kg/day divided q12h.

Adverse effects and comments: See Chlorothiazide.

Hydrocortisone

Indications and use: Acute adrenal insufficiency, congenital adrenal hyperplasia, shock.

Actions: Hydrocortisone is a steroid possessing glucocorticoid activity with some mineralocorticoid effects; most effects probably result from modification of enzyme activity, thus affecting almost all body systems. It promotes protein catabolism, gluconeogenesis, renal excretion of calcium, capillary wall permeability and stability, and red cell production; suppresses immune and inflammatory responses.

Supplied: Injection (acetate, sodium phosphate, sodium succinate), oral suspension (cypionate), topical ointment and cream (acetate).

Route: PO, IV, IM, topical.

Dosage:

- Acute adrenal insufficiency: 1–2 mg/kg/dose IV bolus; then 25–150 mg q24h divided q6h.
- Congenital adrenal hyperplasia: Initial dose, 0.5–0.7 mg/kg/day divided ¼ in AM, ¼ at noon, and ½ at night; maintenance dose, 0.3–0.4 mg/kg/day divided as above.
- Topical (0.5%) apply to area 3 times daily.

Adverse effects and comments: See Dexamethasone. Application to large body surface areas may produce absorption with systemic effects. Avoid facial application.

Indomethacin (Indocin IV)

Indications and use: Pharmacologic closure of patent ductus arteriosus.

Actions: Nonsteroidal anti-inflammatory drug (NSAID) with analgesic and antipyretic properties. Action is principally by inhibition of prostaglandin synthesis, thus inhibiting cyclo-oxygenase, an enzyme that catalyzes the formation of prostaglandin precursors (endoperoxides) from arachidonic acid.

Supplied: Powder for injection, 1-mg vials.

Route: IV.

Dosage: IV at 12–24h intervals. Indocin should be given q12h unless the patient has decreased urinary output.

- Initial dose: 0.2 mg/kg.
- Second dose: < 48 hours, 0.1 mg/kg; 2–7 days, 0.2 mg/kg; > 8 days, 0.25 mg/kg.
- Third dose: < 48 hours, 0.1 mg/kg; 2–7 days, 0.2 mg/kg; > 8 days, 0.25 mg/kg.

Adverse effects: May cause decreased platelet aggregation, transient oliguria (decreased GFR), increased serum creatinine, increased serum concentrations of renally eliminated drugs such as gentamicin, hyponatremia, hyperkalemia, hypoglycemia.

Displaces bilirubin from albumin binding sites, but is not considered clinically significant.

Comments: Contraindicated in NEC or when stool Hematest > 3+, BUN > 30 mg/dL, serum creatinine > 1.8 mg/dL, urine output < 0.6 mL/kg/h for the preceding 8 hours, in thrombocytopenia (< 60,000/mm^3), with active bleeding, or if there has been intraventricular bleeding within the preceding 7 days (*controversial*).

Insulin, Regular

Indications and use: Hyperglycemia, hyperkalemia, increasing caloric intake in infants with glucose intolerance on parenteral nutrition.

Actions: Hormone derived from the beta cells of the pancreas and the principal hormone required for glucose utilization. In skeletal and cardiac muscle and adipose tissue, insulin facilitates transport of glucose into these cells. Stimulates lipogenesis and protein synthesis and inhibits lipolysis and release of free fatty acids from adipose cells. Promotes intracellular shift of potassium and magnesium.

Supplied: Injection, 40 and 100 units/mL. (Iletin I [beef and pork, Beef Regular Iletin II [purified beef], Humulin R [human insulin, recombinant DNA origin], Actrapid [purified pork], Pork Regular Iletin II [purified pork], Velosulin [purified pork]).

Note: Should be diluted by the Pharmacy to 1 Unit/mL in diluent provided by the manufacturer to improve accuracy in measurement and avoid overdose.

Route: IV, SC.

Dosage:

- Hyperglycemia: Loading dose, 0.1 unit/kg/dose infused IV over 15–20 minutes; maintenance dose, 0.02–0.1 units/kg/h by continuous IV infusion (titrate with hourly determinations of blood glucose until stable, then q4h) (dilute insulin as above).
- Hyperkalemia: Give calcium gluconate, 50 mg/kg/dose IV, and sodium bicarbonate IV, 1 meq/kg/dose IV, first; then give dextrose, 600–800 mg/kg/dose, and insulin, 0.2 unit/kg/dose IV (3–4:1 glucose to insulin ratio).
- Increase caloric intake for infants on parenteral nutrition: 0.02–0.1 units/kg/h IV as continuous infusion. Monitor serum glucose q hour until stable, then q4h.

Adverse effects: Hypoglycemia (may cause coma, severe CNS injury), hyperglycemic rebound (Somogyi effect), urticaria, anaphylaxis.

Comments: Human insulin (preferred) is less antigenic than pork-derived insulin, which is less antigenic than beef-derived insulin. Insulin adsorbs to plastic surfaces of IV systems. In concentrations of 10 units/L, approximately 50% of the insulin binds to the tubing. At greater concentrations approximately 5 units/L binds to the IV tubing. Adjust dose as needed.

Isoniazid (Laniazid, Nydrazid)

Classification: Antituberculous agent.

Action and spectrum: Bactericidal effect on growing tubercle bacilli by interfering with lipid and protein synthesis. Spectrum includes *Mycobacterium* spp (*M tuberculosis, M kansasii, M avium*).

Supplied: Injection, syrup, 100 mg/mL; 50 mg/5 mL.

Route: PO, IM.

Dosage:

- Primary tuberculosis: 10–15 mg/kg/day divided q12–24h with rifampin for 9–12 months.
- Skin test conversion: 10–15 mg/kg/day PO q24h for 9 months.

Adverse effects: Peripheral neuropathy, seizures, encephalopathy, blood dyscrasias, allergy.

Isoproterenol (Isuprel, others)

Indications and use: Shock, cardiac arrest, Adams-Stokes syndrome, ventricular arrhythmias due to AV block, bronchospasm.

Actions: Acts on both beta$_1$- and beta$_2$-adrenergic receptors with minimal or no effect on alpha receptors in therapeutic doses. Relaxes bronchial smooth muscle, cardiac stimulation (inotropic and chronotropic), and peripheral vasodilation (reduces cardiac afterload).

Supplied: Injection (1:5000), 0.2 mg/mL; solution for nebulization, aerosol (various strengths).

Route: IV, inhalation.

Dosage: IV: 0.05–0.5 mcg/kg/min (titrate). Inhalation/nebulization: 0.1 mL to max of 0.5 mL/dose. Dilute to 2 mL with normal saline, given q4h prn.

Adverse effects: Tremor, vomiting, hypertension, tachycardia, cardiac arrhythmias.

Comments: Contraindicated in hypertension, degenerative heart disease, hyperthyroidism, tachycardia caused by digoxin toxicity, and preexisting cardiac arrhythmias. Increases cardiac oxygen consumption out of proportion to increase in cardiac oxygen output. Not considered an inotropic agent of choice.

Kanamycin Sulfate (Kantrex)

Classification: Aminoglycoside.

Action and spectrum: Mechanism of action is identical to that of gentamicin. Active primarily against gram-negative aerobic bacteria, including *Escherichia coli,* *Klebsiella, Enterobacter, Serratia, Proteus,* and some *Pseudomonas* sp. Some activity against staphylococci and mycobacteria. Not active against other gram-positive organisms or anaerobes.

Supplied: Injection.

Route: IM or IV (infuse over 30 minutes).

Dosage: Base initial dose on body weight, then monitor levels and adjust using pharmacokinetics.

- < 1.2 kg, 0–4 weeks postnatal age: 7.5 mg/kg/dose q18–24h.
- 1.2–2 kg:
    0–7 days: 7.5 mg/kg/dose q12–18h.
    > 7 days: 7.5 mg/kg/dose q8–12h.
- > 2 kg:
    0–7 days: 10 mg/kg/dose q12h.
    > 7 days: 10 mg/kg/dose q8h.

Elimination and metabolism: Primarily renally excreted by glomerular filtration. Half-life is 4–8 hours.

Adverse effects: See Gentamicin.

Comments: See Gentamicin. Desired serum peak is 25–35 mcg/mL (sample obtained 30 minutes after infusion complete) and serum trough is < 10 mcg/mL (sample obtained 30 minutes to just prior to next dose). In general, a set of serum peak and trough levels should be obtained at about the 4th maintenance dose. Monitor serum creatinine every 3–4 days. Excessive serum peak levels are associated with ototoxicity and excessive trough levels with nephrotoxicity.

Ketoconazole (Nizoral)

Classification: Antifungal agent.

Action and spectrum: A broad-spectrum antifungal agent that acts by disrupting cell membranes. Fungicidal against *Blastomyces dermatitidis, Candida* sp, *Coccidioides immitis, Histoplasma capsulatum, Paracoccidioides brasiliensis,* and *Phialophora* sp. Development of resistance is rare.

Supplied: Oral suspension.

Route: PO.

Dosage: 2.5–5 mg/kg/day q24h.

Elimination and metabolism: Hepatic metabolism.

Adverse effects: Gastric distress is the most common side effect. Hepatic damage is rare.

Comments: Penetration into CSF is poor, which means that ketoconazole should not be used in the treatment of fungal meningitis. Minimum period of treatment for candidiasis is 1–2 weeks, but duration should be based on clinical response. Monitor liver function tests. Limited experience in neonates.

Levothyroxine (T$_4$, Synthroid)

Indications and use: Treatment of congenital hypothyroidism.

Actions: Thyroid hormones increase metabolic rate of body tissues noted by increases in oxygen consumption, respiratory rate, body temperature, cardiac output, heart rate, blood volume, rate of fat, protein, and carbohydrate metabolism, enzyme system activity, growth, and maturation. Thyroid hormones are very important in CNS development. Deficiency in infants results in growth retardation, failure of brain growth and development.

Supplied: Injection, 200 mcg/vial as a lyophilized powder; tablets, 0.025, 0.05, 0.075, 0.088, 0.1, 0.112, 0.125, 0.15, and 0.175 mg scored tablets. Tablets may be crushed and mixed with water or a small amount of infant formula and administered immediately after mixing. Discard unused portion.

Route: IV, IM, PO.

Dosage: **Note:** The parenteral dose should be approximately one-half of the previously established oral dose.

- 0–6 months: 25 to 50 mcg/day PO (8–10 mcg/kg/day).
- 6–12 months: 50–75 mcg/day PO (6–8 mcg/kg/day).
- Alternatively, 8–10 mcg/kg/day PO has been recommended for infants from birth to one year.

Adverse effects: Adverse effects are usually due to excessive dose. If these occur, discontinue and reinstitute at lower dose: tachycardia, cardiac arrhythmias, tremors, diarrhea, weight loss, fever.

Lidocaine (Xylocaine, others)

Indications and use: Intravenous lidocaine is used almost exclusively for the short-term control of ventricular arrhythmias (premature beats, tachycardia, and fibrillation) or for prophylactic treatment of such arrhythmias. Skin infiltration as a local anesthetic.

Actions: Type I antiarrhythmic agent, with most activity related to blockade of the fast sodium channels in Purkinje fibers. Also a CNS depressant with sedative, analgesic, and anticonvulsant properties.

Supplied: IV forms: Injection (premixed) in D5W, 2 mg/mL (500 mL), 4 mg/mL (250 mL), 8 mg/mL (250 mL). Injection (for IV bolus) 10 mg/mL (5 mL). Injection (for IV admixture—must be diluted) 40 mg/mL (25 mL). 0.5% and 1% solution for local anesthesia.

Route: IV, SC, or Intratracheal (IT).

Dosage: 1 mg/kg/dose as IV bolus q5min to maximum total dose of 5 mg/kg, followed by IV infusion of 10–50 mcg/kg/min.

Adverse effects: Adverse effects generally involve the CNS: drowsiness, dizziness, tremulousness, and paresthesias. Muscle twitching, seizures, coma, respiratory depression, and respiratory arrest may also occur.

Comments: Primarily metabolized by the liver; dosage adjustment is necessary in liver failure. Contraindicated in SA or AV nodal block.

Therapeutic levels: 1–5 mcg/mL. Toxicity associated with levels > 5 mcg/mL.

Lorazepam (Ativan)

Indications and use: Treatment of status epilepticus resistant to conventional anticonvulsant therapy (ie, phenobarbital, phenytoin).

Actions: A benzodiazepine, facilitates gamma aminobutyric acid (GABA), which mediates transmission and mimics the actions of glycine at its receptor sites. Penetrates the blood-brain barrier more slowly than diazepam; however, the duration of action of lorazepam in the control of seizure activity in children studied was at least 3 hours in 83% of cases and 24 hours or longer in nearly 59% of cases. Median onset of seizure control is 10 minutes.

Supplied: Oral solution 2 mg/mL; injection, 2 mg/mL.

Route: PO, IM, IV.

Dosage: Status epilepticus:

- Initial dosage: 0.05 mg/kg/dose IV. If no response after 15 minutes, repeat initial dose. May dilute with an equal volume of sterile water, normal saline, or 5% dextrose in water. Infuse dose over 2–3 minutes.
- Sedation, anxiety: 0.05–0.1 mg/kg/dose IV q4–8h prn.

Adverse effects: May cause respiratory depression, apnea, hypotension, bradycardia, cardiac arrest, and seizure-like activity. Paradoxic CNS stimulation may occur, usually early in therapy; the drug should be discontinued if this effect occurs. Lorazepam overdose may be reversed using flumazenil (Romazicon) 5–10 mcg/kg/dose IV.

Magnesium Sulfate

Indications and use: Hypomagnesemia and refractory hypocalcemia.

Actions: May depress CNS and peripheral neuromuscular transmission by decreasing acetylcholine release. Acts on cardiac muscle to slow SA nodal impulse formation and prolong conduction time.

Supplied: Injection, oral.

Route: IM, IV, or PO.

Dosage: Hypomagnesemia or refractory hypocalcemia:

- Initial dosage: 0.2 meq/kg/dose IV or IM q6h until serum Mg level is normal or symptoms resolve or 0.8–1.6 meq/kg/dose PO 4 times daily.
- Maintenance dosage: 0.25–0.5 meq/kg/24h IV (add to infusion or give IV).

Adverse effects: Hypotension, flushing, depression of reflexes, depressed cardiac function, CNS, and respiratory depression.

Comments: Contraindicated in renal failure. Monitor serum magnesium, calcium, and phosphate levels. Infuse IV magnesium sulfate over several hours.

Meperidine (Demerol)

Indications and use: Preoperative medication and for relief of moderate to severe pain.

Actions: Stimulates opiate receptors in CNS. Meperidine produces respiratory depression proportionate to drug dose. Duration of respiratory depression can extend several hours beyond the plasma half-life.

Supplied: Injection 25 mg/mL; syrup 50 mg/mL.

Route: PO, IM, IV, SC.

Dosage: 0.5–1.5 mg/kg. Maximum of 2 mg/kg/dose IV, IM, SC, and 4 mg/kg/dose PO.

Adverse effects: Normeperidine (active metabolite) has excitant effects that may precipitate tremors, myoclonus, or seizures. Other side effects include respiratory and circulatory depression, nausea, vomiting, constipation, and sedation.

Comments: Effects can be reversed by naloxone 0.1 mg/kg IV.

Methicillin Sodium (Staphcillin)

Classification: Penicillinase-resistant penicillin.

Action and spectrum: Mechanism of action identical to that of other beta-lactam antibiotics. Active chiefly against penicillinase-positive and penicillinase-negative staphylococci. Less effective than penicillin G against other gram-positive cocci. No activity against enterococci.

Supplied: Injection.

Route: IM or IV (infuse over 20 minutes).

Dosage:

- Meningitis:
    - < 2000 g and 0–7 days old: 100 mg/kg/day divided q12h.
    - < 2000 g and > 7 days old: 150 mg/kg/day divided q8h.
    - > 2000 g and 0–7 days old: 150 mg/kg/day divided q8h.
    - > 2000 g and > 7 days old: 200 mg/kg/day divided q6h.
- Other diseases:
    - < 2000 g and 0–7 days old: 50 mg/kg/day divided q12h.
    - < 2000 g and > 7 days old: 75 mg/kg/day divided q8h.
    - > 2000 g and 0–7 days old: 75 mg/kg/day divided q8h.
    - > 2000 g and > 7 days old: 100 mg/kg/day divided q6h.

Elimination and metabolism: Renal. Half-life variable (60–120 minutes or longer).

Adverse effects: Nephrotoxicity (interstitial nephritis) occurs more often with methicillin than with other penicillins. May cause hypersensitivity reactions, anemia, leukopenia, thrombocytopenia, phlebitis at infusion site, and hemorrhagic cystitis (in poorly hydrated patients).

Comments: In cases of methicillin resistance, vancomycin becomes the antistaphylococcal drug of choice. Dosage adjustment necessary in renal impairment. Monitor serum urea nitrogen and creatinine. Contains 2.9 meq sodium per gram.

Methyldopa (Aldomet)

Indications and use: Hypertension.

Actions: Mechanism of action is not fully understood. Metabolized to alpha methylnorepinephrine in the CNS, where it lowers arterial pressure by stimulation of central alpha-adrenergic receptors. Reduction of plasma renin may also play a role in its antihypertensive effect.

Supplied: Injection, suspension.

Route: IV, PO.

Dosage: 5–40 mg/kg/day divided q6–8h.

Adverse effects: Most common adverse effect is drowsiness, which occurs within the first 48–72 hours and may cause marked depression, orthostatic hypotension, sodium retention, edema, a positive direct Coombs test reaction in 10–20% of patients (reversible), and drug fever. Causes fluid and sodium retention and should be given with a diuretic.

Comments: Preferred route of administration is oral, but absorption from the gastrointestinal tract is unpredictable (10–15%). Contraindicated with active hepatic disease.

Metronidazole (Flagyl)

Classification: Bactericidal antibiotic.

Action and spectrum: The mechanism of action is not established. Good activity against anaerobic protozoa, including Trichomonas vaginalis, Entamoeba histolytica, Giardia lamblia, and Balantidium coli. Good activity also against gram-positive bacteria (Costridium spp, Peptococcus, Peptostreptococcus, and Veillonella spp) and anaerobic gram-negative bacteria (Bacteroides spp and Fusobacterium spp). Nonsporulating gram-positive bacilli are often resistant (eg, Propionibacterium spp, Actinomyces), and the drug has minimal activity against aerobic and facultative anaerobic bacteria.

Supplied: Tablets (suspension can be compounded by pharmacist), injection.

Route: PO or IV (infuse commercial dilution over 1 hour).

Dosage:

- < 2000 g:15 mg/kg/day divided q12h.
- > 2000 g and 0–7 days old: 15 mg/kg/day divided q12h.
- > 2000 g and > 7 days old: 30 mg/kg/day divided q12h.

Elimination and metabolism: Hepatic metabolism with final excretion via the urine and feces. Large volume of distribution (penetrates into all body tissues and fluids).

Adverse effects: Occasional vomiting, diarrhea, insomnia, weakness, rash, phlebitis at injection site. Rarely leukopenia. Mutagenicity and carcinogenicity may occur, but not established in humans.

Comments: Some texts recommend an initial loading dose of 15 mg/kg, with the first maintenance dose either 48 hours later (for premature infants < 2000 g) or 24 hours later (for the infant > 2000 g at birth). Effectively penetrates into the CSF and therefore indicated for meningitis due to susceptible anaerobic pathogens.

Note: Some centers use empiric coverage with ampicillin and gentamicin for NEC. The use of metronidazole in NEC remains controversial.

Metoclopramide (Reglan, others)

Indications and use: Used in a variety of gastrointestinal disorders. In neonates and infants, the drug has been used investigationally for feeding intolerance and gastroesophageal reflux.

Actions: Dopamine antagonist acting on the CNS and on other organs. Gastrointestinal smooth muscle stimulant. Increases the resting tone of the esophageal sphincter. In neonates, metoclopramide resulted in a significant decrease in gastric aspirate, increased weight gain, shortened GI transit time, and increased food intake.

Supplied: Syrup, injection.

Route: IM, IV, PO.

Dosage: 0.1–0.2 mg/kg/dose given q6hr 20 minutes before feedings.

Adverse effects: CNS effects include restlessness, drowsiness, and fatigue. Extrapyramidal reactions may occur but usually subside 24 hours after discontinuance of the drug, and most patients will respond rapidly to diphenhydramine.

Comments: Contraindicated with bowel obstruction and seizure disorders.

Mezlocillin Sodium (Mezlin)

Classification: Semisynthetic extended-spectrum penicillin.

Action and spectrum: Mechanism of action identical to that of other beta-lactam antibiotics. Effective principally against gram-negative organisms, including *Haemophilus influenzae, Klebsiella pneumoniae, Proteus mirabilis, Escherichia coli, Pseudomonas aeruginosa,* and some *Serratia* spp. Active also against many anaerobes, including *Peptococcus* spp, *Peptostreptococcus* spp, and *Bacteroides* spp (eg, *Bacteroides fragilis*).

Supplied: Injection.

Route: IM or IV (infuse over 30 minutes).

Dosage:

- 0–7 days: 150 mg/kg/day divided q12h.
- > 7 days: 225 mg/kg/day divided q8h.

Elimination and metabolism: Excreted primarily unchanged with urine; less than 10% hepatically metabolized.

Adverse effects: See Carbenicillin and Penicillin G (Aqueous), Parenteral.

Comments: Does not cause platelet dysfunction. Avoid IM use if possible. Adjust dosage in renal impairment. Mezlocillin contains 1.85 meq sodium per gram.

Note: Limited experience in neonates.

Midazolam (Versed)

Indications and use: Antianxiety agent. May be used for infants on assisted ventilation who are agitated and need sedation, or as a sedative prior to procedures.

Actions: Short-acting benzodiazepine.

Supplied: Injection, as 1 mg/mL and 5 mg/mL. Contains 1% benzyl alcohol.

Route: IV, IM, and IV continuous infusion.

Dosage:

- Intermittent: 0.1–0.3 mg/kg/dose IV q2–4h prn.
- Continuous infusion: Loading dose: 0.2 mg/kg IV.
- Infusion: 0.4–0.6 mcg/kg/min.
- Max: 6 mcg/kg/min.

Adverse effects: Respiratory depression and arrest with excessive doses or rapid IV infusions. May cause hypotension. Infuse IV slowly. Use caution, particularly if fentanyl is being used concurrently.

Morphine Sulfate (various)

Indications and use: Analgesia, preoperative sedation, supplement to anesthesia, acute pulmonary edema.

Actions: CNS opiate receptor agonist resulting in analgesia, drowsiness, and alterations in mood and pain perception. Vasodilatory (especially coronary vessels)

Supplied: Injection, oral solution.

Route: IM, IV, SC.

Dosage: 0.1–0.2 mg/kg/dose q2–4h or continuous administration of 0.01–0.1 mg/kg/h.

Adverse effects: Dose-dependent side effects include miosis, respiratory depression, drowsiness, bradycardia, and hypotension. Constipation, sedation, GI upset, urine retention, histamine release, and sweating may occur. Causes physiological dependence; taper dose gradually after long-term use to avoid withdrawal.

Nafcillin Sodium (Unipen)

Classification: Semisynthetic penicillinase-resistant penicillin.

Action and spectrum: Mechanism of action identical to that of other beta-lactam antibiotics. Spectrum identical to that of methicillin (ie, primarily antistaphylococcal).

Supplied: Injection.

Route: IV (infuse over 30 minutes), IM (avoid—very irritating).

Dosage:

- < 2000 g and 0–7 days old: 50 mg/kg/day divided q12h.
- < 2000 g and > 7 days old: 75 mg/kg/day divided q8h.
- > 2000 g and 0–7 days old: 50 mg/kg/day divided q8h.
- > 2000 g and > 7 days old: 75 mg/kg/day divided q6h.

Elimination and metabolism: Hepatic metabolism; concentrated in bile.

Adverse effects: Thrombophlebitis, hypersensitivity, and leukopenia. Severe tissue injury after IV extravasation.

Comments: Avoid IM use. Contains 2.9 meq sodium per gram.

Neomycin Sulfate (Mycifradin, others)

Classification: Aminoglycoside.

Action and spectrum: Mechanism of action identical to that of gentamicin. Indicated in the treatment of diarrhea due to enteropathogenic *Escherichia coli* and as preoperative prophylaxis before intestinal surgery.

Supplied: Oral solution (125 mg/5 mL).

Route: PO

Dosage: 50–100 mg/kg/d divided q4–6h.

Elimination and metabolism: Renal excretion if systemic absorption occurs; otherwise fecally excreted.

Adverse effects: Sensitization with allergic reaction.

Comments: Poorly absorbed from gastrointestinal tract, but significant levels can occur, especially in impaired renal function. Inactive against anaerobic organisms.

Netilmicin Sulfate (Netromycin)

Classification: Aminoglycoside.

Action and spectrum: See Gentamicin.

Supplied: Injection.

Route: IM or IV (infuse over 30 minutes).

Dosage: Monitor and adjust by pharmacokinetics. Initial empirical dosing based on body weight:

- < 7 days postnatal age:
    - < 1 kg and < 28 weeks' gestational age: 2.5 mg/kg/dose q24h.
    - < 1.5 kg and < 34 weeks' gestational age: 2.5 mg/kg/dose q18h.
    - > 1.5 kg and > 34 weeks' gestational age: 2.5 mg/kg/dose q12h.
- > 7 days postnatal age:
    - < 1.2 kg: 2.5 mg/kg/dose q18–24h.
    - > 1.2 kg: 2.5 mg/kg/dose q8h.

Elimination and metabolism: Renal excretion. Half-life is 4–8 hours.

Adverse effects: Ototoxicity associated with serum peak concentrations greater than 12 mcg/mL; nephrotoxicity associated with serum trough concentrations greater than 4 mcg/mL.

Comments: Therapeutic range is 6 and 10 mcg/mL (sample obtained 30 minutes after infusion completed) and serum trough concentrations below 3 mcg/mL (sample obtained 30 minutes to just before next dose). Obtain initial set of serum peak and trough levels at about the 4th maintenance dose. Monitor serum creatinine every 3–4 days. Other comments: see Gentamicin. Limited experience in neonates.

Naloxone (Narcan)

Indications and use: Narcotic reversal and investigationally for the treatment of septic shock.

Actions: A pure opiate antagonist with little or no agonistic activity. It has minimal or no pharmacologic effect, even in high doses, in patients who have not received opiates. Onset of action is within 1–2 minutes after intravenous injection and 2–5 minutes following subcutaneous or intramuscular injection. Duration of action is generally 45 minutes to 4 hours.

Supplied: Injection 0.4 mg/mL, 1.0 mg/mL.

Route: IV, IM, SC, Intratracheal (IT).

Dosage: 0.1 mg/kg. May repeat in 5 minutes.

Comments: Avoid in infants of narcotic-addicted mothers because naloxone may precipitate acute withdrawal syndrome. Infant must be monitored for reappearance of respiratory depression and need for repeated doses.

Neostigmine Methylsulfate (Prostigmin)

Indications and use: Improvement of muscle strength in the treatment of myasthenia gravis. Reversal of nondepolarizing neuromuscular blocking agents (tubocurarine, pancuronium) and occasionally for postoperative distention and urinary retention.

Actions: Neostigmine inhibits hydrolysis of acetylcholine and thus produces generalized cholinergic responses.

Supplied: Injection 0.25 mg/mL, 0.5 mg/mL, and 1 mg/mL.

Route: IM, IV, SC, or PO.

Dosage:

- Myasthenia gravis:
  Diagnosis: 0.04 mg/kg/dose IM × 1 or 0.02 mg/kg/dose IV × 1.
  Treatment: 0.01–0.04 mg/kg/dose IM, IV, or SC q2–3h prn.
- Reversal of nondepolarizing neuromuscular blocking agents:
  Infants: 0.025–0.1 mg/kg/dose. (Use with atropine: Dose 0.01–0.04 mg/kg; or 0.4 mg atropine for each mg of neostigmine.)

Adverse effects: Cholinergic crisis, which may include bronchospasm, increased bronchial secretions, vomiting, diarrhea, bradycardia, respiratory depression, seizures, and coma.

Comments: Antidote is atropine 0.01–0.04 mg/kg/dose. Reversal of blocking agent should not be attempted for at least 30 minutes after a dose of pancuronium or tubocurarine.

Nitroprusside (Nipride, Nitropress)

Indications and use: Severe hypertension and hypertension crisis, congestive heart failure, congenital heart lesions that have resulted in pulmonary hypertension with increased pulmonary vascular resistance.

Actions: Direct-acting vasodilator (arterial and venous) that reduces peripheral vascular resistance (afterload). Venous return is reduced (preload). Acts within seconds to lower blood pressure; when discontinued, the effect dissipates within minutes. Rapidly metabolized to thiocyanate, which is eliminated by the kidneys.

Supplied: Injection.

Route: Continuous IV infusion.

Dosage: 0.5–8 mcg/kg/min (titrate to desired response) by IV infusion.

Adverse effects: Generally related to too-rapid reduction in blood pressure. Thiocyanate may accumulate, especially in patients receiving high doses or those who have impaired renal function. Cyanide toxicity can develop abruptly if large doses are administered rapidly. Cyanide causes early persistent acidosis. Thiocyanate toxicity appears at plasma levels of approximately 5–10 mg/dL levels of 20 mg/dL have been associated with death. Thiocyanate levels should be monitored in any patient receiving 5 mcg/kg/min or more of nitroprusside, especially patients with renal impairment. Toxicity is treated with 20% sodium thiosulfate (10 mg/kg/min for 15 minutes).

Comments: Contraindicated with increased intracranial pressure, hypertension secondary to arteriovenous shunts, or coarctation of the aorta. Reconstitute contents of 50-mg vial in 2–3 mL D5W, then further dilute in D5W for infusion. Protect from light.

Norepinephrine Bitartrate (Levarterenol, Levophen)

Indications and use: Vasoconstriction and cardiac stimulation as adjunctive therapy to correct shock after fluid volume replacement. Prolongation of local anesthetics by decreasing vascular absorption.

Actions: Direct effect on alpha-adrenergic receptors and beta-adrenergic receptors of the heart (beta$_1$) but not those of the bronchi or peripheral blood vessels (beta$_2$). Norepinephrine has less effect on beta$_1$ receptors than does epinephrine or isoproterenol.

Supplied: Injection.

Route: IV infusion.

Dosage: 0.02–0.1 mcg/kg/min initially, titrated to attain desired perfusion.

Adverse effects: Respiratory distress, arrhythmias, bradycardia or tachycardia, hypertension, and vomiting.

Comments: In case of extravasation, use phentolamine 0.1–0.2 mg/kg SC, infiltrated into the area of extravasation within 12 hours.

Nystatin (Mycostatin, Nilstat)

Action and spectrum: Fungistatic and fungicidal in vitro against a wide variety of yeasts and yeastlike fungi. Acts by disrupting cell membranes. Neonatal indications include oral candidiasis (thrush), *Candida* diaper rash, and benign mucocutaneous candidiasis.

Supplied: Oral suspension, 100,000 units/mL; topical cream, powder, and ointment.

Route: PO, topical.

Dosage:

- Oral thrush: 0.5–1 mL to each side of the mouth qid after feedings for 7–10 days.
- Diaper rash: Topical cream applied tid-qid for 7–10 days.

Elimination and metabolism: Poorly absorbed. Most is passed unchanged in the stool.

Adverse effects: Side effects uncommon, but may cause diarrhea.

Oxacillin Sodium (Bactocill, Prostaphlin)

Classification: Semisynthetic penicillinase-resistant penicillin.

Action and spectrum: Mechanism of action is identical to that of other beta-lactam antibiotics. Spectrum of activity is identical to that of nafcillin and methicillin.

Supplied: Injection.

Route: IM or IV (infuse over 30 minutes).

Dosage:

- < 2000 g and 0–7 days old: 50 mg/kg/day divided q12h.
- < 2000 g and > 7 days old: 100 mg/kg/day divided q8h.
- > 2000 g and 0–7 days old: 75 mg/kg/day divided q8h.
- > 2000 g and > 7 days old: 150 mg/kg/day divided q6h.

Elimination and metabolism: Metabolized chiefly in the liver and excreted in bile. Renal excretion is substantial but requires no adjustment in renal failure.

Adverse effects: Hypersensitivity reactions (rash), thrombophlebitis, mild leukopenia, elevation in AST (SGOT).

Comments: Avoid IM injection of oxacillin. This drug contains 2.8 meq sodium per gram.

Pancuronium Bromide (Pavulon)

Indications and use: To increase pulmonary compliance in an uncooperative neonate during mechanical ventilation. To produce skeletal muscle relaxation during surgery.

Actions: Nondepolarizing neuromuscular blocking agent that produces skeletal muscle paralysis mainly by causing a decreased response to acetylcholine at the myoneural junction. Pancuronium may cause an increase in heart rate. The onset of action is generally 30–60 seconds, with a duration of action of about 40–60 minutes, but it may be much longer in neonates.

Supplied: Injection 1 mg/mL.

Route: IV.

Dosage:

- Initial dosage: 0.03 mg/kg IV; repeat prn.
- Maintenance dosage: 0.03–0.09 mg/kg IV q1–4h prn to maintain paralysis.

Adverse effects: Tachycardia may occur.

Comments: Neonates are particularly sensitive to the actions of pancuronium; prolonged paralysis may be noted. Ventilation must be supported during neuromuscular blockade. Many centers place a sign over patient's bedside to alert all medical personnel that the infant is paralyzed. Neostigmine and atropine (see dose p 497) are used for reversal.

Papaverine Hydrochloride (various)

Indications and use: Peripheral arterial spasms.

Actions: Directly relaxes vascular smooth muscle and results in vasodilation.

Supplied: Injection, tablets.

Route: PO, IM, IV (infuse over 1–2 minutes).

Dosage: 6 mg/kg/24h in 4 divided doses.

Comments: Intravenous infusion should be performed under a physician's supervision, since arrhythmias and fatal apnea may result from rapid injection.

Note: Limited experience in neonates.

Paraldehyde (Paral)

Indications and use: Status epilepticus resistant to conventional therapy (ie, phenobarbital, phenytoin, diazepam, lorazepam).

Actions: A rapid-acting hypnotic agent effective against all types of seizures when administered in large doses. Precise mechanism of action is unknown.

Supplied: Oral solution, rectal liquid.

Route: PO, PR.

Dosage: Rectal: 0.3 mL/kg/dose q4–6h. Dilute in equal volume of olive oil.

Adverse effects: Side effects severely limit use. May cause pulmonary edema and hemorrhage, severe coughing, irritation to gastrointestinal mucosa, and thrombophlebitis. Overdose may cause cardiac and respiratory depression. Rectal administration may cause proctitis.

Comments: Routine use in infants is discouraged. Contraindicated in pulmonary or hepatic disease.

Note: Paraldehyde dissolves plastic and reacts with rubber stoppers in bottles and syringes. Do not use plastic equipment for administration. For rectal administration, use glass syringes.

Penicillin G (Aqueous), Parenteral

Action and spectrum: Mechanism of action is identical to that of other beta-lactam antibiotics. Effective mainly against streptococci, some community-acquired staphylococci (except methicillin-resistant and penicillinase-producing strains), *Neisseria gonorrhoeae, Neisseria meningitidis, Bacillus anthracis, Clostridium tetani, Clostridium perfringens, Bacteroides* (oropharyngeal strains), *Leptospira,* and *Treponema pallidum.*

Supplied: Injection, as the potassium or sodium salt.

Route: IM or IV (infuse over 20 minutes).

Dosage:

- Meningitis:
  - < 2000 g and 0–7 days old: 100,000 units/kg/day divided q12h.
  - < 2000 g and > 7 days old: 150,000 units/kg/day divided q8h.
  - > 2000 g and 0–7 days old: 150,000 units/kg/day divided q8h.
  - > 2000 g and > 7 days old: 200,000 units/kg/day divided q6h.
- Other diseases:
  - < 2000 g and 0–7 days old: 50,000 units/kg/day divided q12h.
  - < 2000 g and > 7 days old: 75,000 units/kg/day divided q8h.
  - > 2000 g and 0–7 days old: 50,000 units/kg/day divided q8h.
  - > 2000 g and > 7 days old: 100,000 units/kg/day divided q6h.

Elimination and metabolism: Renal.

Adverse effects: Allergic reactions, rash, fever, change in bowel flora, *Candida* super-infection, diarrhea, hemolytic anemia. Very large doses may cause seizures.

Comments: 1600 units = 1 mg. Some strains of group B streptococci are penicillinase producers, thus requiring the addition of an aminoglycoside antibiotic for synergistic bactericidal effect. Good activity against anaerobes. Drug of choice for tetanus neonatorum. Contains 1.7 meq of sodium or potassium per million units.

Penicillin G Benzathine (Bicillin L-A, Permapen)

Action and spectrum: See Penicillin G (Aqueous), Parenteral. A drug of choice in the treatment of asymptomatic congenital syphilis.

Supplied: Injection.

Route: IM only. (Viscosity requires ≥ 23-gauge needle.)

Dosage: 50,000 units/kg once.

Elimination and metabolism: Renally excreted over a prolonged interval owing to slow absorption from the injection site.

Adverse effects and comments: See Penicillin G (Aqueous), Parenteral. 1211 units = 1 mg. Not often used.

Penicillin G Procaine (Duracillin A.S., Wycillin)

Action and spectrum: See Penicillin G (Aqueous), Parenteral. A drug of choice in the treatment of symptomatic or asymptomatic congenital syphilis.

Supplied: Injection.

Route: IM only. (Viscosity requires ≥ 23-gauge needle.)

Dosage: 50,000 units/kg/dose q24h.

Elimination and metabolism: See Penicillin G (Aqueous), Parenteral.

Adverse effects: See Penicillin G (Aqueous), Parenteral. May also cause sterile abscess formation at injection site. Contains 120 mg procaine per 300,000 units, which may cause allergic reactions, myocardial depression, or systemic vasodilation. There is cause for much greater concern about these effects in the neonate than in older patients.

Comments: 1000 units = 1 mg. Not often used.

Pentobarbital (Nembutal)

Indications and use: Sedative/hypnotic. Used for agitation, preprocedure sedation, or as an anticonvulsant.

Actions: Short-acting barbiturate.

Supplied: Injection, 50 mg/mL; elixir, 18.2 mg/5 mL (18% alcohol), suppositories. (Suppositories could be used for the older, bigger infant only as 30 mg is the smallest size available, and it is recommended that they not be divided.)

Route: PO, PR, IM, IV.

Dosage:

- Sedative: 2–6 mg/kg/day divided tid. Max: 100 mg/d.
- Hypnotic and anticonvulsant: 3–5 mg/kg/dose. Max: 100 mg/dose.

Adverse effects: Inject IV dose slowly in fractional doses. Observe IV site closely during administration as this drug may cause extravasation injury. Tolerance and physical dependence may occur with continued use. May cause somnolence, apnea, bradycardia, rash, pain on IM injection, thrombophlebitis, osteomalacia from prolonged use (rare), excitability. May increase reaction to painful stimuli. Rapid IV administration may cause hypotension and apnea.

Phenobarbital

Indications and use: Tonic-clonic and partial seizures, neonatal withdrawal syndrome, and neonatal jaundice.

Actions: Anticonvulsant that limits the spread of seizure activity and increases the threshold for electrical stimulation of the motor cortex. In neonates, the initial half-life is 100–120 hours or longer, gradually declining to 60–70 hours at about 3–4 weeks of age. Reduction in serum bilirubin levels is attributed to increased levels of glucuronyl transferase and intracellular Y-binding protein. More effective in reducing bilirubin levels in full-term infants than in premature infants and must be administered at least 2 or 3 days before detectable reductions can be observed. Phenobarbital is effective in controlling symptoms of neonatal withdrawal syndrome with the exception of vomiting and diarrhea.

Supplied: Oral elixir, tablets, injection.

Route: IV, IM, PO.

Dosage:

- Seizures:
    Loading dose: 20–30 mg/kg IV or IM over 15–30 minutes. May give in two divided doses.
    Maintenance dose: 2.5–4 mg/kg/day as single dose or divided q12h. For neonates < 30 weeks start 1–3 mg/kg/day.
- Hyperbilirubinemia: Dose not clearly established. Generally 4–5 mg/kg/day.
- Neonatal withdrawal syndrome: 5–10 mg/kg/day in 4 divided doses. Monitor serum phenobarbital concentrations and withdrawal score.

Adverse effects: Sedation, lethargy, paradoxical excitement, gastrointestinal distress, ataxia, and rash.

Comments: Contraindicated in porphyria. Monitor serum levels and adjust dosage to maintain between 15 and 40 mcg/mL for anticonvulsant activity.

Phentolamine (Regitine)

Indications and use: Treatment of extravasation from IV dopamine or norepinephrine (levarterenol, Levophed). Helps prevent dermal necrosis and sloughing.

Actions: Phentolamine is an alpha-adrenergic blocking drug that works to reverse the severe vasoconstriction from extravasation of vasopressors such as dopamine.

Supplied: Injection, 5 mg/mL.

Route: SC.

Dosage: 0.1 to 0.2 mg/kg diluted to 1 mL saline injected into the area of extravasation within 12 hours.

Adverse effects: Hypotension, tachycardia, cardiac arrhythmias, flushing, GI upset.

Phenytoin (Dilantin)

Indications and use: Seizures unresponsive to phenobarbital.

Actions: Raises seizure threshold of the motor cortex to electrical or chemical stimuli. Precise mechanism of anticonvulsant activity has not been determined. Bilirubin displaces phenytoin from albumin-binding sites, increasing the percentage of unbound drug; this may complicate the interpretation of serum levels. Follows zero-order pharmacokinetics, where small dosage adjustments may result in large changes in serum drug concentrations. Neonates and other infants absorb phenytoin poorly from the gastrointestinal tract. Use in the long-term management of seizures in neonates is questionable owing to the difficulty in appropriate dosing.

Supplied: Oral suspension, injection.

Route: PO, IV.

Dosage:

- IV: 15–20 mg/kg as loading dose at a rate not greater than 0.5 mg/kg/min, followed by maintenance dose of 5–8 mg/kg/day divided q12–24h.
- PO: Highly variable—from 5–8 mg/kg/day up to 8 mg/kg/dose q12h.

Adverse effects: Few reports of toxicity in neonates, probably because of the difficulty of physically assessing the common toxic manifestations. In adults and children, adverse effects include nystagmus, ataxia, lethargy, slurred speech, diplopia, headache, hirsutism, behavioral changes, and gum hyperplasia. Hypotension occurs with rapid IV administration.

Comments: Therapeutic levels between 10 and 20 mcg/mL (may be lower in preterm infants). Multiple drug interactions.

Phosphorus

Indications and use: Treatment of hypophosphatemia, provision of maintenance phosphorus in parenteral nutrition solutions, or treatment of nutritional rickets of prematurity.

Actions: Phosphorus is an intracellular ion required for formation of energy-transfer enzymes such as ADP and ATP. Phosphorus is also needed for bone metabolism and mineralization.

Supplied: Injection, Sodium Phosphates, 3 mMol elemental phosphorus/mL and 4 meq sodium/mL; Potassium Phosphates, 3 mMol elemental phosphorus/mL and 4.4 meq potassium/mL.

Route: IV, PO.

Dosage:

- Severe hypophosphatemia: 0.15–0.3 mMol/kg/dose (= 5–9 mg elemental phosphorus/kg/dose). Infuse slowly over several hours or dilute in daily 24–hour maintenance IV solution (preferred).
- Maintenance: 0.5–2 mMol/kg/day (= 16–63 mg elemental phosphorus/kg/day). For oral use, may use parenteral form and give PO in divided doses, diluted in infants's feedings.

Adverse effects: Hyperphosphatemia, hypocalcemia, hypotension. GI discomfort may occur with oral administration. Rapid IV bolus of potassium phosphates can cause cardiac arrhythmias.

Piperacillin Sodium (Pipracil)

Classification: Semisynthetic extended-spectrum penicillin.

Action and spectrum: See Mezlocillin. Good in vivo activity against *Pseudomonas aeruginosa.*

Supplied: Injection.

Route: IM or IV (infuse over 30 minutes).

Dosage:

- < 2000 g and 0–7 days old: 150 mg/kg/day divided q12h.
- < 2000 g and > 7 days old: 225 mg/kg/day divided q8h.
- > 2000 g and 0–7 days old: 225 mg/kg/day divided q8h.
- > 2000 g and > 7 days old: 300 mg/kg/day divided q6h.

Elimination and metabolism: Excreted unchanged in the urine.

Adverse effects: See Mezlocillin. Hypokalemia and leukopenia are less pronounced.

Comments: Avoid IM use where possible. Should be reserved for cases resistant to ticarcillin. Contains 1.85 meq (42.5 mg) sodium per gram.

Polymyxin B Sulfate (Aerosporin)

Action and spectrum: Acts by disrupting the integrity of the bacterial cell wall. Bactericidal against most aerobic gram-negative bacilli. Chiefly useful against *Pseudomonas.* Effective also against *Escherichia coli, Enterobacter,* and *Klebsiella.* Not active against *Proteus.* This drug has been replaced by other safer agents, except for treating organisms resistant to other drugs.

Supplied: Injection.

Route: PO, IV (dilute to final concentration of 1000–2000 units/mL in 5% dextrose and infuse over 1–2 hours).

Dosage:

- IV: 30,000–40,000 units/kg/day divided q8h.
- PO: 10–20 mg/kg/d divided q6–8h for up to 5 days.

Elimination and metabolism: Slow renal excretion.

Adverse effects: May cause reversible renal injury (proteinuria, hematuria, azotemia), rash, fever, neuromuscular blockade (rare), thrombophlebitis at injection site.

Comments: Poor tissue penetration. Does not cross blood-brain barrier. Not absorbed orally. Not often used.

Potassium Chloride (KCl)

Indications and use: Correct hypokalemia, maintenance potassium provision. Also corrects hypochloremia.

Actions: Potassium is essential for maintaining intracellular tonicity, transmission of nerve impulses, contraction of cardiac, skeletal, and smooth muscle, and maintenance of normal renal function.

Supplied: Injection 2 meq/mL; oral liquid, 10, 15, 20, 30, and 40 meq/15 mL.

Route: IV, PO.

Dosage: Maintenance: 2–3 meq/kg/day diluted in 24-hour maintenance IV solution. Higher doses are often required in infants receiving diuretics. Titrate dose with previous day's requirements and daily serum potassium determination. Max rate: Infants on cardiac monitor: 0.5 meq/kg/h; infants not on cardiac monitor: 0.3 meq/kg/h. Dilute bolus doses in 6–8 hours of IV solution, if possible. For oral use, the injectable form of the drug may be given in divided doses PO and diluted in the infant's formula.

Adverse effects: Avoid rapid IV injection. Excessive dose and/or rate may cause cardiac arrhythmias (peaked T waves, widened QRS, flattened P waves, bradycardia, heart block), respiratory paralysis, hypotension with rapid infusion. Potassium accumulates with renal dysfunction. Causes severe vein irritation; do not give undiluted in a peripheral vein. Dilute to 0.08 meq/mL, if possible.

Prazosin (Minipress)

Indications and use: Hypertension and congestive heart failure. Experimental in infants and should be used only when traditional therapy has failed.

Actions: Postsynaptic alpha-adrenergic blocking agent that reduces peripheral vascular resistance and blood pressure.

Supplied: Capsules 1 mg.

Route: PO.

Dosage:

- Test dose: 5–10 mcg/kg PO.
- Maintenance dosage: Up to 25 mcg/kg/dose q6h.

Adverse effects: Dizziness, weakness, fatigue, palpitations, headache, and nausea. The most severe adverse effect in adults is the "first dose phenomenon" in which severe orthostatic hypotension occurs.

Prednisone (Liquid Pred, Prednisone Intensol Concentrate)

Indications and use: Resistant neonatal hypoglycemia, airway edema, weaning infants with bronchopulmonary dysplasia (BPD) from the ventilator. Used chiefly as an anti-inflammatory or immunosuppressive agent. Not indicated for adrenocortical insufficiency because of minimal mineralocorticoid activity.

Actions: An intermediate-acting glucocorticoid. Prednisone has four times the anti-inflammatory potency as hydrocortisone, and one-half the mineralocorticoid potency.

Supplied: Tablets, 1, 2.5, 5, 10 mg (scored); oral solution, 5 mg/5 mL (5% alcohol) and 5 mg/mL (30% alcohol).

Route: PO.

Dosage: 0.1–2 mg/kg/d qd or divided q12h.

Adverse effects: Cataracts, leukocytosis, peptic ulcer, nephrocalcinosis, myopathy, osteoporosis, diabetes, growth failure, hyperlipidemia, hypocalcemia, hypokalemic alkalosis, sodium retention and hypertension, increased susceptibility to infection. Withdraw dose gradually after prolonged therapy to prevent acute adrenal insufficiency.

Procainamide Hydrochloride (various)

Indications and use: As prophylaxis to maintain normal sinus rhythm in paroxysmal atrial tachycardia, atrial fibrillation, premature atrial and ventricular contractions, and ventricular tachycardia.

Actions: Class I antiarrhythmic agent similar to quinidine. Partially metabolized by the liver to the active metabolite N-acetylprocainamide (NAPA).

Supplied: Capsules, tablets, injection.

Route: PO, IM, IV.

Dosage:

- IV (monitor ECG and blood pressure): 1.5–2 mg/kg (dilute to 10 mg/mL) over 10–30 minutes. Repeat as needed to maximum dose of 10–15 mg/kg; then continuous infusion of 20–60 mcg/kg/min.
- PO: 5–15 mg/kg q4–6h.

Therapeutic levels:

- Procainamide: 3–10 mcg/mL, toxicity associated with levels > 12 mcg/mL.
- NAPA: 10–20 mcg/mL; toxicity associated with levels over 30 mcg/mL.

Adverse effects: Serious toxic effects if given rapidly IV, including asystole, myocardial depression, ventricular fibrillation, hypotension, reversible lupus like syndrome. May cause nausea, vomiting, diarrhea, anorexia, skin rash, tachycardia, agranulocytosis, and hepatic toxicity.

Comments: Contraindicated in second- or third-degree heart block, bundle branch block, digitalis intoxication, and allergy to procaine. Do not use in atrial fibrillation or flutter until ventricular rate is adequately controlled, to avoid a possible paradoxic increase in ventricular rate. Quinidine (see p 506) is generally used for long-term therapy because it has less associated toxicity. Phenylephrine should be available to treat severe hypotension caused by IV procainamide. QRS or QT prolongation greater than 35% of baseline is an indication to withhold further doses of procainamide.

Propranolol (Inderal, others)

Indications and use: Hypertension, supraventricular tachycardia, premature ventricular contractions, tachycardia, and tetralogy spells.

Actions: Nonselective beta-adrenergic blocking agent. Inhibits adrenergic stimuli by competitively blocking beta-adrenergic receptors within the myocardium and bronchial and vascular smooth muscle. Decreases heart rate, myocardial contractility, and cardiac output.

Supplied: Oral liquid, injection.

Route: PO, IV.

Dosage:

- Arrhythmias:
  IV: 0.025–0.15 mg/kg/dose to a maximum of 1 mg/dose as slow push.
  PO: 0.5–2 mg/kg/day q6–8h. May increase to 1 mg/kg q6h or more as tolerated.
- Hypertension: 0.5–2 mg/kg/day PO q6–12h. May increase as tolerated.

- Tetralogy spells: 0.15–0.25 mg/kg/dose slow IV. May repeat q15min prn, or 1–2 mg/kg/dose PO q6h prn.

Adverse effects: Generally dose-related hypotension, nausea, vomiting, bronchospasm, heart block, depression, hypoglycemia, and depressed myocardial contractility.

Comments: Contraindicated in obstructive pulmonary disease, asthma, heart failure, shock, second- or third-degree heart block, hypoglycemia. Use with caution in renal or hepatic failure.

Prostaglandin E$_1$: See Alprostadil.

Protamine Sulfate (various)

Indications and use: Reversal of heparin; heparin overdose.

Actions: Combines with heparin, forming a stable salt complex. Devoid of anticoagulant activity. Effect on heparin is almost immediate and persists for approximately 2 hours.

Supplied: Injection.

Route: IV.

Dosage: For every 100 units of heparin estimated to remain in patient, give 1 mg by slow infusion over 3–5 minutes or not greater than 5 mg/min. Maximum dose of 50 mg.

Adverse effects: May cause fall in blood pressure, bradycardia, dyspnea, anaphylaxis. Excessive administration beyond that needed to reverse heparin effect may have anticoagulant effect.

Pyridoxine (vitamin B$_6$) (Hexalpha-Betalin, others)

Indications and use: For treatment of pyridoxine-dependent seizures and to prevent or treat vitamin B$_6$ deficiency.

Actions: Vitamin B$_6$ is essential in the synthesis of GABA, an inhibitory neurotransmitter in the CNS; GABA increases the seizure threshold. Vitamin B$_6$ is also required for heme synthesis and amino acid, carbohydrate, and lipid metabolism.

Supplied: Tablets, injection.

Route: PO, IM, IV.

Dosage: For vitamin B$_6$-dependent seizures, give 100 mg IV as a single test dose, followed by a 30-minute observation period. If a definite response is seen, begin maintenance of 50–100 mg PO daily.

Pyrimethamine (Daraprim)

Action and spectrum: Folic acid antagonist selective for plasmodial dihydrofolate reductase. Activity highly selective for plasmodia (cidal) and *Toxoplasma gondii.*

Supplied: Tablets.

Route: PO.

Dosage: For toxoplasmosis, give 1 mg/kg/d divided q12h for 4 weeks. Combine with sulfadiazine.

Elimination and metabolism: Hepatic metabolism.

Adverse effects: Anorexia, vomiting, megaloblastic anemia, leukopenia, thrombocytopenia, pancytopenia, atrophic glossitis, rash, seizures, shock.

Comments: Give folinic acid (leucovorin), 1 mg orally daily or 3 mg twice weekly, if leukopenia or thrombocytopenia occurs. Administer with feedings if vomiting persists. Give sulfadiazine alone in empirical therapy of toxoplasmosis until the diagnosis is ruled out. Reduced dosage in hepatic dysfunction.

Quinidine Sulfate (various)

Indications and use: Restoration of normal sinus rhythm in atrial flutter or fibrillation once the ventricular rate is controlled by digoxin. Prevention of atrial and ventricular arrhythmias.

Actions: Group I antiarrhythmic agent with cardiac effects similar to those of procainamide. Direct depressant effect on myocardial contractility, conduction velocity, and excitability. Causes increase in PR, QRS, and QT intervals.

Supplied: Capsules, tablets, injection.

Route: PO, IM (quinidine gluconate, polygalaturonate) (IV not recommended).

Dosage: 5–15 mg/kg q6h PO or 2–4 mg/kg q2–4h IM. Total daily dose 10–30 mg/kg.

Therapeutic levels: 3–7 mcg/mL.

Adverse effects: Severe hypotension with IV use. Adverse reactions in about 30% of patients include nausea, vomiting, diarrhea, blood dyscrasias, and drug fever. Overdose may cause cinchonism or respiratory depression.

Comments: Contraindicated with AV nodal block.

Ranitidine (Zantac)

Indications and use: Duodenal and gastric ulcers, gastroesophageal reflux, and hypersecretory conditions (eg, Zollinger-Ellison syndrome).

Actions: Histamine (H_2) receptor antagonist; competitively inhibits the action of histamine on the parietal cells, decreasing gastric acid.

Supplied: Injection, oral liquid.

Route: PO, IV.

Dosage: 0.1–0.8 mg/kg/dose IV q6h; 1–2 mg/kg/dose PO q12h.

Adverse effects: Constipation, diarrhea, sedation, tachycardia rarely.

Notes: Does not interact with other drugs. Injection contains 0.5% phenol. No short-term toxicity noted.

Rifampin (Rifadin, Rimactane)

Action and spectrum: A broad-spectrum antibiotic that exerts its bacteriostatic action by inhibiting DNA-dependent RNA polymerase activity. Effective against mycobacteria, *Neisseria,* and gram-positive cocci (eg, staphylococci). Resistance develops rapidly, so the drug should always be used in combination with other agents for synergistic effect.

Supplied: Capsules (oral liquid can be compounded from the capsules by the pharmacist in 10 mg/mL concentration); injection.

Route: PO, IV.

Dosage: 10–20 mg/kg/day divided q12h.

Elimination and metabolism: Hepatic. Half-life is about 3 hours.

Adverse effects: Gastrointestinal irritation (anorexia, vomiting, diarrhea), hypersensitivity (rash, pruritus, eosinophilia), drowsiness, ataxia, blood dyscrasias (leukopenia, thrombocytopenia, hemolytic anemia), hepatitis (rare), elevation of serum urea nitrogen and uric acid levels. Causes pink to red discoloration of urine.

Comments: Crosses into CSF. When rifampin is used, it should always be used in combination with other agents to provide synergistic effect (eg, vancomycin plus gentamicin with or without rifampin for infection with vancomycin-resistant or tolerant staphylococci).

Note: Rifampin is a potent enzyme inducer of hepatic metabolism. Patients receiving phenytoin, phenobarbital, or theophylline may have a substantial decrease in serum concentration of these drugs after starting rifampin. Careful monitoring of serum drug concentrations is necessary.

Sodium Bicarbonate (various)

Indications and use: Metabolic acidosis. Treatment of certain intoxications (eg, salicylates, phenothiazines) and renal tubular acidosis. Adjunctive treatment of hyperkalemia.

Actions: Alkalinizing agent that dissociates to provide bicarbonate ion.

Supplied: Injection.

Route: PO, IV.

Dosage:

- Cardiac arrest (no longer recommended for routine use):
  Initial dose: 1–2 meq/kg IV slowly over 2 minutes.
  Subsequent doses: Number of meq = $0.3 \times$ wt (kg) $\times$ base deficit
- Renal tubular acidosis:
  Distal: 2–3 meq/kg/day.
  Proximal: 5–10 meq/kg/day as initial dose; adjust prn for maintenance.

Adverse effects: Rapid correction of metabolic acidosis with sodium bicarbonate can lead to intraventricular hemorrhage, hyperosmolality, metabolic alkalosis, hypernatremia, and hypokalemia.

Comments: Use with close monitoring of arterial blood pH.

Sodium Polystyrene Sulfonate (Kayexalate)

Indications and use: Treatment of hyperkalemia.

Actions: Cation exchange resin that releases sodium in exchange for other cations such as potassium. Each gram of resin exchanges 1 meq sodium for each meq potassium removed. Other cations such as calcium, magnesium, and iron are also bound.

Supplied: Powder for suspension, suspension (in 33% sorbitol) (1.25 g/5 mL, containing 4.1 meq sodium ion per gram).

Route: PO, PR (prepare in 20–25% sorbitol solution).

Dosage: 1 g resin will exchange 1 meq potassium. Usual dose is 1 g/kg/dose PO q6h or q2–6h PR.

Adverse effects: Large doses may cause fecal impaction. Hypokalemia, hypocalcemia, hypomagnesemia, and sodium retention may occur.

Spironolactone (Aldactone)

Indications and use: Primarily used in conjunction with a thiazide diuretic in the treatment of hypertension, congestive heart failure, and edema when prolonged diuresis is desirable.

Actions: Mild diuretic with potassium-sparing effects. Competitive antagonist of aldosterone.

Supplied: Tablets 25 mg. (A 4 mg/mL suspension can be compounded by the pharmacist.)

Route: PO.

Dosage: 1.5–3 mg/kg/day divided q12h.

Adverse effects: Hyperkalemia, dehydration, hyponatremia, and gynecomastia (usually reversible).

Comments: Contraindicated in hyperkalemia, anuria, and rapidly deteriorating renal function. Monitor potassium closely when giving potassium supplements. More expensive but more effective than potassium supplements.

Streptokinase (Kabikinase, Streptase)

Indications and use: Deep venous thrombosis and femoral artery thrombosis following cardiac catheterization.

Actions: Thrombolytic enzyme that converts plasminogen to the enzyme plasmin (fibrinolysin). Plasmin degrades fibrin, fibrinogen, and other plasma procoagulant proteins.

Supplied: Powder for injection.

Route: IV.

Dosage:

- Loading dose: 1500–2000 Units/kg infused over 30–60 minutes.
- Maintenance dosage: 1000 Units/kg/h as continuous infusion for 24–72 hours. Titrate dose to maintain thrombin time at 2–5 times normal control value.

Adverse effects: May cause severe spontaneous bleeding, hypersensitivity and anaphylactic reactions, fever (common), and chills.

Comments: Before starting therapy, obtain baseline thrombin time, activated partial thromboplastin time, prothrombin time, hematocrit, and platelet count; repeat all tests every 12 hours. It is desired to maintain thrombin time at 2–5 times normal and prothrombin time and activated partial thromboplastin time as 1.5–2 times normal. Prepare final infusion solution to concentration of 1000 Units/mL in 5% dextrose in water. At the end of streptokinase therapy, begin IV heparin. Antidote: Aminocaproic acid, loading dose 200 mg/kg IV or PO stat followed by maintenance dose of 100 mg/kg/dose IV or PO q6h for up to 10 days after the procedure. ***Note:*** Limited experience in neonates.

Sulfacetamide Sodium (Isopto Cetamide, Sodium Sulamyd, others)

Action and spectrum: Mechanism, see Sulfadiazine. Indicated in acute conjunctivitis. Spectrum includes *Staphylococcus aureus, Streptococcus pneumoniae, Haemophilus influenzae* and *Moraxella* spp.

Supplied: Ophthalmic solution (10%), ophthalmic ointment.

Route: Topical.

Dosage: Instill 1–2 drops into each eye q2h initially, then increase time interval as condition responds or ointment in each eye q4–6h for 7–10 days.

Comments: See Sulfadiazine for adverse effects. May cause local irritation. Ophthalmic solution preferred over neomycin-containing ophthalmic preparation because of decreased incidence of local irritation and allergic response.

Sulfadiazine

Action and spectrum: Acts via competitive antagonism of p-aminobenzoic acid, an essential factor in folic acid synthesis. Spectrum of action includes both gram-positive and gram-negative organisms. In neonatology, used chiefly against *Toxoplasma gondii* in combination with pyrimethamine.

Supplied: Tablets.

Route: PO.

Dosage: For toxoplasmosis, give 120 mg/kg/day divided q6h for 4 weeks. Combine with pyrimethamine.

Elimination and metabolism: Rapid renal excretion.

Adverse effects: Hypersensitivity (fever, rash, hepatitis, vasculitis, lupus-like syndrome), neutropenia, agranulocytosis, thrombocytopenia, aplastic anemia, Stevens-Johnson syndrome, crystalluria (keep urine alkaline and output high). Kernicterus may occur.

Comments: Avoid use in neonates except for treatment of congenital toxoplasmosis. See comments under Pyrimethamine regarding folinic acid use.

Surfactant (Exosurf Neonatal)

Indications and use: Surfactant therapy is indicated for the prophylactic treatment of infants with a birth weight < 1350 g who are at risk for the development of any type of respiratory distress syndrome (RDS), or for infants with a birth weight > 1350 g with coexisting, proven pulmonary immaturity and/or compromise. Exosurf Neonatal is also indicated for neonates with established surfactant deficiency syndrome.

Actions: Surfactant acts to decrease the work of breathing, increase lung compliance, and increase alveolar expansion and stability by decreasing surface tension preventing atelectasis at end expiration. As a result, surfactant directly acts to reverse surfactant deficiency syndrome, prevent or reduce the development of pulmonary interstitial edema (PIE), which may progress to other forms of RDS, and reduce oxygen positive pressure mechanical ventilation requirements. The pharmacologic activity of commercial surfactant results from the combined action of three synthetic components: dipalmitoyl phosphatidylcholine (DPPC), cetyl alcohol, and tyloxapol. DPPC, the major component of natural surfactant rapidly and efficiently acts to dramatically decrease alveolar surface tension. Cetyl alcohol facilitates the dispersion and adsorption of DPPC onto the air:liquid interface of the alveoli. Cetyl alcohol modulates this physiologically essential function without the increased risk or immunogenicity of infectious potential associated with foreign protein substances. Tyloxapol provides the product with a hydrophilic agent that allows for reconstitution of the lyophilized powder. Tyloxapol also plays a minor role in distribution of the active components into the smaller airways.

Supplied: Exosurf Neonatal is supplied in a kit containing a 10-mL vial containing DPPC 108 mg, cetyl alcohol 12 mg, tyloxapol 8 mg and NaCl 46.75 mg (tonicity agent), a 10-mL vial of sterile water for injection, and endotracheal tube adaptors of varying sizes. Prior to reconstitution, the drug requires no special storage requirements. Once reconstituted using exactly 8 mL sterile water, the milky white suspension is stable for up to 12 hours either at room temperature or under refrigeration.

Route: Surfactant can only be administered endotracheally using a special ET tube adaptor supplied with the drug kit, without the interruption of mechanical ventilation and after radiographic confirmation of the location of the endotracheal tube (ET) tip in the trachea unless impractical due to time restraints.

Dosage and administration: Prior to administration of surfactant, the infant should be well suctioned, and suctioning should be withheld for 2 hours following the dose unless clinically necessary. Prophylactic surfactant is administered as a single 5 mL/kg dose as soon as RDS is clinically confirmed after birth. Second and third doses may be subsequently administered if necessary while the infant remains mechanically ventilated and under respiratory distress. Rescue treatment for infants who acutely develop RDS is administered as two 5 mL/kg doses, with the first dose given at the time of diagnosis, and the second 12–24 hours later.

Administration of the dose requires intubation and should be given in half doses with the first half given over 1–2 minutes using the appropriately sized ET adaptor with the infant positioned at the midline position. The adaptor fits into the ventilator line and has a Leur lock syringe port through which the drug is administered while maintaining the closed system of the respirator. The infant's head and torso are then rotated 45 degrees to the right and held in that position for 30 seconds. The infant is then returned to midline and the remaining drug administered in the same manner with the head and torso rotated to the left for 30 seconds.

Adverse effects: Significant adverse effects associated with Exosurf Neonatal during clinical use to this point include increased incidence of pulmonary hemorrhage, apnea, and methylxanthine dosage requirements. Other adverse effects associated with the use of the drug involve increased risk of patent ductus arteriosus (PDA), thrombocytopenia, and acute changes in respiratory status; the latter of which may be a direct result of the pharmacologic activity of the drug and require rapid adjustment of mechanical ventilatory parameters.

Comments: Administration of surfactant requires close and continuous monitoring during and 30 minutes after administration of the dose to ensure maximum safety, efficacy, and benefit. This should include blood gas monitoring, adjustments of mechanical ventilatory parameters, and monitoring of changes in clinical signs and symptoms consistent with changes in oxygenation and pulmonary function.

Theophylline (various)

Indications and use: Apnea of prematurity. There is evidence that theophylline can improve lung compliance and aid in weaning infants from respiratory support in diseases such as bronchopulmonary dysplasia.

Actions: A methylxanthine. Theophylline probably acts by virtue of adenosine antagonism. Neonates have the unique ability to convert theophylline to caffeine in a ratio of 1:0.3, respectively, and caffeine may approach 50% of theophylline serum levels. Thus, it is impossible to distinguish the pharmacodynamic effects of theophylline from those of caffeine in the neonate. Theophylline produces excitation throughout all levels of the CNS; produces modest decreases in peripheral vascular resistance, and increases cardiac output; relaxes pulmonary airway smooth muscle, with resultant increase in vital capacity; decreases diaphragmatic fatigue; and may cause marked increases in cerebrovascular resistance, resulting in decreased cerebral blood flow. In premature infants at risk for ventricular hemorrhage, the latter effect may be deleterious.

Supplied: Oral solution, injection.

Route: IV, PO.

Dosage:

- Apnea of prematurity: 5–6 mg/kg PO or IV (infused over 15–30 minutes) as loading dose, followed by maintenance dose of 2 mg/kg q12h starting 12 hours after loading dose.
- Ventilator weaning: 6.5 mg/kg PO or IV as loading dose, followed by maintenance dose of 3–4 mg/kg q12h.

Adverse effects: Side effects and toxicity include hyperglycemia, diuresis, dehydration, feeding intolerance, tachycardia and other arrhythmias, hyperreflexia, jitteriness, and seizures.

Comments: Levels for apnea are 6–11 mcg/mL. Toxicity is associated with levels greater than 15–20 mcg/mL. Monitor serum levels on day 4 of therapy: peak level 1 hour after an IV dose is completed or 2 hours after an oral dose, and trough level 30 minutes before next dose. Levels of caffeine and theophylline should ideally be monitored any time toxicity is suspected or when apnea spells appear to be increasing in frequency.

Ticarcillin Disodium (Ticar)

Classification: Semisynthetic extended-spectrum penicillin.

Action and spectrum: See Mezlocillin.

Supplied: Injection.

Route: IM or IV (infuse over 30 minutes).

Dosage:

- < 2000 g and 0–7 days old: 150 mg/kg/day divided q12h.
- < 2000 g and > 7 days old: 225 mg/kg/day divided q8h.
- > 2000 g and 0–7 days old: 225 mg/kg/day divided q8h.
- > 2000 g and > 7 days old: 300 mg/kg/day divided q6h.

Elimination and metabolism: Renally excreted.

Adverse effects: See Mezlocillin. Hypokalemia pronounced.

Comments: Drug of first choice when considering an extended-spectrum penicillin. Avoid IM use if possible. Contains 5.2 meq sodium per gram.

Ticarcillin Disodium and Clavulanate Potassium (Timentin)

Classification: Combination antibiotic of ticarcillin (a carboxypenicillin) and clavulanic acid (beta-lactamase inhibitor).

Spectrum: Good antipseudomonal activity similar to ticarcillin except additional coverage of lactamase-producing species, particularly gram-positive cocci (eg, *Staphylococcus aureus*, *Streptococcus pneumoniae* and group B streptococcus). Good coverage against gram-negative organisms, including *E coli, Klebsiella,* and *Proteus.* Also demonstrated activity against anaerobes like *Clostridium* and *Peptostreptococcus.*

Supplied: Injection.

Route: IV.

Dosage:

- < 2000 g and 0–7 days old: 150 mg/kg/day divided q12h.
- < 2000 g and > 7 days old: 225 mg/kg/day divided q8h.
- > 2000 g and 0–7 days old: 225 mg/kg/day divided q8h.
- > 2000 g and > 7 days old: 300 mg/kg/day divided q6h.

Elimination: Ticarcillin, renal (tubular secretion); clavulanic acid, hepatic and renal.

Adverse effects: See Ticarcillin Disodium (Ticar).

Tobramycin Sulfate (Nebcin)

Classification: Aminoglycoside.

Action and spectrum: Mechanism of action and spectrum identical to those of gentamicin.

Supplied: Injection, ophthalmic drops, ophthalmic ointment.

Route: IM or IV (infuse over 30 minutes), topical (ophthalmic).

Dosage:

- IM or IV: Monitor and adjust by pharmacokinetics. Initial empirical dosing based on body weight:
    - < 7 days postnatal age:
    - < 1 kg and < 28 weeks' gestational age: 2.5 mg/kg/dose q24h.
    - < 1.5 kg and < 34 weeks' gestational age: 2.5 mg/kg/dose q18h.
    - > 1.5 kg and > 34 weeks' gestational age: 2.5 mg/kg/dose q12h.
    - > 7 days postnatal age:
    - < 1.2 kg: 2.5 mg/kg/dose q18–24h.
    - > 1.2 kg: 2.5 mg/kg/dose q8h.
- Ophthalmic: Instill 1 or 2 drops into each eye 2–6 times a day or more often as needed; or apply a small amount of ointment into each eye q3–4h.

Elimination and metabolism: Renal.

Adverse effects: See Gentamicin.

Comments: Reserve for cases resistant to gentamicin. Obtain serum peak and trough concentrations at about the 4th maintenance dose. Desired serum peak concentration is 4–10 mcg/mL (sample obtained 30 minutes after infusion complete); desired serum trough concentration is < 2 mcg/mL (sample obtained 30 minutes to just before the next dose).

Tolazoline (Priscoline)

Indications and use: Hypoxia caused by persistent pulmonary hypertension (PPH).

Actions: Alpha-adrenergic blocking agent with histaminergic properties. Results in pulmonary and systemic vasodilator effects. Histaminic effects stimulate gastric secretion and peripheral vasodilation and increase salivary, lacrimal, respiratory tract, and pancreatic secretions. Response to tolazoline is marked by cutaneous flushing followed by increased PaO_2.

Supplied: Injection.

Route: IV.

Dosage: 1–2 mg/kg IV as initial dose (infused over 5–10 minutes) followed by a continuous infusion of 0.3–0.6 mg/kg/h. Some infants respond rapidly; others may require 30 minutes or more.

Adverse effects: Tachycardia, nausea, vomiting, diarrhea, gastrointestinal bleeding, increased gastrointestinal secretions, increased pilomotor activity, sweating, thrombocytopenia, agranulocytosis, and hypotension.

Comments: Contraindicated in renal failure, hypotension shock, and intraventricular hemorrhage. Dopamine and dobutamine are often used to support systemic pressure in neonates with PPH; both drugs may have adverse effects on peripheral vascular resistance, especially at higher dosages. For severe hypotension use ephedrine (0.2 mg/kg/dose) to increase peripheral vascular resistance or dopamine (< 10 mcg/kg/min) to improve cardiac output. Epinephrine administered with tolazoline may cause a paradoxical reduction in blood pressure followed by an exaggerated rebound blood pressure elevation.

Tromethamine (THAM)

Indications and use: Metabolic acidosis when sodium bicarbonate is contraindicated because of elevated serum sodium (eg, metabolic acidosis in persistent fetal circulation treated with multiple doses of sodium bicarbonate).

Actions: Alkalinizing agent that acts as a proton (hydrogen ion) acceptor; combines with hydrogen ions and their associated anions of acids (lactic, pyruvic, carbonic, and other metabolic acids). The resulting salts are then renally excreted.

Supplied: Injection, 0.3 Molar solution (36 mg/mL).

Route: IV.

Dosage:

- Loading dose: 3–5 mL/kg of undiluted solution infused over 1 hour, or dose = wt in kg × 1.1 × base deficit in meq/L.
- Maintenance dosage: 3 mL/kg/h (undiluted solution) as continuous infusion. Titrate dose to desired response via frequent blood gas monitoring.

Adverse effects: Respiratory depression, thrombophlebitis, venospasm, alkalosis, transient hypocalcemia or hypoglycemia, and hyperkalemia. Extravasation may cause sloughing of the skin.

Comments: Contraindicated in anuria, uremia, and chronic respiratory acidosis. Do not administer for periods longer than 24 hours. Hyperkalemia is a problem especially with decreased renal function.

Tubocurarine (Curare)

Indications and use: To improve oxygenation in the uncooperative neonate during mechanical ventilation. To provide muscle relaxation during general anesthesia.

Actions: Nondepolarizing (competitive) neuromuscular blocking agent. Rapid IV administration may cause hypotension, bradycardia, and possibly circulatory collapse. Atropine is an effective prophylactic agent. Onset of paralysis is generally 1–2 minutes after IV administration. Duration of paralysis depends on the number of doses and the total dosage delivered and may persist for 20 to 90 minutes.

Supplied: Injection 3 mg/mL.

Route: IV; IM only if IV access is not available.

Dosage: Infuse undiluted over 1 minute or more to minimize cardiovascular effects.

- Initial dosage: 0.25–0.5 mg/kg IV.
- Maintenance dosage: 0.15 mg/kg/dose IV prn.

Adverse effects: Hypotension, bradycardia, possibly circulatory collapse and allergic reactions.

Comments: For reversal, give neostigmine, with atropine, IV. See dose p 497.

Vancomycin Hydrochloride (Vancocin, others)

Action and spectrum: Bactericidal action by interference with bacterial cell wall synthesis. Active against most gram-positive cocci and bacilli, including streptococci, staphylococci (including methicillin-resistant staphylococci), clostridia (including *Clostridium difficile*), *Corynebacterium,* and *Listeria monocytogenes.* Bacteriostatic against enterococci. No cross-resistance between vancomycin and other antibiotics has been reported. The drug of choice against methicillin-resistant staphylococci and *C difficile*.

Supplied: Injection, oral solution.

Route: IV, PO.

Dosage:

- IV: Monitor and adjust by pharmacokinetics. Initial empirical dosing based on body weight:
  - < 1.2 kg, 0–4 weeks postnatal age: 15 mg/kg/dose q 24h.
  - 1.2–2 kg:
    - 0–7 days: 15 mg/kg/dose q12–18h.
    - > 7 days: 15 mg/kg/dose q8–12h.
  - > 2 kg:
    - 0–7 days: 15 mg/kg/dose q12h.
    - > 7 days: 15 mg/kg/dose q8h.
- PO: To treat pseudomembranous colitis due to *C difficile* or staphylococcal enterocolitis. 20–40 mg/kg/day divided q6h for 5–7 days.

Elimination and metabolism: Renally excreted. Half-life 7–9 hours.

Adverse effects: Allergy (rash, fever), ototoxicity (with serum peak levels > 40 mcg/mL), thrombophlebitis at site of injection. Too rapid infusion may cause rash, chills, and fever (red-man syndrome) mimicking anaphylactic reaction. Rapid infusion may cause apnea and bradycardia without other signs of "red-man syndrome." Infuse dose over at least 60 minutes.

Comments: Therapeutic range: 20–40 mcg/mL (sample drawn 60 minutes after infusion complete) and serum trough levels of 5–10 mcg/mL (sample drawn 30 minutes to just before next dose). In general, draw serum peak and trough levels at about the 4th maintenance dose. Monitor serum creatinine. If staphylococci exhibit vancomycin tolerance, combine vancomycin and an aminoglycoside with or without rifampin. Oral doses are poorly absorbed. Powder for injection, diluted and flavored, is the most economical means of oral dosing.

Varicella-Zoster Immune Globulin (VZIG)

Indications and use: For protection of infants of mothers with varicella-zoster infections (chicken pox) within 5 days before or 48 hours after delivery; of postnatally exposed preterm infants under 1000 g or under 28 weeks regardless of maternal history; and of postnatally exposed premature infants whose maternal history is negative for varicella.

Actions: Passive immunity through infusion of IgG antibody. Protection lasts 1 month or longer. VZIG does not reduce the incidence but acts to decrease the risk of complications.

Supplied: Injection, 125 units/1.25 mL vial.

Route: IM only.

Dosage: 0–10 kg: 125 units IM as a single dose injected at one site.

Adverse effects: Pain, erythema, swelling, and rash at the site of injection; rarely, anaphylaxis.

Comments: Best results are achieved if VZIG is given within 96 hours after exposure. It is obtained through the American Red Cross Blood Services. ***Note:*** Do not give IV.

Vecuronium Bromide (Vecuronium)

Indications and use: Skeletal muscle relaxation and paralysis in infants requiring mechanical ventilation.

Actions: Nondepolarizing muscle relaxant that competitively antagonizes autonomic cholinergic receptors. Onset of action is 1–2 minutes with a duration that varies with dose and age.

Supplied: Powder for injection.

Route: IV.

Dosage: 0.03–0.15 mg/kg IV push q1–2h to maintain paralysis.

Adverse effects: May cause hypoxemia.

Comments: Causes less tachycardia than pancuronium bromide. When used with narcotics, decreases in heart rate and blood pressure have been observed.

Vidarabine (Vira-A)

Action and spectrum: Antiviral agent for treatment of herpes encephalitis. Inhibits viral DNA formation. Good activity against herpes simplex type 1, poor activity against adenoviruses or RNA viruses. Activity against varicella-zoster virus unconfirmed.

Supplied: Injection (monohydrate), 200 mg/mL, equivalent to 187.4 mg vidarabine; ophthalmic ointment, 3%.

Route: Ophthalmic, IV (dilute to 1 mg/2.2 mL and infuse over 12–24 hours).

Dosage:

- Ophthalmic: Instill a small amount into each eye q3h.
- IV:
    < 1 month: 15–30 mg/kg/day as a 18–24h infusion.
    > 1 month: 10–15 mg/kg/day as a 12-hour or longer infusion.

Adverse effects: Rash, pain at injection site. Decreased reticulocyte count, white cell count, and platelet count. Elevated total bilirubin and AST (SGOT).

Comments: Rarely used. Volume necessary for IV infusion may cause fluid overload. Acyclovir is usual agent of choice. Must filter final solution (use 0.45-micron filter).

Vitamin D$_2$ (Ergocalciferol, Calciferol, Drisdol)

Indications and use: To prevent or treat rickets and to manage hypocalcemia due to vitamin D deficiency.

Actions: Regulation of plasma calcium and phosphate, supporting normal mineralization of bone.

Supplied: Oral solution (8000 Units/mL); Injection (500,000 Units/mL for IM use only).

Route: PO, IM.

Dosage: 400–800 Units/day.

Comments: Excessive doses may lead to hypervitaminosis D, manifested by hypercalcemia and its associated complications.

Vitamin E (dl-alpha-tocopherol Acetate, Aquasol E)

Indications and use: Investigational for treatment or prevention of anemia of prematurity, retinopathy of prematurity, bronchopulmonary dysplasia, and intraventricular hemorrhage.

Actions: A potent free radical scavenger. An antioxidant to prevent destruction of unsaturated fatty acids and cell membranes by uncontrolled free radicals. At birth, tissue stores of alpha-tocopherol (active form) are low.

Supplied: Drops, 50 Units/mL.

Route: PO.

Dosage:

- Requirements: The following recommendations are currently followed in infant formulas.
    Full-term infants: 0.3 Units/100 kcal or 0.7 Units/g linoleic acid.
    Premature infants: 1 Unit/g of linoleic acid.
- Anemia of prematurity: Prevention or treatment requires only adequate nutritional intake of vitamin E.
- Alternative: Prophylaxis: 25–50 Units/day PO until 2–3 months of age. Treatment: 50–200 Units/day PO for 2 weeks.

Comments: Physiologic serum levels for premature infants are 1–3 mg/dL. Serum levels should be monitored when pharmacologic doses of vitamin E are administered. Liquid preparation is very hyperosmolar (3000 mOsm/L) and should be diluted. (1 mg of dl-alpha-tocopherol acetate = 1 Unit).

Vitamin K₁ (Phytonadione, AquaMephyton, Mephyton)

Indications and use: Prevention and treatment of hemorrhagic disease of the newborn, vitamin K deficiency.

Actions: Required for the synthesis of blood coagulation factors II, VII, IX, and X. Because vitamin K_1 may require 3 hours or more to stop active bleeding, fresh-frozen plasma, 10 mL/kg, may be necessary when bleeding is severe. The drug has no antagonistic effects against heparin.

Supplied: Tablets, injection.

Route: PO, IM, IV. (For IV use, dilute in 5% dextrose in water and infuse over 30 minutes or longer.)

Dosage:

- Neonatal hemorrhagic disease:
    Prevention: 1 mg IM at birth; if infant < 1500 g, give 0.5 mg IM at birth. Treatment: 1 mg as single dose.
- Deficiency state: 1 mg/dose PO, IM, or slowly IV.
- Oral anticoagulant overdose: 1–2 mg/dose IV q4–8h prn. (Follow serial prothrombin time and partial thromboplastin time for response.)

Adverse effects: Relatively nontoxic. Hemolytic anemia and kernicterus have been reported in neonates given menadiol sodium disphosphate (vitamin K_3; Synkayvite); however, vitamin K_1 has not been associated with toxic symptoms or hypersensitivity. No association between exposure to vitamin K at birth and an increased risk of any childhood cancer or of all childhood cancers combined were found using data from the Collaborative Perinatal Project, although a slightly increased risk could not be ruled out.

74 Effects of Drugs and Substances on Lactation and Breast-Feeding

The drugs and substances listed below are those for which reliable data on their effect during lactation have been compiled. This listing is undoubtedly incomplete as it is impossible to list every possible medication. Clinical judgment about the possible effects of maternal drug intake while nursing must always be exercised.

Drug or Substance	Compatability with Breast-Feeding, Effect on Lactation and Adverse Effects on Infant
Acetaminophen	Generally compatible with breast-feeding.
Albuterol	Generally compatible with breast-feeding. Monitor for agitation and spitting up. Use inhaled form to decrease maternal absorption.
Alcohol	Generally compatible with breast-feeding. Monitor for drowsiness, diaphoresis, weakness, and failure to thrive. Intake of 1 g/kg/d may decrease maternal milk ejection reflex.
Amantadine	Contraindicated. Causes release of levodopa in central nervous system.
Amikacin	Generally compatible with breast-feeding. Low concentrations in breast milk because of poor oral absorption.
Aminoglycosides	Generally compatible with breast-feeding. All antibiotics are excreted in breast milk in limited amounts. Apparently safe, not absorbed in newborn gastrointestinal tract. Monitor for diarrhea.
Aminophylline	Generally compatible with breast-feeding. Monitor for irritability.
Amiodarone	Breast-feeding is not recommended because of iodine contained in each dose and possible accumulation of amiodarone in the infant.
Amitriptyline	Generally compatible with breast-feeding.
Amoxapine	Generally compatible with breast-feeding.
Amoxicillin	Generally compatible with breast-feeding. Monitor for diarrhea.
Amphetamine	Generally compatible with breast-feeding. Monitor for irritability, poor sleeping patterns.
Ampicillin	Generally compatible with breast-feeding. Monitor for diarrhea.
Aspartame	Generally compatible with breast-feeding. Use cautiously in carrier of phenylketonuria.
Aspirin	Generally compatible with breast-feeding. Monitor for spitting up or bleeding. Increased risk with high doses used for rheumatoid arthritis (3–5 g/day).
Atenolol	Generally compatible with breast-feeding.
Atropine	Generally compatible with breast-feeding. No adverse effects reported.
Bethanechol	Generally compatible with breast-feeding. May cause abdominal pain and diarrhea.

Drug or Substance	Compatability with Breast-Feeding, Effect on Lactation and Adverse Effects on Infant
Bromides	Breast-feeding not recommended because of possible drowsiness and rash.
Bromocriptine	Contraindicated. Suppresses lactation.
Brompheniramine	Generally compatible with breast-feeding. Monitor for agitation, poor sleeping pattern, feeding problems.
Butorphanol	Generally compatible with breast-feeding.
Caffeine	Generally compatible with breast-feeding. Monitor for irritability, poor sleeping patterns.
Calcitonin	May inhibit lactation.
Captopril	Generally compatible with breast-feeding.
Carbamazepine	Generally compatible with breast-feeding. Risk of bone marrow suppression if taken chronically.
Carbimazole	Generally compatible with breast-feeding. Monitor for goiter.
Cascara sagrada	Generally compatible with breast-feeding. Monitor for diarrhea.
Cefaclor	Generally compatible with breast-feeding. Monitor for diarrhea.
Cefadroxil	Generally compatible with breast-feeding. Monitor for diarrhea.
Cefamandole	Generally compatible with breast-feeding. Monitor for diarrhea.
Cefazolin	Generally compatible with breast-feeding. Monitor for diarrhea.
Cefonicid	Generally compatible with breast-feeding. Monitor for diarrhea.
Cefoperazone	Generally compatible with breast-feeding. Monitor for diarrhea.
Ceforanide	Generally compatible with breast-feeding. Monitor for diarrhea.
Cefotaxime	Generally compatible with breast-feeding. Monitor for diarrhea.
Ceftizoxime	Generally compatible with breast-feeding. Monitor for diarrhea.
Ceftriaxone	Generally compatible with breast-feeding. Monitor for diarrhea.
Cefuroxime	Generally compatible with breast-feeding. Monitor for diarrhea.
Cephalexin	Generally compatible with breast-feeding. Monitor for diarrhea.
Cephalosporins	Generally compatible with breast-feeding. All antibiotics are excreted in breast milk in limited amounts. Monitor for rash; sensitization possible.
Cephalothin	Generally compatible with breast-feeding. Monitor for diarrhea.
Cephapirin	Generally compatible with breast-feeding. Monitor for diarrhea.
Cephradine	Generally compatible with breast-feeding. Monitor for diarrhea.
Chloral hydrate	Generally compatible with breast-feeding. Monitor for sedation, rash.
Chloramphenicol	Discontinue during breast-feeding. Risk of bone marrow toxicity. Nurse after 24 hours off the drug.
Chloroform	Generally compatible with breast-feeding.
Chloroquine	Generally compatible with breast-feeding.

Drug or Substance	Compatability with Breast-Feeding, Effect on Lactation and Adverse Effects on Infant
Chlorothiazide	Generally compatible with breast-feeding but may suppress lactation, especially in first month of lactation. Adverse effects have not been reported, but infant's electrolytes and platelets should be monitored.
Chlorpheniramine	Generally compatible with breast-feeding. Monitor for agitation, poor sleeping pattern, feeding problems.
Chlorpromazine	Generally compatible with breast-feeding. Monitor for sedation.
Chlorpropamide	Contraindicated. Excreted in breast milk and may cause hypoglycemia.
Chlortetracycline	Generally compatible with breast-feeding. Monitor for diarrhea.
Chocolate	Generally compatible with breast-feeding. Irritability or increased bowel activity if mother consumes excessive amounts (> 16 oz/day).
Cimetidine	Contraindicated. May suppress gastric acidity in infant, inhibit drug metabolism, and cause CNS stimulation.
Clindamycin	Discontinue during breast-feeding. Risk of gastrointestinal bleeding. Nurse after 24 hours off the drug.
Clonazepam	Generally compatible with breast-feeding. Monitor for respiratory and CNS depression.
Clonidine	Contraindicated. Excreted in breast milk.
Cloxacillin	Generally compatible with breast-feeding. Monitor for diarrhea.
Cocaine	Contraindicated. Causes cocaine intoxication in infant from maternal intranasal use (hypertension, tachycardia, mydriasis, apnea) and from topical use on mother's nipples (apnea and seizures).
Codeine	Generally compatible with breast-feeding. Monitor for sedation. Milk ejection reflex (letdown) may be inhibited.
Contraceptives, oral	Contraindicated. Can cause breast enlargement and proliferation of vaginal epithelium in infants.
Coumadin (warfarin, dicumarol)	Generally compatible with breast-feeding.
Cyclophosphamide	Contraindicated. Possible immune suppression. Unknown effect on growth or association with carcinogenesis.
Cyproheptadine	Generally compatible with breast-feeding. Monitor for agitation, poor sleeping pattern, feeding problems.
Desipramine	Generally compatible with breast-feeding.
Dextroamphetamine	Contraindicated. May cause infant stimulation.
Diazepam	Contraindicated. May cause infant sedation.
Diazoxide	Contraindicated. May case hyperglycemia.
Dicumarol	See Coumadin.
Digoxin	Generally compatible with breast-feeding. Monitor for spitting up, diarrhea, heart rate changes.
Diphenhydramine	Generally compatible with breast-feeding. Monitor for agitation, poor sleeping pattern, feeding problems.
Dipyridamole	Generally compatible with breast-feeding.
Disopyramide	Generally compatible with breast-feeding.
Ephedrine	Generally compatible with breast-feeding. Monitor for agitation.
Ergotamine	Contraindicated. Causes vomiting, diarrhea, convulsions.
Erythromycin	Generally compatible with breast-feeding. Monitor for diarrhea.

Drug or Substance	Compatability with Breast-Feeding, Effect on Lactation and Adverse Effects on Infant
Ethambutol	Generally compatible with breast-feeding.
Ethanol	See Alcohol.
Ethosuximide	Generally compatible with breast-feeding. Rare occurrence of bone marrow suppression and gastrointestinal upset.
Fava beans	Generally compatible with breast-feeding. Hemolysis in patients with G6PD deficiency.
Fenoprofen	Excreted in breast milk in small quantities.
Folic acid	Generally compatible with breast-feeding.
Furosemide	Generally compatible with breast-feeding.
Gallium-69	Discontinue during breast-feeding. Radioactivity can remain in breast milk for 2 weeks.
Gentamicin	Generally compatible with breast-feeding. Monitor for diarrhea, bloody stools.
Gold salts	Contraindicated. May cause rash, inflammation of kidney and liver.
Guanethidine	Generally compatible with breast-feeding.
Haloperidol	Generally compatible with breast-feeding.
Halothane	Generally compatible with breast-feeding.
Heparin	Generally compatible with breast-feeding.
Heroin	Generally compatible with breast-feeding. Monitor for depression, withdrawal.
Hydralazine	Generally compatible with breast-feeding.
Hydrochlorothiazide	Generally compatible with breast-feeding. See Chlorothiazide.
Hydromorphone	Generally compatible with breast-feeding. Monitor for sedation. Milk ejection reflex (letdown) may be inhibited.
Ibuprofen	Generally compatible with breast-feeding. Effects unknown.
Imipramine	Generally compatible with breast-feeding.
Insulin	Generally compatible with breast-feeding.
Iodine-125	Contraindicated. Risk of thyroid cancer. Radioactivity present in milk for 12 days.
Iodine-131	Contraindicated. Radioactivity in milk for 2–14 days.
Isoniazid	Generally compatible with breast-feeding. Monitor for rash, diarrhea, constipation.
Isoproterenol	Generally compatible with breast-feeding. Monitor for agitation, spitting up. Use aerosol form to decrease maternal absorption.
Isotretinoin	Contraindicated.
Kanamycin	Generally compatible with breast-feeding. Low concentrations in breast milk due to poor oral absorption. Monitor for diarrhea.
Labetalol	Generally compatible with breast-feeding. Monitor for hypotension, bradycardia.
Levodopa	Contraindicated. Inhibitory effect on prolactin release.
Levothyroxine (T_4)	Generally compatible with breast-feeding. Probably does not interfere with neonatal thyroid screening.
Liothyronine (T_3)	Generally compatible with breast-feeding. Probably does not interfere with neonatal thyroid screening.
Lithium	Contraindicated during breast-feeding. Milk levels average 40% of maternal serum concentration. Monitor infant for cyanosis, hypotonia, bradycardia, and other lithium toxicities.
Lorazepam	Generally compatible with breast-feeding. Monitor for sedation.

Drug or Substance	Compatability with Breast-Feeding, Effect on Lactation and Adverse Effects on Infant
Magnesium sulfate	Generally compatible with breast-feeding.
Meperidine	Generally compatible with breast-feeding. Monitor for sedation. Milk ejection reflex (letdown) may be inhibited.
Mepindolol	Generally compatible with breast-feeding. Monitor for hypotension, bradycardia.
Meprobamate	Generally compatible with breast-feeding but excreted in milk in high amounts. Monitor for sedation.
Metaproterenol	Generally compatible with breast-feeding. Monitor for agitation, spitting up. Use aerosol form to decrease maternal absorption.
Methadone	Generally compatible with breast-feeding. Monitor for sedation, depression, withdrawal on cessation of methadone treatment.
Methimazole	Contraindicated. Potential for interfering with thyroid function.
Methotrexate	Contraindicated. Possible immune suppression. Its effect on growth and association with carcinogenesis are unknown.
Methyldopa	Generally compatible with breast-feeding. Risk of hemolysis, increased liver enzymes.
Methyprylon	Generally compatible with breast-feeding. Monitor for drowsiness.
Metoclopramide	Generally compatible with breast-feeding. Increases milk production.
Metoprolol	Generally compatible with breast-feeding.
Metronidazole	Discontinue during breast-feeding. Do not nurse until 12–24 hours after discontinuing to allow excretion of drug.
Minoxidil	Generally compatible with breast-feeding. Monitor for hypotension.
Monosodium glutamate	Generally compatible with breast-feeding.
Morphine	Generally compatible with breast-feeding. Monitor for sedation. Milk ejection reflex (letdown) may be inhibited.
Nadolol	Generally compatible with breast-feeding.
Naproxen	Generally compatible with breast-feeding. Adverse effects unknown.
Nicotine	Generally compatible with breast-feeding. Excessive amounts may cause diarrhea, vomiting, tachycardia, irritability, and decreased milk production.
Nitrofurantoin	Generally compatible with breast-feeding. Excreted in milk in small amounts. Monitor infants with G6PD deficiency for hemolytic anemia.
Oral contraceptives	See Contraceptives, oral.
Oxacillin	Generally compatible with breast-feeding. Monitor for diarrhea.
Oxazepam	Generally compatible with breast-feeding. Monitor for sedation, depression.
Oxprenolol	Generally compatible with breast-feeding. Monitor for hypotension, bradycardia.
Oxycodone (Percodan, Percocet)	Generally compatible with breast-feeding. Monitor for drowsiness.
Penicillins	Generally compatible with breast-feeding. All antibiotics are excreted in breast milk in limited amounts. Monitor for rash, diarrhea, spitting up.
Phencyclidine	Contraindicated. Excreted in high amounts in breast milk.

Drug or Substance	Compatability with Breast-Feeding, Effect on Lactation and Adverse Effects on Infant
Phenindione	Contraindicated. Causes hemorrhage in infants.
Phenobarbital	Generally compatible with breast-feeding. Monitor for sucking problems, sedation, rashes.
Phenylbutazone	Generally compatible with breast-feeding.
Phenylpropanolamine	Generally compatible with breast-feeding. Monitor for agitation.
Phenytoin	Generally compatible with breast-feeding. Monitor for methemoglobinuria (rare).
Pindolol	Generally compatible with breast-feeding. Monitor for hypotension, bradycardia.
Potassium iodide	Contraindicated. Goiter and allergic reactions may be seen.
Prednisone	Generally compatible with breast-feeding. Safety of long-term therapy has not been established. If maternal dose is more than 2 times physiologic, avoid breast-feeding.
Primidone	Generally compatible with breast-feeding. Monitor for irritability.
Prochlorperazine	Generally compatible with breast-feeding.
Propoxyphene	Generally compatible with breast-feeding. Monitor for withdrawal after long-term high-dose maternal use.
Propranolol	Generally compatible with breast-feeding. Monitor for hypotension, bradycardia.
Propylthiouracil	Generally compatible with breast-feeding.
Pseudoephedrine	Generally compatible with breast-feeding. Monitor for agitation.
Pyridoxine	Generally compatible with breast-feeding.
Pyrimethamine	Generally compatible with breast-feeding.
Quinidine	Generally compatible with breast-feeding. Monitor for rash, anemia, arrhythmias. Risk of optic neuritis with chronic use.
Radiopharmaceuticals (generally)	Discontinue during breast-feeding. Consult nuclear medicine physician for selection of radionuclide with shortest excretion time.
Ranitidine	Generally compatible with breast-feeding. May increase the infant's gastric pH.
Reserpine	Generally compatible with breast-feeding. Monitor for infantile galactorrhea.
Riboflavin	Generally compatible with breast-feeding.
Rifampin	Generally compatible with breast-feeding.
Saccharin	Generally compatible with breast-feeding.
Secobarbital	Generally compatible with breast-feeding.
Sulfamethoxazole, sulfonamide	Contraindicated. Highly bound drugs can displace bilirubin from protein, increasing risk of kernicterus, without effect on serum bilirubin.
Technitium-99m	Contraindicated. Radioactivity present in breast milk for 15 hours to 3 days.
Terbutaline	Generally compatible with breast-feeding. Monitor for agitation and spitting up. Use inhaled form to decrease maternal absorption if available.
Tetracyclines	Contraindicated. Causes staining of teeth and growth inhibition.
Theophylline	Generally compatible with breast-feeding. Monitor for irritability.
Thiamine	Generally compatible with breast-feeding.
Thioridazine	Generally compatible with breast-feeding.

Drug or Substance	Compatability with Breast-Feeding, Effect on Lactation and Adverse Effects on Infant
Thiouracil	Contraindicated. Causes decreased thyroid function. (Does not apply to propylthiouracil.)
Ticarcillin	Generally compatible with breast-feeding. Monitor for diarrhea.
Timolol	Generally compatible with breast-feeding. Monitor for hypotension, bradycardia.
Tobramycin	Generally compatible with breast-feeding. Poor oral absorption. Monitor for diarrhea.
Tolbutamide	Generally compatible with breast-feeding. Monitor for jaundice.
Trifluoperazine	Generally compatible with breast-feeding.
Trimethoprim	Generally compatible with breast-feeding.
Valproic acid	Generally compatible with breast-feeding but carries risk of hepatitis, hemorrhagic pancreatitis.
Vegetarian diet	Generally compatible with breast-feeding. Monitor for vitamin B_{12} deficiency (failure to thrive, psychomotor retardation, megaloblastic anemia).
Vitamin B_{12}	Generally compatible with breast-feeding.
Vitamin D	Generally compatible with breast-feeding. Monitor for increased calcium levels.
Vitamin K	Generally compatible with breast-feeding.
Warfarin	See Coumadin.

75 Effects of Drugs and Substances Taken During Pregnancy

The drugs listed below include a fetal-risk category to indicate a systemically absorbed drug's potential for causing birth defects or neonatal disorders. Regardless of the designated risk category or presumed safety, no drug or substance should be used during pregnancy unless it is clearly needed. Please refer to the manufacturer's product literature or reference listed at the end of the chapter for further information.

FDA Fetal-Risk Categories

Category A   Adequate studies in pregnant women have not demonstrated a risk to the fetus in the first trimester of pregnancy; there is no evidence of risk in the last 2 trimesters.

Category B   Animal studies have not demonstrated a risk to the fetus, but there are no adequate studies in pregnant women.
or
Animal studies have shown an adverse effect, but adequate studies in pregnant women have not demonstrated a risk to the fetus during the first trimester of pregnancy and there is no evidence of risk in the last 2 trimesters.

Category C   Animal studies have shown an adverse effect on the fetus, but there are no adequate studies in humans. The benefits from the use of the drug in pregnant women may be acceptable despite its potential risks.
or
There are no animal reproduction studies and no adequate studies in humans.

Category D   There is evidence of human fetal risk, but the potenial benefits from the use of the drug in pregnant women may be acceptable despite its potential risks.

Category X   Studies in animals or humans or adverse reaction reports, or both, have demonstrated fetal abnormalities. The risk of use in pregnant women clearly outweighs any possible benefit.

Drug or Substance	FDA Fetal Risk Category, Adverse Effects, and Clinical Comments
Acebutolol	Category B. May cause bradycardia and hypotension in infants exposed near term. Carefully monitor blood pressure and heart rate.
Acetaminophen	Category B. Safe for short-term use in therapeutic doses. If medication is required to treat fever or pain, use acetaminophen rather than aspirin.
Acetazolamide	Category C. No reports of fetal risk available.
Acetohexamide	Category D. Pregnant diabetics should be managed with insulin, not oral hypoglycemics. Causes symptomatic hypoglycemia due to hyperinsulinemia in the newborn. Monitor

Drug or Substance	FDA Fetal Risk Category, Adverse Effects, and Clinical Comments
	infant's serum glucose for 5 days after birth. (See Chap 41 for treatment of hypoglycemia.)
Acetophenazine	Category C. No reports of fetal risk available.
Acetylcholine	Category C. No reports of fetal risk available.
Acyclovir	Category C. Report of 2 infants exposed in utero exhibited no toxicity.
Albumin	Category C. No known problems associated with its use in pregnancy.
Albuterol	Category C. Used to prevent premature labor, as is terbutaline and ritodrine. May cause fetal tachycardia (> 160 beats/min) and hypoglycemia in the newborn. Decreases incidence of neonatal respiratory distress syndrome.
Alcohol	Category D or X if used excessively. Causes multiple congenital anomalies. Causes fetal alcohol syndrome (prenatal and postnatal growth deficiency, facial dysmorphogenesis, CNS abnormalities, impairment in mental and motor functioning), spontaneous abortion, renal anomalies, alcohol withdrawal syndrome, and other abnormalities.
Alteplase (TPA tissue-type plasminogen activator)	Category C. No information available.
Amantadine	Category C. Teratogenic in animals in high doses. In one reported case, exposure to amantidine in the first trimester may have caused a single ventricle with pulmonary atresia.
Ambenonium	Category C. No reports of fetal risk available. Intravenous anticholinesterases could potentially induce premature labor.
Amikacin	Category C. No reports of adverse effects in the fetus. Testing for ototoxicity is recommended because other aminoglycosides, kanamycin and streptomycin, have been associated with eighth cranial nerve damage.
Amiloride	Category B. No reports of fetal risk available.
Aminocaproic acid	Category C. No reports of fetal risk available.
Aminoglutethimide	Category D. Possible virilization when given throughout pregnancy.
Aminophylline	Category C. At birth, transient tachycardia, irritability, and vomiting may occur, especially if mother's serum concentrations are above the therapeutic range. No congenital defects have been reported.
Aminopterin	Category X. Several reports have described fetal malformations when the drug has been used unsuccessfully to induce abortion in the first trimester.
Para-aminosalicylic acid (PAS)	Category C. In one study, congenital defects were found in 5 infants; other studies have reported no fetal risk.
Amiodarone	Category C. Transient bradycardia reported in one newborn. Since this drug contains iodine, there is potential concern regarding the fetal thyroid gland. Thyroid function testing of newborns of mothers who have taken the drug during pregnancy is recommended.
Amitriptyline	Category D. Malformations, neonatal withdrawal, and urinary retention in the neonate are potential problems.
Ammonium chloride	Category B. Three possible malformations (inguinal hernia if the drug was taken during the first trimester, cataracts,

Drug or Substance	FDA Fetal Risk Category, Adverse Effects, and Clinical Comments
	and benign tumors) have been reported. Acidoses may occur in the mother and fetus when the drug is taken near term.
Amobarbital	Category D. Increased incidence of congenital defects reported. May cause withdrawal syndrome.
Amoxapine	Category C. No reports of fetal risk available.
Amoxicillin	Category B. No evidence of fetal or neonatal risk.
Amphetamines	Category C. With amphetamine abuse, there is an increased incidence of preterm labor, placental abruption, fetal distress, postpartum hemorrhage, intrauterine growth retardation, feeding difficulty, drowsiness, and lassitude that may last several months.
Amphotericin B	Category B. No reports of fetal risk available.
Ampicillin	Category B. No reports of fetal risk available.
Amyl nitrite	Category C. Insufficient data to draw conclusions regarding the safety of this agent during pregnancy.
Anileridine	Category B. Potential risk of withdrawal syndrome and respiratory depression from maternal use of this narcotic analgesic.
Anisindione	Category D. This drug is a coumadin (warfarin) derivative; there is significant risk of congenital defects. May cause the fetal warfarin syndrome (nasal hypoplasia with a flattened, upturned appearance, stippled epiphyses, and possibly other features such as low birth weight, eye defects, developmental retardation, congenital heart disease, and death). May also cause hemorrhage. If anticoagulation is required during pregnancy, heparin is a safer choice.
Antacids	Category C. No teratogenic effects reported. Avoid chronic use of high doses.
Antazoline	Category C. No data available for this antihistamine.
Aspirin	Category C. May cause increased risk of hemorrhage, closure of the ductus arteriosus, and prolonged labor. First-trimester use does not increase risk of congenital heart defects. Risk is greatest in the last 3 months of pregnancy. High doses may cause increased perinatal mortality and intrauterine growth retardation. If medication is required to treat fever or pain, use acetaminophen rather than aspirin.
Atenolol	Category C. May cause bradycardia and hypotension in infants exposed near term. Monitor blood pressure and heart rate carefully.
Atropine	Category C. No reports of fetal risk available.
Aurothioglucose	Category C. No reports of fetal risk available; however, experience with its use during pregnancy limited.
Azathioprine	Category D. Most investigators have found azathioprine to be relatively safe. In a few cases, however, abnormalities have been reported, including leukopenia and thrombocytopenia, immunosuppression, transient chromosomal aberrations, and congenital defects. Interferes with effectiveness of an intrauterine contraceptive device.
Bacampicillin	Category B. No reports of fetal risk available.
Bacitracin	Category C. No reports of fetal risk available.
BCG vaccine	Category C. Animal studies have not been done. If possible, avoid use in pregnancy.
Belladonna	Category C. Associated with fetal malformations of varying

Drug or Substance	FDA Fetal Risk Category, Adverse Effects, and Clinical Comments
	severity in general and with minor malformations when used in the first trimester.
Benzocaine	Category C. No adverse effects reported.
Benzoyl peroxide	Category C. No adverse effects reported.
Benzthiazide	Category D. Thiazide-related diuretics may cause increased risk of congenital defects if taken during the first trimester. May also cause hypoglycemia, thrombocytopenia, hyponatremia, hypokalemia, and death. May inhibit labor. Use during pregnancy only if required for patients with heart disease. Carefully monitor infant's electrolytes, platelet count, and serum glucose after birth.
Benztropine	Category C. May cause decreased intestinal motility in the infant.
Beta carotene.	Category C. No reports of fetal risk available.
Betamethasone	Category C. Stimulates fetal lung maturation, thus reducing incidence and severity of respiratory distress syndrome. No reports of congenital defects associated with human use of corticosteroids in pregnancy.
Bethanechol	Category C. No reports of fetal risk available, but data limited.
Biperiden	Category C. No reports of fetal risk available.
Bisacodyl	Category C. Bulk-forming (methylcellulose) or surfactant (docusate) laxatives preferred for use in pregnancy over this stimulant laxative.
Bismuth subsalicylate (Pepto-Bismol)	Contains salicylates. See Aspirin.
Bleomycin	Category C. If possible, avoid during pregnancy. Two normal infants were born to mothers receiving bleomycin and other antineoplastic agents in the 2nd and 3rd trimesters.
Bretylium	Category C. No reports of fetal risk available; however, may cause maternal hypotension, with potential risk to the fetus from reduced uterine blood flow and hypoxia.
Bromides	Category D. Possible association with polydactyly, GI malformations, clubfoot, and congenital dislocation of hip. May cause neonatal bromism (poor suck, diminished Moro's reflex, hypotonia). Monitor serum bromide concentrations in the newborn.
Bromocriptine	Category C. Does not pose significant risk to the fetus.
Brompheniramine	Category C. Increased risk of fetal malformations if taken during the first trimester.
Buclizine	Category C. Possible increased risk of fetal malformations.
Busulfan	Category D. Use during pregnancy associated with fetal malformations and low birth weight.
Butalbital	Category C. No association with fetal malformations reported. However, withdrawal syndrome may occur; observe infant for 48 hours after birth.
Butorphanol	Category B. No association with fetal malformations reported; however, respiratory depression and withdrawal syndrome may occur.
Caffeine	Category B. Moderate consumption of caffeine probably does not pose a risk to the fetus; even so, it is prudent to avoid or limit its consumption. Consumption of 6–8 cups

Drug or Substance	FDA Fetal Risk Category, Adverse Effects, and Clinical Comments
	of coffee per day may be associated with decreased fertility, spontaneous abortion, and low birth weight.
Calcifediol	Category A for RDA amounts; category D for therapeutic and higher doses. Calcifediol is a vitamin D analog. High doses of vitamin D are teratogenic in animals but not in humans. Because vitamin D raises calcium levels, it may be associated with supravalvular aortic stenosis syndrome, which is often associated with hypercalcemia of infancy.
Calcitonin	Category B. No reports of fetal risk available.
Calcitriol	Category A for RDA amounts; category D for therapeutic and higher doses. High doses of vitamin D are teratogenic in animals but not in humans. Because vitamin D raises calcium levels, it may be associated with supravalvular aortic stenosis syndrome, which is often associated with hypercalcemia of infancy.
Camphor	Category C. No reports of fetal risk with topical application available. May cause fetal death and respiratory failure with maternal ingestion.
Captopril	Category C. Fetal malformations and intrauterine growth retardation have been associated with the use of captopril during pregnancy in 2 cases. Is embryocidal in animals. Data are limited, but it is recommended that this drug be avoided during pregnancy.
Carbachol	Category C. No reports of fetal risk available.
Carbamazepine	Category C. May cause craniofacial defects, fingernail hypoplasia, developmental delay (similar to fetal hydantoin syndrome).
Carbarsone	Category D. Contains arsenic, which has been associated with lesions of the CNS. If possible, avoid during pregnancy.
Carbenicillin	Category B. This drug has been used in a large number of pregnancies; no malformations have been associated with its use.
Carbimazole	Category D. May cause aplasia cutis (scalp defects). For the treatment of hyperthyroidism during pregnancy, use propylthiouracil rather than carbimazole or methimazole.
Carbinoxamine	Category C. No reports of fetal risk available, but data limited.
Carphenazine	Category C. No reports of fetal risk available, but data limited.
Casanthranol	Category C. No reports of fetal anomalies reported in 109 infants exposed to this drug during pregnancy.
Cascara Sagrada	Category C. Higher than expected risk for benign tumors in one study, but confirmation needed.
Castor oil	Category C. May cause premature labor.
Cefaclor	Category B. No reports of fetal risk available.
Cefadroxil	Category B. No reports of fetal risk available.
Cefamandole	Category B. Data are limited, but no abnormalities noted in one infant exposed to this drug in the first trimester.
Cefazolin	Category B. No reports of fetal risk available.
Cefonicid	Category B. No reports of fetal risk available.
Cefoperazone	Category B. No adverse newborn effects noted when administered to the mother at term.

Drug or Substance	FDA Fetal Risk Category, Adverse Effects, and Clinical Comments
Ceforanide	Category B. No reports of fetal risk available.
Cefotaxime	Category B. No reports of fetal risk available.
Cefoxitin	Category B. No adverse newborn effects noted when administered to the mother at term.
Ceftizoxime	Category B. No adverse newborn effects noted when administered to the mother at term.
Ceftriaxone	Category B. No adverse newborn effects noted when administered to the mother at term.
Cefuroxime	Category B. No adverse newborn effects noted.
Cephalexin	Category B. No adverse newborn effects noted.
Cephalothin	Category B. No adverse newborn effects noted.
Cephapirin	Category B. No data available.
Cephradine	Category B. No adverse newborn effects noted.
Chloral hydrate	Category C. No adverse effects reported.
Chlorambucil	Category D. Reports of unilateral agenesis of kidney and ureter, cardiovascular anomalies. May cause low birth weight.
Chloramphenicol	Category C. No congenital defects reported. Avoid at term because of the risk for gray syndrome (cardiovascular collapse).
Chlordiazepoxide	Category D. Some studies have found increased risk of fetal malformations; however, others have not confirmed this. When given at term, neonatal depression with hypotonia persisting for up to a week has been reported. Neonatal withdrawal syndrome may occur.
Chloroquine	Category C. Generally considered safe, but there may be a small increased risk of birth defects.
Chlorothiazide	Category D. Thiazide-related diuretics may cause increased risk of congenital defects if taken during the first trimester. May also cause hypoglycemia, thrombocytopenia, hyponatremia, hypokalemia, and death. May inhibit labor. Use in pregnancy only if required for patients with heart disease. Monitor infant's electrolytes, platelet count, and serum glucose carefully after birth.
Chlorpheniramine	Category B. Possible association with fetal malformations reported, but statistical significance unknown.
Chlorpromazine	Category C. Probably safe and effective for treatment of vomiting and nausea of pregnancy when used occasionally at low doses. Avoid administration at term because it may cause hypotension. May cause extrapyramidal syndrome (tremors, increased muscle tone) in the infant when administered near term.
Chlorpropamide	Category D. Pregnant diabetics should be managed with insulin, not oral hypoglycemics. Causes symptomatic hypoglycemia due to hyperinsulinism in the newborn. Monitor the infant's serum glucose for 5 days after birth (see p 211 for treatment of hypoglycemia).
Chlortetracycline	Category D. Tetracyclines should be avoided during pregnancy because they may cause adverse effects, including yellow staining of teeth, inhibition of bone growth, maternal liver toxicity, and congenital defects.
Chlorthalidone	Category D. Thiazide-related diuretics may cause increased risk of congenital defects if taken during the first trimester.

Drug or Substance	FDA Fetal Risk Category, Adverse Effects, and Clinical Comments
	May also cause hypoglycemia, thrombocytopenia, hyponatremia, hypokalemia, and death. May inhibit labor. Use in pregnancy only if required for patients with heart disease. Carefully monitor infant's electrolytes, platelet count, and serum glucose after birth.
Cholecalciferol	Category A for RDA amounts; category D for therapeutic and higher doses. Calcifediol is a vitamin D analog. High doses of vitamin D are teratogenic in animals but not in humans. Because vitamin D raises calcium levels, it may be associated with supravalvular aortic stenosis syndrome, which is often associated with hypercalcemia of infancy.
Cholera vaccine	Category C. Inactivated bacterial vaccine. May be given in pregnancy to meet travel requirements.
Cholestyramine	Category C. Not systemically absorbed but may bind fat-soluble vitamins in GI tract and cause vitamin deficiency in the fetus, although this effect has not been reported.
Ciclopirox	Category B. No adverse effects reported.
Cimetidine	Category B. One report of transient liver impairment in the newborn has not been confirmed by other investigators.
Cisplatin	Category D. Data limited to one case report in which no adverse effects to the fetus were reported.
Citrate and citric acid (Shohl's, Bicitra, Polycitra)	Category C. Avoid sodium citrate in toxemic patients (contains 1 mEq/mL sodium).
Clemastine	Category C. No data available.
Clindamycin	Category B. No adverse effects reported.
Clofibrate	Category C. No adverse effects reported; however, data limited. Avoid administration near term, especially in preterm infants, because of their limited capacity for glucuronidation of this compound.
Clomiphene	Category X. May cause neural tube defects and other fetal malformations.
Clomipramine	Category D. Three cases of infant lethargy, hypotonia, cyanosis, jitteriness, irregular respirations, respiratory acidosis, and hypothermia have been reported.
Clonazepam	Category C. May cause apnea.
Clonidine	Category C. Data limited; however, no adverse effects reported.
Clotrimazole	Category B. No adverse effects reported.
Cloxacillin	Category B. No adverse effects reported.
Coal tar	Category C. No adverse effects reported.
Cocaine	Category C. Or Category X for nonmedicinal use. May cause withdrawal syndrome, multisystem abnormalities due to the vasoconstrictive properties of the drug including urogenital anomalies, prematurity, spontaneous abortions, fetal growth retardation, neurobehavioral deficits, EEG abnormalities, cerebral infarctions, cardiorespiratory pattern abnormalities, and abruptio placentae.
Codeine	Category C. May cause malformations, respiratory depression, and withdrawal syndrome.
Colchicine	Category C. Use by the father prior to conception associated with atypical Down's syndrome; however, not confirmed by other investigators.

Drug or Substance	FDA Fetal Risk Category, Adverse Effects, and Clinical Comments
Colestipol	Category C. Not systemically absorbed but may bind fat-soluble vitamins in GI tract and cause vitamin deficiency in the fetus, although this effect has not been reported.
Colistimethate	Category B. No adverse effects reported.
Contraceptives, oral	Category X. May affect development of sexual organs and may cause hyperbilirubinemia in the newborn.
Corticotropin	Category C. No adverse effects reported.
Cortisone	Category D. No association with congenital malformations found in one large study; however, other studies reported abnormalities including cataracts, cyclopia, interventricular septal defect, gastroschisis, and other abnormalities.
Coumadin	Category D. Significant risk of congenital defects. May cause fetal warfarin syndrome (hypoplastic, flattened nasal bridge, stippled epiphyses, and possibly other features such as low birth weight, eye defects, development retardation, congenital heart disease, and death). May also cause hemorrhage. If anticoagulation is required during pregnancy, heparin given at the lowest effective dose is probably a safer choice.
Cromolyn	Category B. Generally considered safe for use in pregnancy.
Crotamiton	Category C. No adverse effects reported. It is one of the preferred drugs for treatment of scabies in pregnant women.
Cyclacillin	Category B. Has been used in a large number of pregnancies and has not been associated with malformations.
Cyclamate	Category C. No adverse effects reported.
Cyclizine	Category B. Teratogenic in animals but not in humans.
Cyclophosphamide	Category D. May cause fetal malformations from first-trimester exposure, possible pancytopenia, low birth weight. Paternal use of the drug prior to conception may cause malformations in the infant.
Cyproheptadine	Category B. No adverse effects reported.
Cytarabine	Category D. May cause chromosomal abnormalities and congenital anomalies with maternal or paternal use prior to conception, and low birth weight; however, normal infants have been delivered.
Dacarbazine	Category C. No information available.
Dactinomycin	Category C. Stillbirth and low birth weight may occur; however, normal infants have been delivered.
Danthron	Category C. One study reported a higher than expected risk of benign tumors, but confirmation of this is needed.
Daunorubicin	Category D. Successful pregnancies with normal infants reported; however, abnormalities such as low birth weight, anemia, hypoglycemia, intrauterine death, and myocardial necrosis may occur. Paternal use may result in congenital defects in the infant.
Deferoxamine	Category C. No abnormalities reported.
Demeclocycline	Category D. Tetracyclines should be avoided during pregnancy because they may cause adverse effects, including yellow staining of teeth, inhibition of bone growth, maternal liver toxicity, and congenital defects.
Desipramine	Category C. Withdrawal syndrome reported.
Desmopressin	Category B. No adverse effects reported.
Dexamethasone	Category C. No known congenital defects reported. Given in premature labor to stimulate fetal lung maturation.

Drug or Substance	FDA Fetal Risk Category, Adverse Effects, and Clinical Comments
Dextroamphetamine	Category C. May cause congenital defects such as cardiac abnormalities, biliary atresia, and eye defects; may cause withdrawal syndrome.
Diatrizoate	Category D. Monitor thyroid function because this drug may suppress the fetal thyroid gland when administered by intra-amniotic injection.
Diazepam	Category D. May cause hypotonia, lethargy, sucking difficulties, and withdrawal syndrome. May also cause craniofacial abnormalities, sullen and expressionless face, low Apgar scores, apneic spells, delayed motor development, and hypotonia.
Diazoxide	Category C. May cause transient fetal bradycardia and hyperglycemia.
Dicloxacillin	Category B. No adverse effects reported.
Dicumarol	Category D. This drug is a coumadin (warfarin) derivative; there is significant risk of congenital defects. May cause fetal warfarin syndrome (hypoplastic, flattened nasal bridge, stippled epiphyses, and possibly other features such as low birth weight, eye defects, developmental retardation, congenital heart disease, and death). May also cause hemorrhage. If anticoagulation is required during pregnancy, heparin given at the lowest effective dose is probably a safer choice.
Dienestrol	Category X. Contraindicated during pregnancy. May lead to high estrogen concentrations in the blood leading to fetal malformations.
Diethylstilbestrol	Category X. May result in complications of the reproductive system, including carcinoma of the cervix and vagina. Hirsutism and irregular menses may result, but this is controversial. GU abnormalities, including neoplasms, may also occur in male offspring.
Digitalis	Category C. No congenital defects reported. Neonatal death has resulted from maternal overdose.
Digitoxin	Category C. No congenital defects reported.
Digoxin	Category C. No congenital defects reported.
Dihydrotachysterol	Category A for RDA amounts; category D for therapeutic and higher doses. Calcifediol is a vitamin D analog. High doses of vitamin D are teratogenic in animals but not in humans. Because vitamin D raises calcium levels, it may be associated with supravalvular aortic stenosis syndrome, which is often associated with hypercalcemia of infancy.
Dimenhydrinate	Category B. Has not been associated with major or minor fetal malformations. May have oxytocic effect.
Diphenhydramine	Category C. May be associated with fetal malformations such as GU malformations, inguinal hernia, club foot, ventricular septal defect, and other abnormalities such as oral clefts and withdrawal syndrome.
Diphenoxylate (combined with atropine, Lomotil)	Category C. No abnormalities reported.
Diphtheria and tetanus toxoids	Category C. No data available on safety of diphtheria toxoid; therefore, the manufacturer does not recommend use of the combination product in pregnancy.
Dipyridamole	Category C. No abnormalities reported.

Drug or Substance	FDA Fetal Risk Category, Adverse Effects, and Clinical Comments
Disopyramide	Category C. No abnormalities reported.
Disulfiram	Category X. Causes fetal malformations and spontaneous abortion.
Dobutamine	Category C. No adverse effects reported, but data limited.
Docusate	Category C. No fetal malformations reported. Possible hypomagnesemia with use throughout pregnancy.
Dopamine	Category C. No adverse effects reported.
Doxepin	Category C. Possible decrease in GI motility if given at term.
Doxorubicin	Category D. Normal pregnancies have occurred in mothers treated with this drug; however, fetal malformations have also been reported.
Doxycycline	Category D. Tetracyclines should be avoided during pregnancy because they may cause adverse effects, including yellow staining of teeth, inhibition of bone growth, maternal liver toxicity, and congenital defects.
Doxylamine	Category B. Probably not associated with malformations.
Droperidol	Category C. No adverse effects reported.
Echothiophate	Category C. No information available, but transplacental passage not likely due to its chemical structure.
Edrophonium	Category C. No adverse effects reported. May cause premature labor.
Enalapril	Category C. May cause renal malformations, hypotension, and renal failure at birth. If oligohydramnios occurs, change mother to another antihypertensive agent.
Ephedrine	Category C. Minor fetal malformations may possibly be associated with its use during the first trimester. May cause fetal tachycardia.
Epinephrine	Category C. May cause fetal malformations with first-trimester use and inguinal hernia with use anytime during pregnancy.
Ergocalciferol	Category A for RDA amounts; category D for therapeutic and higher doses. Calcifediol is a vitamin D analog. High doses of vitamin D are teratogenic in animals but not in humans. Because vitamin D raises calcium levels, it may be associated with supravalvular aortic stenosis syndrome, which is often associated with hypercalcemia of infancy.
Ergotamine derivatives	Category X. May cause intrauterine fetal death from drug-induced increase in uterine motility and placental vasoconstriction.
Erythromycin	Category B. No abnormalities reported.
Estradiol	Category X. Estrogenic hormones contraindicated during pregnancy. In utero exposure may cause developmental changes in psychosexual performance of boys, less heterosexual experience, and fewer masculine interests.
Estrogens (conjugated)	Category X. Estrogenic hormones contraindicated during pregnancy. May cause fetal malformations.
Ethacrynic acid	Category D. May decrease placental perfusion, ototoxicity. Not recommended for use in pregnancy.
Ethambutol	Category B. No abnormalities reported.
Ethinyl estradiol	Category X. Use of estrogenic hormones during pregnancy contraindicated. In utero exposure may cause developmental changes in psychosexual performance of boys, less heterosexual experience, and fewer masculine interests.

Drug or Substance	FDA Fetal Risk Category, Adverse Effects, and Clinical Comments
Ethiodized oil	Category D. May cause neonatal hypothyroidism.
Ethisterone	Category D. Possible association with congenital anomalies.
Ethosuximide	Category C. May cause congenital anomalies, spontaneous hemorrhage in the neonate.
Ethynodiol	Category D. May cause modified development of sexual organs and hyperbilirubinemia of the newborn.
Famotidine	Category B. No adverse effects reported, but data limited.
Fenoprofen	Category B; category D if used near term. No congenital malformations reported. May cause constriction of ductus arteriosus in utero, persistent pulmonary hypertension of the newborn, and inhibition of labor.
Fenoterol	Category B. No malformations reported. Inhibits uterine activity at term.
Fentanyl	Category B; category D with prolonged high doses. No malformations reported. May cause respiratory depression and withdrawal syndrome.
Ferrous sulfate	Category B. No adverse effects reported.
Flecainide	Category C. No congenital defects reported.
Flucytosine	Category C. No defects reported, although its metabolite (flurouracil) may produce fetal malformations.
Fludrocortisone (Florinef)	Category C. Observe infant for signs of adrenocortical insufficiency and treat if required.
Fluoride	Category C. Crosses the placenta. No information available on fetal effects.
Fluorouracil	Category D. May cause fetal malformations (first-trimester use), cyanosis and jerking extremities (third-trimester use), and low birth weight (used at any time during pregnancy).
Fluphenazine	Category C. Extrapyramidal effects; possible congenital malformations in one infant.
Folic acid	Category A. Folate deficiency may result in congenital anomalies.
Formaldehyde	No FDA fetal risk category established. Increased risk of spontaneous abortion and small-for-gestational-age infants.
Furazolidone	Category C. No congenital defects reported.
Furosemide	Category C. No congenital defects reported. Generally not indicated in pregnancy except in patients with cardiovascular disorders.
Gentamicin	Category C. No congenital defects reported. Potentiation of magnesium sulfate-induced neuromuscular weakness. Monitor infant for ototoxicity as this has occurred with other aminoglycosides (kanamycin and streptomycin).
Gentian violet	Category C. Fetal malformations may possibly occur, but confirmation needed.
Glycopyrrolate	Category B. Minor fetal malformations may possibly occur but are unlikely.
Gold sodium thiomalate	Category C. Probably no risk to the fetus, but experience limited.
Griseofulvin	Category C. Teratogenic in animals, but no data available for humans.
Guaifenesin	Category C. May cause inguinal hernias with first-trimester use.
Haloperidol	Category C. Limb reductions reported in 2 reports, but other studies have not confirmed this.

Drug or Substance	FDA Fetal Risk Category, Adverse Effects, and Clinical Comments
Heparin	Category C. No reports of congenital defects reported. Heparin preferred over oral anticoagulants during pregnancy.
Hepatitis B immune globulin (HBIG)	Category B. No adverse effects reported.
Hepatitis B vaccine	Category C. No adverse effects reported.
Heroin	Category B; category D with prolonged high-dose use. May cause congenital malformations, jaundice, respiratory distress syndrome, low Apgar scores, withdrawal, low birth weight, and increased perinatal mortality.
Hexachlorophene	Category C. Increased risk of anomalies with excessive first-trimester use.
Hexamethonium	Category C. No congenital abnormalities reported.
Homatropine	Category C. Possible association with minor malformations.
Hyaluronidase	Category C. No adverse effects reported.
Hydralazine	Category C. No congenital abnormalities reported.
Hydrochlorothiazide.	Category D. See Chlorothiazide.
Hydrocodone	Category B; category D with prolonged high-dose use. No malformations reported; however, respiratory depression or withdrawal syndrome may occur.
Hydromorphone	Category B; category D with prolonged high-dose use. No malformations reported; however, respiratory depression or withdrawal syndrome may occur.
Hydroxyprogesterone	Category D. May cause ambiguous genitalia. In males, may cause less heterosexual experience and fewer masculine interests.
Hydroxyzine	Category C. Possible relation between fetal malformations and use during first trimester, but statistical significance not known.
Ibuprofen	Category B; category D in third trimester. No congenital anomalies reported. May cause closing of the ductus arteriosus in utero, persistent pulmonary hypertension of the newborn, and inhibition of labor.
Idoxuridine	Category C. No data available on use in human pregnancy.
Imipramine	Category D. May cause fetal malformations, withdrawal syndrome, and urine retention.
Indomethacin	Category B; category D if taken after 34 weeks' gestation. May cause delayed labor, premature closure of the ductus arteriosus, persistent pulmonary hypertension of the newborn, renal failure, intestinal perforation, and death.
Insulin	Category B. Insulin rather than oral hypoglycemics should be used to control diabetes. Poorly controlled diabetes associated with an increased risk of congenital defects.
Intravenous fat emulsion	Category C. No adverse effects reported.
Iodine	Category D. Topical use may result in significant absorption of iodine, resulting in transient hypothyroidism in the newborn. See also Povidone iodine and Potassium iodide.
Iron (ferrous sulfate)	Category B. No adverse effects reported.
Isocarboxazid	Category C. Increased risk of fetal malformations.
Isoetharine	Category C. Use in the first-trimester associated with a possible increased risk of minor fetal malformations.
Isoniazid	Category C. Increased risk of fetal malformations found in one study but not confirmed by other studies.

Drug or Substance	FDA Fetal Risk Category, Adverse Effects, and Clinical Comments
Isoproterenol	Category C. Use in the first-trimester associated with a possible increased risk of minor fetal malformations.
Isosorbide dinitrate	Category C. Possible association of fetal malformation with first-trimester exposure to vasodilators.
Isotretinoin (Accutane, retinoic acid)	Category X. With first-trimester use, causes severe birth defects including external ear, CNS, craniofacial, cardiac, and thymic anomalies. Prevent pregnancy during use and discontinue the drug 1 month prior to conception.
Isoxuprine	Category C. No congenital defects reported; however, fetal tachycardia and neonatal ileus may occur, and infants with cord levels exceeding 10 ng/mL may have respiratory distress syndrome, hypotension, hypocalcemia, and death.
Kanamycin	Category D. May cause eighth cranial nerve damage.
Labetalol	Category C. May cause hypotension and bradycardia. Monitor infant for 48 hours after birth.
Lactulose	Category B. No information available.
Laetrile	Category C. Theoretical risk of cyanide poisoning.
Levallorphan	Category D. May cause neonatal respiratory depression.
Levarterenol	Category D. No fetal malformations reported but may cause reduction of uterine blood flow.
Levorphanol	Category B with therapeutic doses; category D if used at high doses for prolonged periods of time. May cause respiratory depression and withdrawal syndrome.
Levothyroxine	Category A. First-trimester use possibly associated with cardiovascular anomalies, Down's syndrome and polydactyly, but confirmation needed.
Lidocaine	Category C. No association with malformations were found.
Lincomycin	Category B. No congenital anomalies or other problems reported.
Lindane (Kwell)	Category C. May cause neurotoxicity and aplastic anemia. Use pyrethrins with piperonyl butoxide rather than lindane to treat lice during pregnancy.
Liothyronine	Category A. No adverse effects reported.
Liotrix	Category A. First-trimester use possibly associated with cardiovascular anomalies, Down's syndrome, and polydactyly, but confirmation needed.
Lithium	Category D. May cause cardiac congenital defects when used in the first trimester and toxicity in the newborn (cyanosis, hypotonia, bradycardia, nephrogenic diabetes insipidis, and other disorders) when used near term. Reduce risk by using lowest dose possible, monitoring serum concentrations, and avoiding sodium-restricted diets and sodium-wasting diuretics.
Loperamide	Category B. No adverse effects reported.
Lorazepam	Category C. May cause neonatal respiratory depression and hypotonia.
LSD	Category C. Available data indicate that pure LSD does not cause chromosomal abnormalities, spontaneous abortions, or congenital malformations.
Lynestrenol	Category D. Use of progestogens not recommended during pregnancy.
Lypressin	Category B. No adverse effects reported.
Magnesium salts	Category B. May cause neonatal respiratory depression and muscle weakness if used just prior to delivery and congeni-

Drug or Substance	FDA Fetal Risk Category, Adverse Effects, and Clinical Comments
	tal rickets with prolonged infusion. Possible respiratory arrest when gentamicin given to newborns with high magnesium levels. Inhibits indomethacin effect for ductal closure.
Mandelic acid	Category C. Possible association with fetal malformations, but confirmation needed.
Mannitol	Category C. No adverse effects reported.
Maprotiline	Category B. No adverse effects reported.
Marijuana	Category C. May cause impaired fetal growth.
Measles vaccine	Category X. Not for use during pregnancy because of risk of fetal malformations.
Mechlorethamine	Category D. Possible fetal malformations with first-trimester use and low birth weight with use any time during pregnancy.
Meclizine	Category B. Possible fetal malformations reported, but confirmation needed.
Meclofenamate	Category B; category D if taken in third trimester. May cause delayed labor, premature closure of the ductus arteriosus, and persistent pulmonary hypertension of the newborn.
Medroxyprogesterone	Category D. Not recommended for use in pregnancy because of risk of fetal malformations associated with use of female sex hormones.
Melphalan	Category D. May cause low birth weight.
Menadione	Category C; category X if given at term. May cause hyperbilirubinemia with increased risk of kernicterus if given at term. Use phytonadione (vitamin K_1), not menadione or menadiol (Synkayvite), at birth for prevention of hemorrhagic disease of the newborn.
Meperidine	Category B; category D with prolonged use of high doses. May cause respiratory depression and withdrawal syndrome. First-trimester use possibly associated with inguinal hernia, but confirmation needed.
Mephentermine	Category C. No adverse effects reported.
Mephenytoin	Category C. No adverse effects reported.
Mephobarbital	Category D. May cause withdrawal and hemorrhagic disease of the newborn.
Mepindolol	Category C. May cause bradycardia and hypotension in infants exposed near term. Carefully monitor blood pressure and heart rate.
Meprobamate	Category D. May be associated with fetal malformations when used in the first trimester. Avoid during pregnancy.
Mercaptopurine	Category D. May cause fetal malformations, pancytopenia, and low birth weight.
Mercury	Category not established. May be associated with increased risk of cerebral palsy.
Mesoridazine	Category C. No adverse effects reported.
Mestranol	Category X. May cause fetal malformations. Avoid estrogenic hormones during pregnancy.
Metaproterenol	Category C. Prevents premature labor. May cause fetal tachycardia and neonatal hypoglycemia.
Metaraminol	Category D. May reduce uterine blood flow.
Methadone	Category B; category D with prolonged use of high doses. May cause withdrawal syndrome, low birth weight, and death.
Methamphetamine	Category C. With amphetamine abuse, there is an increased

Drug or Substance	FDA Fetal Risk Category, Adverse Effects, and Clinical Comments
	incidence of preterm labor, placental abruption, fetal distress, postpartum hemorrhage, intrauterine growth retardation, feeding difficulty, drowsiness, and lassitude that may last several months.
Methantheline	Category C. Possibly associated with minor fetal malformations.
Methaqualone	Category D. Possible fetal malformations reported.
Methenamine	Category C. Associated with fetal malformations, but confirmation needed.
Methicillin	Category B. No adverse effects reported.
Methimazole	Category D. May cause aplasia cutis (scalp defects). Use propylthiouracil rather than carbimazole or methimazole to treat hyperthyroidism during pregnancy.
Methotrexate	Category D. Associated with fetal malformations and low birth weight.
Methsuximide	Category C. No adverse effects reported.
Methyldopa	Category C. Probably not associated with fetal malformations. Monitor neonate for hypotension for 48 hours after delivery.
Methylene Blue	Category C. Possibly associated with fetal malformations, but confirmation needed. May cause hemolytic anemia, hyperbilirubinemia, and methemoglobinemia with intra-amniotic injection of large doses.
Methylergonovine	Category C. Stimulates contractions of uterus. Indicated only for postpartum use and in the second stage of labor.
Methylphenidate	Category C. No adverse effects reported.
Methysergide	Category not established. Do not use in pregnancy due to oxytocic properties.
Metoclopramide	Category B. No adverse effects reported, but data limited.
Metolazone	Category D. Thiazide-related diuretics may cause increased risk of congenital defects if taken during the first trimester. May also cause hypoglycemia, thrombocytopenia, hyponatremia, hypokalemia, and death, and may inhibit labor. Use during pregnancy only if required for patients with heart disease. Carefully monitor infant's electrolytes, platelet count, and serum glucose after birth.
Metoprolol	Category B. Hypotension and bradycardia may occur. Monitor infant for 48 hours after birth.
Metrizamide	Category D. Monitor the infant's thyroid function at birth (see p 000, Thyroid Diseases). A related drug, diatrizoate, has suppressed the fetal thyroid gland when administered by intra-amniotic injection.
Metronidazole	Category B. Possible fetal malformations with first-trimester use.
Miconazole	Category B. No adverse effects reported.
Mineral Oil	Category C. No adverse effects reported, but may inhibit maternal absorption of fat-soluble vitamins (ADEK).
Minocycline	Category D. Tetracyclines should be avoided during pregnancy because they may cause adverse effects, including yellow staining of teeth, inhibition of bone growth, maternal liver toxicity, and congenital defects.
Minoxidil	Category C. No adverse effects reported.
Mithramycin (Plicamycin)	Category X. May cause fetal harm. Avoid during pregnancy.

Drug or Substance	FDA Fetal Risk Category, Adverse Effects, and Clinical Comments
Molindone	Category C. No adverse effects reported.
Morphine	Category B; category D with prolonged use of high doses. May cause respiratory depression and withdrawal syndrome. First-trimester use possibly associated with inguinal hernia, but confirmation needed.
Moxalactam	Category C. No adverse effects reported.
Mumps virus vaccine	Category X. Not for use in pregnancy because of risk of malformations.
Nadolol	Category C. May cause bradycardia and hypotension in infants exposed near term. Carefully monitor blood pressure and heart rate.
Nafcillin	Category B. No adverse effects reported.
Nalbuphine	Category B. May cause respiratory depression and withdrawal syndrome.
Naldixic acid	Category B. No adverse effects reported.
Naloxone	Category B. No adverse effects reported.
Naproxen	Category B; category D if given near term. May cause closure of the ductus arteriosus, with resulting pulmonary hypertension of the newborn. Avoid use near term.
Neomycin	Category C. No fetal malformations reported. May cause ototoxicity, which has been reported with use of other aminoglycosides.
Neostigmine	Category C. No fetal malformations reported.
Niacin/niacinamide	Category A for RDA doses; category C with excessive intake. No adverse effects reported.
Nicotine	Category X. May cause dose-related low birth weight, decreased placental blood flow, increased risk of stillborn or neonatal death, and sudden infant death syndrome (SIDS).
Nifedipine	Category C. No adverse effects reported, but experience limited.
Nitrofurantoin	Category B. No adverse effects reported. May theoretically cause hemolysis if given near term in patients with glucose-6-phosphate dehydrogenase (G6PD) deficiency.
Nitroglycerin	Category C. No adverse effects reported; however, fetal malformations have been reported with first-trimester use of other vasodilators.
Nitroprusside	Category C. May cause fetal bradycardia.
Norethindrone	Category D. May cause masculinization of female infants.
Norethynodrel	Category D. May cause masculinization of female infants.
Nortriptyline	Category D. May possibly cause fetal malformations, but confirmation needed. May cause urine retention in the newborn.
Novobiocin	Category C. No adverse effects reported, but may cause hyperbilirubinemia if used near term.
Nystatin	Category B. No adverse effects reported.
Oleandomycin	Category C. No adverse effects reported.
Opium	Category B for therapeutic doses; category D for prolonged use of high doses. May cause respiratory depression and withdrawal syndrome. May also cause inguinal hernia, but confirmation needed.
Oral contraceptives	See Contraceptives, oral.
Oxacillin	Category B. No adverse effects reported.
Oxazepam	Category C. No adverse effects reported.

Drug or Substance	FDA Fetal Risk Category, Adverse Effects, and Clinical Comments
Oxprenolol	Category C. May cause bradycardia and hypotension in infants exposed near term. Carefully monitor blood pressure and heart rate.
Oxtriphylline	Category C. No adverse effects reported.
Oxycodone	Category B for therapeutic doses; category D for prolonged use of high doses. May cause withdrawal syndrome and respiratory depression. No congenital malformations reported.
Oxymorphone	Category B for therapeutic doses; category D for prolonged use of high doses. May cause withdrawal syndrome and respiratory depression. No congenital malformations reported.
Oxytetracycline	Category D. Tetracyclines should be avoided during pregnancy because they may cause adverse effects, including yellow staining of teeth, inhibition of bone growth, maternal liver toxicity, and congenital defects.
Pantothenic acid	Category A for RDA doses; category C for excessive doses. No adverse effects reported.
Paraldehyde	Category C. Easily diffuses across placenta and may cause neonatal respiratory depression when used at term.
Paramethadione	Category D. Increased risk of spontaneous abortion and other abnormalities, including tetralogy of Fallot, mental retardation, and failure to thrive.
Paregoric	Category B for therapeutic doses; category D for prolonged use of high doses. May cause withdrawal syndrome and respiratory depression. No congenital malformations reported.
Parenteral nutrition (TPN)	Category C. No adverse effects reported.
Penicillamine	Category D. May cause connective tissue abnormalities (cutis laxa).
Penicillin G/Penicillin G, benzathine/ Penicillin V	Category B. Association with adverse effects very unlikely.
Penicillin G, Procaine	Category B. Association with congenital malformations unlikely.
Pentazocine	Category B for therapeutic doses; category D for prolonged use of high doses. May cause withdrawal syndrome and respiratory depression. No congenital malformations reported.
Pentobarbital	Category D. May cause withdrawal syndrome and hemorrhage in the newborn.
Perphenazine	Category C. No adverse effects reported.
Phenacetin	Category B. May cause fetal malformations (musculoskeletal malformations, kidney and adrenal anomalies), but confirmation needed.
Phenazopyridine	Category B. No adverse effects reported.
Phencyclidine (PCP)	Category X. May cause dysmorphic features, nystagmus, hypertonicity, respiratory distress, and withdrawal syndrome.
Phenelzine	Category C. May cause fetal malformations.
Phenindione	Category D. There is significant risk of congenital defects. If anticoagulation is required during pregnancy, heparin is a safer drug choice.

Drug or Substance	FDA Fetal Risk Category, Adverse Effects, and Clinical Comments
Pheniramine	Category C. First-trimester use possibly associated with fetal malformations.
Phenobarbital	Category D. May cause withdrawal syndrome, hemorrhagic disease in the newborn, and minor fetal malformations.
Phenylephrine	Category C. Fetal malformations reported, but confirmation needed. May cause constriction of uterine vessels.
Phenylpropanolamine	Category C. May cause constriction of uterine vessels. May also cause malformations, but confirmation needed.
Phenytoin	Category D. May cause fetal hydantoin syndrome (craniofacial—broad nasal bridge, low set hairline, short neck, microcephaly; limbs—hypoplasia of nails and distal phalanges; impaired growth; and many other abnormalities). May also cause tumors and hemorrhage in the newborn at delivery.
Phytonadione	Category C. No adverse effects reported.
Pilocarpine	Category C. No adverse effects reported.
Pindolol	Category B. May cause bradycardia and hypotension in infants exposed near term. Carefully monitor blood pressure and heart rate.
Piperazine	Category B. No adverse effects reported.
Pneumococcal vaccine	Category C. No adverse effects reported; however, use during pregnancy for high-risk patients only.
Poliovirus vaccine, inactivated (Salk, injection, IPV) and Poliovirus vaccine (live, oral, OPV)	Category C. No adverse effects reported; however, use during pregnancy for patients with high risk of exposure only. IPV is preferred over OPV except for patients who need immediate protection.
Polymyxin B	Category B. No adverse effects reported.
Potassium chloride/potassium citrate/potassium acetate/potassium gluconate	Category A. No adverse effects reported.
Potassium iodide	Category D. May cause hypothyroidism and goiter with prolonged use; however, the 10-day preparation for thyroid surgery is safe.
Povidone-iodine	Category D. Topical use may result in significant absorption of iodine, resulting in transient hypothyroidism with goiter in the newborn.
Prazosin	Category C. No adverse effects reported.
Prednisone/prednisolone	Category B. May possibly cause immunosuppression and cataracts; carries a small risk of fetal malformations.
Primaquine	Category C. No adverse effects reported. May theoretically cause hemolysis if given near term in patients with glucose-6-phosphate dehydrogenase (G6PD) deficiency.
Primidone	Category D. Possible risk of fetal malformations similar to those associated with phenytoin and of tumors and hemorrhage of the newborn at birth.
Probenecid	Category B. No adverse effects reported.
Procarbazine	Category D. May cause fetal malformations and low birth weight.
Prochlorperazine	Category C. Fetal malformations reported rarely.
Promazine	Category C. Fetal malformations reported rarely.

Drug or Substance	FDA Fetal Risk Category, Adverse Effects, and Clinical Comments
Promethazine	Category C. Not a teratogen; however, may cause respiratory depression when given at term.
Propantheline	Category C. No adverse effects reported.
Propoxyphene	Category C. May possibly cause fetal malformations and has caused neonatal withdrawal syndrome.
Propranolol	Category C. May cause low birth weight, fetal depression at birth, prolonged labor, neonatal hypoglycemia, hypotension, and bradycardia. Carefully monitor blood pressure, respirations, and heart rate in infants exposed near term.
Propylthiouracil	Category D. Fetal malformations reported, but association with this drug unclear. May cause reversible hypothyroidism and goiter in the infant. Drug of choice to use to treat hypothyroidism during pregnancy.
Protamine	Category C. No adverse effects reported.
Pseudoephedrine	Category C. May cause minor fetal malformations with first-trimester use.
Psyllium (Metamucil)	Category B. Psyllium or another bulk-producing laxative is preferred if a laxative is needed during pregnancy.
Pyrantel pamoate	Category C. No adverse effects reported.
Pyrethrins with piperonyl butoxide	Category C. No adverse effects reported.
Pyridostigmine	Category C. May cause premature labor when given near term.
Pyridoxine	Category A. Probably does not cause fetal malformations.
Pyrilamine	Category C. May cause fetal malformations and benign tumors.
Pyrimethamine	Category C. Probably does not cause birth defects. Administer with folinic acid supplementation.
Pyrvinium pamoate	Category C. No adverse effects reported.
Quinacrine	Category C. May cause fetal malformations with first-trimester use.
Quinidine	Category C. May cause neonatal thrombocytopenia.
Quinine	Category X. Has caused malformations of the limbs, CNS, heart, and GI tract as well as deafness, and other abnormalities.
Rabies immune globulin	Category B. No adverse effects reported.
Ranitidine	Category B. No adverse effects reported, but data limited.
Reserpine	Category C. May cause fetal malformations, increased respiratory secretions, cyanosis, hypothermia, lethargy, and anorexia.
Ribavirin	Category X. Teratogenic in animals. No abnormalities were seen, however, in the one human exposure reported.
Rifampin	Category C. Probably not a teratogen. May cause hemorrhagic disease of the newborn; prevent with vitamin K administration.
Rubella vaccine	Category X. This live virus vaccine should not be used during pregnancy because of risk of congenital rubella syndrome.
Scopolamine	Category C. May cause tachycardia, fever, and lethargy.
Secobarbital	Category D. May cause hemorrhagic disease of the newborn. Prevent with vitamin K administration.
Selenium sulfide	Category C. No adverse effects reported.

Drug or Substance	FDA Fetal Risk Category, Adverse Effects, and Clinical Comments
Simethicone	Category C. No adverse effects reported.
Sodium iodide (1 131)	Category X. Has caused fetal malformations, damage to fetal thyroid gland, and hypothyroidism.
Sodium polystyrene sulfonate (Kayexalate)	Category C. No adverse effects reported.
Spectinomycin	Category B. No adverse effects reported.
Spironolactone	Category D. No adverse effects reported; however, there is a potential risk of antiandrogenic effects.
Streptokinase	Category C. No adverse effects reported.
Streptomycin	Category D. May cause eighth cranial nerve damage.
Sucralfate	Category B. No adverse effects reported.
Sulfasalazine	Category B. May increase risk of kernicterus when given near term.
Sulfonamides	Category B. May increase risk of kernicterus when given near term.
Sulindac	Category B; category D if used during last trimester. No congenital anomalies reported. May cause closing of the ductus arteriosus in utero, persistent pulmonary hypertension of the newborn, and inhibition of labor.
Terbutaline	Category B. May cause fetal tachycardia and neonatal hypoglycemia.
Tetanus immune globulin	Category B. No adverse effects reported.
Tetanus toxoid	Category C. No adverse effects reported.
Tetracycline	Category D. Tetracyclines should be avoided during pregnancy because they may cause adverse effects, including yellow staining of teeth, inhibition of bone growth, maternal liver toxicity, and congenital defects.
Theophylline	Category C. May cause transient tachycardia, irritability, and vomiting at birth, especially if mother's serum concentrations are above the therapeutic range. No congenital defects reported.
Thiabendazole	Category C. No adverse effects reported, but data limited.
Thiethylperazine	Category C. Do not use during pregnancy because of risk of fetal malformations.
Thioguanine	Category D. May cause fetal malformations and chromosomal abnormalities.
Thioridazine	Category C. Probably safe for use in pregnancy.
Thiotepa	Category D. No adverse effects reported, but data limited.
Thiothixene	Category C. No information available.
Thyroid	Category A. Probably safe for use in pregnancy.
Ticarcillin	Category B. No adverse effects reported.
Timolol	Category C. May cause bradycardia and hypotension in infants exposed near term. Carefully monitor blood pressure and heart rate.
Tobacco	Category X. Dose-related risk of low birth weight, decreased placental blood flow, decreased fetal breathing movements, stillbirth, neonatal death, and sudden infant death syndrome (SIDS).
Tobramycin	Category D. No congenital defects have been reported. Potentiation of magnesium sulfate-induced neuromuscular weakness. Monitor infant for ototoxicity, as it has occurred with other aminoglycosides (eg, kanamycin and streptomycin).

Drug or Substance	FDA Fetal Risk Category, Adverse Effects, and Clinical Comments
Tolazamide	Category C. May cause prolonged neonatal hypoglycemia when given near term.
Tolazoline	Category C. May cause fetal malformations.
Tolbutamide	Category C. May cause prolonged neonatal hypoglycemia when given near term.
Tolmetin	Category B; category D if given near term. No congenital anomalies reported. May cause closing of the ductus arteriosus in utero, persistent pulmonary hypertension of the newborn, and inhibition of labor.
Tolnaftate (Tinactin)	Category C. No information available.
Tranylcypromine	Category C. May cause fetal malformations.
Tretinoin	Category B. When used topically, teratogenic risk is thought to be close to zero.
Triamterine	Category D. No adverse effects reported.
Trifluoperazine	Category C. Probably safe for use in pregnancy.
Trihexyphenidyl	Category C. May cause congenital defects.
Trimeprazine	Category C. Has been associated with congenital defects, but confirmation needed.
Trimethadione	Category D. Causes adverse effects on the fetus, including intrauterine growth retardation, mental and physical retardation, impaired hearing, cardiac defects, abnormally set ears, oral clefts, fetal demise, urogenital malformations, skeletal abnormalities, and other abnormalities.
Trimethapan	Category C. No adverse effects reported.
Trimethobenzamide	Category C. May cause congenital defects and extrapyramidal dysfunction in the neonate.
Trimethoprim	Category C. This drug is a folate antagonist so there is a risk of fetal malformations; however, none attributable directly to trimethoprim have been reported.
Tripelennamine	Category B. No adverse effects reported.
Triprolidine	Category C. No adverse effects reported.
Tromethamine	Category C. No information available.
Urokinase	Category B. No adverse effects reported.
Valproic acid	Category D. Increases risk of spina bifida and fetal malformations similar to those caused by phenytoin.
Vancomycin	Category C. May cause hypotension if given near term. Infuse over 1 hour and monitor blood pressure.
Vasopressin	Category B. No fetal malformations reported. May cause uterine contractions.
Verapamil	Category C. May cause decreased urine blood flow, hypotension, and fetal bradycardia.
Vidarabine	Category C. Insufficient data available.
Vincristine	Category D. Congenital defects such as atrial septal defect, kidney malformation, pancytopenia, and low birth weight have been reported.
Vitamin A	Category A. Probably safe for use in pregnancy when used at the RDA dose, but congenital defects have been reported with excessive doses.
Vitamin B_{12}	Category A. No adverse effects reported.
Vitamin C	Category A. No reports directly linking this vitamin to congenital defects in humans. May cause scurvy in infants if it is used at high doses during pregnancy.
Vitamin D	Category A for RDA dose; category D for therapeutic and higher doses. High doses of vitamin D are teratogenic in animals but not in humans. Because vitamin D raises cal-

Drug or Substance	FDA Fetal Risk Category, Adverse Effects, and Clinical Comments
	cium levels, it may be associated with supravalvular aortic stenosis syndrome, which is often associated with hypercalcemia of infancy.
Vitamin E	Category A. No adverse effects reported.
Vitamin K	See Phytonadione; Menadione.
Warfarin	Category D. There is significant risk of congenital defects. May cause fetal warfarin syndrome (hypoplastic, flattened nasal bridge, stippled epiphyses; and other features such as low birth weight, eye defects, development retardation, congenital heart disease, and death). May also cause hemorrhage. If anticoagulation is required during pregnancy, heparin given at the lowest effective dose is probably a safer choice.
Zinc sulfate	Category C. No information available. Manufacturer recommends that supplementation not be given during pregnancy.

REFERENCES

Briggs GG, Freeman RK, Yaffe SJ: *Drugs in Pregnancy and Lactation,* 3rd ed. Williams & Wilkins, 1990.
Gilstrap LC, Little BB: *Drugs and Pregnancy.* Elsevier, New York, 1992.
Manufacturer's product information for medication listed.

Appendices

AFP. Alpha-fetoprotein
AGA. Appropriate for gestational age
ARC. AIDS-related complex
ASD. Atrial septal defect
ATN. Acute tubular necrosis
BG. Babygram (x-ray that includes the chest and abdomen)
BPD. Biparietal diameter
  Bronchopulmonary dysplasia
BW. Birth weight
  Body weight
CBG. Capillary blood gases
CDH. Congenital diaphragmatic hernia
CHD. Congenital hip dislocation
  Congenital heart disease
CID. Cytomegalovirus inclusion disease
CLD. Chronic lung disease
CPIP. Chronic pulmonary insufficiency of prematurity
CST. Contraction stress test
DDST. Denver Developmental Screening Test
ECMO. Extracorporeal membrane oxygenator
EDC. Estimated date of confinement
FBS. Fasting blood sugar
  Fetal blood sample
FHR. Fetal heart rate
FHT. Fetal heart tones
GA. Gestational age
  General anesthesia
GDM. Gestational diabetes mellitus
$G_xP_xAb_xLC_x$. Shorthand for gravida/para/abortion/living children
G_xP_x0000. First zero, full term; second zero, premature; third zero, abortion; fourth zero, living children
HC. Head circumference
HCM. Health care maintenance
HDON. Hemolytic disease of the newborn
HLHS. Hypoplastic left heart syndrome
HMD. Hyaline membrane disease
IDAM. Infant of a drug-addicted mother
INF. Intravenous nutritional feedings
IODAM. Infant of a drug-addicted mother
IODM. Infant of a diabetic mother
IUGR. Intrauterine growth retardation
IVH. Intraventricular hemorrhage
LBW. Low birth weight
LBWL. Low birth weight "lytes"
LGA. Large for gestational age
L/S ratio. Lecithin:sphingomyelin ratio
MAS. Meconium aspiration syndrome
MCA. Multiple congenital abnormalities
MCT. Medium-chain triglycerides

MSUD. Maple syrup urine disease
NEC. Necrotizing enterocolitis
NICU. Neonatal intensive care unit
NST. Nonstress test
OCT. Oxytocin challenge test
OFC. Occipital frontal circumference
P&PD. Percussion and postural drainage
PBLC. Premature birth, living child
PDA. Patent ductus arteriosus
PFC. Persistent fetal circulation
PIE. Pulmonary interstitial emphysema
PLAST. Percussion, lavage, suction, turn
PPH. Persistent pulmonary hypertension
PROM. Premature rupture of membranes
RDS. Respiratory distress syndrome
RLF. Retrolental fibroplasia
ROM. Range of motion
   Rupture of membranes
ROP. Retinopathy of prematurity
RT. Rubella titer
RVH. Right ventricular hypertrophy
Sao$_2$. Oxygen saturation of arterial blood
SEH. Subependymal hemorrhage
SGA. Small for gestational age
SIDS. Sudden infant death syndrome
SVD. Spontaneous vaginal delivery
TAR. Thrombocytopenia-absent radii (a syndrome)
TBLC. Term birth, living child
TD$_x$FLM. TD$_x$ fetal lung maturity
TEF. Tracheoesophageal fistula
THAM. Trishydroxymethylaminomethane (tromethamine)
THAN. Transient hyperammonemia of the newborn
TOF. Tetralogy of Fallot
TORCH. Toxoplasmosis, other, rubella, cytomegalovirus, herpes simplex
TORCHS. The same plus syphilis
TTN. Transient tachypnea of the newborn
UAC. Umbilical artery catheter
UVC. Umbilical vein catheter
VBG. Venous blood gas
VLBW. Very low birth weight

APPENDIX B. APGAR SCORING

Apgar scores are a numerical expression of the condition of a newborn infant on a scale of 0–10. The scores are usually recorded at 1 and 5 minutes after delivery and become a permanent part of the health record. They have clinical usefulness not only during the nursery stay but at later child health visits also, when clinical status at delivery may have a bearing on current diagnostic assessments. The system was originally described by Virginia Apgar, MD, an anesthesiologist, in 1953.

Sign	0	1	2
*A*ppearance (color)	Blue or pale	Pink body with blue extremities	Completely pink
*P*ulse (heart rate)	Absent	Slow (< 100/min)	> 100/min
*G*rimace (reflex irritability)	No response	Grimace	Cough or sneeze
*A*ctivity (muscle tone)	Limp	Some flexion	Active movements
*R*espirations	Absent	Slow, irregular	Good, crying

APPENDIX C. BLOOD PRESSURE DETERMINATIONS

APPENDIX TABLE C-1. NORMAL BLOOD PRESSURE IN PREMATURE INFANTS[a]

	600–999g		1000–1249 g	
Day	Systolic (SD)[b]	Diastolic (SD)	Systolic (SD)	Diastolic (SD)
1	37.9 (17.4)	23.2 (10.3)	44 (22.8)	22.5 (13.5)
3	44.9 (15.7)	30.6 (12.3)	48 (15.4)	36.5 (9.6)
7	50.0 (14.8)	30.4 (12.4)	57 (14.0)	42.5 (16.5)
14	50.2 (14.8)	37.4 (12.0)	53 (30.0)	
28	61.0 (23.5)	45.8 (27.4)	57 (30.0)	

[a] Based on data from Ingelfinger JR, Powers L, and Epstein MF: Blood pressure norms in low birth weight infants: Birth through four weeks. *Pediatr Res* 1983;**17**:319A.
[b] SD = standard deviation (plus or minus).

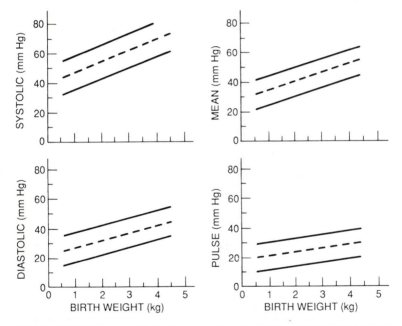

APPENDIX FIGURE C-1. Typical systolic, diastolic, mean aortic, and pulse pressure measured through umbilical artery catheters in healthy newborns up to 12 hours of age. (Reproduced, with permission, from Versmold HT et al: Aortic blood pressure during the first 12 hours of life in infants with birth weight from 610 to 4220 grams. *Pediatrics* 1981;**67**:611.)

APPENDIX D. CEREBROSPINAL FLUID NORMAL VALUES

OPENING PRESSURE	
Newborn	80–110 mm water
Infant	< 200 mm water
Glucose	
Premature	24–63 mg/dL (CSF:blood ratio 55–105%)
Term	44–128 mg/dL (CSF:blood ratio 44–128%)
PROTEIN	
Premature	65–150 mg/dL
Term	20–170 mg/dL
WHITE CELL COUNT	
Premature	0–25/mm^3 (57% PMNs)
Term	0–22/mm^3 (61% PMNs)

APPENDIX E. CHARTWORK

ADMISSION HISTORY
   A. Identification (ID). State the name, age, sex, and weight of the infant. Include whether the patient or mother was transported from another facility or if he was born at home or within the hospital.
   Infant James, a 3-hour-old 1800-gram white male, is an inborn patient from Baltimore, Maryland.
   B. Chief complaint (CC). The major problems of the patient are usually listed in the order of severity of disease process or occurrence.
   1. Respiratory distress syndrome.
   2. Suspected neonatal sepsis.
   3. Premature birth living child (PBLC).
   C. Referring physician. Include the name, address, and phone number of the referring physician.
   Dr. Nick Pavona, Grove Lane Medical Center, Baltimore, Maryland telephone (301) 446–6631.
   D. History of present illness (HPI). The history of the present illness is more helpful if it is divided into 4 separate paragraphs.
   1. Initial statement. This part of the HPI includes the patient's name, gestational age, birth weight, sex, age of the mother, and the number of times she has been pregnant along with the number of living children she has.
   2. Prenatal history. Discuss the maternal prenatal care and record the number of prenatal clinic visits. Include any medications the mother was taking, any pertinent prenatal tests done, and the results.
   3. Labor and delivery. Include a detailed history of the labor and delivery: type of delivery, type of anesthesia, any medication used, and any fetal monitoring (including results).
   4. Infant history. Discuss the initial condition of the infant and the need for resuscitation and write a detailed description of what occurred. Include the Apgar scores and discuss when the infant became symptomatic or when problems were first noted.
   Infant James is a 1800-g white male delivered to a 19-year-old G2 now P2, LC2 married white female.
   The mother had excellent prenatal care. She had her first prenatal visit at approximately 8-weeks' gestation and then saw her obstetrician routinely. She was on no medications nor has any history of ethanol or cigarette abuse.

She had rupture of membranes (ROM) at 33 weeks with some mild contractions. At that time, she was seen by her obstetrician, who confirmed the premature rupture of the membranes. She was admitted to the hospital and started on IV ritodrine in an attempt to stop the labor. She was also closely observed for signs of infection. After 4 days of hospitalization, fever developed, with an increase in her white cell count. Because of suspicion of chorioamnionitis, ritodrine was stopped and pitocin was begun to induce labor. Ampicillin and gentamicin were started after cervical cultures were obtained; results are pending. External fetal monitoring had been normal until 4 hours after the pitocin induction, at which time it showed late decelerations. At this point, an emergency cesarean section was performed. General anesthesia was used, and the infant was delivered within 6 minutes.

The infant was delivered depressed at birth, with 1-minute Apgar of 4. He required bag-mask ventilation with 100% oxygen. No medications were needed. The 5-minute Apgar was 7. The infant appeared poorly perfused and had poor color without oxygen. He was stabilized and transported on 100% oxygen to the NICU.

E. Family history (FH). The family history should include any previous complicated births and their history, miscarriages, neonatal deaths, or premature births. Also include any major family medical problems (eg, hemophilia, sickle cell disease).

Mrs. James had one prior uncomplicated vaginal delivery that went to term. There is a history of myelodysplasia in infant James' maternal first cousin.

F. Social history (SH). In the social history, include a brief statement discussing the parent's age, marital status, siblings, occupation, and where they are from.

The parents are separated and both live in Baltimore. Mother is a 19-year-old factory worker and cares for their 2-year-old daughter; the father is 24 and works as a custodial engineer.

G. Laboratory data. List the admission laboratory and radiology results.

H. Assessment. State your evaluation of the infant's problems. It can include a list of suspected and potential problems, as well as a differential diagnosis.

  1. Respiratory distress syndrome: Since the infant is premature, hyaline membrane disease must be considered. Pneumonia is also a likely cause because of the maternal history of suspected chorioamnionitis.

  2. Suspected neonatal sepsis: Because of the high suspicion of chorioamnionitis and the premature onset of labor, there is an increased septic risk in this infant. Certain pathogens need to be ruled out. Group B streptococcus is the most common pathogen in this age group, but Listeria monocytogenes *and gram-negative pathogens should be considered.*

  3. Premature birth living child: The infant is a 33 weeks' gestation by Ballard examination.

  I. Plan. Include the therapeutic and diagnostic plans for the infant. (See section "Admission Orders," p 550.)

PROGRESS NOTES

The most commonly used format for daily progress notes is the *SOAP* method. *SOAP* is an acronym in which *S* = subjective, *O* = objective, *A* = assessment, and *P* = plan. Each problem should be discussed in this format. First, state the problems you are to discuss in the order of severity or occurrence and assign a number to them. Then discuss each problem in the *SOAP* format as outlined below.

A. Subjective (S). Include an overall subjective view of the patient by the physician.

B. Objective (O). Include data that can be objectively gathered, usually in 3 areas:

  1. Vital signs (temperature, respiratory rate, pulse, blood pressure).

2. Pertinent physical examination.

3. Laboratory data and other test results.

C. Assessment (A). Include evaluation of the above data.

D. Plan (P). Discuss the medication changes, laboratory orders, and any other new orders, as well as the treatment plan.

E. Example. Below is an example of part of a progress note using the *SOAP* format.

Problem 1. Respiratory distress syndrome
Problem 2. Suspected neonatal sepsis
Problem 3. Premature birth living child (PBLC)

Problem 1. Respiratory distress syndrome

S Infant James is now 4 days old and doing much better. He has been able to wean down to 30% oxygen with good arterial gases.

O Vital signs: temperature 98.7, respirations 52, pulse 140, blood pressure 55/35.

Physical examination: The peripheral perfusion appears good with no obvious cyanosis. There is no grunting or nasal flaring, but the infant has mild substernal and intercostal retractions. The chest sounds slightly wet.

Laboratory data and other test results: Arterial blood gases on 30% oxygen—pH 7.32, CO_2 48, O_2 67, 97% saturation. Chest x-ray shows mild haziness in both lung fields.

A Infant James has resolving mild hyaline membrane disease.

P The plan is to wean the oxygen as long as his arterial Pao_2 is greater than 55.

ADMISSION ORDERS

The following format is useful for writing admission orders. It involves the mneumonic *A.D.C. VAN DISSEL.* This stands for *A*dmit, *D*iagnosis, *C*ondition, *V*ital signs, *A*ctivity, *N*ursing procedures, *D*iet, *I*nput and *O*utput, *S*pecific drugs, *S*ymptomatic drugs, *Ex*tras, and *L*aboratory data.

A. Admit. Specify the location of the patient (neonatal intensive care unit, newborn nursery) and the attending physician in charge and house officer along with their paging numbers.

B. Diagnosis. List the admitting diagnoses.

1. Respiratory distress syndrome.
2. Suspected neonatal sepsis.
3. Premature birth living child.

C. Condition. Note if the patient is in stable or critical condition.

D. Vital signs. State the desired frequency of monitoring of vital signs. Specify rectal or axillary temperature. Rectal temperature is usually done initially to obtain a core temperature and also to rule out imperforate anus. Then, follow axillary temperature. Other parameters include blood pressure, pulse, respiratory rate. Weight, length, and head circumference should also be obtained on admission.

E. Activity. All are at bed rest but one can specify "minimal stress or hands-off protocol" here. This notation is used for infants who react poorly to stress by dropping their oxygenation as in patients with persistent pulmonary hypertension. At most centers, it means handle the infant as little as possible and record all vital signs off the monitor.

F. Nursing procedure. Respiratory care (ventilator settings, chest percus and postural drainage orders, endotracheal suctioning with frequency). Also require that a daily weight and head circumference be recorded. The frequency of Dextrostix (or Chemstrip-bG) testing is included in this section, since it is a bedside procedure.

G. Diet. All infants admitted to the neonatal intensive care unit are usually made NPO (nothing by mouth) for at least 6 to 24 hours until they are accessed and stabilized. When appropriate, write specific diet orders.

H. Input and output (I and O). Request that the nursing staff record accurate input and output of each baby. This record is especially important for infants on intravenous fluids and those just starting oral feedings. Specify how often you want the urine tested for specific gravity and glucose.

I. Specific drugs. State drugs to be administered, giving specific dosages and routes of administration. It is useful to also include the milligrams-per-kilogram-per-day dose of the drug to allow cross-checking and verification of the dose ordered. An example is:

Ampicillin 150 mg IV q12h (300 mg/kg/d divided q12h).

For all infants, order the following medications at the time of admission.

1. Vitamin K (see Chap 73) is given to prevent hemorrhagic disease of the newborn.

2. Erythromycin eye drops (see Chap 73) is given to prevent gonococcal ophthalmia.

J. Symptomatic drugs. These drugs are not routinely used in a neonatal intensive care unit and would include such items as pain and sleep medications.

K. Extras. Any other orders required but not included above, such, as roentgenograms, electrocardiography, and ultrasonography.

L. Laboratory data. Include laboratory data drawn on admission, plus routine laboratory orders with frequency (eg, arterial blood gases q2h, sodium and potassium bid).

DISCHARGE SUMMARY

The following information is written at the time of discharge and provides a summary of the infant's illness and hospital stay.

A. Date of admission.

B. Date of discharge.

C. Admitting diagnosis.

D. Discharge diagnosis. List in order of occurrence or severity.

E. Attending physician and service caring for the patient.

F. Referring physician and address.

G. Procedures. Include all invasive procedures.

H. Brief history, physical examination, and laboratory data on admission. Use the admission history, physical examination, and laboratory data as a guide.

I. Hospital course. The easiest way to approach this section of the discharge summary is to discuss each problem in paragraph form.

J. Condition at discharge. A complete physical examination is done at the time of discharge and is included in this section. It is important to include the discharge weight, head circumference, and length so that growth can be assessed at the time of the patient's initial checkup. Also include the type and amount of formula the patient is on and any pertinent discharge laboratory values.

K. Discharge medications. Include the name(s) of medication(s), the dosage(s), and length of treatment. If the patient is being sent home on an apnea monitor, it is helpful to include the monitor settings and the planned course of treatment.

L. Disposition. Note where the patient is being sent (outside hospital, home, foster home).

M. Discharge instructions and follow-up. Include instructions to the parents on medications and when the patient is to return to clinic (and exact location). It is helpful to indicate tests that need to be done on follow-up and any results that need to be rechecked (eg, bilirubin, repeat phenylketonuria screen).

N. Problem list. Same list as the discharge diagnosis list.

APPENDIX F. GROWTH CHARTS

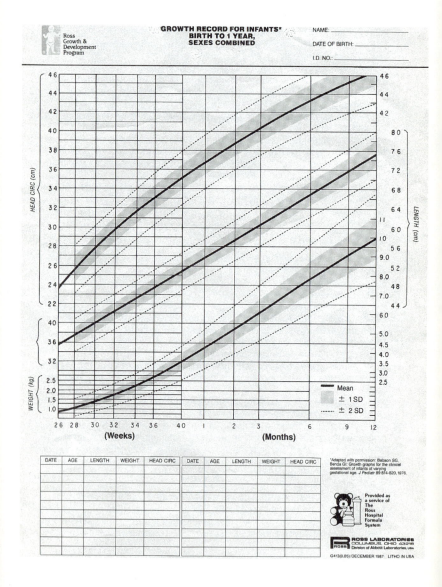

APPENDIX FIGURE F–1. Growth charts for infants. *(Reprinted with the permission of Ross Laboratories.)*

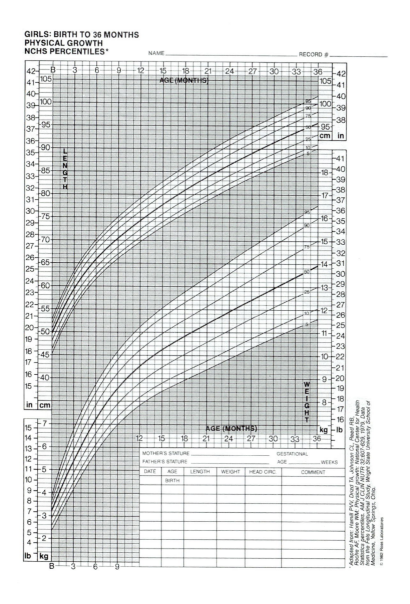

GIRLS: BIRTH TO 36 MONTHS
PHYSICAL GROWTH
NCHS PERCENTILES*

APPENDIX FIGURE F–2. Growth chart for girls; weight and length: birth to 36 months. *(Reprinted with the permission of Ross Laboratories.)*

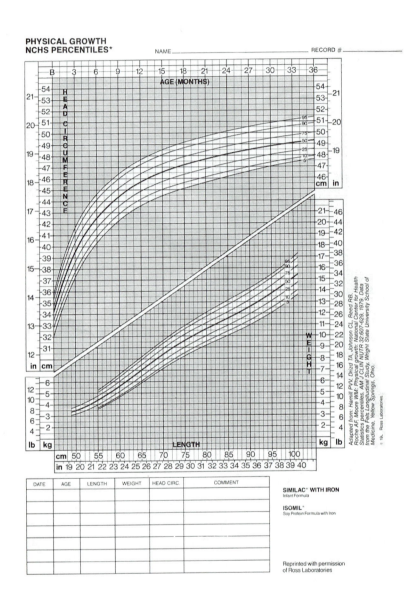

APPENDIX FIGURE F–3. Growth chart for girls; head circumference and weight: birth to 36 months. *(Reprinted with the permission of Ross Laboratories.)*

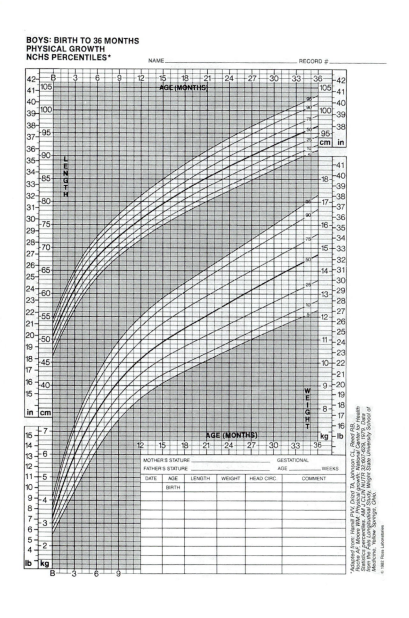

APPENDIX FIGURE F–4. Growth chart for boys; weight and length: birth to 36 months. *(Reprinted with the permission of Ross Laboratories.)*

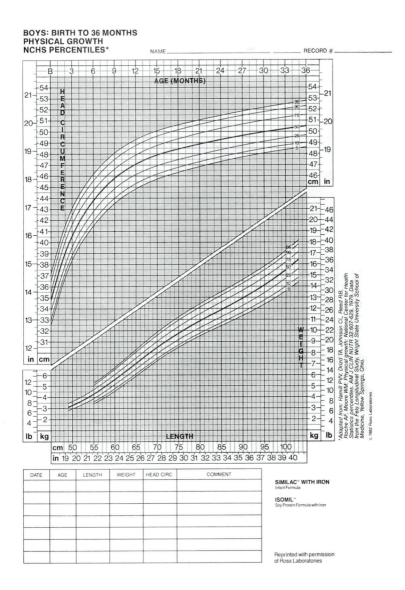

APPENDIX FIGURE F–5. Growth chart for boys; head circumference and weight: birth to 36 months. *(Reprinted with the permission of Ross Laboratories.)*

APPENDIX G. ISOLATION GUIDELINES

PRECAUTIONS FOR PERINATAL PATIENTS IN CONJUNCTION WITH UNIVERSAL BODY SUBSTANCE PRECAUTIONS

INFECTION/DISEASE	MATERNAL PRECAUTIONS	NEONATAL PRECAUTIONS	ROOM-IN	MOTHER MAY VISIT IN NURSERY	BREAST-FEEDING	ADDITIONAL CONSIDERATIONS
AIDS/HIV Positive			Yes	Yes	No, HIV may be transmitted through breast milk.	Recommend PPD and anergy testing for Mother. Report AIDS to Public Health Department via Infection Control Practitioner.
CHICKEN POX (see VARI-CELLA)						
CYTOMEGALOVIRUS (CMV)		Careful handwashing after contact with urine or respiratory secretions	Yes	Yes	Yes	
CHLAMYDIA TRACHOMATIS			Yes	Yes	Yes	Prophylactic use of topical erythromycin at birth prevents inclusion conjunctivitis.
DIARRHEA			Yes	Yes	Yes	Cohort infants and staff.
GONOCOCCAL OPHTHALMIA NEONATORIUM			Yes, after 24 hours of maternal treatment with antibiotics.	Yes, after 24 hours of maternal treatment with antibiotics.	Yes, after 24 hours of maternal treatment with antibiotics	

(continued)

INFECTION/DISEASE	MATERNAL PRECAUTIONS	NEONATAL PRECAUTIONS	ROOM-IN	MOTHER MAY VISIT IN NURSERY	BREAST-FEEDING	ADDITIONAL CONSIDERATIONS
HEPATITIS–A, B, C			Yes	Yes	Yes	May give Immune Globulin for Hepatitis A. All newborns to receive Hepatitis B vaccine before discharge. Infants born to HBsAg positive mothers should also receive Hepatitis B Immune Globulin. Report to Public Health Department via Infection Control Practitioner.
HERPES SIMPLEX –Maternal Genital (Active primary or recurrent; or positive culture in last 2 weeks)			Yes	Yes	Yes, unless vesicular lesions involve breast.	Scalp monitors should be avoided when possible for infants of women suspected of having genital herpes.
HERPES SIMPLEX –Neonatal Neonatal infection or positive culture in absence of disease			No	Yes	Yes	Culture obtained from conjunctiva, oral pharynx, or skin lesion 48 hours or later after birth are more likely to identify neonatal infection. A positive culutre obtained $\geq$ 24 hours after birth needs immediate antiviral treatment, even in absence of symptoms.

(continued)

Disease						
LICE (see section on PEDICULOSIS)						
MEASLES	Labor & Delivery and Postpartum recovery in private room. Mask within 3 feet of patient.	Private room. Mask in close contact.	No	No	Not until mother is judged to be noncontagious.	Contagious during prodrome and up to 4 days of rash illness. Report to public Health Department via Infection Control Practitioner.
MUMPS (INFECTIOUS PAROTITIS)	Private room. Mask within 3 feet of patient.	Private room	No	No	Not until mother is judged to be noncontagious.	Contagious for 9 days after onset of swelling. Report to Public Health Department via Infection Control Practitioner.
PEDICULOSIS (LICE)			Not until 24 hours after start of effective therapy, then may room-in or visit.	Not unitl 24 hours after start of effective therapy, then may visit.	Not until 24 hours after start of effective therapy.	Contacts should be examined and treated if infected.
PERTUSSIS (WHOOPING COUGH)	Private room. Mask within 3 feet of patient	Private Room. Mask in close contact.	No	No	Not until mother is judged to be noncontagious.	Contagious for 7 days after start of effective therapy. Report to Public Health Department via Infection Control Practitioner.
RESPIRATORY SYNCYTIAL VIRUS (RSV)		Transfer to ICU or Pediatric Ward	Yes	Yes, in ICU or Pediatric patient room.	Yes	

(continued)

INFECTION/DISEASE	MATERNAL PRECAUTIONS	NEONATAL PRECAUTIONS	ROOM-IN	MOTHER MAY VISIT IN NURSERY	BREAST-FEEDING	ADDITIONAL CONSIDERATIONS
RUBELLA (GERMAN MEASLES) –Maternal	Private room. Mask within 3 feet of patient.	Mask in close contact.	Yes	No	No	Isolate for 7 days after onset of rash. Persons who have had Rubella do not need to wear a mask. Susceptible persons stay out of room, if possible. Report to Public Health Department via Infection Control Practitioner.
RUBELLA (GERMAN MEASLES) –Congenital			Yes	Yes	Yes	Rubella is contagious until 1 year of age unless nasopharyngeal and urine cultures after 3 months of age are negative for Rubella virus. Day care providers should be made aware of the potential hazard to susceptible pregnant contacts. Susceptible persons stay out of room, if possible. Report to Public Health Department via Infection Control Practitioner.

(continued)

SCABIES	No contact until 24 hours after start of effective therapy, then may room-in or visit in nursery.	No contact until 24 hours after start of effective therapy, then may room-in or visit in nursery.	Not until 24 hours after start of effective therapy.	Treatment of household contact is recommended.
STAPHYLOCOCCUS AUREUS	No	Yes	Yes	Two or more concurrent cases of impetigo related to a nursery or single case of breast abscess in a nursing mother or infant is presumptive evidence of an epidemic, report immediately to attending physician and Infection Control Department.
SYPHILIS	Yes, after 24 hours of treatment with antibiotics.	Yes, after 24 hours of treatment with antibiotics.	Yes, after 24 hours of treatment with antibiotics.	Report to Public Health Department via Infection Control Practitioner.
TUBERCULOSIS 1. Mother with +PPD and no evidence of current disease.	Yes	Yes	Yes	Infant should be tested: PPD at 4 to 6 weeks of age, at 3 to 4 months of age, and 12 months of age.

(continued)

INFECTION/DISEASE	MATERNAL PRECAUTIONS	NEONATAL PRECAUTIONS	ROOM-IN	MOTHER MAY VISIT IN NURSERY	BREAST-FEEDING	ADDITIONAL CONSIDERATIONS
TUBERCULOSIS (cont'd) 2. Mother with untreated (newly diagnosed) minimal disease, or disease has been treated for 2 or more weeks AND is judged to be noncontagious at delivery.			Yes	Yes	Yes	Infant should have CXR and PPD at 4 to 6 weeks of age; if negative retest at 3 to 4 and 6 months of age. Recommend HIV testing for mother. Report to Public Health Department via Infection Control Practitioner.
3. Mother with current pulmonary TB. Suspected of being contagious at time of delivery.	Labor and Delivery and Postpartum care in private room with negative pressure, non-recirculating air, keep door closed. Mask required at all times.		No contact until mother is judged non-contagious.	No contact until mother is judged non-contagious.	Not until mother is judged non-contagious.	Infant should be given INH until 6 months of age, then repeat PPD. If PPD+, continue INH for a total of 12 months. Recommend HIV testing for mother. Report to Public Health Department via Infection Control Practitioner.
4. Mother has extra-pulmonary spread of TB (ie, miliary, bone, meningitis, etc)			No contact until mother is judged non-contagious.	No contact until mother is judged non-contagious.	Not until mother is judged non-contagious.	Infant should be given INH until 6 months of age, then repeat PPD. If PPD+, continue INH for a total of 12 months. Report to Public Health Department via Infection Control Practitioner.

(continued)

VARICELLA (CHICKEN POX) OR VARICELLA ZOSTER in immunocompromised patient or if disseminated —Maternal/Neonate	Labor and Delivery and Postpartum care in private room with negative pressure, non-recirculating air, keep door closed. Gown, mask, and gloves required. Continue precautions until all lesions are crusted.	Private room with negative pressure, non-recirculating air. Gown, mask, and gloves required. If they must be hospitalized beyond 10 days of age, continue precautions until 21 days of age. If VZIG given, keep on precautions until 28 days after exposures.	Yes, after lesions have crusted.	Yes, may visit in private room after mother's lesions have crusted.	Yes, after lesions have crusted.	May be contagious 1–2 days before the onset of rash. Persons who have had Chickenpox do not need to wear a mask. Hospitalized patients should be discharged prior to the 10th day following exposure, if possible. Exposed susceptible patients should be placed on precautions beginning 10 days after exposure and continue until 21 days after last exposure, or until 28 days if VZIG given.

Revised: October 1993

NEONATOLOGY

APPENDIX H. PHOTOTHERAPY TABLE

The initial table (now revised and updated) was developed at the University of Kentucky Medical Center to help decide when to begin patients on phototherapy. The birth weight is plotted against the age of the baby in days. If the indirect bilirubin level, expressed in mg/dL, exceeds the number listed in the table, then phototherapy should be seriously considered. As always, clinical judgment should be exercised when interpreting this table. New guidelines have been recommended for phototherapy for **full term infants.** Levels for well, term infants with no hemolysis are now recommended at 17.5–22.0 mg/dL for phototherapy. For full-term infants that are sick or with hemolytic disease, levels are 13–17.5 mg/dL. This table applies to well infants with no evidence of hemolysis; however, if the infant is sick or there is hemolysis, phototherapy should be initiated at lower levels than shown in the table.

Birth Weight (g)	Days						
	1	2	3	4	5	6	7
< 1000	> 5	> 5	> 5	> 5	> 7	> 7	> 10
1000–1249	> 5	> 5	> 5	> 8	> 8	> 10	> 12
1250–1499	> 8	> 8	> 8	> 10	> 12	> 12	> 12
1500–1749	> 10	> 10	> 10	> 12	> 12	> 13	> 13
1750–1999	> 10	> 10	> 12	> 13	> 13	> 13	> 13
2000–2499	> 10	> 12	> 12	> 15	> 15	> 15	> 15
> 2500	> 10	> 12	> 13	> 15	> 18	> 18	> 18

APPENDIX I. TEMPERATURE CONVERSION TABLE

Celcius	Fahrenheit	Celcius	Fahrenheit
34.0	93.2	37.6	99.6
34.2	93.6	37.8	100.0
34.4	93.9	38.0	100.4
34.6	94.3	38.2	100.7
34.8	94.6	38.4	101.1
35.0	95.0	38.6	101.4
35.2	95.4	38.8	101.8
35.4	95.7	39.0	102.2
35.6	96.1	39.2	102.5
35.8	96.4	39.4	102.9
36.0	96.8	39.6	103.2
36.2	97.1	39.8	103.6
36.4	97.5	40.0	104.0
36.6	97.8	40.2	104.3
36.8	98.2	40.4	104.7
37.0	98.6	40.6	105.1
37.2	98.9	40.8	105.4
37.4	99.3	41.0	105.8

Celsius = (Fahrenheit − 32) × 5/9
Fahrenheit = (Celsius × 9/5) + 32

APPENDIX J. UMBILICAL ARTERY CATHETER MEASUREMENTS

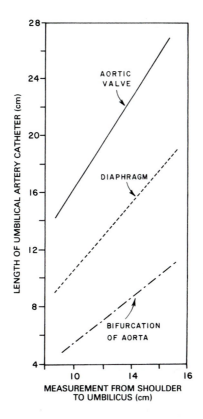

APPENDIX FIGURE J–1. The umbilical artery catheter can be placed in one of 2 positions. The "low" catheter is placed below the level of L3 to avoid the renal and mesenteric vessels. The "high" catheter is placed between the thoracic vertebrae from T6 to T9. The graph is used as a guide to help determine the catheter length for each position. The "low" line corresponds to the aortic bifurcation in the graph, whereas a "high" line corresponds to the diaphragm. To determine catheter length: Measure (in centimeters) a perpendicular line from the top of the shoulder to the umbilicus. This determines the shoulder-umbilical length. Plot this number on the graph to determine the proper catheter length for the umbilical artery catheter. It is helpful to add the length of the umbilical stump to the catheter length. *(Data from Dunn PM: Localization of the umbilical catheter by post-mortem measurement. Arch Dis Child 1966;**41**:69.)*

APPENDIX K. UMBILICAL VEIN CATHETER MEASUREMENTS

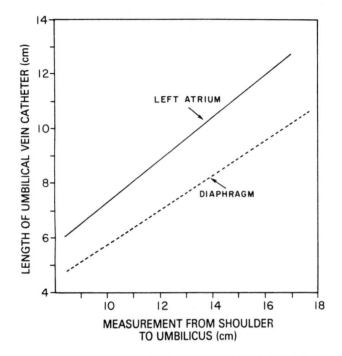

APPENDIX FIGURE K–1. The umbilical venous catheter is placed above the level of the diaphragm. Determine the shoulder-umbilical length as for the umbilical artery catheter. Use this number and determine the catheter length using the graph. Remember to add the length of the umbilical stump to the length of the catheter. *(Data from Dunn PM: Localization of the umbilical catheter by post-mortem measurement.* Arch Dis Child *1966;**41**:69.)*

APPENDIX L. WEIGHT CONVERSION TABLE

Ounces	1 lb	2 lb	3 lb	4 lb	5 lb	6 lb	7 lb	8 lb
				Grams				
0	454	907	1361	1814	2268	2722	3175	3629
1	482	936	1389	1843	2296	2750	3204	3657
2	510	964	1418	1871	2325	2778	3232	3686
3	539	992	1446	1899	2353	2807	3260	3714
4	567	1021	1474	1928	2381	2835	3289	3742
5	595	1049	1503	1956	2410	2863	3317	3771
6	624	1077	1531	1985	2438	2892	3345	3799
7	652	1106	1559	2013	2466	2920	3374	3827
8	680	1134	1588	2041	2495	2948	3402	3856
9	709	1162	1616	2070	2523	2977	3430	3884
10	737	1191	1644	2098	2552	3005	3459	3912
11	765	1219	1673	2126	2580	3033	3487	3941
12	794	1247	1701	2155	2608	3062	3515	3969
13	822	1276	1729	2183	2637	3090	3544	3997
14	851	1304	1758	2211	2665	3119	3572	4026
15	879	1332	1786	2240	2693	3147	3600	4054

To convert from kilograms to pounds, multiply kg by 2.2.
To convert from pounds to grams, multiply lb by 454.

APPENDIX M. WHITE BLOOD COUNT GRAPH

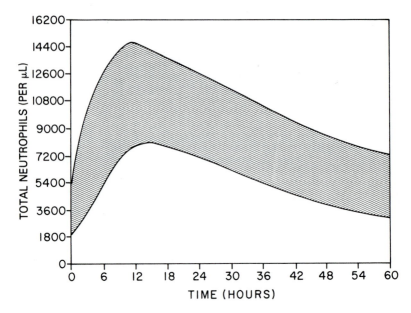

APPENDIX FIGURE M-1. Reference range for total neutrophil count in the first 60 hours of life. The total number of neutrophils is calculated as follows:

$$\frac{(\text{No. of segs} + \text{No. of stabs/bands}) \times \text{Total white blood cell count}}{100}$$

The heavy lines denote the range of neutrophil counts of normal healthy infants. A neutrophil count that falls below the curve suggests bacterial infection. A count that falls above the curve also suggests bacterial infection but less strongly. (After Manroe BL et al: The neonatal blood count in health and disease: I. Reference values for neutrophilic cells. *J Pediatr* 1979;**95**:89.)

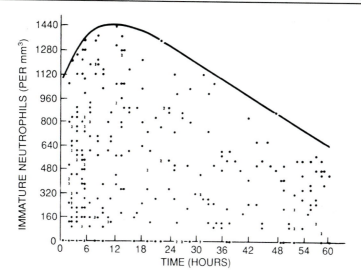

APPENDIX FIGURE M-2. Reference range for immature neutrophils in the first 60 hours of life. An immature neutrophil count above the curve suggests bacterial infection. See also p. 000. (After Manroe; see Fig M-1.)

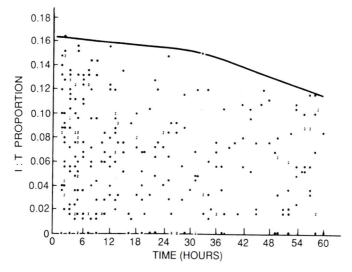

APPENDIX FIGURE M-3. Reference range for the proportion of immature to total neutrophils (I:T) in the first 60 hours of life. An immature to total neutrophil (I:T) proportion above the curve suggests bacterial infection. See also p. 000. (After Manroe; see Fig M-1.)

Index

NOTE: Page numbers in bold face type indicate a major discussion. A *t* following a page number indicates tabular material and an *i* following a page number indicates an illustration. Drugs are listed under their generic names. When a drug trade name is listed, the reader is referred to the generic name.